Dr. David L. Moore

9780801606601

# Improving dental practice through preventive measures

# Improving dental practice through preventive measures

*Edited by*

## Joseph L. Bernier
**D.D.S., M.S., F.A.C.D., F.D.S., R.C.S.(Eng.)**

Professor and Chairman, Department of Oral Pathology, Georgetown University; Major General, United States Army Dental Corps (Ret.); formerly Assistant Surgeon General and Chief of the Dental Corps, Department of the Army, Washington, D. C.

*and*

## Joseph C. Muhler
**D.D.S., Ph.D., F.A.C.D.**

Professor of Research, Department of Biochemistry, School of Medicine; Chairman, Department of Preventive Dentistry, Indiana University School of Dentistry; Director, Preventive Dentistry Research Institute, Indianapolis, Indiana

**SECOND EDITION**

*With 228 illustrations*

## The C. V. Mosby Company
Saint Louis    1970

**Second edition**

Copyright © 1970 by **The C. V. Mosby Company**

All rights reserved. No part of this book may be reproduced in any manner without written permission of the publisher.

Previous edition copyrighted 1966

Printed in the United States of America

Standard Book Number 8016-0660-8

Library of Congress Catalog Card Number 75-137114

Distributed in Great Britain by Henry Kimpton, London

# Contributors

**JOSEPH L. BERNIER, D.D.S., M.S., F.D.S., R.C.S.(Eng.)**

Professor and Chairman, Department of Oral Pathology, Georgetown University; Major General, United States Army Dental Corps (Ret.); formerly Assistant Surgeon General and Chief of the Dental Corps, Department of the Army, Washington, D. C.

**DAVID BIXLER, D.D.S., Ph.D.**

Associate Professor of Dental Sciences and Medical Genetics, Indiana University School of Dentistry, Indianapolis, Indiana

**CHARLES J. BURSTONE, D.D.S., M.S.**

Professor and Head, Department of Orthodontics, The University of Connecticut School of Dental Medicine, Farmington, Connecticut

**SIMON CIVJAN, B.Ch.E., D.D.S., M.S.**

Lieutenant Colonel, United States Army Dental Corps; Chief, Department of Dental Materials, United States Army Institute of Dental Research, Washington, D. C.

**THOMAS K. CURETON, Jr., B.S., B.P.E., M.A., Ph.D.**

Professor of Physical Education and Director of the Physical Fitness Research Laboratory, University of Illinois, Chicago, Illinois

**IRVING GLICKMAN, B.S., D.M.D.**

Professor and Chairman, Department of Periodontology; Research Professor of Oral Pathology, Tufts University School of Dental Medicine, Boston, Massachusetts

**WAYNE L. HARVEY, D.D.S.**

Associate Professor of Dentistry and Chairman of Removable Partial Denture Department, University of Missouri at Kansas City School of Dentistry, Kansas City, Missouri

**FRANK C. JERBI, D.D.S.**

Associate Professor of Removable Prosthodontics, University of Maryland School of Dentistry, Baltimore, Maryland

**SIMON KATZ, D.D.S., Ph.D.**

Assistant Professor of Preventive Dentistry, Department of Preventive Dentistry, Indiana University School of Dentistry, Indianapolis, Indiana

## Contributors

**VICTOR H. MERCER, D.D.S., M.S.D.**

Instructor, Department of Preventive Dentistry, Indiana University School of Dentistry; Assistant Director, Division of Dental Health, Indiana State Board of Health, Indianapolis, Indiana

**DAVID L. MOORE, D.D.S.**

Professor, Department of Operative Dentistry, University of Missouri at Kansas City, Kansas City, Missouri

**JOSEPH C. MUHLER, D.D.S., Ph.D., F.A.C.D.**

Professor of Research, Department of Biochemistry, School of Medicine, and Chairman, Department of Preventive Dentistry, Indiana University School of Dentistry, Indianapolis, Indiana

**HAMILTON B. G. ROBINSON, D.D.S., M.S.**

Dean and Professor of Dentistry, University of Missouri at Kansas City School of Dentistry, Kansas City, Missouri

**JAMES R. ROCHE, D.D.S.**

Professor, Graduate Pedodontics, Indiana University School of Dentistry, Indianapolis, Indiana

**JAMES H. SHAW, M.S., Ph.D.**

Professor of Nutrition, Harvard School of Dental Medicine, Boston, Massachusetts

**ROBERT B. SHIRA, D.D.S.**

Major General, United States Army Dental Corps; Assistant Surgeon General and Chief of the Army Dental Corps, Department of the Army, Washington, D. C.

**GEORGE K. STOOKEY, M.S.D.**

Assistant Professor of Basic Sciences, Department of Preventive Dentistry, Indiana University School of Dentistry, Indianapolis, Indiana

**RUSSELL W. SUMNICHT, D.D.S., M.P.H.**

Professor of Preventive Dentistry, University of Missouri at Kansas City School of Dentistry, Kansas City, Missouri

# Preface

The second edition of *Improving Dental Practice Through Preventive Measures* reflects the change in attitude of practicing dentists toward the concepts of preventive dentistry. Two new chapters have been added to the contents of the first edition. One concerns current concepts of enamel structure and its role in the initiation and extension of dental caries, while the second concerns preventive operative dentistry. Dr. James R. Roche has replaced Dean Ralph E. McDonald as contributor for the chapter on pedodontics, and as a result of the untimely death of Dr. Margetis, his chapter has been revised by Dr. Simon Civjan. All of the chapters have been modified to reflect the changing concepts in preventive dentistry. The chapters on fluoride therapy, the role of dentifrices in oral health, and preventive periodontics have been completely revised to incorporate the most recent concepts in these fields.

The contributors to any dental text always feel, perhaps ambitiously, that their work will in some way modify dental practice so as to reflect a reduction in oral disease for the population. We hold no claims that this text will make such a dramatic impact on oral health. However, as the result of numerous conversations and discussions with our colleagues since the first edition appeared, we believe that the incorporation of current concepts in preventive dentistry for the general practitioner has helped organize the practice of more preventive dentistry in dental offices throughout the country.

Many research workers are beginning to suggest that the control of dental caries is soon to be accomplished. No portion of the book reflects this hypothesis, but the authors do take note of the important fact that both the research worker and the general practitioner will have many more sound teeth to consider for treatment for longer periods of time, as people live longer and preventive care improves. If this occurs, the preservation of the soft tissues will become more important. The revision considers this aspect of preventive dentistry.

The revision of any text is often more difficult to prepare than is a new volume. Any omissions or inaccuracies rest solely with the editors, and we hope our readers will continue to correspond with us so as to provide us with their knowledge concerning new concepts which can be incorporated into subsequent editions.

Joseph L. Bernier
Joseph C. Muhler

# Contents

1 Preventive dentistry—a philosophy of dental practice, 1
**Joseph L. Bernier**

2 Incorporation of preventive dentistry into office practice, 7
**Victor H. Mercer**

3 Preventive nutrition, 31
**James H. Shaw**

4 Enamel and dental caries, 59
**Simon Katz**

5 Control of rampant dental caries, 80
**Russell W. Sumnicht**

6 Fluoride therapy, 92
**George K. Stookey**

7 Dentifrices and oral hygiene, 157
**Joseph C. Muhler**

8 Preventive pedodontics, 177
**James R. Roche**

9 Preventive periodontics, 208
**Irving Glickman**

10 Preventive orthodontics, 229
**Charles J. Burstone**

11 Preventive operative dentistry, 248
**David L. Moore**

12 Preventive prosthodontics (complete dentures), 273
**Frank C. Jerbi**

13  Preventive adult space maintainers (partial dentures), 297
    **Wayne L. Harvey**

14  Preventive oral surgery, 328
    **Robert B. Shira**

15  Preventive oral pathology, 345
    **Hamilton B. G. Robinson**

16  Radiation biology in dental practice, 355
    **David Bixler**

17  The role of dental materials in preventive dentistry, 370
    **Simon Civjan**

18  Physical fitness and dynamic health, 397
    **Thomas K. Cureton, Jr.**

# Improving dental practice through preventive measures

# Chapter 1 Preventive dentistry—a philosophy of dental practice

## Joseph L. Bernier

Introduction
Philosophy of preventive dentistry
Philosophy in action—treatment plan
    Urgent
    Gingival and periodontal therapy
    Prophylaxis and anticaries therapy
    Occlusal adjustment
    Counselling in self-care
Attitudes of the dental profession
Conclusion

## INTRODUCTION

During the past two decades many significant changes have occurred in various fields in science—for example, the humanities, and dentistry—and in the society of which we are an integral part. The present application of the scientific knowledge that has accrued to the practice of dentistry during this time is a problem to which many are directing their attention. Some of the factors that have had significant impact are favorable support of research by the federal government, changes in the attitudes of patients, the advent of specialization, and greater emphasis on graduate education. In the midst of these changes it is hardly surprising that dentistry and dental education have undergone an unprecedented period of self-scrutiny, reappraisal, and definition of objectives. From these soul-searching efforts has come the realization that new views in many areas are necessary if the responsibilities of the profession are to be met.

One need only peruse the dental journals and note the content of scientific programs of dental groups to be aware of the growing interest in preventive dental practice. This is true not because preventive dentistry is the "fashion of the moment," but rather because dental research has provided extremely useful tools and knowledge to prevent much oral disease. The most effective of these are the anticariogenic compounds; also, better approaches to diagnosis have added greatly to our ability to prevent oral diseases, particularly gingival and periodontal disease. To these must be added the knowledge that preventive dental practice has been shown to be economically feasible in a number of private practices. Furthermore, organized programs such as those in the military services have proved to be highly successful; the results of these programs have had a deep impact on those who have been involved.

This combination of growing interest and economic feasibility has brought preventive dentistry to the forefront of dental thinking; as a result, many dentists and dental groups are seeking scientific help and advice as to how to become involved in such a program and practice.

The quality of dental education and dental service and the continuing contributions to better dental practice in the United States justify American dentistry's reputation for progress and excellence. Remarkable achievements have been made in the manner in which the profession provides dental care. However, until a few years ago the most significant achievements contributed more to dentistry's growth as an art rather than a science. Recent developments promise to change the entire complexion of dental practice and to far outshadow the progress of the past. These new developments offer the means for professional growth through practical and profitable application of the preventive philosophy that dentistry has sought for so long. The day is in sight when the handpiece and the forceps will be no more than incidental symbols of the profession. If American dentistry is to continue its leadership it cannot fail to note and make adjustments to meet the potential of these developments.

Farsighted dentists predict the day when oral disease will be largely eliminated or controlled through preventive means. More skeptical members of the profession consider effective prevention of dental disease an unrealistic goal; still others have become so concerned with attempting to roll back the tide of oral disease through corrective and reparative therapy that to them any approach to dental health care other than the curative approach would be a neglect of professional responsibility.

## PHILOSOPHY OF PREVENTIVE DENTISTRY

It is clear that few specific preventive measures are available to the dentist, as compared with those that can be used by the physician. This is due in part to the chronicity of the two principal oral diseases—dental caries and periodontal disease—and in part to the fact that the exact nature of neither disease is well understood. Therefore the practice of preventive dentistry, being a philosophy of intent designed to guide every therapeutic action as a measure of prevention, differs somewhat from the practice of preventive medicine, even though the goals are the same.

Certainly it is obvious that every dentist, whether he is a general practitioner or a specialist, must be an exponent of the preventive concept. Let us first discuss the philosophy behind preventive dentistry before considering its application to dental practice.

Most would agree it is self-evident that all our actions follow some analysis of the problem that is to be affected by such actions. Sometimes such an analysis is superficial. On other occasions it is deep and penetrating. In either circumstance its intent, whether realized or not, is to rationalize the actions to follow. This, then, is one way to develop a philosophy—a reason for actions.

The proper care of the oral health of a patient requires a series of actions. Sometimes many actions are necessary, other times only a few. It is the coupling of these procedures into a plan designed to reach a single goal that is the basis for a philosophy of preventive dentistry. Without an orderly commingling of individual efforts there is no assurance that any final goal will be achieved.

Because of a seemingly inescapable aspect of its educational pattern dentistry has caused itself to become fragmented. We do not refer to the matter of specialization but to the attitudes instilled in all dentists while in dental school. This will be discussed in some detail later in the chapter.

If one considers the insertion of a restoration, the replacement of missing teeth, or the extraction of a tooth as an individual accomplishment—an end in itself—then the total health of the patient is not being served. This means that the operator is concerned with the reparative procedure itself and not with its long-range effect in preventing disease.

The philosophy of preventive dentistry gives meaning to the practice of dentistry. It brings to the forefront the science of dentistry without detracting from the art involved. In assessing the oral health problem of a patient, the dentist need only ask this question of himself, "What will be the total oral health status in 10 years, after I have finished the multiple procedures that must be performed now?"

Because of the specificity of this philosophy some have suggested that the type of practice it espouses would better be termed comprehensive dentistry. There is much merit in this suggestion since it is obvious that we are thinking in terms of the problems of individual patients and how these problems can be solved in the best interests of the patient.

Public health dentistry and social dentistry are referred to by some as preventive dentistry. Since they deal largely with the problems of groups and populations it seems best to consider this as a necessary and separate aspect of patient care. Coupled with the philosophy of preventive dentistry, however, they constitute a formidable program to ensure proper oral health of the individual and the general population.

## PHILOSOPHY IN ACTION—TREATMENT PLAN

As necessary as a philosophy, or reason for action, may be, there is a firm requirement that its implementation be practical and feasible. As a means of providing guidance for clinical practice in conformance with the philosophy of preventive dentistry a procedural sequence to constitute the basis for treatment planning is suggested. It consists of the following five phases.

Phase 1. Urgent
Phase 2. Gingival and periodontal therapy
Phase 3. Prophylaxis and anticaries therapy
Phase 4. Occlusal adjustment
Phase 5. Counselling in self-care

A special form should be designed for the treatment plan for those for whom complex treatment is required. This form should provide space for recording consultations, if they are required. The treatment plan becomes a part of the patient's dental health record to serve as a guide for all of the treatment procedures to follow.

**Urgent.** Treatments of an emergency nature, or those deemed necessary to prevent early development of an emergency condition, are of course performed first. Some thought must be given to the decision as to what is urgent. This is basically a professional question and will vary considerably. Obviously, existing pain must be controlled, using whatever method is deemed desirable by the dentist. Extraction may be indicated, or perhaps pulp removal, followed by endodontic therapy. In other instances drug therapy may be necessary.

Furthermore, the immediate problem may be a painful gingivitis or periodontitis, in which case other specific therapy is required. As to the treatment of urgent conditions deemed necessary to prevent early development of an emergency condition, a wide possibility of circumstances must be considered. Some might decide that a relatively small but deep carious lesion was a potential source of pain; others might not. Assuming the former, it might follow that the insertion of a restoration, either temporary or permanent, would be indicated. So it is clear that considerable flexibility must be inherent in developing the treatment plan.

**Gingival and periodontal therapy.** Treatment of existing gingival or periodontal disease is then initiated, and in general no surgical, restorative, or other corrective treatments other than those deemed urgent are attempted until all soft tissue disease is controlled. Here again the obvious need to recognize the possibility of various professional decisions is apparent. Indeed, this could be the first element of the treatment plan if the gingival or periodontal inflammation were considered to be urgent.

In phase 2 the entire plan of therapy is evolved. It could be that extractions are indicated as part of the periodontal therapy. Furthermore, it is conceivable that some gingival surgery might be necessary. The need for flexibility and variance of professional opinion is again obvious. Assessment of the patient's general physical state and dietary status takes place during this phase of treatment. These matters are dealt with in detail in other chapters of the book.

**Prophylaxis and anticaries therapy.** Periodic dental prophylaxis is considered an important therapeutic measure for all dentulous patients; the relegation of such treatment to a "nice-to-have" or a "cosmetic" category is unrealistic. The application of a stannous fluoride preparation, together with dental prophylaxis, take place during the third phase of treatment. Either compatible lava-pumice or zirconium silicate may be mixed with the stannous fluoride. (Details for this technic may be found in Chapter 6.)

However, prophylaxis and fluoride therapy do not tell the whole story. It is important that the scaling and polishing not be considered an exclusive anticariogenic measure. True, it serves that purpose when the technic referred to previously is followed. Equally important, however, is its role in the arrestment and prevention of gingival disease—the precursor to periodontitis.

With the introduction of effective anticariogenic chemicals, the role of prophylaxis has shifted somewhat from what was once a procedure for establishing a healthy relationship between the tooth and the periodontium to a tooth-polishing technic designed to prepare the tooth for fluoride application. Emphasis on both roles is important, but they must be kept in balance since the objectives of both can be achieved if a proper technic is followed. It does not appear that self-application of fluoride compounds can serve this purpose.

**Occlusal adjustment.** During the fourth phase of treatment all obvious discrepancies in occlusion are corrected as an important step in the prevention of periodontal disease. (Surgery, restorative procedures, and construction of prostheses are then performed.)

You will note that reference is made to "all obvious discrepancies." This is important since it is not implied that complete occlusal adjustment must be accomplished in each instance. Rather, obvious prematurities should be eliminated and unobstructed guide planes established. Care must be taken in such adjustments to avoid developing other discrepancies of equal or greater severity.

The insertion of restorations and the construction of indicated prostheses are the next steps in the treatment plan. Indeed, this is a most important phase of the treatment plan since it is here that true prevention is practiced. Every operative or prosthetic procedure must be viewed as a part of the whole plan in which all efforts blend together to ensure good oral health in the future. This point is emphasized in the various chapters to follow.

**Counselling in self-care.** Since evidence of inadequate self-care practices is an indication of a need for early instruction and motivation for improvement, this phase receives continuous attention throughout the course of treatment.

It is not possible to place too much emphasis on this aspect of the treatment plan. The patient must be carefully and diligently carried through a complete educational program in oral health. It must begin with the first visit and continue throughout the entire period of patient care, even into the recall period.

The counselling given the patient should be somewhat tailored to the individual person and his problems. But the underlying concept of diligent home care must be a continuing thread in the entire program.

Individual home kits are available that serve this purpose very well. They contain all the necessary items for achieving good oral home care, including disclosing wafers, which are most useful in assessing the patient's accomplishments.

## ATTITUDES OF THE DENTAL PROFESSION

The reactions of members of the dental profession to this philosophy of preventive dentistry are, of course, varied. Among the established practitioners this is to be expected since significant changes in the format of such a practice are difficult to make. However, many are making the effort and succeeding.

This core of professional practitioners constitutes the major group that must be convinced if preventive practice is to become a meaningful reality. Of equal importance, however, are the recent graduates of our dental schools and the faculty members who teach them.

The school of dentistry, where the future dentist receives his philosophy of dental practice, obviously must have its entire teaching effort permeated with this concept of preventive dentistry. Thus all activities should be consistent in this approach or the student may become confused and enter dental practice not knowing the true value of prevention. The basic beliefs, the mental perspective, and the guiding principles of activity derived from this philosophy must be thoroughly believed in and practiced by the members of the faculty if the student is expected to do the same.

Ideally one might hope that the philosophy and practice of prevention in dentistry would naturally permeate all segments of the dental profession, and it is possible that this could happen. However, it is likely that this would take far too long, during which time much oral disease could have been prevented. One might identify the important segments of the profession as the dental students, dental faculties, and practicing profession; therefore to complete the picture it is necessary to add the vast lay population, an integral element, from whence the patients emerge. Each element of the profession has particular interests in the preventive concept together with its own problems that must first be solved.

The dental student is flexible in his learning experience. He will carry away what has been presented to him if he is convinced of its beneficial effects. It is therefore imperative that he be exposed to an organized and well-delineated program course if he is to place prevention in its proper perspective.

There is an ever-increasing number of individuals in all aspects of the dental profession who believe in the concept of preventive practice and who seek advice on how it can be developed in private practice, in communities, and in the dental schools.

## CONCLUSION

The need for recognizing the importance of prevention in dental practice is seemingly obvious. Many dentists now practicing in accordance with this philosophy are proving that it is feasible and practical.

More emphasis must be placed on prevention in the dental school curriculum. This trend is evident, but there is much remaining to be accomplished.

Graduating dentists have an awareness of the preventive aspects of dental practice, but this awareness does not parallel that which exists for the well-established areas of dentistry. A far better balance is essential.

# Chapter 2 Incorporation of preventive dentistry into office practice

Victor H. Mercer

Introduction
Caries activity testing
Nutritional counselling
Patient education
    Direct education
    Indirect education
        Electronic programming
        Pamphlets
        Slides
        Motion pictures
Use of fluoride in the dental office
Recall
Conclusion

## INTRODUCTION

The measure of our knowledge concerning preventive dentistry is the extent to which our patients benefit from its use. The ultimate benefits of preventive dentistry are attained through our knowledge, the communication of our knowledge through treatment and education, and our ability to enable the patient to utilize this information.

We cannot confine preventive dentistry to any unique list of dental services or procedures; neither can we limit prevention to areas of dental caries or periodontal disease. Preventive dentistry encompasses all phases of dental disease and treatment. It is as vitally concerned with the principles of tooth extraction as with the need for preserving teeth. It resists the necessity of resorting to artificial dentures and yet is involved with the technics of denture construction. It is as concerned with community opportunities to improve dental health as with singular services we perform for individual patients. It attempts to prevent disease entities, and yet, when disease entities exist, it is involved with their correction and prevention of complications.

Preventive dentistry is further concerned with human relations and with motivation; it requires management of our time so that we may utilize to the best advantage our opportunities to serve patients. The successful practice of preventive dentistry requires the ability to put our knowledge and skills to the best possible use in the promotion and improvement of dental health.

Preventive dentistry is a positive approach to the practice of dentistry. It energizes our understanding of everyday treatment situations; it promotes good will with our patients and encourages their maximum acceptance of dental health principles; and it gives us the satisfaction that comes from putting forth our best efforts and provides challenge and enjoyment in our practice of dentistry.

There are certain established practices of preventive dentistry that are accepted by every dentist. Such services as dental prophylaxis and topical fluoride treatments are familiar practices of preventive dental care that we accept in principle and use to advantage with most patients. In addition, there are preventive practices that are less familiar, less frequently used, and not as well understood—for example, caries activity testing and diet counselling. Because procedures such as these have less established precedence of use we often tend to overlook their very real potential for contribution to the practice of dentistry. It is with some of these lesser known practices, as well as with new and dynamic aspects of familiar preventive practices, that this chapter will be primarily concerned. The reader is asked to consider constructively and to study carefully the considerations and challenges presented here and to carefully weigh them in the light of his own opportunities to prevent dental disease. These programs are not intended to constitute the whole of an office preventive dentistry program, but rather to provide new and positive avenues of approach to the challenges of modern dental practice.

## CARIES ACTIVITY TESTING

Every dentist appreciates the importance of both visual examination and radiographic examination in determining the presence of dental caries. Both means of diagnosis are usually essential in arriving at an accurate estimation of a carious condition. Realizing what these examinations do *not* reveal is also important in terms of total patient care and prevention.

Regardless of how well we have performed visual and radiographic examinations in diagnosing caries, we still have not determined in most cases why the problem exists. Whether caries is caused by or is precipitated by such factors as excessive oral populations of acid-producing organisms, conditions of inadequate oral buffering and prolonged clearance of acid in the plaque, salivary insufficiency or high viscosity, food retention and morphologic problems, or problems of poor oral hygiene has not been clearly established. If we are to deal effectively with preventing the recurrence of dental caries we should understand the reasons for the initial occurrence of the problem. The primary purpose for conducting caries activity testing is to determine those oral factors that may be responsible for the occurrence and recurrence of the carious process. These factors are usually not discovered in the initial diagnosis of caries. Therefore caries activity testing helps provide the "why" in caries diagnosis.

An equally important feature of caries activity testing is the educational benefit to the patient. The tests provide highly motivating experiences and ones that carry dramatic and lasting impact. The patient who undergoes caries activity testing usually responds energetically to suggested home care programs, educational programs, and recall programs. This is especially true if the patient is impressed with the fact that the laboratory tests will evaluate his cooperation at home.

In my personal clinical experience more than 70 percent of patients with rampant caries have responded favorably to office preventive programs based on caries activity testing. In virtually all such cases patient education has been strengthened through such programs.

Two cases of actual patient caries activity testing are presented as examples of clinical use of this type of testing. The patients referred to are among three hundred who have undergone this program.

*Patient B. P.,* 17-year-old male
   Decayed, missing, and filled surfaces: 79
   Active caries surface involvement: 59
   Caries history: Rampant since 2 years of age
   Repeated attempts by other dentists to restore mouth unsuccessful because of recurrent caries
   Results of caries activity testing: Extremely low resting and stimulated salivary flow; stimulated flow averaged 2 to 4 ml. per 15 minutes; patient had excessive materia alba accumulation despite satisfactory brushing habits (use of disclosing wafer[1]); oral clearance notably prolonged (glucose clearance test[2]); reduced buffering capacity (modified Wach test,[3] modified Dreizen test[4]); other tests (Snyder test,[5] salivary viscosity,[6] plaque pH determination[7]) showed little deviation from normal
   Treatment: Medical history negative; patient placed on saliva-stimulating drug (pilocarpine) prior to meals for 1 month under guardian's supervision; salivant (saliva-stimulating) foods prescribed during course of meals
   Results of treatment: Stimulated salivary flow averaged 20 ml. per 15 minutes after 1 month, 16 ml. per 15 minutes after 2 months, 18 ml. per 15 minutes after 1 year, and 21 ml. per 15 minutes after 2 years; there was a noticeable reduction of materia alba after 2 months, 1 year, and 2 years; no new caries after 1 and 2 years (mouth initially restored)

In this case the treatment was combined with full-mouth restorative procedures, office audiovisual education, diet counselling (with both patient and parent), and individualized home care. The patient was placed on a stringent recall program. The fact that there was no recurrence of caries after 2 years was a welcome and encouraging departure from the patient's previous caries history.

*Patient A. S.,* 17-year-old female
   Decayed, missing, and filled surfaces: 76
   Active caries surface involvement: 42
   Caries history: Rampant since 10 years of age
   Results of caries activity testing: Saliva extremely high in acidogenic and aciduric microorganisms and in acid production (Snyder test,[5] modified Wach test[3]); diet analysis showed 76 percent carbohydrate by weight in total diet and 55 percent of carbohydrate being partaken between meals; average eating frequency per day of 12.5 times; other caries activity tests were normal or near normal; brushing habits were poor
   Treatment: Patient and parent received extensive nutritional counselling; nutritional and oral hygiene counselling covered a 4-month, 12-visit period; counselling and operative dentistry were performed simultaneously; repeat of Snyder test and Wach test after 6 and 12 months, along with follow-up diet survey after 12 months, impressed patient with concern of problem and resulted in significant improvement in food habits and reduction in acidogenic and aciduric bacterial population
   Results of treatment: Marked improvement in oral health; patient attitude and general enthusiasm for good dental health showed remarkable improvement (no new caries observed after 1 year; one new surface after 18 months; no new caries after 24 and 30 months)

Again the result was highly encouraging; the patient was able to look forward to the future with the confidence that she would continue to achieve good dental health through preventive dentistry.

Although these are typical examples of the various problems and situations encountered in caries activity testing, it would not be totally accurate to give the impression that complete success is invariably obtained. In considering the 70 percent success of caries activity testing in terms of patient response it must be remembered that each case presented challenging and undeterminable problems before testing was begun. These for the most part were patients with major and rampant caries conditions, and the results often reflected major revisions in habits and practices of many years. Frequently the diet patterns of an entire family needed to be changed.

It is not suggested that caries activity testing be used for each patient. The cost may be prohibitive in some cases, and in others the patient may not be sufficiently motivated to undergo the rigors and demands of the program. With selected patients, however, the results more than justify the time and cost. Patients for whom caries activity testing may be particularly rewarding are classified as follows.
 1. Patients with a high or rampant caries condition who exhibit genuine concern for their problem
 2. Patients with active caries conditions or histories of high caries who are to receive fixed or removable partial dentures, orthodontic treatment, or esthetic rehabilitation
 3. Patients who do not respond to routine office education and home care programs

A few statements are in order concerning the patient education aspects of caries activity testing. Perhaps more than with any other procedure available to the dentist, such a program individualizes and personalizes patient education. It expresses in a meaningful way our concern for the patient and his dental problems and brings about a closer coordination of purpose with the patient in all aspects of care and treatment. It further emphasizes that we are actively working toward promoting good and continued patient dental health.

The experiences of caries activity testing provide much satisfaction to the dentist as well as to the patient. Basically the dentist is enhancing the success of his treat-

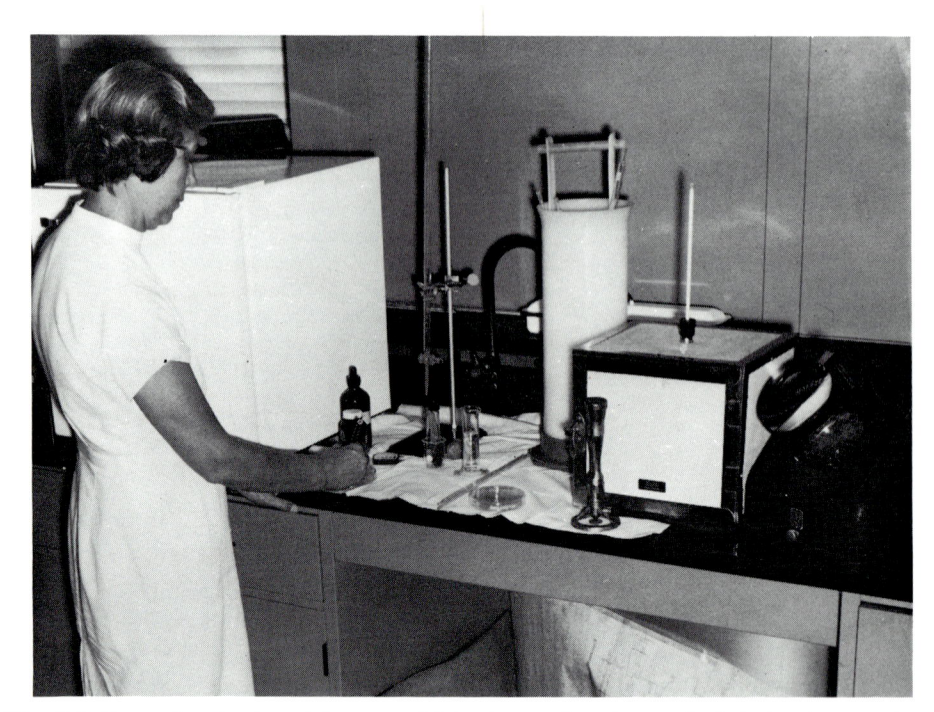

**Fig. 2-1.** Preventive dentistry laboratory. Major items of equipment include incubator, colony counter, refrigerator, and burette.

ment by concerning himself with the correction of those conditions that are likely to result in recurrence of the caries problem. Perhaps most important, he is contributing substantially toward the success of his patient's overall education and preventive dental programs.

It is generally agreed that multiple caries activity testing is significantly more diagnostic than the use of any single test. Suggested tests include disclosing wafer test,[1] glucose clearance test,[2] modified Wach test,[3] modified Dreizen test,[4] Snyder test,[5] salivary flow and viscosity test,[6] and plaque pH determination.[7] This combination of procedures provides a well-coordinated program of office caries activity testing with maximum simplicity of procedure and minimum involvement of time and expense.

A preventive dentistry laboratory is shown in Fig. 2-1. Such a facility is compact, inexpensive to equip, and adaptable to a minimum space requirement.

## NUTRITIONAL COUNSELLING

This section will present a practical clinical approach to patient situations involving diet and nutrition. The dentist who is interested in nutritional counselling, however, must first have a fundamental knowledge of nutrition as it applies to dental health and dental disease. For a background concerning the principles of nutrition the reader is referred to Chapter 3.

Food habits are personal and intimate subjects with our patients. Proper foundations of trust and confidence must be established before we may expect our patients to accept our suggestions for diet revision and change. If nutritional counselling is to be successful, constructive and understanding approaches to the subject are needed. In no other area of patient education is the concept of good personal relations more important in order to derive a cooperative response. The satisfactions of nutritional counselling make the effort challenging and worthwhile.

The degree to which we succeed in nutritional counselling is proportional to the desire to understand the patients and to be understood by them. To some degree, as patients realize our concern for their problems, they will tend to build good habits. We must realize, however, that practices of diet and nutrition are a composite of many physical and social influences and as such are not changed easily. Recommendations, if not compatible with developed practices, may be very difficult for the patient to maintain. Recommended revisions must be personalized according to our understanding of the individual and of the environmental factors that influence his ability to cooperate. If certain foods are to be eliminated from the diet we must help the patient to find acceptable substitutes. If we do not believe that the patient is able to accept major and radical changes we must tailor the recommendations toward progressive revisions in his food habits.

Effective nutritional counselling requires both energy and time. Follow-up counselling is important if the patient is to understand and absorb the instructions. It is most difficult for the patient to coordinate the recommendations provided at a single interview. Because the success of the instruction depends on a clear understanding of procedures to be followed, continued counselling is imperative to a successful outcome. In addition, follow-up counselling makes possible greater emphasis on the importance of proper eating habits to good dental health and helps strengthen the recommendations.

Technics of counselling also need to be adjusted to the needs of the individual. It is helpful to talk not only with the patient but also with the person who plans, pur-

## 12  *Improving dental practice through preventive measures*

chases, and prepares his food. When the patient is a child, it is useful to consult with both child and parent. In all interviews the positive and constructive form of approach is the most effective form of persuasion.

Nutritional counselling may be coupled with caries activity testing with excellent coordination of both procedures. Although this usually takes place at the early appointments, it is sometimes psychologically more effective to carry out these programs

**PATIENT NUTRITION SURVEY**

Patient _____

Date _____

Recordings on alternate days   Include all foods; e.g., sugar, salt, butter,
For a 12-day period            margarine,—Specify amount according to direction

|   | Breakfast | Amt. | Lunch | Amt. | Dinner | Amt. | Between meals | Amt. |
|---|-----------|------|-------|------|--------|------|---------------|------|
| 1 |           |      |       |      |        |      |               |      |
| 2 |           |      |       |      |        |      |               |      |
| 3 |           |      |       |      |        |      |               |      |

**Fig. 2-2.** Patient diet survey sheet. Diets are recorded on alternate days for a 12-day period.

*Incorporation of preventive dentistry into office practice* 13

further along in the course of treatment. Much of the success of the program depends on the early personal relationship that is established with the patient. As with caries activity testing, nutritional counselling results in a lasting and loyal relationship between dentist and patient.

The use of a diet survey sheet (Fig. 2-2) and diet survey instructions (Fig. 2-3) accentuates the meaning of the program to the patient and provides a basis for recommendations. It is helpful to the patient's understanding of dental health for the dentist to go over these survey sheets item by item and to point out areas in which

**DIET SURVEY INSTRUCTIONS**

Please record food intake for 6 days. Include everything that is consumed; except, water, coffee, or tea, unless cream or sugar is used.

Show the kind and amount of each meal item. For example: 1 glass (8 oz.) whole milk; 1 average serving (3 oz.) roast beef; ½ cup (4 oz.) fresh fruit salad; 2 medium oatmeal cookies; coffee with 1 teaspoon sugar.

Brand names of cereal or special food products may be included to help clarify the exact food item eaten. If any between-meal foods are eaten, show this in the appropriate column.

To assist in keeping accurate records, use common household measuring cups and spoons. If a household food scale is available, use it to weigh meat servings.

**USEFUL INFORMATION**

8 tablespoons = ½ cup
1 cup = 8 oz.
1-3 oz. meat serving = 1 medium roast beef slice-¼" thick, or 1 small fish, 1 hamburger pattie, 2 medium-sized pieces of fried chicken, or 3 slices of cold cuts.

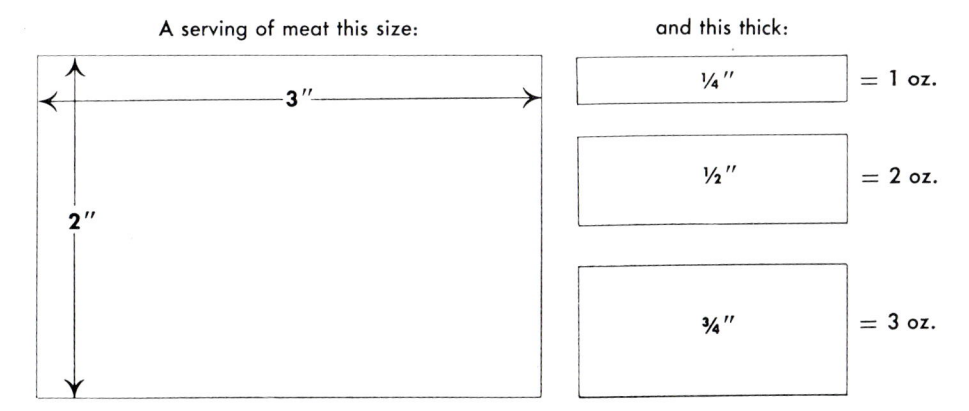

A serving of meat this size:      and this thick:

3"
2"

¼" = 1 oz.

½" = 2 oz.

¾" = 3 oz.

**Fig. 2-3.** Diet survey instruction sheet aids the patient in preparing diet survey sheet.

## NUTRITION SURVEY
### Foods for good health and foods to avoid

Patient_____

Date_____

**BUILD HABITS AROUND THESE FOODS!**

**Milk group**

Milk (_____glasses daily)
Cheese
Cottage cheese
Ice cream

**Meat group** (_____ servings daily)

Meat (beef, pork, lamb, liver,
    heart, kidney)
Fish
Poultry
Eggs
Peanut butter
Dried nuts and beans

**Vegetables and fruits** (_____ servings)

Dark green vegetables (spinach, asparagus, broccoli, etc.)
Yellow vegetables (carrots, cauliflower, squash, etc.)
Citrus fruits and juices
Tomatoes
Apples

**Breads and cereals**

(Use only enriched and whole
grain products. Check label)
Bread
Cooked cereal*
Ready to eat cereal*

**Snacks**

Fruit juices
Raw vegetables (carrots, celery, radishes, tomatoes,
    cauliflower, etc.)
Raw fruits (apples, pears, plums, oranges, etc.)

**Special foods**

*Select those items as low in sucrose as possible.

**AVOID THESE FOODS!**

Brownies
Bubble gum
Cakes
Candy
Candied fruit
Chewing gum
Chocolate milk
Chocolate sauce
Cinnamon breads
Cookies
Cream puffs
Doughnuts
Dried fruits*
Fruits canned in syrup
Honey
Jams
Jellies
Pastries
Pies
Raisin bread
Soda pop
Sugar
Sundaes
Syrups

**Fig. 2-4.** Composite food list of desirable and undesirable foods. Colored pencils are used to underline special emphasis foods.

dietary revisions will be helpful. In most cases personalized, printed recommendations should be given to the patient to study at his leisure.

The recommended revisions should be reasonably suited to the patient's habits and should be simple in directions. A follow-up survey 1 to 2 months later will provide the patient with further opportunity to direct his attention toward his food habits. As with the initial survey, sitting down with the patient and reviewing the survey findings will help provide the proper emphasis. This is also an excellent time for reviewing earlier recommendations and discussing problems or questions that may have arisen.

There are presently available in the literature excellent source materials concerning proper foods for good health.[8-10] In addition, there are sources that provide the sucrose content of various foods and beverages.[11, 12] These combined lists are helpful in designing and implementing diet programs for patients. It is a simple task to alter and tailor these lists to a composite list of foods that may be used as a starting point for nutritional education (Fig. 2-4). For example, as each undesirable food is underlined on the patient survey form, this food and a desirable substitute are underlined in contrasting colors on the composite printed list. When we have completed going over the individual diet survey form with the patient we have an acceptable list of substitute foods underlined on the printed form. The patient may help select the substitute foods according to his likes and tastes. It is then easy to take a second form sheet (Fig. 2-5) and to prepare individual recommendations for foods or food groups

**NUTRITION SURVEY**

Patient____________________

Date____________________

Home care plan____________________

____________________

Foods to especially include____________________

____________________

____________________

Foods to particularly avoid____________________

____________________

____________________

**Fig. 2-5.** Individualized patient diet form should be posted in food preparation area with composite food list.

that the patient should especially avoid or include. When the counselling is completed we have two forms to give the patient; the first is a printed list of foods with underlined emphasis on certain foods and the second is a list of specific and individual recommendations for the patient's personal dietary practices. The two forms that the patient takes home should be posted in a convenient place in the kitchen as a reminder and guide during mealtime and when preparing food.

It has been shown that combining the personal intimacy of direct counselling with the printed form approach is a reasonable and effective means to attain good patient nutrition education.

## PATIENT EDUCATION

The primary objective of patient education is to motivate each patient to assume positive and responsible attitudes toward establishing good dental health. One important means of accomplishing this is to provide satisfying experiences for our patients through the practice of preventive dentistry. The patient who is exposed to caries activity testing and diet counselling, for example, experiences the best in preventive dentistry procedure and is likely to respond in a manner paralleling the depth and scope of his experience. In a like manner, the patient who has undergone dental office audiovisual programming may be expected to react in relation to the extent of his educational experiences. Each practice and procedure of preventive dentistry is vitally charged with opportunity for education, and patient education is the core of our total preventive program.

As preventive dentistry is based soundly on patient education, so is patient education based on good public relations. Goals of patient education cannot be accomplished without developing sincere attitudes of concern, understanding, and friendliness. This involves winning the respect of patients through presenting ourselves and our work at their best. The more that we make good public relations a habit, the more satisfaction and enthusiasm we and our patients derive from our efforts. Favorable patient experiences lead to favorable attitudes and positive responses.

Methods of providing patient education are divided into two categories. The first will be referred to as a direct approach to patient education—meaning that direct contact is employed between the dentist (or auxiliary office personnel) and the patient. The second is an indirect approach to patient education—learning and motivation through the use of modern electronic equipment, pamphlets, and dental photography.

### Direct education

Direct patient education is considered by most workers to be the most effective form of patient education. Face-to-face contact and eye-to-eye contact give us tremendous advantages over other forms of communication. Because our practices are geared to a specific tempo, however, and because direct patient education represents use of premium practice time this approach must be carefully planned and oriented with the patient treatment program. This involves using specific procedures of education at specific times during the treatment schedule. It also involves considering the use of our own and our auxiliaries' time to the best possible advantage in determining which direct education procedures will be used.

Among the most important and most effective means of direct patient education practices are caries activity testing and diet counselling. We already have discussed the mechanics of these programs and how they contribute to the total care and education program provided for the patient. There are other specific direct forms of patient education that may be used to advantage with the majority of patients. Treatment conferences or case presentations are an indispensable part of office practice because they help to convey the treatment that will best benefit the patient as well as help to explain the nature of the involved costs.

Other direct patient education opportunities such as instruction in toothbrush technic or demonstration of the use of dental irrigators may be invaluable means of relating office treatment and experience to the patient's home care program.

With each of these direct patient education experiences the use of models, photographs, and visual aids in general provides understanding and clarity to our communications. Among the most important visual aids are the patient's own radiographs, study models, and photographs, as well as visual histories of other work we have accomplished.

The direct method of patient education should be programmed in advance for each patient. We must decide in which areas the patient most needs education assistance and then must make every effort to coordinate counselling with the related or corresponding treatment procedure. This permits education at the right psychologic moment and makes possible the best utilization of time. Advance planning further ensures that we will have sufficient time to carry out our intended instructional programming.

A word should be said about random patient education practices in the dental office. All of us and our staffs have the opportunity to discourse with the patient at chairside or during "in-between" moments in the office. When possible these moments should be used constructively, with the entire office team aware of its role in providing a continuous office atmosphere of learning and motivation. It should be standard office procedure that the dentist or the auxiliary uses discussion time to talk to a patient about his understanding of good dental health; the patient grows to appreciate this more than discussions concerning the stock market or other nondental subjects.

**Indirect education**

Indirect patient education combines a variety of electronic devices to provide an impressive and highly effective means of audiovisual instruction. While indirect patient education is basically supplemental education, it is an important and often indispensable part of the total office preventive and education program.

Consider a situation with which some dentists are faced almost daily—emergency tooth extraction. Because the patient is brought in on an emergency basis, there is invariably too little time for the dentist to counsel the patient in the importance of having a replacement tooth or of continuing dental treatment. One means of overcoming this problem is to use indirect patient education. After extracting the tooth the dentist explains that he would like the patient to remain in the office for a few moments to view a series of especially prepared slides or filmstrips that cover a subject of particular concern and importance to the patient; the dentist may also explain that this will provide the patient with a few moments of rest and composure prior to returning to outside activities. The patient is taken to a recovery area, which may be a recovery room, business office, laboratory, or operatory not in use, and the program is prepared by an assistant or receptionist. The patient may be left alone to view the slides or filmstrips; after viewing, he turns the machine off and returns to the reception area. The receptionist determines the response of the patient and, if the patient desires, arranges an appointment for further examination.* Thus a situation that began as a negative rather than a positive implication results in a valuable learning experience for the patient.

This is but one of the many dental office situations in which indirect patient education may serve to take the place of the dentist. Providing office educational programs with the aid of electronics is a new and fascinating field and one that is limited only by lack of inventiveness and imagination. Let us consider the types of programs presently possible by this means.

**Electronic programming.** One very effective method of providing indirect dental office patient education is with an automatic filmstrip projector (Figs. 2-6 and 2-7); such a projector is used primarily with professionally prepared filmstrip programs and consists of a projector and a speaker within a single unit. Either a record or a cassette tape provides the sound portion of the program. Filmstrip programs are available from several sources and contain fifty to one hundred color slides printed on a single strip of 35 mm. film. The sound track and pictures are in complete synchronization and a period of only a few seconds is needed to prepare a program for a viewer. Filmstrips are available dealing with a variety of dental health subjects and are prepared skillfully with the aid of dental educators and teaching psychologists. Programs usually run from 7 to 12 minutes.

A recent innovation patterned after the automatic filmstrip projector is the automatic motion picture projector that employs super 8 film cartridges to which coordinated sound has been added. This projector may be used with professional movie films; it employs a speaker and a screen within a single unit. The American Dental Association is presently providing a patient education service using the automatic motion picture projector and professionally prepared film programs; the service may be obtained on a monthly rental basis.

Professional automatic filmstrip or motion picture programs offer factual and instructive information in a manner that is pleasing and interesting to the patient. The use of a professional speaker to provide the oratory often presents some advantages from the patient's viewpoint by having a third party provide authoritative substantiation to the dentist's own recommendations.

Professional patient education programs serve a highly useful purpose in dental office education, but it also is possible for the dentist to provide his own indirect patient education programming. With the use of tape recording, for example, it is possible to project one's own voice into color slides. It is further possible to make these programs entirely automatic with the use of an automatic slide projector and push-button sound synchronization (Fig. 2-8). In designing these programs we may use both our own slides and slides available from such sources as the American Dental Association. If our tape recording and projection equipment does not permit sound synchronization we may design our programs to operate manually. In this instance we may indicate on the tape when we wish the patient to change the slide.

I have found that the cassette recorders are superior to the reel-to-reel recorders in facilitating the preparation, storing, and presentation of taped programs. Modern

---

*An easy-to-read dental health education book written in lay terms is: Muhler, J. C.: Fifty-two pearls and their environment, Bloomington, 1966, Indiana University Press.

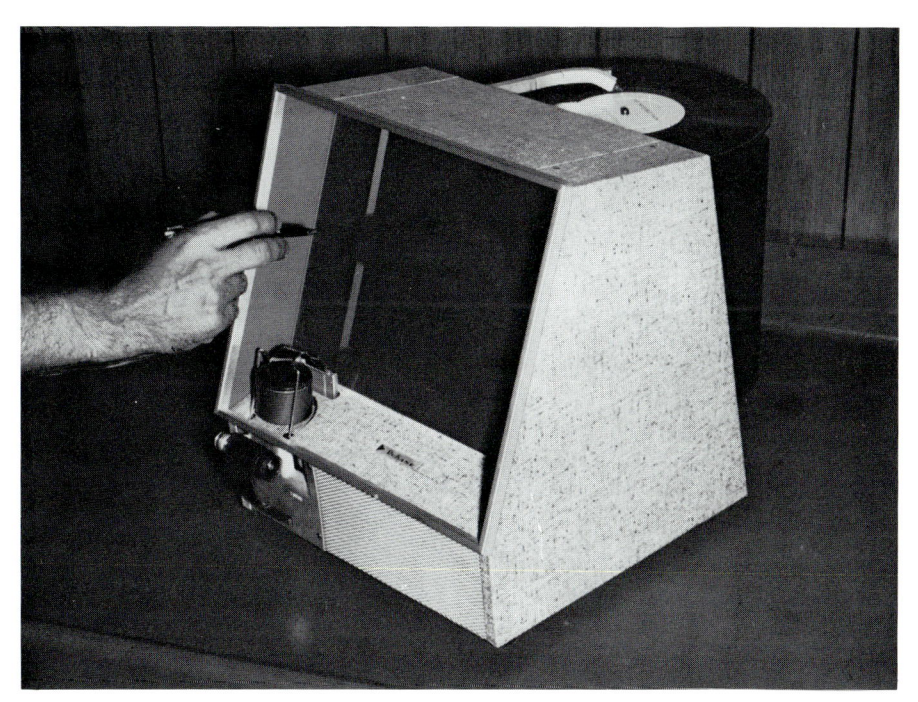

*Incorporation of preventive dentistry into office practice* 19

**Fig. 2-6.** Sound filmstrip projector for indirect patient education. Projector, sound, and picture contained in single unit.

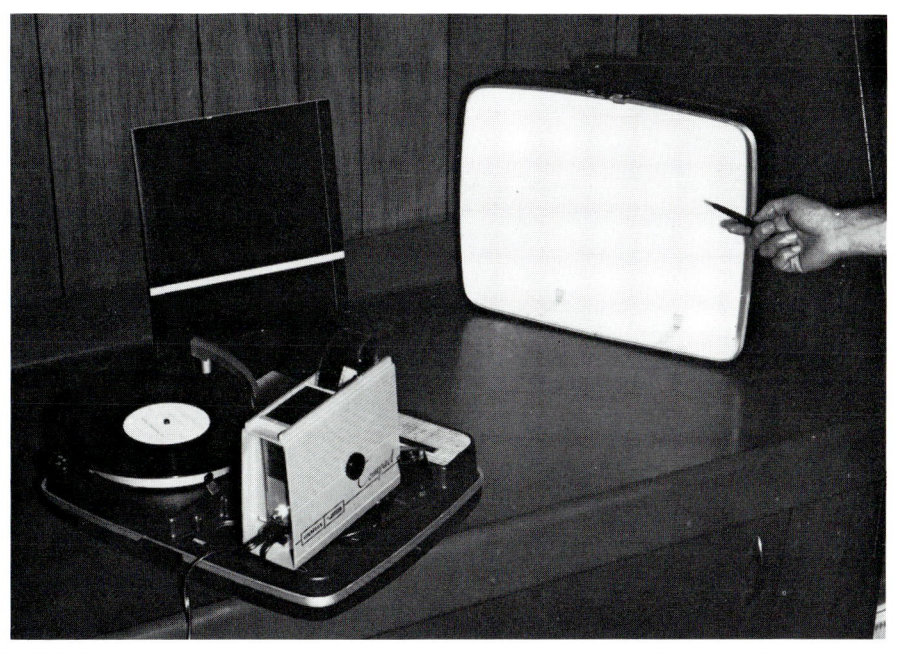

**Fig. 2-7.** Sound filmstrip projector for indirect patient education. Sound and projector contained in single unit. Picture may be projected into inside of cover or on wall or screen. Filmstrip projector may be used independently.

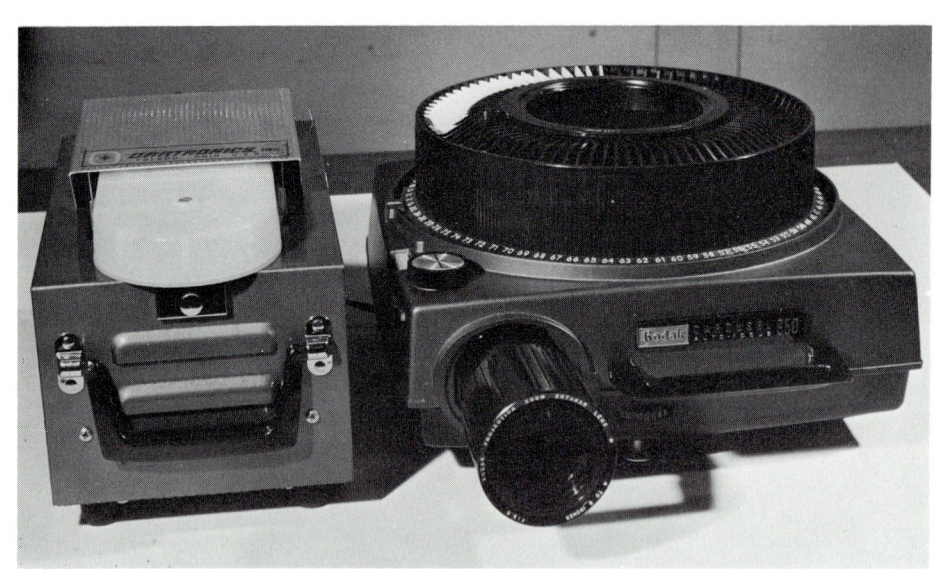

**20** *Improving dental practice through preventive measures*

**Fig. 2-8.** Indirect patient education employing casette tape recorder and automatic slide projector.

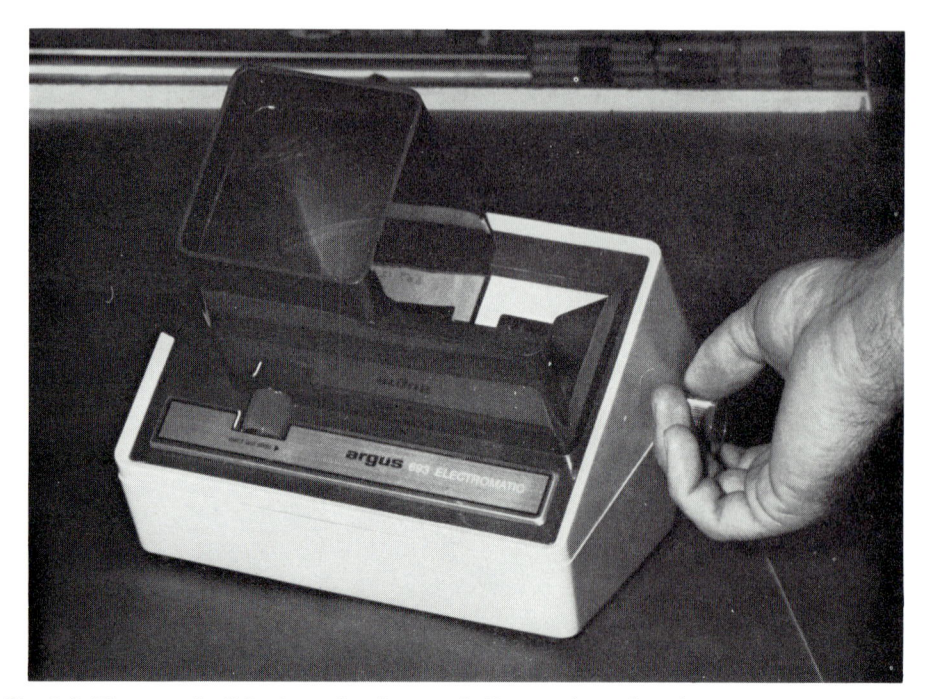

**Fig. 2-9.** Electromatic slide viewer for direct or indirect patient education.

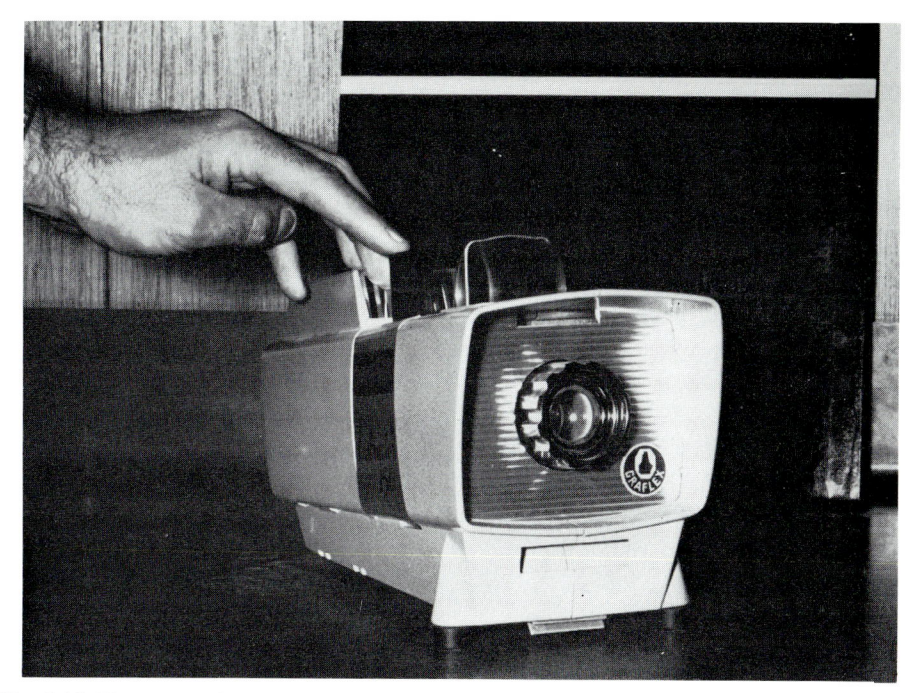

**Fig. 2-10.** Nonautomatic filmstrip projector.

casette tapes may be used identically to reel-to-reel recorders in synchronizing sound programs with an automatic slide projector.

An interesting and inexpensive innovation for viewing color slides is the electromatic slide viewer (Fig. 2-9). Simple to operate, this viewer permits slides to be changed automatically or with a stop-and-go switch. The unit is completely self-contained and is an excellent visual aid for direct or indirect patient education. The viewer may be operated manually for indirect programming.

The dentist may use filmstrips instead of slides when preparing his own patient education program. A single strip of 35 mm. film with each picture permanently in proper sequence is used. Special cameras are available as well as several excellent filmstrip programs from the American Dental Association. If desired, a nonautomatic filmstrip projector (Fig. 2-10) may be used for either direct or indirect patient education.

The use of tape recording and/or professional slide film programming is a fascinating and rewarding experience in setting forth the best efforts to educate patients. These procedures, when combined with direct patient education practices, provide an interesting, varied, and highly successful means of contributing to the patient's dental health through preventive dentistry.

**Pamphlets.** Before we leave the subject of visual education a few words should be said about the use of pamphlets in the dental office—pamphlets should be used discriminately and only when the patient is properly oriented. A pamphlet should be issued for a specific purpose and to serve an individual need. Seldom should more than a single pamphlet be given at one time. The patient should be given only the information that he will utilize. The American Dental Association is an excellent source of dental health literature; its catalogue is mailed yearly to members. Other sources for pamphlets are state health departments, food and dairy associations, and some professional service divisions of commercial dentifrice companies. The dentist should of course review and study all of these pamphlets before providing them for home reading for his patients.

In selecting direct and indirect means of patient education it is good practice to enter on the patient's record the program and procedure used, along with the date of the health education presentation. Education programming often may be outlined to the patient in advance, similar to the manner in which we present our treatment program. This points out to the patient that we are providing a well-coordinated plan of treatment and prevention and stresses the role of dental health education in the overall office care program.

**Slides.** Dental photography is a useful and rewarding means of providing patient education. Photographs on 35 mm. or No. 127 film may be used to excellent advantage in 2 by 2 inch slides. If desired, a single-frame camera in which the film relationships are suitable to the program format may be used to provide filmstrip pictures. We have already discussed how slides and filmstrips may be programmed with a tape recorder.

The dentist who has had little or no experience with dental photography will be impressed with the simplicity and low cost with which these procedures may be carried out. It is recommended that a dealer or salesman be consulted, but a few comments may be made here.

If a 35 mm. camera is used, it should be a single lens reflex type. A ring flash unit and auxiliary lenses to allow closeup photographs will be needed. It is a further advantage to have a camera with an automatic lens. Three excellent low-cost cameras for dental photography are the Kodak Startech, Kodak Instatech, and Superba Progrex. For the dentist preferring photographic prints to color slides, the Polaroid CU-5 camera is inexpensive, is simple to operate, and provides instant color pictures.

**Motion pictures.** For the dentist who may prefer motion pictures to slides for patient education, there is presently excellent photographic and projection equipment available at minimum cost. Super 8 movie equipment is quite prevalent and provides several modern advantages in operation and convenience to the amateur photographer. With certain pieces of super 8 equipment sound may be added directly to a magnetic strip on the film and played back automatically through the projector. With other super 8 systems sound may be programmed with the movie by synchronization with an external tape recorder. Again, it is recommended that a dealer be consulted to determine which equipment will best suit the dentist's needs.

## USE OF FLUORIDE IN THE DENTAL OFFICE

A dental office involved in preventive dentistry is a busy and a productive office. Maximum time utilization is of the essence. The priority practices of preventive dentistry should be those that will most significantly benefit the patients and that will best justify the time used; these criteria should be used to decide the role that fluoride should play in any office program of caries prevention.

The dental practitioner should want to know about the following important points regarding the uses of fluoride.

1. Which fluoride compound and technic have proved most effective for the dental office?

2. How will the use of these procedures benefit a total office preventive program?
3. Does the result justify the dentist's time and the patient's expense?
4. Which patients will benefit from the use of fluoride?

If the use of patient fluoride procedures is to be justified careful consideration must be provided for each of these four questions. In doing this we will use a consensus of the total topical fluoride literature as reference.

The first question to be considered is "Which compound and technic have proved most effective?" In the light of all available evidence and considering the extent and amount of research that have gone into evaluating all fluoride compounds it must be concluded that stannous fluoride is the compound presently available that has "proved most effective." (See Chapter 5 for a more complete discussion of this topic.) This is a far-reaching conclusion and is supported by the number of studies conducted, the number of investigators involved, the number of subjects involved in the research, and the total benefits obtained.

Although considerable attention in recent years has been directed to the fluoride-phosphate compounds,[13-19] the bulk of evidence, both clinical and laboratory, supports stannous fluoride as an effective, safe, and useful compound for dental office use.[20-25, 30-34]

A third compound, sodium fluoride, also lacks versatility (not useful for adults or for children whose teeth developed in an area with optimal fluoride in the water) and requires a series of four treatments, compared to a single treatment for stannous fluoride.

Regarding the latter part of the first question ("Which technic is most effective?"), there is evidence that the use of multiple stannous fluoride therapy (Fig. 2-11) is more effective than any single patient fluoride procedure.[20-23] By multiple procedure is meant the use of either a stannous fluoride–lava pumice or stannous fluoride–zirconium silicate compound for administering a prophylaxis, followed by a topical application of a stannous fluoride aqueous solution and followed further by the use of an approved fluoride dentifrice in the home care program. Present evidence indicates that the use of these multiple stannous fluoride procedures will result

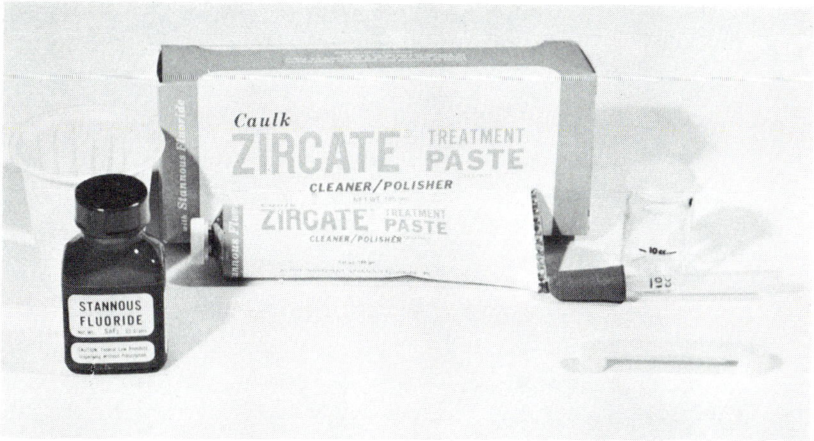

**Fig. 2-11.** Stannous fluoride–zirconium silicate prophylaxis paste plus stannous fluoride and measuring devices for aqueous topical treatment.

in caries reductions of approximately 70 percent in both children's and adults' permanent teeth.

The second question ("How will the use of these procedures benefit a total office preventive program?") is important in coordinating our recall programs, home care programs, and patient education activities into a carefully planned curriculum.

In answering this question it should be pointed out that, for adequate protection against caries for the patient with a low level of caries or with inactive caries, the stannous fluoride–zirconium silicate prophylaxis (or stannous fluoride–lava pumice prophylaxis, although this is less palatable to the patient) should be administered every 6 months for a total of at least 18 months. For the child or adult who has experienced or is presently experiencing an active caries problem the stannous fluoride–zirconium silicate prophylaxis (Zircate Treatment Paste with stannous fluoride) should be accompanied by the stannous fluoride liquid topical treatment. If there is no new caries after the initial three prophylaxis treatments (or prophylaxis plus topical) the stannous fluoride–zirconium silicate prophylaxis may be given once yearly as a booster treatment until the patient returns with one or more active carious lesions. If new caries occurs it may be prudent to step up the fluoride protection program. It should be emphasized also that each period of prophylaxis is a good opportunity to administer the stannous fluoride–zirconium silicate prophylaxis paste. This will usually enable treatments to correlate closely with the recall program that will be prescribed for most patients. Because the success in recalling patients determines to a great extent the effectiveness of a patient education program we must provide the patient with sufficient stimuli to regard recall as an important part of his total education experience. As the patient becomes aware of the relationship between office fluoride procedures and his dental health his enthusiasm for recall is stimulated.

Similarly, from a standpoint of home care, stannous fluoride helps to emphasize good procedure. There is considerable evidence, for example, that use of an approved stannous fluoride dentifrice (the third procedure of multiple stannous fluoride therapy) will prolong the protective effects of the stannous fluoride prophylaxis and topical application.[21-25] In effect, we provide a topical treatment each time we brush our teeth with the dentifrice by replacing those protective ions that are lost through attrition and abrasion. This means that we are providing our patient with a tangible means of caries prevention and one with which he may work to implement a successful home care program. Through the use of multiple stannous fluoride therapy we are thus helping the patient to understand his role in the home care program.

Multiple dental office fluoride procedures also help to implement the office programs of patient education. Thoroughness in dealing with a caries problem tells the patient that we are vitally interested in his dental well-being. In addition, the thoroughness of our efforts impresses on the patient the measure of his own responsibility in caring for his mouth.

The third question ("Does the result justify the dentist's time and patient's expense?") must also be answered in the affirmative. We have already discussed the contributions to recall, home care, and office education and from these standpoints alone we have considerable justification for administering fluoride treatment. When in addition we consider significant caries reductions it is not difficult to justify the time, energy, and cost involved with these treatments.

The answer to the final question ("Which of my patients will benefit?") depends on the choice of fluoride compound. If one of the fluoride-phosphate compounds or sodium fluoride is used as the fluoride compound we may anticipate that the maximum caries preventive benefit will occur with children's permanent teeth in a suboptimum fluoride area.[14-19, 26-29] If we use stannous fluoride, however, we are assured of effectiveness for the teeth of both children and adults[21-23, 30, 31] as well as benefit regardless of the water fluoride content.[22, 32] Therefore with stannous fluoride we expand our benefits to the great majority of patients in our practice.

• • •

I have attempted in this section to present an objective and accurate view of the current status of fluoride in relationship to dental practice. There is no question that stannous fluoride presents by far the most convincing evidence of effectiveness of any fluoride compound available. However, further clarification needs to be made. Because stannous fluoride in liquid topical form has a disagreeable taste to some and results in pigmentation of demineralized enamel, there are those who would question the good judgment of its use. It should be remembered that enamel which becomes pigmented from stannous fluoride represents arrested development of caries.[33, 34] Experience has shown that pigmentation is a highly favorable sign; as long as pigmentation is present caries either will be arrested completely or will progress very slowly. Also, although the taste of topical stannous fluoride is disagreeable, this slight unpleasantness may be minimized by warning the patient of the taste and by telling him to avoid excessive contact of the substance with his tongue. When patients are advised of the benefits to be gained from the use of topical stannous fluoride (where indicated), few will object to a temporary taste inconvenience, but will respond favorably to receiving the best that dentistry has to offer. It should be stressed that I am referring here only to the liquid topical treatment; the stannous fluoride–zirconium silicate prophylaxis paste has a pleasant taste.

• • •

## RECALL

A recall program should reflect a total office preventive dentistry program. It is an important measure of the effectiveness of communication with our patients. If the approach to office education and prevention is meaningful patients will welcome recall as an integral and important part of treatment. If we are haphazard in our preventive approach to patient care we can anticipate a poor response to recall.

A good recall program offers distinct advantages to both patient and dentist. From the patient's viewpoint it helps assure good health by regular examination and prophylactic treatment, if required, and is an economical approach to dental treatment. For the dentist it is an important means of equalizing the distribution of patients and income and of establishing a permanency of patients in his practice.

If recall is to be effective the patient's relationship with the dental office must be established in a manner that will provide maximum incentive for him to return. This positive relationship is based on an understanding of the meaning of prevention in terms of his own needs. It is established and built upon throughout our initial programs of care and treatment.

There are three basic methods for recalling a patient: (1) scheduling the appointment in advance, (2) reminding the patient by telephone, and (3) using reminder cards. A successful method will usually employ a combination of two of the three technics.

```
                    VICTOR H. MERCER, D.D.S.
                       1051 E. Raymond Street
                        Indianapolis, Indiana

                                              Date:_____

        Dear_____,

            The calendar tells us that you are due for your recall ex-
        amination. As you know, this is an important part of your total
        preventive dentistry program.

        Reason for recall:_____
        _____

            We will contact you within the next few days to arrange
        an appointment.
                                    Sincerely,

                                    VICTOR H. MERCER, D.D.S.
```

Fig. 2-12. Recall reminder card.

Patients respond better to an actual appointment than to a telephone call or a card; however, the telephone is more effective than the reminder card when the appointment is not scheduled in advance. The most effective means of recall is scheduling the appointment in advance and following this with a duplicate of the appointment card or a telephone reminder 1 week before the appointment. Because it is not always practical to schedule an appointment several months in advance, an alternative is to send the reminder card (Fig. 2-12) and follow up with a telephone call 1 week later. The actual appointment is best scheduled by telephone.

If a reminder card is used to initially notify a patient of recall, it should be personalized to the extent of writing in the patient's name and reason for recall. A personal salutation also helps to informalize and individualize the message. The use of a personal note instead of the card lends directness and individuality to the recall message. A further personal touch to the recall reminder is to have the patient address the card or letter prior to being placed on recall. This works especially well with children, who enjoy receiving mail addressed to them in their own handwriting.

Reference filing is of the utmost importance in establishing an active and successful recall program. This may be accomplished in several ways. One of the simplest is the recall list, which is indexed on a monthly basis. Generally the recall list works reasonably well, although it may be more time consuming than some other methods.

A method of recall that is more precise than the recall list is the recall card file system (Fig. 2-13), which involves placing a recall card in an index file according to the month of recall. Cards are removed at the beginning of the month and the pa-

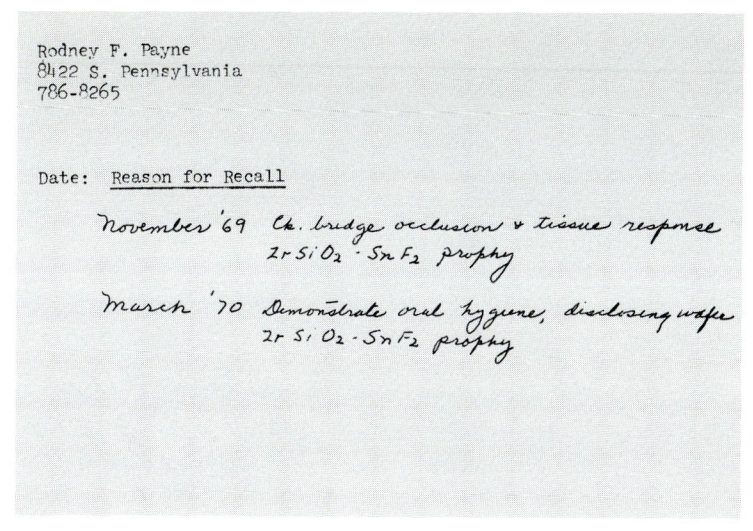

**Fig. 2-13.** Recall card used in recall card file system.

tients are sent reminder cards and called. When an advance appointment is made a duplicate of the appointment card is attached to the recall card, which informs the receptionist or assistant of the appointment. Preaddressed postal cards or envelopes may also be attached to the patient's card. The cards used in the card file system are permanent and may be reindexed.

Other programs of recall utilize the patient's treatment record and thus eliminate the need for a special recall card file. One method is to maintain two file drawers designated "active" and "recall," respectively. When a patient is finished with active treatment his chart is placed in the recall file in alphabetical order, with an attached color tab corresponding to the month of recall. At the designated time charts bearing a certain color tab are removed and the patients are contacted. This method is more confusing than the recall card file system.

Regardless of the reference method used to recall patients, the important features of a recall program are that it be simple, occupy a minimum of office procedure, and provide maximum motivation to the patient. The recall program that is effective is one that works.

Definite and routine procedures should be carried out at the recall appointment. Thorough examination (both clinical and radiographic), prophylaxis, and stannous fluoride treatment should be performed for most patients. In addition, time should be allotted for counselling patients in matters of oral hygiene, diet, and home care. Audiovisual education should be used in emphasizing certain aspects of care and treatment. Often selective caries activity testing needs to be repeated to check thoroughness of home care or diet. It is good procedure to check oral hygiene with a disclosing wafer before the prophylaxis.

Operative procedures, if needed, should usually be deferred to a subsequent appointment; this allows the dentist to better utilize his time and allows the patient to prepare psychologically for operative treatment. A wet reading of the radiographs while the patient is in the office is good practice in arranging for future appointments and for advising the patient of needed treatment. With proper utilization of time and coordination by auxiliary personnel the recall appointment can and should be completed in 1 hour or less.

## CONCLUSION

Preventive dentistry in the most complete sense encompasses all efforts in the dental office and in the community to improve dental health. Its overall contribution is concerned with treatment, education, and public relations, and it employs positive and practical means of influencing dental health.

Because preventive dentistry is concerned with people, the purpose of this chapter has been to outline, in terms of practical employment, those practices that will enhance our approach to people's dental problems. Some of these practices have been familiar to the reader; others have no doubt been relatively unfamiliar. In all instances they have been chosen because they represent a vital and usable means of preventing dental disease. These include caries activity testing, nutritional counselling, direct and indirect patient education practices, use of office fluoride, and patient recall.

There are of course many additional preventive dental services that have not been specifically covered or have received only brief mention here. The use of the disclosing wafer in the patient home care program, for example, is becoming more important in developing good oral hygiene practices. Proper management of problems of morphology and occlusion is also of utmost concern in providing total preventive care. Excellent discussions of these and other opportunities of preventive dentistry may be found in other parts of this text. The dentist who is concerned with prevention will search out and utilize this information to good advantage for his patients. Prevention is the cornerstone of good patient care, and tremendously rewarding experiences are possible for both the patient and dentist through its use.

## REFERENCES

1. Arnim, S. S., and Williams, Q. E.: How to educate patients in oral hygiene, Dent. Radiogr. Photogr. 32:61, 1959.
2. Cox, G. J., Draus, F. J., and Entress, C. P.: How long does sugar remain in the mouth? D. Progress 3:152, 1963.
3. Wach, E. C., and others: Testing caries activity by acid production in saliva, J. Dent. Res. 22:415, 1943.
4. Dreizen, S., and others: Buffer capacity of saliva as a measure of dental caries activity, J. Dent. Res. 25:213, 1946.
5. Snyder, M. L.: A simple colorimetric method for the estimation of relative numbers of *Lactobacillus* in saliva, J. Dent. Res. 19:349, 1940.
6. McDonald, R. E.: Human saliva—a study of the rate of flow and viscosity and its relationship to dental caries, Indianapolis, 1950, Indiana University (Master's thesis).
7. Stephan, R. M.: Intra-oral hydrogen ion concentrations associated with dental caries activity, J. Dent. Res. 23:257, 1944.
8. Jay, P.: Dietary program for the control of dental caries, Ann Arbor, Michigan, 1951, The Overbeck Co., Publishers.
9. Nizel, A. E.: Nutrition in clinical dentistry, Philadelphia, 1960, W. B. Saunders Co.
10. American Medical Association: Handbook of nutrition, ed. 2, New York, 1951, McGraw-Hill Book Co.
11. Home and Garden Bulletin No. 72, Washington, D. C., 1964, Superintendent of Documents, Government Printing Office.
12. American Dental Association: Diet and dental health, Chicago, 1963, The Association.
13. Brudevold, F., and others: Study of acidulated fluoride solutions: in vitro effects on enamel, Arch. Oral Biol. 8:167, 1963.

14. Wellock, W. D., and Brudevold, F.: Study of acidulated fluoride solutions, II, the caries inhibiting effect of single annual topical applications of an acidic fluoride and phosphate solution: a two-year experience, Arch. Oral Biol. 8:179, 1963.
15. Pameijer, J. H. N., Brudevold, F., and Hunt, E. E.: Study of acidulated fluoride solutions, III, cariostatic effect of repeated topical sodium fluoride applications with and without phosphate: a pilot study, Arch. Oral Biol. 8:183, 1963.
16. Wellock, W. D., and others: Caries increments, tooth discoloration and state of oral hygiene in children given single annual applications of acid phosphate fluoride and stannous fluoride, Arch. Oral Biol. 10:453, 1965.
17. Averill, H. M., and others: A two year comparison of three topical fluoride agents, Amer. J. Public Health 57:1627, 1967.
18. Cartwright, H. V., Lindahl, R. L., and Bawden, J. W.: Clinical findings on the effectiveness of stannous fluoride and acid phosphate fluoride as caries reducing agents in children, J. Dent. Child. 35:36, 1968.
19. Horowitz, H. S.: Effect on dental caries topically applied acidulated phosphate fluoride: results after two years, J.A.D.A. 78:568, 1969.
20. Mercer, V. H., and Gish, C. W.: Stannous fluoride versus sodium fluoride and acid phosphate as a topical agent, J. Indiana Dent. Ass. 45:15, 1966.
21. Bixler, D., and Muhler, J. C.: Effect on dental caries in children in nonfluoride area of combined use of three agents containing stannous fluoride: a prophylactic paste, a solution and a dentifrice, J.A.D.A. 68:792, 1964.
22. Gish, C. W., and Muhler, J. C.: Effect on dental caries in children in a natural fluoride area of combined use of three agents containing stannous fluoride: a prophylactic paste, a solution and a dentifrice, J.A.D.A. 70:914, 1965.
23. Scola, F. P., and Ostrom, C. A.: Clinical evaluation of stannous fluoride when used as a constituent of a compatible prophylactic paste, as a topical solution, and in a dentifrice in naval personnel, II, report of findings after two years, J.A.D.A. 77:594, 1968.
24. Muhler, J. C.: The combined anticariogenic effect of a single stannous fluoride treatment and the unsupervised use of a stannous fluoride dentifrice, J. Dent. Res. 38:994, 1959.
25. Mercer, V. H., and Muhler, J. C.: Laboratory studies concerning the synergistic effect of a single topical stannous fluoride treatment and the use of a stannous fluoride-containing dentifrice, J. Dent. Res. 40:712, 1961.
26. Downs, R. A., and Pelton, W. J.: Effect of topically applied fluorides in dental caries experience on children residing in fluoride areas, J. Dent. Child. 18:2, 1951.
27. Kutler, B., and Ireland, R. L.: Effect of sodium fluoride application on dental caries in adults, J. Dent. Res. 31:493, 1952.
28. Ast, D. B.: Sodium fluoride dental caries prophylaxis, New York Dent. J. 16:441, 1950.
29. Galagan, D. J., and Vermillion, J.: Effect of topical fluorides on teeth matured on fluoride bearing water, Dent. Abstr. 1:230, 1956.
30. Protheroe, D. H.: Study to determine the effect of topical application of stannous fluoride on dental caries in young adults, Roy. Canad. D. Corps Quart. 1:18, 1961.
31. McDonald, R. E., and Muhler, J. C.: The superiority of topical application of stannous fluoride on primary teeth, J. Dent. Child. 24:84, 1957.
32. Muhler, J. C.: The anticariogenic effectiveness of a single application of stannous fluoride in children residing in an optimum fluoride area, J.A.D.A. 61:431, 1960.
33. Muhler, J. C.: Stannous fluoride enamel pigmentation—evidence of caries arrestment, J. Dent. Child. 27:157, 1960.
34. Mercer, V. H., and Muhler, J. C.: The clinical demonstration of caries arrestment following topical stannous fluoride treatments, J. Dent. Child. 32:65, 1965.

# Chapter 3 Preventive nutrition

## James H. Shaw

Need for good nutrition
The dentist and the application of nutritional knowledge
What constitutes the ideal diet?
    Milk group
    Meat group
    Vegetable-fruit group
    Bread-cereal group
Nutritional relationships to oral cavity
    Soft tissues
    Mineralized tissues
        Nutritional influences during tooth development
        Nutritional influences during tooth maturation
        Postdevelopmental relationships to the teeth
    Nutrition and periodontal disease
    Nutrition and congenital errors of development
Evaluation of nutritional status
Recommendations for dietary improvement
    Protein, vitamins, and minerals
    Energy and fat and carbohydrate consumption
    Dietary supplementation
    Dietary recommendations for patients after surgery or denture insertion
Communication of recommendations to the patient
Conclusion

## NEED FOR GOOD NUTRITION

The goal of good nutrition is to provide daily an adequate and well-balanced supply of all nutrients throughout the various periods of life with appropriate adjustments during times of altered need, such as pregnancy, lactation, diarrhea, wound healing, and so on. For maintenance of optimal nutriture each individual must be considered and provided for on the basis of his background, preferences, way of life, and specific needs. Fulfillment of this goal requires the availability of appropriate high quality food; in addition, the food should be selected carefully, prepared adequately to conserve nutritional values, and served in palatable and esthetically attractive fashion with special attention to the provision of varied menus.

The ideal is to anticipate altered needs with changing circumstances on a preventive basis rather than to force the patient to adopt more heroic and less effective procedures to correct existing deficiencies that may have existed for long periods and may have left indelible records. Inadequacy of fluoride or deficiencies of calcium, phosphorus, or vitamin D during tooth development are typical examples of nutritional problems with sequelae that cannot be erased by later addition of these food factors to the diet. The chemical composition and the histologic integrity of the teeth indelibly reflect the circumstances during mineralization and serve as physiologic kymographs. In all probability the nutritional relationships to atherosclerosis have comparably long-standing and involved features that are not wholly reversible by a return to optimal diets.

Of all the facets of our physical environment probably the most important is the food that we obtain from it. Literally we are in large measure what we eat. While optimal nutriture does not automatically guarantee that we will be free from infections and degenerative diseases, it does ensure that our bodies will be better able to cope with the rigors of our environment and with the disease problems to which we are subjected.

The nutritional needs of a person ultimately depend on the requirements and responsibilities of the myriad cells that compose the body. Our individual cells are incredibly complex and efficient engines that are capable of liberating stored chemical energy to do work either within themselves, within the body, or on the surrounding environment. The kind of work varies from one cell type to another and covers a multitude of energy transformations. The work may be mechanical, as in the muscular contraction for walking, talking, or pumping blood; it may be transportal and concentrative, as in the establishment and maintenance of high intracellular potassium concentrations and high extracellular sodium concentrations and in the elaboration of the high hydrogen ion concentration of gastric juice; it may be electrical, as in the transmission of neural impulses; or it may be chemical, as in the synthesis of macromolecules for continued cellular function, growth, multiplication, and replacement, repair, and mineralization of bones and teeth.

An analogy may help to illustrate the need of these cells to be adequately nourished constantly. Just as the motor of a car requires gasoline as its stored energy source to perform the work needed for operation of the car, cells require chemically stored energy in the form of fats and carbohydrates (and less desirably in proteins) for conversion through oxidation to utilizable forms of energy with which the cells are able to power their work requirements. The most precise and high-powered gasoline engine of a modern car is required basically to do only two kinds of work, propel the car and generate electricity, which it performs in simple fashion through combustion (oxidation) at wholly unphysiologic temperatures and very inefficiently. In contrast, cells have a far greater number and variety of work responsibilities, which they perform efficiently under the very demanding requirement of minimal deviation from body temperature. Whereas the gasoline engine requires gasoline and oxygen as the sole consumable nutrients, cells require not only fuel as their energy source and oxygen for its oxidation but also a variety of other chemicals to enable them to liberate energy and to provide the building blocks for synthesis of macromolecules. The cells' requirements in addition to oxygen and an energy source are water, one or more polyunsaturated fatty acids, and at least twenty amino acids, thirteen vitamins, and thirteen minerals.

Just as the motor of a car dies when all the gasoline has been burned, so the activities of cells stop when their energy source or the supply of any one of their other required nutrients has been exhausted. Cessation of one or more types of cellular activity may not be as conspicuous and dramatic as that of a gasoline engine because of conservation measures or storage of some nutrients in the body. Nonetheless, the end result is eventually no different. Furthermore, cells faced with metabolic disorders or poor absorption of nutrients from the intestine behave similarly to a gasoline engine with a dirty carburetor, an improper fuel-oxygen mixture, or poor timing of the spark plugs.

The preceding analogy may serve to underline the imperative need for good nutrition on a meal-by-meal and day-by-day basis. Indeed, the food that we eat is undoubtedly the most important single determinant of our general state of health and well-being throughout life, of our useful productivity in society, and of our enjoyment of leisure time. Adequate nutrition cannot guarantee freedom from all illnesses and accidents. However, ample evidence indicates that the well-nourished individual responds more readily during recovery. The need for special attention to the provision of the best diet possible during illness and after accidents and surgery is obvious because of the increased nutritional requirements for the synthesis of the components used in repair.

## THE DENTIST AND THE APPLICATION OF NUTRITIONAL KNOWLEDGE

Happily there is an increasing emphasis on the prevention of disease in all the health professions, and the dentist has heretofore unparalleled opportunities to participate in the prevention of disease as well as in its treatment. Simultaneously, evidence for the benefits of good nutrition continues to accrue. Each member of the health professions needs to know what constitutes a good diet for a specific individual under a given physiologic circumstance. Equally important, each member of the health professions needs to seek ways and means to effectively apply his knowledge of good nutrition for the benefit of each individual under his care and supervision.

In view of these developments the dentist has major responsibilities, as well as real opportunities to follow through in the nutritional phase of patient care. He is well respected in his community, which means that appropriate, thoughtful recommendations will have a high likelihood of acceptance. The dentist in many cases sees a wider variety of patients than the physician because of the universality of the need for dental care in otherwise outwardly healthy individuals. In a pedodontic practice the dentist will often find that he is the only member of the health professions who has any significant contact during the long period of growth and development when nutritional demands are high—after termination of pediatric care and before the onset of physical problems associated with the middle-aged and older patient.

The dentist should create opportunities during the course of diagnostic and treatment procedures that may be turned to discussions of nutritional practices and requirements instead of to sports, politics, and the stock market. The dentist's auxiliary staff can be educated to provide supporting help in the collection of dietary information from patients and in the evaluation of diet histories. The waiting room can and should be used very effectively for the display of attractive posters emphasizing various phases of good nutrition, as well as other phases of preventive dentistry. Well-designed booklets dealing with nutrition should also be made available to all patients. A shelf of elementary nutrition textbooks for loan between visits may often prove to be popular when coordinated with the total preventive care program provided by the dentist. Probably no one in the health professions has more opportunity than the dentist to observe the results of poor dietary and nutritional practices, which are evidenced in the varied tissues of the oral cavity. Nor has any other member of the health team a greater opportunity to see the benefits resulting from improved practices.

The dentist increasingly needs to understand the fundamentals of the science of nutrition and their application in the dental profession. This knowledge should not be narrowly limited to those nutritional influences on oral tissues only, important as they are, but should encompass the entire body. Axiomatically, what is good nutrition for oral tissues is good nutrition for all other body tissues. The amounts and distribution of nutrients necessary to provide systemic optimal health will at the same time provide optimal health for the varied tissues of the oral cavity. There is no evidence that the oral tissues during development or maintenance have quantitatively different requirements for nutrients than comparable tissues elsewhere in the body. However, the dentist would in addition be concerned to ensure more careful attention to those dietary components likely to promote undesirable collections of food debris on and between the tooth surfaces. The dentist should also be concerned about providing an adequate source of fluoride ingestion, especially during tooth development. Normally his recommendations for nutritional well-being would be accompanied by specific advice of other kinds to encourage optimal oral hygiene.

It is imperative that the dietary recommendations given by a dentist not conflict with those provided to the same individual at some earlier or later occasion by a member of another health profession. When both recommendations are based on sound nutritional information, there is little likelihood of dissonance unless there has been some major intervening change in the patient's health and needs. Whenever appropriate, there should be nutritional consultation between the dentist and the physician.

The dentist, and indeed all members of the health professions, must be careful not to espouse fads or to encourage faddism, either in the form of promotion of unnecessary, high-concentration multivitamin, multimineral preparations for routine use or of exorbitant specially grown or prepared foods or in the form of overusage of "special" individual foodstuffs for which panacea claims are made. Very large amounts of money are being spent annually in the United States to purchase many items of this nature. All too frequently the elderly with modest incomes are easy prey for the cure-all, prevent-all advertising of the food faddists and quacks. Ordinarily the same amount of money spent for the purchase of a good distribution of food items can be expected to provide an adequate and better balanced diet. Undue consumption of one or two special items, even though they may be very good in themselves, often leads to lack of concern for provision of a good distribution of all foodstuffs. This trend often occurs when there is a dependence on a multivitamin, multimineral preparation on the basis that this preparation provides all the essential nutrients. Therefore the rest of the food consumed is merely for energy and to appease hunger.

## WHAT CONSTITUTES THE IDEAL DIET?

The ideal diet for a given individual will provide him with an adequate amount of each nutrient as described in Table 3-1.[1] These allowances have been developed through extensive consultation of the members of the Food and Nutrition Board on the basis of the best available clinical studies; the allowances are considered to be generous for the average normal individual. The generosity of the allowances should be taken into account when confronted by the biologic variations within a national population. For any nutrient the variation in requirement from one individual to another through a large population may differ by 50 percent or more.

**Table 3-1.** *Recommended daily dietary allowances, revised 1968, designed for the*

|  | Age† (years) | Weight (Kg., lbs.) |  | Height (cm.; in.) |  | Calories | Protein (Gm.) | Fat-soluble vitamins |  |  |
|---|---|---|---|---|---|---|---|---|---|---|
|  |  |  |  |  |  |  |  | Vitamin A activity (I.U.) | Vitamin D (I.U.) | Vitamin E activity (I.U.) |
| Infants | 0-1/6 | 4 | 9 | 55 | 22 | Kg. × 120 | Kg. × 2.2‡ | 1,500 | 400 | 5 |
|  | 1/6-1/2 | 7 | 15 | 63 | 25 | Kg. × 110 | Kg. × 2.0‡ | 1,500 | 400 | 5 |
|  | 1/2- 1 | 9 | 20 | 72 | 28 | Kg. × 100 | Kg. × 1.8‡ | 1,500 | 400 | 5 |
| Children | 1- 2 | 12 | 26 | 81 | 32 | 1,100 | 25 | 2,000 | 400 | 10 |
|  | 2- 3 | 14 | 31 | 91 | 36 | 1,250 | 25 | 2,000 | 400 | 10 |
|  | 3- 4 | 16 | 35 | 100 | 39 | 1,400 | 30 | 2,500 | 400 | 10 |
|  | 4- 6 | 19 | 42 | 110 | 43 | 1,600 | 30 | 2,500 | 400 | 10 |
|  | 6- 8 | 23 | 51 | 121 | 48 | 2,000 | 35 | 3,500 | 400 | 15 |
|  | 8-10 | 28 | 62 | 131 | 52 | 2,200 | 40 | 3,500 | 400 | 15 |
| Males | 10-12 | 35 | 77 | 140 | 55 | 2,500 | 45 | 4,500 | 400 | 20 |
|  | 12-14 | 43 | 95 | 151 | 59 | 2,700 | 50 | 5,000 | 400 | 20 |
|  | 14-18 | 59 | 130 | 170 | 67 | 3,000 | 60 | 5,000 | 400 | 25 |
|  | 18-22 | 67 | 147 | 175 | 69 | 2,800 | 60 | 5,000 | 400 | 30 |
|  | 22-35 | 70 | 154 | 175 | 69 | 2,800 | 65 | 5,000 | — | 30 |
|  | 35-55 | 70 | 154 | 173 | 68 | 2,600 | 65 | 5,000 | — | 30 |
|  | 55-75+ | 70 | 154 | 171 | 67 | 2,400 | 65 | 5,000 | — | 30 |
| Females | 10-12 | 35 | 77 | 142 | 56 | 2,250 | 50 | 4,500 | 400 | 20 |
|  | 12-14 | 44 | 97 | 154 | 61 | 2,300 | 50 | 5,000 | 400 | 20 |
|  | 14-16 | 52 | 114 | 157 | 62 | 2,400 | 55 | 5,000 | 400 | 25 |
|  | 16-18 | 54 | 119 | 160 | 63 | 2,300 | 55 | 5,000 | 400 | 25 |
|  | 18-22 | 58 | 128 | 163 | 64 | 2,000 | 55 | 5,000 | 400 | 25 |
|  | 22-35 | 58 | 128 | 163 | 64 | 2,000 | 55 | 5,000 | — | 25 |
|  | 35-55 | 58 | 128 | 160 | 63 | 1,850 | 55 | 5,000 | — | 25 |
|  | 55-75+ | 58 | 128 | 157 | 62 | 1,700 | 55 | 5,000 | — | 25 |
| Pregnancy |  |  |  |  |  | + 200 | 65 | 6,000 | 400 | 30 |
| Lactation |  |  |  |  |  | +1,000 | 75 | 8,000 | 400 | 30 |

*From Food and Nutrition Board, National Academy of Sciences, National Research Council. The allowance levels environmental stresses. The recommended allowances can be attained with a variety of common foods, providing other and of nutrients not tabulated.
†Entries on lines for age range 22-35 years represent the reference man and woman at age 22. All other entries repre
‡Assures protein equivalent to human milk. For proteins not 100 percent utilized factors should be increased propor
§The folacin allowances refer to dietary sources as determined by *Lactobacillus casei* assay. Pure forms of folacin
‖Niacin equivalents include dietary sources of the vitamin itself plus 1 mg. equiv. for each 60 mg. of dietary try

There is no guarantee that an individual with a very low requirement for one nutrient will not have a very high requirement for one or more other nutrients. Thus the term allowance was deliberately chosen instead of requirement, hopefully to ensure that even an individual with a higher than average requirement would be adequately provided for within the allowance. At the same time the minor excess for an individual with lower daily needs would not be undesirable to him, except possibly for calories, in which case excess can be readily discerned by frequent use of a scale. These recommended allowances are easily obtained from foods that are routinely available in normal commerce without need for supplementation with proprietary preparations. The abundance and variety of foodstuffs available today makes possible the planning of a wide diversity of diets, all of which would easily *maintenance of good nutrition of practically all healthy people in the United States**

| | | Water-soluble vitamins | | | | | Minerals | | | | |
|---|---|---|---|---|---|---|---|---|---|---|---|
| Ascorbic acid (mg.) | Folacin (mg.)§ | Niacin (mg. equiv.)‖ | Riboflavin (mg.) | Thiamine (mg.) | Vitamin $B_6$ (mg.) | Vitamin $B_{12}$ (μg) | Calcium (Gm.) | Phosphorus (Gm.) | Iodine (μg) | Iron (mg.) | Magnesium (mg.) |
| 35 | 0.05 | 5 | 0.4 | 0.2 | 0.2 | 1.0 | 0.4 | 0.2 | 25 | 6 | 40 |
| 35 | 0.05 | 7 | 0.5 | 0.4 | 0.3 | 1.5 | 0.5 | 0.4 | 40 | 10 | 60 |
| 35 | 0.1 | 8 | 0.6 | 0.5 | 0.4 | 2.0 | 0.6 | 0.5 | 45 | 15 | 70 |
| 40 | 0.1 | 8 | 0.6 | 0.6 | 0.5 | 2.0 | 0.7 | 0.7 | 55 | 15 | 100 |
| 40 | 0.2 | 8 | 0.7 | 0.6 | 0.6 | 2.5 | 0.8 | 0.8 | 60 | 15 | 150 |
| 40 | 0.2 | 9 | 0.8 | 0.7 | 0.7 | 3 | 0.8 | 0.8 | 70 | 10 | 200 |
| 40 | 0.2 | 11 | 0.9 | 0.8 | 0.9 | 4 | 0.8 | 0.8 | 80 | 10 | 200 |
| 40 | 0.2 | 13 | 1.1 | 1.0 | 1.0 | 4 | 0.9 | 0.9 | 100 | 10 | 250 |
| 40 | 0.3 | 15 | 1.2 | 1.1 | 1.2 | 5 | 1.0 | 1.0 | 110 | 10 | 250 |
| 40 | 0.4 | 17 | 1.3 | 1.3 | 1.4 | 5 | 1.2 | 1.2 | 125 | 10 | 300 |
| 45 | 0.4 | 18 | 1.4 | 1.4 | 1.6 | 5 | 1.4 | 1.4 | 135 | 18 | 350 |
| 55 | 0.4 | 20 | 1.5 | 1.5 | 1.8 | 5 | 1.4 | 1.4 | 150 | 18 | 400 |
| 60 | 0.4 | 18 | 1.6 | 1.4 | 2.0 | 5 | 0.8 | 0.8 | 140 | 10 | 400 |
| 60 | 0.4 | 18 | 1.7 | 1.4 | 2.0 | 5 | 0.8 | 0.8 | 140 | 10 | 350 |
| 60 | 0.4 | 17 | 1.7 | 1.3 | 2.0 | 5 | 0.8 | 0.8 | 125 | 10 | 350 |
| 60 | 0.4 | 14 | 1.7 | 1.2 | 2.0 | 6 | 0.8 | 0.8 | 110 | 10 | 350 |
| 40 | 0.4 | 15 | 1.3 | 1.1 | 1.4 | 5 | 1.2 | 1.2 | 110 | 18 | 300 |
| 45 | 0.4 | 15 | 1.4 | 1.2 | 1.6 | 5 | 1.3 | 1.3 | 115 | 18 | 350 |
| 50 | 0.4 | 16 | 1.4 | 1.2 | 1.8 | 5 | 1.3 | 1.3 | 120 | 18 | 350 |
| 50 | 0.4 | 15 | 1.5 | 1.2 | 2.0 | 5 | 1.3 | 1.3 | 115 | 18 | 350 |
| 55 | 0.4 | 13 | 1.5 | 1.0 | 2.0 | 5 | 0.8 | 0.8 | 100 | 18 | 350 |
| 55 | 0.4 | 13 | 1.5 | 1.0 | 2.0 | 5 | 0.8 | 0.8 | 100 | 18 | 300 |
| 55 | 0.4 | 13 | 1.5 | 1.0 | 2.0 | 5 | 0.8 | 0.8 | 90 | 18 | 300 |
| 55 | 0.4 | 13 | 1.5 | 1.0 | 2.0 | 6 | 0.8 | 0.8 | 80 | 10 | 300 |
| 60 | 0.8 | 15 | 1.8 | +0.1 | 2.5 | 8 | +0.4 | +0.4 | 125 | 18 | 450 |
| 60 | 0.5 | 20 | 2.0 | +0.5 | 2.5 | 6 | +0.5 | +0.5 | 150 | 18 | 450 |

are intended to cover individual variations among most normal persons as they live in the United States under usual nutrients for which human requirements have been less well defined. See text for more detailed discussion of allowances

sent allowances for the midpoint of the specified age range.
tionately.
may be effective in doses less than a fourth of the recommended daily allowance.
ptophan.

provide the recommended daily dietary allowances. The previously accepted minimum daily requirements should not be utilized; they do not adequately allow for the biologic variations among human beings, and they should not be permitted to appear on food packages.

The ideal diet for an individual will provide adequate amounts of the nutrients and will do so within a category of foods that are both desirable and attractive to him and that will not violate his various cultural, ethnic, religious, and psychologic preferences. Again the abundance and variety of foods and the diversity of food patterns to be derived from them help to set the stage for acceptance of the dietary recommendations when changes are needed.

No single dietary formulation can be considered to be ideal for all individuals

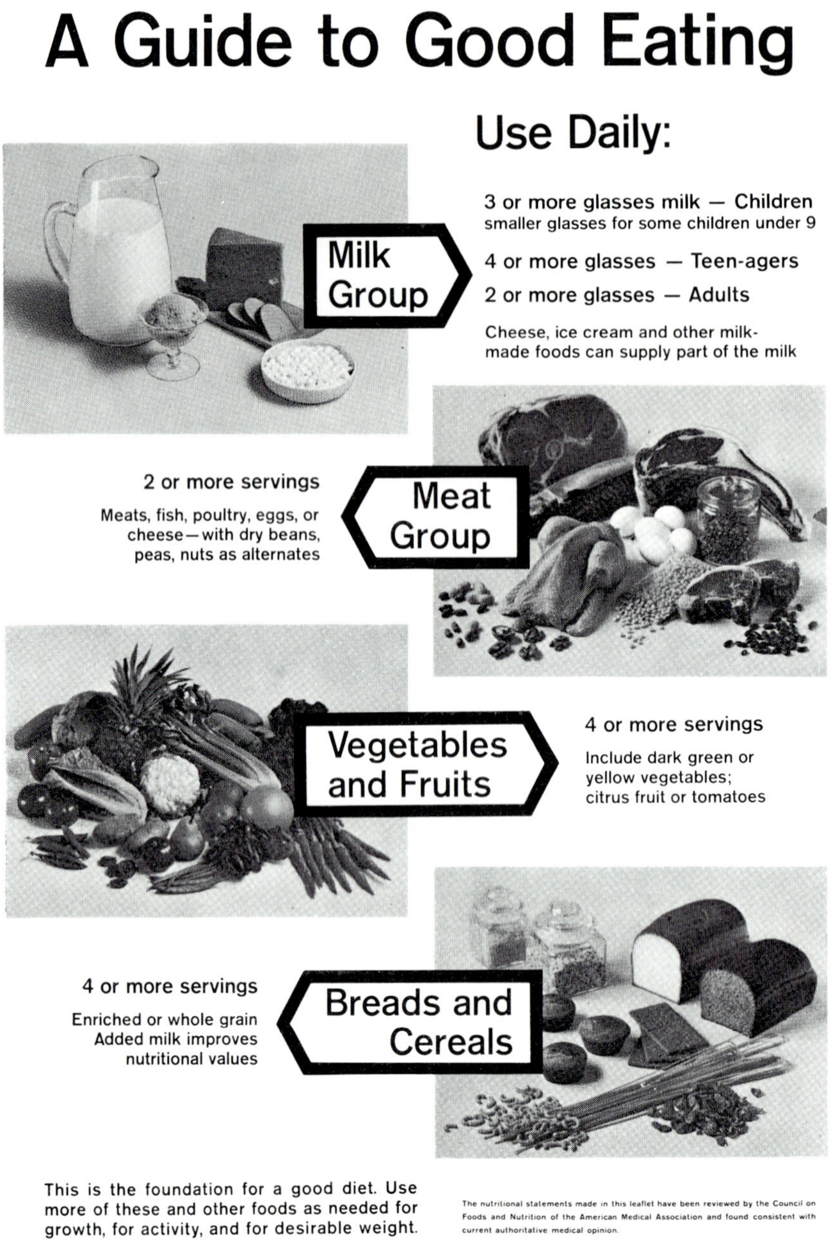

# A Guide to Good Eating

## Use Daily:

**Milk Group**
3 or more glasses milk — Children
smaller glasses for some children under 9
4 or more glasses — Teen-agers
2 or more glasses — Adults
Cheese, ice cream and other milk-made foods can supply part of the milk

**Meat Group**
2 or more servings
Meats, fish, poultry, eggs, or cheese—with dry beans, peas, nuts as alternates

**Vegetables and Fruits**
4 or more servings
Include dark green or yellow vegetables; citrus fruit or tomatoes

**Breads and Cereals**
4 or more servings
Enriched or whole grain
Added milk improves nutritional values

This is the foundation for a good diet. Use more of these and other foods as needed for growth, for activity, and for desirable weight.

The nutritional statements made in this leaflet have been reviewed by the Council on Foods and Nutrition of the American Medical Association and found consistent with current authoritative medical opinion.

**Fig. 3-1.** The four basic food groups shown in the suggested amounts form the foundation of a good diet with the provision for a wide variety of food preferences. (From: A guide to good eating, ed. 3, Chicago, 1965, National Dairy Council.)

even in a limited geographic area. Where food supplies are abundant and varied, literally thousands of adequate and well-balanced menus can be designed, of which many will be suitable for a given individual no matter what his cultural, ethnic, or religious food preferences may be. This circumstance makes possible dietary recommendations that will be appropriate for the individual and greatly increases the likelihood that he will accept and apply them.

In order to aid in menu planning and in the overall examination and evaluation of a diet, the United States Department of Agriculture[2] has suggested that nutritious foods can conveniently and rationally be divided into four basic food categories: milk group, meat group, vegetable-fruit group, and bread-cereal group (Fig. 3-1).

## Milk group

The milk group is composed of the various foods of dairy origin—whole milk, skim milk, cheese, butter, cream, and ice cream. Moderate use of these foods will provide a high percentage of the daily calcium requirements, as well as a good contribution to the daily requirement of high quality protein, riboflavin, and vitamin A. Most whole milk and skim milk and all skim milk powder are now enriched commercially with vitamin D and serve as the best source in the diet for this vitamin. Skim milk powder is also enriched with vitamin A to replace that lost when the butter fat is removed.

The following are suggested levels for use of the milk group by various age and interest categories.

| | |
|---|---|
| Children | 3 to 4 eight-ounce cups per day |
| Teen-agers | 4 or more cups per day |
| Adults | 2 or more cups per day |
| Pregnant women | 4 or more cups per day |
| Nursing mothers | 6 or more cups per day |

Cheese or ice cream can replace part of the recommended amounts of milk in any age group. While whole milk is ordinarily used for the younger ages, skim milk can be used instead in any group for whom caloric supplies need to be reduced or for whom reductions in fat consumption are desired. Oleomargarine can be used interchangeably with butter. When replacement of saturated by polyunsaturated fats is desired, an oleomargarine manufactured to preserve the concentration of polyunsaturated fats in the original oils is best.

## Meat group

The meat group consists of beef, veal, pork, lamb, poultry, fish, and eggs as the principal representatives in most diets. Alternatives are dry beans and other legumes and nuts. These foods provide the major supply of protein of high biologic value, iron, thiamine, and niacin, as well as other members of the vitamin B complex and of the mineral nutrients.

Two or more daily servings of the meat group are highly desirable. Ordinarily no reduction should be made below two daily servings in view of the need for an adequate amount of high-quality protein. A serving of liver once a week is a highly desirable supplement for provision of the vitamin B complex. When meat is not used, as in vegetarian diets, the two servings should include eggs and legumes; probably consumption in the milk group should be increased beyond the suggested levels as a further provision for receiving adequate protein of high biologic value.

**Vegetable-fruit group**

The vegetable-fruit group includes all the leafy green and yellow vegetables, potatoes, and citrus and other fruits. This group supplies important amounts of the minerals and vitamins, especially vitamins A and C.

Four or more servings daily of the vegetable-fruit group should be consumed, including one serving of a citrus fruit, tomato, or raw cabbage to provide adequate vitamin C; three or more servings of other vegetables and fruits, including potatoes, should be included according to individual preference and caloric demands.

When caloric needs are to be reduced, replacement of potatoes and other starchy vegetables with salads or leafy vegetables is desirable. The latter are low in calories, satisfying, and good sources of various minerals and vitamins.

**Bread-cereal group**

The bread-cereal group includes all foods made from the cereal grains—wheat, rye, oats, corn, rice. Many states and other governmental subdivisions require that the major cereal products consumed in their areas be enriched to provide adequate amounts of the nutrients whose concentration has been reduced in the various food preparation processes. The cereals provide generous amounts of thiamine, niacin, and iron. The cereals also provide some protein, although the quality is lower than for those foods in the meat group. Ordinarily a wide variety of vegetable proteins would be needed to provide adequate protein of desirable quality. Usually in the American diet the vegetable proteins are supplemented by proteins of animal source.

For the bread-cereal group, four or more servings daily is a customary recommendation for normal conditions. When caloric needs are low, this recommendation can be reduced and consumed without spreads.

Daily dietary plans based on these suggestions provide the recommended daily dietary allowances simultaneously with varied distribution of foods among the four major groups.

Evaluation of typical diets reveals many items that do not fit into any of these four categories of nutritious food items. Such items as candy, soft drinks, pastries, and alcoholic beverages supply large amounts of calories but in most cases without a proportional contribution to the protein, vitamin, and mineral requirements of the body. Many of these items are ones of dental concern. In the evaluation of a diet these items should be tabulated in a fifth group of basically nonessential food items that are distinctively not parallel in food value to the foregoing four basic food categories.

Usually three meals per day without between-meal snacks is the most desirable arrangement. From a dental standpoint in particular, the additional frequency of food in the mouth and the nature of most between-meal snacks indicate the desirability of reduction in number or complete elimination of snacks. Exception to the latter is sometimes mandatory during recovery from illness, postoperatively—for example, after reduction of a fractured jaw—or when individuals are excessively underweight. In these cases judicious selection of the kind of snacks to minimize the use of highly fermentable and readily retained carbohydrates and appropriate accompanying oral hygiene measures will help to reduce the oral environmental problems.

Experience has shown that a fairly equitable distribution of the foods among the three meals is preferable, especially in order to provide optimal supplementation of proteins by one another. Breakfast in particular should be commented upon, as it is the most frequently neglected meal. Various studies have shown the desirability of a substantial breakfast after a night without food. An inadequate breakfast, such as coffee and doughnut, or omission of breakfast leads to a decreased working efficiency in the late morning. Even in weight reduction schedules, three small appropriately planned meals are more compatible physiologically than the boom-or-bust philosophy of one big meal a day with only one or two snacks at other mealtimes.

## NUTRITIONAL RELATIONSHIPS TO ORAL CAVITY

In any consideration of nutritional relationships to the oral cavity the varied nature of the tissues requires the discussion to be subdivided into the influences related to the soft tissues—oral mucosa, periodontal membrane, sensory papilla, tongue, and so on—and those related to the mineralized tissues—enamel, dentin, and cementum. The discussion of the mineralized tissues will be further subdivided into three intervals with respect to the time of the tooth's life history: the developmental preeruptive period, the maturation period, and the maintenance period.

### Soft tissues

The soft tissues reflect the current metabolic status of the body, often in quicker and more dramatic ways than comparable tissues located elsewhere in the body. Part of this response may result from the fact that oral tissues are subjected to varied traumatic situations because of their position and functon. Stresses such as wide variations in temperature, particle size and harshness, hydrogen ion concentration, dehydrating ability, and osmotic gradients of the food and drink consumed may be sufficiently demanding environmental influences to require the more frequent renewal of soft tissues than would otherwise be necessary. The temperature, humidity, and food available to the oral cavity also promote the prolific growth of widely varied types of microorganisms with varied sequelae.

Scurvy, pellagra, ariboflavinosis, and deficiencies of the vitamin B complex in general are all states for which classic descriptions of the oral signs have been widely published in textbooks on nutrition and on oral medicine.[3] While nutritional deficiencies with oral signs are still very common in underdeveloped countries, they do not occur frequently in countries with high economic standards except in certain population groups with extenuating circumstances. The chronic alcoholic, the mentally deficient, and the aged person with economic or housing problems are especially prone to utilize diets with inadequate attention to distribution among the several food groups and therefore many develop overt nutritional deficiencies. While the dentist in private practice may never see recognizable evidence of any of these classic nutritional deficiency syndromes, the dentist in the clinics of metropolitan hospitals, homes for the aged, or mental institutions will invariably observe occasional cases with all the typical signs. The occasional case of scurvy and of rickets will still be seen among infants who have been neglected. At the other end of the spectrum the occasional case of vitamin A or vitamin D toxicity may also be observed where overly zealous parents have given excess dosages of liver oil concentrates.

**Mineralized tissues**

**Nutritional influences during tooth development.** The systemic environment of the developing tooth controls the tooth's histologic structure, its chemical composition, and even its general size, shape, and cuspal design. In turn, the systemic environment is controlled by the genetic composition, by the health and well-being of the individual, and by the availability of the nutrients required for the adequate growth, development, and mineralization of the tooth. Vitamin A, vitamin C, and vitamin D deficiencies, as well as deficiencies and imbalanced ratios of calcium and phosphorus, cause characteristic malformations in the histologic structure of the developing tooth.[4, 5] Typical of vitamin A's action elsewhere in the body in the development and maintenance of epithelial structures of ectodermal origin, this vitamin is required for the normal differentiation and function of the ameloblasts. Inadequate vitamin A in experimental diets during tooth development results in atrophy of the ameloblasts and inadequate development of the enamel matrix. Vitamin C deficiency during the development of the teeth results in odontoblasts of reduced size that produce the dentin matrix at a reduced rate. The relation of this vitamin to the odontoblasts and to the dentin is typical of its mechanism of action in other tissues of the body, with its primary responsibility in the formation and maintenance of cells of mesodermal origin and in the elaboration of collagen.

Inadequate amounts of vitamin D, of calcium, or of phosphorus, or imbalanced ratios of calcium and phosphorus result in imperfect calcification of the mineralizing enamel matrix and dentin matrix. Only vitamin D deficiency during development is believed to result in an increased caries susceptibility of the tooth in human populations,[6] although grossly imbalanced levels of calcium and phosphorus, especially with regard to high calcium–low phosphorus, may also result in increased caries susceptibility in experimental animals.[7] Vitamins A and C have not been tested adequately in this regard, but there does not seem to be any suggestion that these deficiencies have a relationship to caries susceptibility.

Undoubtedly the fluoride ion plays the most important role of all nutrients during tooth development insofar as promotion of the formation of teeth with different levels of caries resistance is concerned.[8, 9] Chapter 6 is devoted to the relationship of fluorides to preventive dentistry, but it is important to point out here the very strong relationship that this element has to the formation of teeth. Surveys from many parts of the world indicate that teeth suffering from inadequate amounts of fluoride during development are much more susceptible to carious lesions than teeth in adjoining localities where optimal amounts of fluoride are consumed during development. As far as tooth development and mineralization are concerned, the fluoride ion is as vital a component of the hydroxyapatite crystals deposited in the organic matrix as are calcium, phosphorus, magnesium, and others. Fluoride evidently contributes its beneficial effect through the formation of more perfect crystals of somewhat larger size and lower acid solubility.[10] Optimal fluoride levels in the crystals may also be related to a reduction in the crystals' carbonate content.

Other nutritional studies with experimental animals during tooth development are interesting, although known relationships to man have not been demonstrated. Protein deficiency during the development of the teeth of rats results in delayed tooth eruption, smaller molar teeth, higher caries susceptibility, and lack of formation of some of the minor cusps.[11] Delay in tooth eruption is known to occur in populations where protein intake is borderline or inadequate[12] and has also been reported in the Scandinavian countries in times of food shortages, such as during World War II.[13] In the latter case the delayed tooth eruption may not have been attributable to protein deficiency but may have been related to other variables in food rationing.

Trace elements other than fluoride have been suggested as being important in determining caries resistance.[14] Molybdenum and vanadium have been reported to be potential agents for increasing caries resistance during tooth development, whereas selenium has been suggested as an element with the opposite influence. At present there seems to be no clear evidence that these three elements do play a specific role in this regard. Further studies will be necessary to determine whether any trace element other than fluoride is related to caries resistance in man.

**Nutritional influences during tooth maturation.** The maturation period is not well defined. Two specific experimental observations suggest that there is an important period immediately after eruption of the tooth when significant changes are taking place in enamel that may be nutritional in nature. In the recently erupted tooth a much higher incorporation of radioisotope occurs than after the tooth has been in the oral cavity for even a short period of time.[15] For example, incorporation of radiophosphorus in the outer layers of the enamel is almost as high in the immediate posteruptive period as it was in the period just prior to tooth eruption. First, these data suggest that a considerable amount of mineralization continues to take place immediately after eruption. Second, radiographic observations indicate that the newly erupted teeth of the rat has incompletely mineralized areas of the enamel.[16] If the diet provided during this early posteruptive period is a noncariogenic one these areas appear to mineralize and to become resistant to tooth decay. If the diet is one with a strong cariogenic potential, however, further mineralization of these areas does not occur, and they appear to be particularly susceptible to tooth decay.

Neither of these studies has been extended from the experimental animals to man, but they are of such a nature that clinical studies are warranted. The exact metabolic pathway has not been defined, although there are strong suggestions from these data that it is motivated through a typical nutritional pathway operating through the saliva or by direct contact of the food with tooth surfaces.

The long-standing clinical impression that teeth become more resistant to tooth decay after they have been in the oral cavity for months or years may be related to reactions taking place during the maturation period. The continued increase of fluoride in surface enamel in human teeth in both low fluoride and optimal fluoride areas for the decade after tooth eruption may also be indicative of a maturing process and undoubtedly is related to the increased caries resistance with longer exposure to the fluids in the oral cavity.[17]

**Postdevelopmental relationships to the teeth.** Strict evidence of nutritional benefits to the teeth after they are fully erupted in the oral cavity is sparse. Many studies with vitamin D supplementation of otherwise partially inadequate diets have suggested that adequate vitamin D metabolism does promote a lower level of initiation and progression of carious lesions.[6] However, the degree of protection in all these studies was small and totally inadequate to cope with the high caries activity in modern populations. Evidence for immediate nutritional relationships to the maintenance of teeth is otherwise lacking.

Once the teeth have erupted into the oral cavity the relationships of the food that we eat are dietary rather than nutritional. Studies begun decades ago indicated that fermentable carbohydrates retained on tooth surfaces were necessary for the initiation and progression of carious lesions.[18] These early studies have been expanded and made more precise in clinical trials and are fully supported by a great variety of assays in caries-susceptible experimental animals.[19] From the standpoint of clinical studies the most informative data were collected at a mental institution in Vipeholm, Sweden, by Gustafson and his associates.[20] Rather than attempt to eliminate all carbohydrates from the diet, they attempted to determine which were the most harmful with respect to the teeth. Carbohydrate supplements were fed in solution,

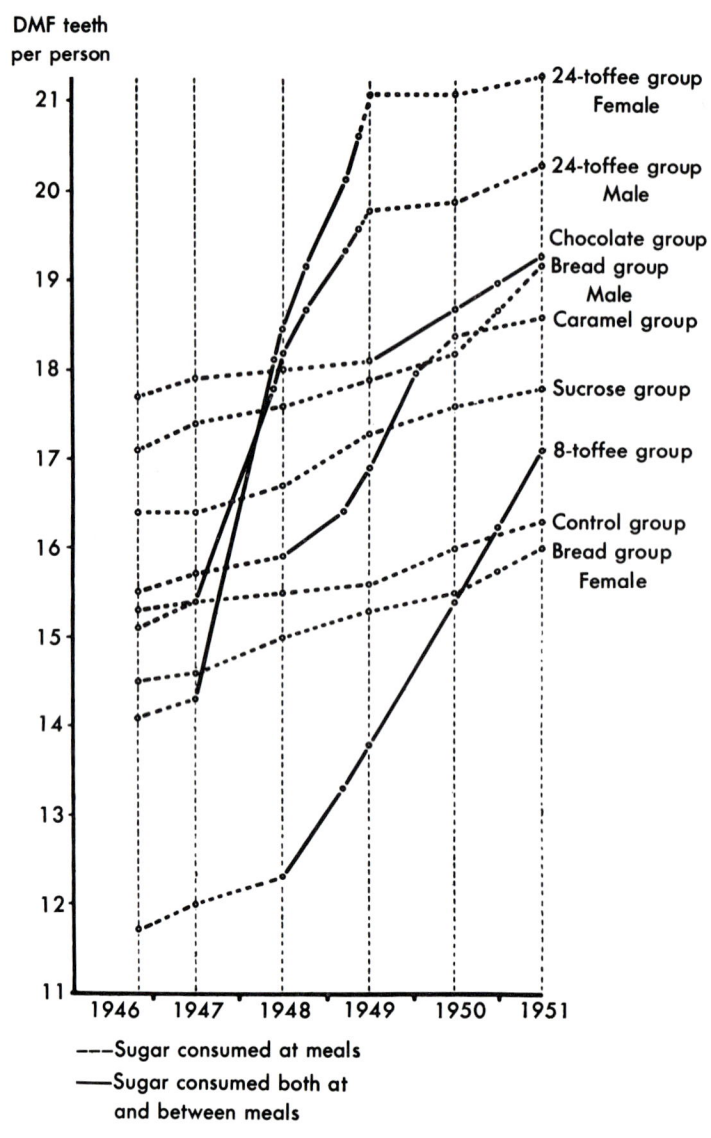

**Fig. 3-2.** Effect of different forms of carbohydrates on dental caries activity of 436 individuals observed over a 5-year period in Vipeholm, Sweden. (From Gustafsson, B. E., and others: Acta Odont. Scand. **11:**232, 1954.)

in bread, and in popular forms of candy. In addition, the supplements were tested at mealtime and between mealtimes. Fig. 3-2 indicates the extent to which carbohydrates from these various sources caused different amounts of tooth decay. In general, all supplements were less harmful at mealtime than when given between meals. Sugar in aqueous solution or sugar in firm Swedish bread was relatively harmless. However, when the sugar was consumed in the form of caramels and toffees, which adhere readily to the tooth surfaces, major increases in the amount of tooth decay occurred during the observation periods. In every group of subjects variations in individual caries activity were observed. Even in the groups in which major increases in the average number of new decayed, missing, and filled teeth were observed, some individuals remained almost or totally free of new carious lesions. This observation can probably be explained by the wide variations in individual susceptibility to tooth decay and in habits of oral hygiene. Whenever high caries activity was observed during the feeding of the supplements, return to the control diet led to the lower caries activity typical of the preexperimental observation period.

Many additional studies of this type need to be performed in order to give the dentist a more adequate ability to determine those foodstuffs that are most cariogenic and to differentiate them from ones of less ability to produce tooth decay.[21, 22] Several intensive programs are under way to attempt to develop in vitro tests for evaluation of the cariogenicity of foods. Most of these tests are based on procedures for estimation of (1) the amount of acid produced when the food is incubated with oral microorganisms and (2) the degree of retention of the foodstuff in the oral cavity. As yet no in vitro test or combination of tests has been shown to have good predictive ability. While satisfactory tests in the laboratory would be of tremendous assistance in screening food items, acceptance of the validity of such tests can be based only on adequate clinical evaluations.

In experimental animals starches and dextrins appear to be retained in only minor amounts on the oral surfaces and have a low caries-producing potential.[23] In early studies most simple monosaccharides and disaccharides all seemed to be equally capable of producing carious lesions in experimental animals. Lactose was the only exception that seemed to be less able to cause the initiation and progression of carious lesions. In some experimental conditions carious lesions occur with diets containing starch but no monosaccharides or disaccharides. More recently, as caries assays have become more refined, there have been suggestions that sucrose (in some, but not all, laboratory conditions) may be more cariogenic than glucose.[24] The latter observation has not been tested adequately in animal populations and not at all in human populations.

Much interest in recent years has centered around the ability of dietary phosphate supplements to cause major reductions in the incidence of experimental dental caries.[25] Widely different phosphates have been shown to have this ability, although effectiveness varies widely for different salts. Among commonly available phosphates the calcium salts are much less efficient than the sodium and potassium salts. The cyclic trimetaphosphate is especially active. Some organic phosphates such as the phytates are also active. The mode of action is thought to be a local influence on the tooth surfaces, although a systemic influence has not been completely ruled out.

Several trials in human populations of phosphate supplementation of flour and sugar have resulted in less promising data than the animal studies. However, in all the human trials a calcium phosphate ($CaHPO_4$) was used as the supplement, that is, one of the least effective on the basis of animal studies. This salt was chosen largely because of the concern that a sodium or potassium phosphate at the level required would reduce the calcium-phosphorus ratio beyond a desirable level. Probably this concern was not fully warranted. In addition, incorporation of a sodium or potassium phosphate in flour and sugar would have altered the hydrogen ion concentration of dough in which these were used as ingredients sufficiently to alter the textures of the final baked goods unless specific alterations of baking formulas and procedures were designed. Appropriate clinical tests need to be conducted with supplementation of flour and sugar, and perhaps even other foodstuffs, by more suitable phosphates to determine if the results in animals are applicable to man.

**Nutrition and periodontal disease**

Various nutritional deficiencies in experimental animals have been shown to adversely influence the integrity of the tissues of the periodontium: protein, tryptophan, calcium, phosphorus, magnesium, vitamin A, the vitamin B complex, vitamin C, and vitamin D.[26] Indeed the maintenance of each structural component has been demonstrated in laboratory studies to be influenced by one or more acute or chronic states of nutritional deficiency. Much uncertainty exists whether any of these experimental deficiencies produce syndromes that closely parallel either periodontitis or periodontosis in man. The histopathology of chronic vitamin C deficiency probably has more similarities to periodontosis than do any of the other deficiencies. However, there is no clear clinical evidence that vitamin C supplementation is helpful in the relief of any periodontal abnormality other than possibly simple gingivitis.

From an epidemiologic standpoint, surveys in many different underdeveloped areas have indicated a high prevalence of periodontal disease and of nutritional deficiencies. Whether there is a causal relationship in these populations between nutritional deficiency and periodontal disease is open to speculation. The almost complete lack of dental care in developing areas undoubtedly contributes to the high prevalence of periodontal disease. However, the presence of widespread nutritional deficiency in these populations may contribute underlying systemic problems that permit earlier and more rapid progression of periodontal diseases.

Much meticulous and prolonged clinical investigation will be necessary before there is a full understanding of the relationship between the nutriture of an individual and periodontal health. Numerous studies conducted under inadequately controlled situations in clinics and private offices have reported substantial benefit from protein, vitamin B complex, and vitamin C therapy during prolonged periodontal treatment. These data are interesting, but at present the results are far from conclusive. While the dentist cannot expect miraculous support from such supplementation during periodontal treatment, he should encourage optimal nutritional habits on the premise that the well-nourished patient will respond more favorably with respect to healing, restoration of blood loss, and other reparative processes than the poorly nourished patient.

**Nutrition and congenital errors of development**

In a variety of experimental situations, investigators have demonstrated in laboratory animals that congenital errors can be produced as a result of nutritional deficiencies at critical times during pregnancy.[27] These errors have included cleft palate, harelip, missing and malpositioned teeth, and underdevelopment of the jaws and of the limbs. Such situations as anoxia, vitamin A, riboflavin, and folic acid deficiency have precipitated such abnormalities. The effect seems to operate through nonspecific pathways rather than through specific ones, which differ from one experimental situation to another. Whether such abnormalities in man ever have a nutritional origin cannot be specified at present. However, adequate studies of other types have indicated that the nutriture of the mother is related to the weight of the newborn infant and to the degree of development and mineralization of the skeleton, including the teeth.[28]

## EVALUATION OF NUTRITIONAL STATUS

Ideally the evaluation of the nutritional status of an individual would be based on clinical examination, appraisal of the diet, and appropriate laboratory tests. Sometimes balance studies would be necessary when the ingested amount of a nutrient such as calcium is analytically determined and compared to the amount excreted. The dentist should be aware in each case how much information needs

**MONDAY**

| Breakfast — Food | Amount | Left over |
|---|---|---|
|  |  |  |
| Noon meal — Food | Amount | Left over |
|  |  |  |
| Night meal — Food | Amount | Left over |
|  |  |  |
| In-between-meals — Food | Amount | Left over |
|  |  |  |

**Fig. 3-3.** Form for home record of food consumption.

**INSTRUCTIONS FOR RECORDING YOUR FOOD DAILY**

**Record each food for the proper meal.**

1. **Meat, fish, poultry,** and **cheese:** Record by size, thickness, and method of preparation.
    Example: Roast Beef 3 in. × 5 in. × ½ in.
    Juice 1 tablespoon

2. **Eggs:** Record by number and how prepared.
    Example: Eggs, scrambled 2

3. **Vegetables:** Record amount. If mixed as in salad, record kinds of vegetables, and salad dressing if used.
    Example: Mixed vegetable salad 1 cup
    Lettuce, celery, carrots and ½ tomato.

4. **Fresh** or **canned fruit:** Record whole, half or quarter pieces eaten. Record juice used over canned fruit. Record sugar added to fruit also.
    Example: Canned peaches 2 halves
    Juice 2 tablespoons

5. **Baker's sliced bread:** Record by slice. If slicing your own bread, record in slices corresponding to baker's bread.

6. **Bread rolls, sweet rolls, cakes:** Record by number and size. Record if frosted.
    Example: Sweet roll 2 in × 3 in. × 2 in.
    Frosting and nuts on top.

7. **Pie:** Record by size. Record kind and one or two crust.
    Example: Apple pie ¼ pie
    Two crust

8. **Butter, margerine,** and **other fats:** Record by teaspoons.
    Example: Bread 1 slice
    Butter ½ teaspoon

9. **Vegetable soup** or **broth** containing **noodles,** or **rice.** Record only vegetables or rice.
    Example: Vegetable soup 1 cup
    Vegetables ½ cup
    (Potatoes, carrots, peas)

10. **Cream soups:** Record amount and if prepared with milk or water.
    Example: Cream of soup 1 cup
    (½ milk and ½ water)

*(Continued.)*

Fig. 3-4. Instructions for use in preparing home record of food consumption.

*Preventive nutrition* 47

11. **Mixed dishes:** Record by amount. Record foods in it and method of preparing. Record approximate quantity of meat.
    Example: Beef stew 1 cup
    (Potatoes, carrots, peas, celery and beef — about ½ beef)

12. **Gravies** and **sauces:** Record by amount.
    Example: Roast pork 2 in. × 3 in. × ¼ in.
    Gravy ¼ cup

13. **Milk, cocoa:** Record by cup and not glass. Record method of preparing cocoa.
    Example: Cocoa 1 cup
    (½ water and ½ milk, 1 tsp. cocoa)

14. **Soft drinks:** Record by bottle.

15. **Coffee** and **tea:** Record only what is used in them.

16. **Cereals:** Record amount and milk and sugar used.
    Example: Cornflakes 1 cup
    Milk ½ cup
    Sugar 2 teaspoons

17. **Leftovers:** If all food is not eaten, record leftovers in leftover column after appropriate food.

18. **Between meals:** Record all food or beverage eaten between meals.

**NIGHT MEAL**

| Food | Amount | Left over |
| --- | --- | --- |
| Hamburg, fried | 2 patties<br>3 in. across<br>¼ in. thick | |
| Mashed potato | ½ cup | |
| Gravy | ¼ cup | |
| Beets | ½ cup | 2 tablespoons |
| Butter | 1 teaspoon | |
| White roll | 1 | |
| Butter | 1 teaspoon | |
| White cake<br>Chocolate frosting | 2 in. × 3 in. × 2 in. | |

Fig. 3-4, cont'd. For legend see opposite page.

**48** *Improving dental practice through preventive measures*

to be collected for an adequate evaluation. Often a few simple questions will indicate the real need that a patient has for nutritional counselling as an aid to improved oral health. In other cases the same leading questions will indicate a more complex situation. The dentist should be discerning enough to recognize when consultation with the patient's physician is appropriate.

In the course of a routine clinical examination of his patient the dentist should be alert to note any signs of nutritional inadequacy, undesirable dietary habits, and striking changes in prevalence of oral diseases since the preceding visit. In the case history should be included questions about the dietary habits of the patient and about his food likes and dislikes. Whenever there are indications of dietary or nutri-

**Fig. 3-5.** Form for recording and calculating amounts of specific nutrients.

tional problems the general history and the clinical examination should be followed at a convenient time by an interview (or interviews) specifically about dietary practices. The patient may be asked to keep a record at home of all foods eaten during a 7-day period. A typical format for such a record is shown in Fig. 3-3. Accompanying instructions, such as those described in Fig. 3-4, are very helpful as a guide to the patient's accurate collection of the data. The reader is referred to Chapter 2 for an additional format on diet surveys.

From such diet surveys several forms of appraisal may be made. One precise but rather time-consuming method is a calculation of the amounts of the various nutrients contained in the diet record. In this case the various foods and their amounts are grouped by basic food categories into the format shown in Fig. 3-5. Then the amounts of the specific nutrients can be calculated from food tables such as those of Bowes and Church.[29] Computer programs are now available for the mechanical handling of data. The amounts are totaled and compared with the recommended daily dietary allowances for an individual of comparable age and sex (Table 3-1).

Another procedure of appraisal is more qualitative in nature and is based on the number and frequency of the basic four food categories and the amounts of undesirable food items (pp. 33 to 39). While this method lacks the precision of the more exacting calculation method, it is a good guide to the food habits of the patient and is practical for the busy dental office.

Throughout all these dietary considerations the patient should be made fully aware that this is an important part of the overall care program provided by the dentist as a means to cope with problems of oral disease and to provide better general health. Appropriately trained auxiliary personnel can be of tremendous assistance to the dentist in the technical aspects of dietary evaluations.

## RECOMMENDATIONS FOR DIETARY IMPROVEMENT

These evaluation data, including the clinical condition of the patient, the degree to which the recommended daily dietary allowances for individual nutrients are being met by the current diet, the distribution of this diet among the basic four food groups, and the frequency and amount of snacks of orally undesirable nature, must all be considered in the light of the cultural, religious, psychologic, and economic preferences and restrictions of the specific patient. The recommendations must be specifically designed for a given patient at a given time in his life and for his present mental and physical circumstances. Generalizations are not appropriate and are not likely to be accepted and applied by the patient. Each recommendation must be carefully explained to the patient to ensure that he understands it and its value to his health.

In all dietary prescriptions the dentist should encourage the use of milk products enriched with vitamin D, whole-grain or enriched white flour in all cereal products, and iodized salt. During growth and development an appropriate supplement of fluoride should be provided if the dentist has assured himself that the patient is not receiving another source of dietary fluorides in the water supply or by prescription from the pediatrician. These considerations along with the development of a good distribution among the major food groups and reduction or elimination of undesirable items from the diet will readily lead to the planning of a dietary program that easily meets the recommended daily dietary allowances in all nutrients.

### Protein, vitamins, and minerals

Within the frame of reference just given, the current diet should be considered first with regard to the extent to which the allowances for protein, vitamins, and minerals are being provided. The goal should be to attain the amounts suggested by the recommended daily dietary allowances. However, it should be remembered that modest decreases of an existing diet for prolonged periods below these allowances will not necessarily be accompanied by overt signs of nutritional deficiency.

Protein is a particularly relevant nutrient to use as an example in a discussion of how recommendations for all nutrients are developed. If the protein intake is low or if an excessively high percentage is provided by a limited number of plant proteins, appropriate changes should be recommended that will correct either problem. In the case of an overall low intake, one or more extra servings of protein-rich foods that the patient enjoys and can afford would be suggested as supplements or in place of less desirable items in the diet. Ideally a recommendation of specific foods would be made which would simultaneously help to balance the distribution among the four basic food groups, be economically feasible, and not violate a preference or dislike of the patient. If there was an economic problem, the recommendation would likely involve the use of dried peas and beans, the less expensive cuts of meat, fish, and skim milk. On the other hand, if the protein intake involved too high a percentage of plant proteins along with a limited variety of sources, the problem might be one of encouraging the use of more proteins of animal origin in place of plant sources or of increasing the variety of plant proteins used. Often the limited intake of animal proteins is associated with economic problems. In this case the patient needs guidance to understand both the need for animal proteins and the fact that the inexpensive sources mentioned previously are nutritionally as desirable as the more expensive ones. In other instances the patient may be a partial vegetarian; he should be encouraged to use additional eggs, cheese, and milk. When the individual is a strict vegetarian and all foods of animal origin are avoided, special care is needed to ensure adequate protein from sufficiently varied sources to supplement each other.

The diet should be similarly considered with respect to the adequacy with which it supplies vitamins and minerals in abundant amounts. Appropriate recommendations should be designed that will encourage consumption of adequate numbers of servings of these foods and at the same time a good distribution among the basic four food groups.

After the various protein, vitamin, and mineral needs have been considered individually and collectively and appropriate additions and substitutions made to care for the patient's needs within his food preference limitations, most dietary descriptions will have a good distribution among the four food groups. If a good distribution has not been attained, further modification should be made to achieve roughly the balance among the food groups suggested previously.

Up to this point no mention has been made of caloric needs or of the amounts of orally undesirable diet components. Fundamentally the needs for protein, vitamins, and minerals should be planned first and these two phases considered secondly. This sequence is necessary because caloric needs and the way that they are supplied are variable and depend on the individual to a greater extent than the requirement for proteins, vitamins, and minerals. The latter nutrients have relatively absolute requirements that are largely irrespective of activity, occupation, or other individual factors. In the sedentary and older age groups, when caloric needs are low, a diet that has been carefully designed to provide adequate protein, vitamins, and minerals will approximate the caloric needs. In other groups in which the caloric needs are higher because of growth and/or greater activity, additional foods will be needed to provide the extra calories. These foods will usually be composed primarily of fats and carbohydrates as energy sources.

**Energy and fat and carbohydrate consumption**

Energy requirements vary strikingly with the period of life, with the size of the individual, and with the level of physical activity. Whereas the rapidly growing, vigorously athletic teenage boy may seem to his parents to eat excessively without a body weight problem, his sedentary middle-aged father may have to leave the table after each meal slightly hungry to maintain an ideal weight.

Energy needs are increased during growth and development and during pregnancy and lactation, since major caloric requirements for synthesis of new tissues and of milk components are superimposed then upon the customary ones for maintenance and physical activity. Energy requirements fall after maturity because of greatly reduced synthetic needs and all too frequently excessive restrictions in physical activity.

The total intake of fats and carbohydrates, that is, calories, should rise and fall in close proportion to energy demands. Unfortunately, man does not have the built-in automatic mechanisms for weight regulation which make possible the precise weight maintenance seen in experimental animals. For maintenance of ideal weight, total consumption of fats and proteins should be regulated carefully and adjusted as frequently as necessary to hold an individual's body weight in the ideal range. Even minor amounts of excess calories from fats or carbohydrates or a combination of the two over prolonged periods will lead to the deposition of excess fat and to obesity. Probably the tendency to minor or extreme degrees of obesity is our most prevalent and serious nutritional problem in North America as a sequelae to abundant food supplies, high standard of living, and inadequate exercise. In the long run prevention of obesity by frequent checking of body weight on scales and adjustment of food consumption and activity levels appropriately is far easier than weight reduction. In the latter case major or even drastic reductions in caloric intake must be begun and maintained for long periods while care is simultaneously taken to provide adequate daily supplies of vitamins, minerals, and proteins to meet all the continuing cellular needs. When weight reduction requires drastic and prolonged caloric restriction the patient should be carefully supervised to ensure the adequacy of all other components of the diet. Unfortunately the psychologic motivation for weight reduction is not sufficiently strong in many people to enable them to adhere to the strict diets necessary for prolonged periods. If the desirable level of weight is achieved continued vigilance must be maintained in order to offset the subtle return of creeping obesity.

Inspection of the table of recommended daily dietary allowances will indicate no suggested values for carbohydrate and fat. Unlike the other nutrients, wide and reciprocal variations in these two major stored energy sources in the diet are possible. In the Orient a very high percentage of the caloric needs is provided by the carbohydrates of rice and other cereal grains. Fat consumption in these populations would vary between one-fifth and one-tenth the typical consumption levels in affluent Western societies. At the other extreme the Eskimo in native environs consumes most of his calories from fats and relatively little from carbohydrate sources. The optimum appears to lie between these extremes and undoubtedly permits considerable variation.

In recent years a great deal of interest has centered around the possibility of a relationship between the level of fat ingested, the degree of unsaturation of the fat ingested, and the incidence of atherosclerosis and coronary heart disease. While no final answer is yet available, the prudent approach to the problem, especially for the middle-aged male, supports the restriction of saturated fat consumption and the provision of adequate amounts of the polyunsaturated fats. Simple restriction of the saturated fats alone is probably not the complete answer. Despite appreciable advertising to the contrary, the addition of polyunsaturated fats such as safflower oil or corn oil to the diet without simultaneous restriction in the intake of saturated fat sources most certainly is not the full answer either. Undoubtedly the current high incidence of coronary heart disease among males is more complex than many discussions of fat consumption would suggest. Undoubtedly genetic constitution, pressures of modern life, limited physical activity, and other factors contribute to the etiology. Other nutrients, smoking, and other factors may possibly be involved in presently undefined ways.

Since the carbohydrates of cereal grains such as corn, rice, wheat, and rye are the most economically produced and yield the greatest amount per unit of land, they will within the foreseeable future constitute man's most plentiful food supply as well as his least expensive one. The design of diets that are largely devoid of carbohydrates and consist of high protein and fat concentrations is possible but will rarely be feasible for widespread human use. Diets that contain very little carbohydrate are expensive beyond the resources of most families and in general do not permit desirable menu variation or optimal palatability for long-term use. Any widespread use of such diets would result in acute shortages and higher prices for those food items necessary for their preparation.

Unquestionably some carbohydrate-containing foods contribute to undesirable oral environments and to increased proneness to oral disease. The incidence of dental caries has been shown repeatedly in clinical studies and laboratory trials to be closely related to the retention of carbohydrate-containing residues on caries-susceptible areas of the teeth. While the extent to which dental caries occurs will vary, depending on the structure and composition of the tooth, genetic constitution, and other factors, carbohydrate-containing residues as substrates for appropriate caries-producing oral microorganisms form the foci without which dental caries does not develop. Complete elimination of all carbohydrates from the diet would prevent dental caries. Perfect oral hygiene, if attainable, would likewise prevent dental caries.

The widespread use of carbohydrate-free diets or diets that contain very little carbohydrate is impossible for the reasons mentioned in the preceding paragraph. However, elimination or drastic restriction of those dietary items that contain carbohydrates and that are readily fermentable and readily retained on and about the protected surfaces of the teeth is a goal to be impressed upon every patient. The patient should be encouraged further to develop good toothbrushing habits (brushing after meals) and to occasionally use a discoloring tablet to evaluate the quality of his oral hygiene.

Many food items have been tested under a variety of in vitro situations to determine if an evaluation of their potential caries-producing properties could be ascertained; this method of testing is much simpler and less laborious than clinical trials. These studies have largely revolved around determination of carbohydrate content and the ability of the food items to produce acid when incubated under standardized conditions with suitable microorganisms. In some studies the investigators have also tried to evaluate the stickiness of the food items and thereby the readiness with which they adhere to teeth. One of the interesting facets of the findings in these investigations is that the carbohydrate content of the food item is not necessarily predictive of the acid production, as might be expected if the carbohydrate were readily available for fermentation. This observation has led to the hypothesis that some food items contain "natural" inhibitors of fermentation that reduce the carbohydrate utilization and the acid production. The inference is made that food items containing such an inhibitor would be less capable of initiating the carious process even if retained on the susceptible tooth surfaces. If such inhibitors exist and if they can be identified and added to foods that do not contain them in adequate amounts, clinical control of dental caries might be possible without major restriction in the kinds and quantities of carbohydrate-containing foods consumed. At present this concept is unfortunately at the early hypothesis stage and must be demonstrated in clinical studies that substantiate in vitro findings in the laboratory. Certainly there is absolutely no shred of evidence as yet indicative of the first half of an often-stated fallacy that the natural sugar in honey is not conducive to caries because of natural inhibitors, whereas the same amount of the same sugar in a commercial candy is harmful.

Presently, guidance with respect to oral environment of the patient with regard to carbohydrate intake must be made according to several rules of thumb rather than absolute dicta. Consumption of foodstuffs that contain high amounts of readily fermentable carbohydrate and are retained on the tooth surfaces should be kept to a minimum, especially between meals. Most cookies, cakes, crackers, presweetened cereals, icing, pastries, soft bread, and candy fall into the undesirable category. When a patient has a high potential for the development of carious lesions these items should be eliminated as completely as possible from the diet; when a patient is less susceptible a greater frequency for consumption of these items may be tolerated. Fresh fruits, vegetables, and hard breads will ordinarily not be expected to contribute adversely to oral health; these foods should be recommended as substitutes when between-meal snacks are necessary. Caramels and raw carrots are at the opposite poles of the undesirable-desirable oral health spectrum. In addition to being advised to maintain low consumption of these undesirable items, the patient should be encouraged to maintain optimal hygiene at all times, but especially after consumption of carbohydrate-containing items.

From a dental standpoint, recommendations to reduce the intake of those types of dietary items that contribute to undesirable oral environmental conditions are designed to correct a dietary problem rather than a strictly nutritional one orally. However, in all probability a secondary nutritional benefit will accrue automatically. If the eliminated items have to be replaced to supply caloric needs, replacement from the basic four food categories with items that are comparable in caloric value will almost invariably contribute substantially to the protein, vitamin, and mineral requirements. On the other hand, if caloric needs can be provided adequately from the remaining foods already in the diet, a substantial amount of surplus calories with their inevitable contribution to obesity will have been eliminated.

**Dietary supplementation**

Ordinarily the healthy individual with a consistently well-balanced and varied diet has no need for supplementary use of protein concentrates or of vitamin and mineral preparations. With wise menu planning, good food preparation procedures, and varied food consumption, routinely available foods through normal sources will provide adequate supplies of all the nutrients for good health. If an individual's daily requirements are being met and there is no deficit from a preceding period, no evidence is available of any benefit to be gained from an additional one or more days' allowance as a supplement. Often the use of a proprietary preparation is a screen for paying little attention to diet planning and to good procedures of food preparation. In this circumstance supplementation is not only undesirable but may be contrary to the best interests of the patient. However, it would be extreme and unjustifiable to take the position that supplementation is never required.

Supplementation during infancy is appropriate, provided that the level is adjusted to approximate the recommended daily dietary allowances. As the child's diet becomes more varied the need for supplementation decreases, so that by the time the child is eating with the family the need is nil. Likewise in older age groups supplementation frequently becomes advisable as the problems of gastrointestinal disease, prolonged use of dentures, malabsorption syndrome, and metabolic abnormalities such as hypothyroidism become more prevalent. Special care and supervision are likely to be needed when the elderly person lives alone, has a limited economic resource, and has poor food storage facilities, all of which tend to result in limited food choices and food faddism. Loss of teeth with inadequate replacement frequently contributes to a decreasing variety of food choices and malnutrition.

When there is evidence of a prolonged deficit supplementation is in order. The level of supplementation should be proportional to the degree and the duration of the deficit based on evaluation of the patient's diet and clinical condition. If the deficit has been small and for a short period, routine use of a preparation that daily provides the equivalent of an extra day's requirement of the necessary vitamins, minerals, or whatever is appropriate. If the deficit had been more severe, more concentrated preparations providing several days' requirements per day would be in order for an appropriate period of repletion. However, care should be taken whenever high levels are provided that they not be used longer than necessary. With both vitamin A and vitamin D, toxic manifestations as serious as their deficiency syndromes can ensue. Lavish claims for high levels of vitamin A for treatment of acne, of vitamin D for arthritis, and of other vitamins for other diseases have been made without justification. Excesses beyond the daily allowance of ten times for vitamin A or one hundred times for vitamin D have been promoted, both of which cause toxicity over prolonged periods.

### Dietary recommendations for patients after surgery or denture insertion

Brief or prolonged periods of masticatory insufficiency after surgery or denture insertion are prime occasions when dietary recommendations are needed and appreciated by the patient. Good prescriptions will prevent the development of nutritional problems even in such areas as fluid balance and will aid in maintenance of the patient's feeling of well-being and in the healing of the oral tissues. In addition, the inculcation of good dietary habits during even the initial brief period of emergency will be especially needed and helpful to denture wearers over the protracted period of more limited masticatory ability occasioned by dentures in comparison to the natural dentition.

Dentists must be prepared to give nutritional advice that is appropriate to patients at the time of oral and periodontal surgery, after reduction and fixation of jaw fractures, and when immediate, transitional, or permanent dentures are inserted. The nature of the recommendations will vary in proportion to the physical condition of the patient and the length of time that reduced ability to masticate will be experienced (or has already been experienced by long-term denture wearers). For any patient believed to be malnourished the recommendations must include specific supplementation of proteins, vitamins, and minerals as needed to the general recommendations that follow.

In the case of the well-nourished patient with minor surgery, the recommendations involve the prescription of adequate fluids and a soft or semisoft diet with chewing on the opposite side of the mouth until sufficient healing and pain relief occur to return to the normal varied diet. When oral or periodontal surgery is extensive a liquid diet for the first day or two is appropriate, followed by a gradual return to a normal diet as soon as healing permits. During accommodation to the use of dentures the patient should be encouraged to consume a liquid diet for only the length of time necessitated by acute pain and to begin to consume soft dietary items and small bite-size pieces of solid foods as soon as tissue tolerance permits. The amount of chewing required and the variety of foods should be increased as rapidly as the education process in the use of dentures permits.

All patients should have been prepared in advance of the insertion of dentures to realize that even the most perfectly designed and constructed dentures are going to be much less adequate than the well-maintained natural dentition. The anatomic and functional interrelationships of natural teeth, the periodontal membrane, and the alveolar bone constitute an apparatus that is capable of withstanding great force during biting and chewing and of reducing a wide variety of food items to dimensions that can be conveniently swallowed and digested. In contrast, the interrelationship of ideally fitted dentures to the soft tissues of the oral cavity is at best a much less desirable substitute for the tooth–periodontal membrane–alveolar bone apparatus. Less masticatory stress can be sustained and the ability to bite into various objects is greatly reduced. The denture wearer should be encouraged to bite and chew at the maximum levels that are physiologically appropriate but he should be urged not to grossly exceed these levels, even for the bravado demonstration to his friends of how well his dentures fit. In addition, the patient receiving dentures should be prepared in advance for the reduced taste perception that will be experienced and also for the reduced awareness of the heat of food items resulting from coverage of the palate. The latter point must be emphasized to reduce the likelihood that the patient will swallow excessively hot fluids with resultant scalding. The tendency of the denture wearer to attempt to swallow too large chunks of food that he has become tired of chewing needs to be discussed with the patient in order to make him aware of the possibility of aspiration and obstruction of the trachea.

The soft tissues upon which the dentures are supported tend to change in their contours and physiologic characteristics as the length of denture use increases. The rate of change varies greatly among individuals. The denture wearer needs to be counselled not to exceed the amount of biting and chewing stress that is comfortable lest more severe stress increase the rate of deterioration of the soft tissues. At the same time he should be cautioned to consume a varied diet that requires as much mastication as can be comfortably tolerated. As the denture wearer becomes aware that his dentures fit less well than at their original insertion, he should be urged to return to his dentist to have the denture either relined or remade. Characteristically the denture wearer gradually and often unconsciously increasingly restricts the variety of his diet to accommodate to ill-fitting dentures instead of seeking to have them suitably altered or replaced to maintain the original level of food selection. When this process of increasing dietary restriction is allowed to persist for years or even decades the dietary choices often become extremely limited. Nutritional deficiencies are prevalent sequelae of this increasing restriction of dietary choices and are especially evident among the elderly and those who live alone, becoming exaggerated when there is apathy, disinterest, or economic restraint. The length of time between episodes of denture relining or replacement will vary, depending on the physiologic condition of the patient and his oral tissues. Each patient should be counselled to be observant about his food habits and to return to the dentist for professional evaluation regularly every 2 years, or sooner if he detects any deterioration in his ability to masticate or improper fitting of his dentures.

The period when a liquid or soft diet is needed is brief after oral or periodontal surgery or during the accommodation to the use of dentures; therefore the emergency is minor and the principal needs are for a reasonable distribution of calories, proteins, and other substances and, even more importantly, for a feeling of well-being and satiety on the part of the patient. Time is too brief for the development of a nutritional deficiency or serious imbalance. In contrast, the period of recovery after jaw fracture or more serious facial injury will be several weeks, which is sufficiently long for more serious nutritional problems to develop. A complete and highly nutritious liquid diet is required when the mandible or maxilla has been fixed to permit fracture healing. If interarch fixation has been employed the diet must be capable of passing distal to the most posterior teeth that are present or through any spaces that are created by missing teeth.

The patient needs to be helped to realize the varieties of nutritious foods that are available and that can be prepared simply for a brief or prolonged period of emergency feeding during limited or negligible ability to masticate. Increasing amounts of advice will be needed in proportion to the length of the emergency in order to assure that no nutritional deficiency develops and that the patient's appetite and well-being are maintained by the nutritional quality, the palatability, and the variety of the dietary items prepared. Traditional foods like milkshakes and eggnogs are usually familiar to the patient. These items may be liberally supplemented during preparation by the addition of skim milk powder or by a larger quantity of ice cream or eggs than is customarily used and may be flavored in the ways most suitable for the individual patient. Soups are also familiar and valuable items for extensive use. In addition, the nutritious quality of strained foods and of chopped foods that have been prepared for the pediatric period of life are often overlooked in the preparation of adult diets at times of masticatory inadequacy. While many adults shun the use of such foods by reason of the implied or imagined implications of baby food consumption, these food products can and do have a vital place in the adult diet at appropriate times. Often these products need to be seasoned more highly to appeal to the individual adult's taste. When an individual lives alone during the need for special liquid diets, the small size of the pediatric food containers is also helpful to provide variety without leftovers and without the need for extensive cold storage facilities. Another procedure of great utility is the use of a blender; almost any food can be reduced by a blender to a form that can be handled readily when a liquid diet is appropriate. After reduction and interarch fixation of jaw fractures, diets that are composed of "blenderized" foods from the four basic food categories will be the most likely method to provide adequate amounts of all nutrients for the prolonged period of masticatory inability.

## COMMUNICATION OF RECOMMENDATIONS TO THE PATIENT

Possibly the most critical point in the sequence of nutritional care for the patient is at the time when the recommendations are provided to him. (See more concerning this topic on p. 49.) This should be performed in person by the dentist and should include a conversation on the importance of nutrition and the ways in which the recommendations will correct the problems and provide the nutrients for optimal nutriture, both generally and with respect to the oral cavity. The patient should be helped to see how the recommendations provide adequate nutrients including water to fulfill the recommended daily dietary allowances, a good distribution among the four major food groups, and a minimum of the orally undesirable items. One or more sample menus should be made available, along with information on what food items can be exchanged for others to maintain the quality of the diet and to give opportunity for variety. These materials should be accompanied by a personal letter in which a brief summary of the content of this conversation is recorded for the patient's later perusal. The patient should be made aware that the recommendations have been designed especially for him and his current needs.

At later appointments pertinent follow-up questions, encouragement, and advice should be given as indicated. It is especially important that the patient realize your continued interest as well as your recognition by encouragement and/or advice of his progress or lack of progress in following the recommendations.

## CONCLUSION

The recognition of nutritional problems, the evaluation of diets, and the design of appropriate recommendations for nutritional improvement are among the most important phases of professional preventive care that a dentist can provide for his patients. In many ways he is uniquely placed in the health professions to provide this type of service. The advice offered can result in the material improvement of the nutriture of the individual as well as in improved oral health and more rapid and desirable response to technical procedures. However, opportunity for service brings the added responsibility to be well informed in the fundamentals of the science of nutrition and to utilize skillfully these facts for specifically designed recommendations for individual patients.

## REFERENCES

1. Food and Nutrition Board: Recommended daily dietary allowances, revised 1963, Pub. 1146, Washington, D. C., 1964, National Academy of Sciences, National Research Council.
2. Essentials of an adequate diet, Agriculture Information Bulletin 160, Washington, D. C., 1956, United States Department of Agriculture.
3. Joliffe, N., editor: Clinical nutrition, ed. 2, New York, 1962, Harper & Row, Publishers.
4. Follis, R. H., Jr.: The pathology of nutritional disease, Springfield, Illinois, 1948, Charles C Thomas, Publisher.
5. Shaw, J. H.: Effect of nutritional factors on bones and teeth, Ann. N. Y. Acad. Sci. **60:**733, 1955.
6. Shaw, J. H.: Nutrition and dental caries. In Toverud, G.: Survey of the literature of

dental caries, Pub. 225, Washington, D. C., 1952, National Academy of Sciences, National Reseach Council.
7. Sobel, A. E., and others: Calcification XXVI; caries susceptibility in relation to diet and composition of teeth, J. Dent. Res. **39:**462, 1960.
8. McClure, F. J., editor: Fluoride drinking waters, Pub. 825, Washington, D. C., 1962, United States Department of Health, Education, and Welfare.
9. Shaw, J. H., editor: Fluoridation as a public health measure, Washington, D. C., 1954, American Association for the Advancement of Science.
10. Eanes, E. D., and others: Small angle x-ray diffraction analysis of the effect of fluoride on human bone apatite, Arch. Oral Biol. **10:**161, 1965.
11. Shaw, J. H., and Griffiths, D.: Dental abnormalities in rats attributable to protein deficiency during reproduction, J. Nutrition **80:**123, 1963.
12. Sweeney, E. A., and Guzman, M.: Oral conditions in children from three highland villages in Guatemala, Arch. Oral Biol. **11:**687-698, 1966.
13. Toverud, G.: The influence of war and the post-war conditions on the teeth of Norwegian school children, Milbank Mem. Fund Quart. **34:**354, 1956; **35:**127, 373, 1957.
14. Hadjimarkos, D. M.: Trace elements and tooth decay, Discovery **26:**36, 1965.
15. Sognnaes, R. F., Shaw, J. H., and Bogoroch, R.: Radiotracer studies on bone, cementum, dentin and enamel of rhesus monkeys, Amer. J. Physiol. **180:**408, 1955.
16. Briner, W. W., Francis, M. D., and Rosen, S.: Rate of development and regression of hypomineralized areas (HMA) in rat molars, 43rd general meeting, I.A.D.R. Abstract 210, 1965.
17. Brudevold, F., Steadman, L. T., and Smith, F. A.: Inorganic and organic components of tooth structure, Ann. N. Y. Acad. Sci. **85:**110, 1960.
18. Cox, G. J.: Oral environment and dental caries. In Toverud, G.: Survey of the literature of dental caries, Pub. 225, Washington, D. C., 1952, National Academy of Sciences, National Research Council.
19. Sognnaes, R. F., editor: Advances in experimental caries research, Washington, D. C., 1955, American Association for the Advancement of Science.
20. Gustafsson, B. E., and others: The Vipeholm dental caries study; the effect of different levels of carbohydrate intake on caries activity in 436 individuals observed for five years, Acta Odont. Scand. **11:**232, 1954.
21. Lundquist, C.: Oral sugar clearance: its influence on dental caries activity, Odont. Rev. (supp. 1) **13:**35, 1952.
22. Ludwig, T. G., and Bibby, B. G.: Acid production from different carbohydrate foods in plaque and saliva, J. Dent. Res. **36:**56, 1957.
23. Schweigert, B. S., and others: Dental caries in the cotton rat, VIII, further studies on the dietary effects of carbohydrate, protein and fat on the incidence and extent of carious lesions, J. Nutrition **32:**405, 1946.
24. Krasse, B.: The effect of caries-inducing streptococci in hamsters fed diets with sucrose or glucose, Arch. Oral Biol. **10:**223, 1965.
25. Nizel, A. E., and Harris, R. S.: The effects of phosphates on experimental dental caries: a literature review, J. Dent. Res. **43:**1123, 1964.
26. Shaw, J. H.: The relation of nutrition to periodontal disease, J. Dent. Res. **41:**264, 1962.
27. Warkany, J.: Production of congenital malformations by dietary measures; experiments in mammals, J.A.M.A. **108:**2020, 1958.
28. Stuart, H. C.: Findings in examinations of newborn infants and infants during the neonatal period which appear to have a relationship to the diets of their mothers during pregnancy, Fed. Proc. **4:**271, 1945.
29. Bowes, A. deP., and Church, C. F.: Food values of portions commonly used, ed. 9, Philadelphia, 1963, J. B. Lippincott Co.

# Chapter 4 Enamel and dental caries

## Simon Katz

Characteristics of enamel in relation to dental caries
    Chemical composition
    The crystallographic nature of the inorganic components of dental enamel
The structure of enamel
    Surface enamel
Pathogenesis of the carious process
Possible mechanisms of caries formation
    The dissolution of the mineral components
        Acid dissolution
        Chelation
    The dissolution of the organic matrix
    The simultaneous dissolution of organic and inorganic matrices
Theories of dental caries
    Exogenous theories
        The chemicoparasitic theory of Miller
        Proteolytic theories
        The proteolysis chelation theory
    Endogenous theories
Dental factors affecting the susceptibility of the teeth to decay
    Anatomic factors
    Chemical factors
        The reactions of enamel with fluoride
        Other chemical factors
    Crystallographic factors
    Structural factors
Conclusion

Dental caries is an infectious disease characterized by a series of complex chemical and microbiologic reactions that result in the destruction of the tooth if the process remains unchecked. It is almost universally agreed that this destruction, which progresses from the surface of the tooth to the interior, results from chemical substances produced in the immediate tooth environment.

From a preventive dentistry viewpoint, then, two entities have to be considered in the etiology of dental caries: (1) the tooth, which is destroyed; and (2) the tooth environment, where the destructive agents are formed.

Much is known about the characteristics and likelihood of occurrence of cariogenic factors in the tooth environment. Much less information is available concerning the factors responsible for the susceptibility or resistance of the teeth themselves to dental decay. Inasmuch as caries is primarily a lesion of enamel we will review in this chapter the modern concepts concerning the relationships between incipient dental caries and different characteristics of enamel, in the hope of finding some clues applicable to the prevention and/or control of the initial lesion.

## CHARACTERISTICS OF ENAMEL IN RELATION TO DENTAL CARIES
### Chemical composition

Enamel, the hardest and most mineralized tissue of the animal economy, is composed of three different substances: minerals, organic matrix, and water (Table 4-1).

The mineral portion of the enamel is a basic calcium phosphate with small proportions of carbonate and magnesium and trace amounts of fluoride, lead, aluminum, strontium, iron, and other elements. Table 4-2 presents average values for the mineral composition of both sound and carious human enamel.

The organic components of human enamel compose several fractions (Table 4-3).

According to the data in Table 4-2, sound enamel and carious enamel are practically identical. However, from the point of view of dental caries resistance the simple mention of the chemical composition of the enamel is misleading because it does not reflect accurately the true composition of the tissue at the point of initiation

**Table 4-1.** *Percentage of minerals, organic matter, and water in human enamel, by weight and volume*

|  | Weight | Volume* |
|---|---|---|
| Minerals | 97 | 91 |
| Organic matter | 1 | 3 |
| Water | 2 | 6 |

*The density of whole human enamel is approximately 3.0, while that of its organic components is 1.2. The density of water is of course 1.0.

**Table 4-2.** *Inorganic components of sound and carious human enamel*

|  | Percent dry weight | |
|---|---|---|
| Component | Sound | Carious* |
| Water | 2.0 | 3.1 |
| Calcium | 36.7 | 36.0 |
| Phosphorus | 17.4 | 17.0 |
| Magnesium | 0.5 | 0.4 |
| Carbon dioxide | 2.4 | 1.6 |
| Calcium/phosphorus | 2.1 | 2.1 |
| Fluoride† | 90-130 (p.p.m.) | 490-580 (p.p.m.) |

*Enamel attacked by dental caries.
†The process of dental caries chemically encompasses a two-way reaction: dissolution and reprecipitation. During reprecipitation the fluoride ion is concentrated; this explains its higher concentration in caries as compared to sound enamel. Sound enamel from carious teeth contains, on the average, less fluoride than sound enamel from sound teeth.

**Table 4-3.** *Organic components of enamel*

| Component | Percent dry weight |
|---|---|
| Insoluble protein | 0.25 |
| Soluble protein* | 0.25 |
| Lipids | 0.60 |
| Citrate | 0.10 |

*Includes mucoproteins.

of the carious process, that is, the enamel surface. Layer by layer analysis of enamel, beginning at the outermost surface and proceeding inward, demonstrates that surface enamel contains more fluoride, phosphate, and total nitrogen and less carbonate than subsurface enamel. The importance of these differences in terms of dental caries susceptibility will be discussed subsequently.

**The crystallographic nature of the inorganic components of dental enamel**

The chemical composition of teeth and bones was recognized at the end of the eighteenth century, when Hatchett[1] reported that they were composed of calcium phosphate in addition to small amounts of calcium carbonate. Inasmuch as the ratio of calcium to phosphorus closely approached that for calcium phosphate, it was assumed that the mineral component of bones and teeth was chiefly tricalcium phosphate—$Ca_3(PO_4)_2$—with a small amount of calcium carbonate plus much smaller quantities of other elements such as magnesium, sodium, potassium, and fluorine. More detailed concepts concerning the nature of the calcium phosphate composition of the teeth and bones had to wait until better knowledge of the chemistry of the alkaline earth phosphate was available and new tools were applied to investigate their structural nature; in 1917 Bassett[2] provided new information on the subject. He showed experimentally that when calcium phosphate precipitates in slightly acid, neutral, or slightly alkaline solutions—a range within which the reaction of body fluids is comprised—the most stable form for the precipitate is a basic phosphate to which the formula $3\ Ca_3(PO_4)_2 \cdot Ca(OH)_2$ was attributed. This is the formula of a number of widely dispersed minerals called apatites, particularly one of them, hydroxyapatite. In view of these considerations and in view of his analytical findings, Bassett[2] concluded that "the mineral constituents of bone and teeth consist in the main of hydroxyapatite mixed with a certain amount of calcium carbonate and containing small amounts of sodium, potassium and magnesium bicarbonate, which appear to be merely absorbed by the phosphate-carbonate aggregate."[3]

Correct as they basically are, Bassett's ideas indicate attempts to force a formulation of the bone and teeth minerals to fit the concepts of exact chemical structure prevalent at that time. These attempts reached their peak with the formula proposed by Gassman[3] in 1928; his formula represented bone salts chemically as a calcium phosphate–carbonate whose formula was given as

$$\left[ Ca \left( \begin{array}{c} OPO_3\ Ca \\ \\ \\ OPO_3\ Ca \end{array} \right) Ca \right]_3 CO_3$$

where $CO_3$ could be replaced by chloride or fluoride ions. This and similar formulations demonstrated that the crystalline nature of the biologic apatites was unknown. In fact, Bassett[2] speaks of "possibly amorphous phosphate" in his description of the bone minerals. The definite proof of the crystalline nature of the biologic apatites was established only when more sophisticated techniques, particularly x-ray diffraction, were added to the analytical procedures currently in use. In 1926 Gross[4] reported that x-ray diffraction patterns obtained from enamel and dentin minerals were similar to those found in mineral apatites. The same year de Jong[5] arrived at the same conclusion about bone. The apatitic nature of the mineral components of bone and teeth has been confirmed by every work performed in this field since these early studies.

These early reports provided only a comparison between the x-ray diffraction pattern of bone and teeth apatites and those mineral apatites but did not contribute to the elucidation of the intimate structure of the apatite crystal. It remained to Mehmel[6] and Naray-Szabo[7] to define the crystal structure of fluorapatite as representative of the group. They calculated, independently, the atomic positions within the crystal from x-ray diffraction data; both published their respective reports in 1930. Their model is currently accepted by practically all crystallographers, and only very small refinements of the apatite atomic positions have been introduced.

The structure of hydroxyapatite is considered to be basically the same as that of fluorapatite, with the two hydroxyl ions occupying very closely the same fluoride sites. According to this model, the unit cell of hydroxyapatite—the smallest structural unit that repeats in the three-dimensional pattern of the crystal lattice—is a small four-sided prism (about 9.41 cm.$^{-8}$ by 6.86 cm.$^{-8}$) containing ten atoms of calcium, six phosphate tetrahedra, and two hydroxyl ions. These figures include the total content of the unit cell, that is, atoms that are entirely within its limits, and the proportional part of atoms which, being in boundary positions, are shared by more than one unit cell. With these limitations the chemical formula currently accepted for hydroxyapatite is $Ca_{10}(PO_4)_6(OH)_2$.

Of the ten calcium ions contained in the unit cell, four (Ca I) are stacked in two columns in the interior of the cell on the threefold rotation axis parallel to the c-axis, coordinating with oxygen atoms from the phosphate groups surrounding them. The other six (Ca II), which are coordinated with both oxygen atoms and hydroxyl groups, are located around the screw axis that runs through the corners of the unit cell, parallel to the c-axis. There are twenty-four oxygen atoms, all bonded to phosphorus atoms to form six phosphate tetrahedral groups. These oxygen atoms are divided into O I, O II, and O III, according to their relationships with the other components of the cell. Finally, the two hydroxyls occupy the corners of the unit cell, with the OH axis almost superimposed with the direction of the c-axis. Fig. 4-1 shows a stereoscopic model of fluorapatite. Apatites belong to the hexagonal crystallographic system and their symmetry symbol is $P6_3/m$.

One of the most striking properties of the apatite series is the frequency of ionic substitutions within their formula with practically no change of the crystallographic parameters, that is, the so-called isomorphic substitutions. Gruner and associates[8] reported that fluorapatite, chloroapatite, hydroxyapatite, carbonate-apatite, and oxyapatite form an isomorphous series capable of solid solution in one another. Klement[9] showed that lead can replace calcium in natural and synthetic apatites; he and Lagergren and Carlstrom[10] reported the substitution of strontium for calcium. McDonald[11] and associates were able to observe the same types of substitutions in bone apatite after injecting experimental animals with lead and strontium. Replacement of calcium by magnesium or sodium in bone and tooth minerals has been frequently reported, as well as substitution of carbonate for hydroxyl and/or phosphate groups. McConnell[12] has postulated also the substitution of $(O_4H_4)^{-4}$ (the so-called tetrahedral hydroxyls) for $PO_4^{-3}$ apatite tetrahedra. Klement and Hasselbach,[13] and McConnell and Foreman,[14] reported the synthesis of stannous-calcium apatites. Klement and Hasselbach prepared a stannous-calcium chloroapatite with eight calcium ions

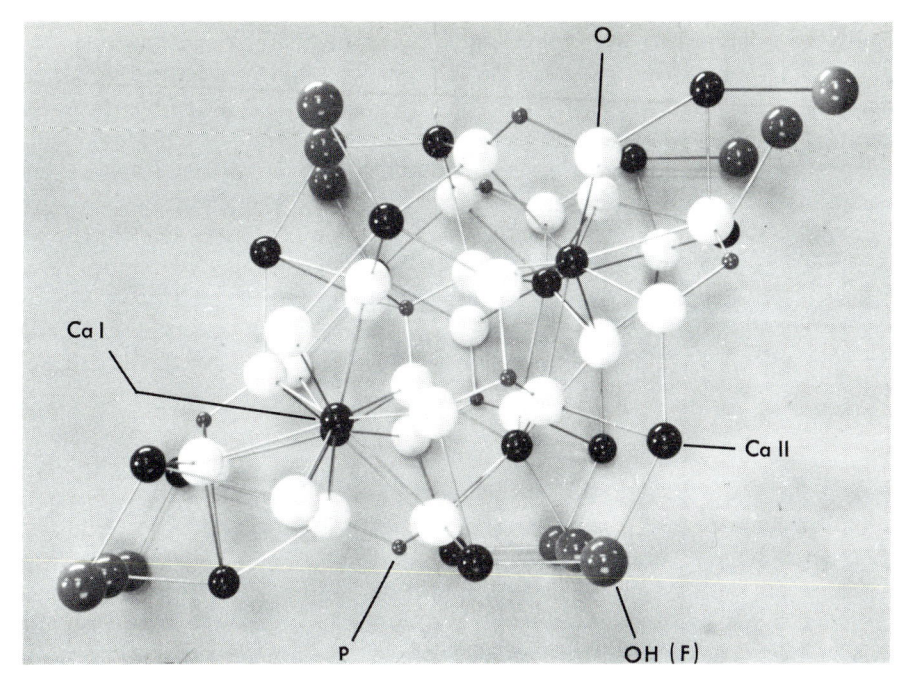

Fig. 4-1. Atomic model of the fluoroapatite unit cell. (Model prepared by J. R. Wolsieffer and J. C. Schaefer.)

replaced by tin (II) and a stannous-calcium fluorapatite with five calcium ions replaced by tin (II). McConnell and Foreman's preparation appears to be a tin-calcium hydroxy-fluorochloroapatite in which tin (II) ions have substituted for nine calcium ions.

Apatite is not the name of a definite compound; it is the name of a crystallographic structure. Even the phosphate tetrahedra, which are considered to be the foundation of apatites, can and are substituted, at least in certain proportion, by $AsO_4$, $VO_4$, $SiO_4$, or $SO_4$ tetrahedra, with provisions to balance the differences in electrical charges, when needed. Trautz[15] has been able to prepare in the laboratory "a sulphateapatite, which contains no phosphate," represented by the formula $Ca_4Na_6(SO_4)_6F_2$. Its x-ray diffraction pattern and unit cell dimensions are similar to those of fluorapatite.

From a dental point of view, the substitutions that have received the most attention are those of fluoride for hydroxyl, resulting in fluorapatite, and of carbonate for phosphate and/or hydroxyl, resulting in the formation of carbonate-apatite. The first yields crystallographically more perfect apatites; they have been shown to be more acid-resistant (and thus more caries-resistant) than nonsubstituted apatites. Carbonate, on the other hand, interferes with the crystallization of apatites, thus resulting in less perfect specimens. The significance of carbonate substitution, in terms of dental caries etiology and/or prevention, is still a controversial matter.

In biologic systems the substitution of fluoride for hydroxyl is never complete. The surface layer of enamel from teeth of persons living in communities having an average of 1 $\mu$g fluoride/ml. in their drinking water contains an average of 800 to 900 p.p.m. fluoride. Assuming isomorphic substitution of fluoride for hydroxyl, this is equivalent to 2.0 to 2.5 percent of the total possible isomorphic substitution. Of all the layers of enamel the surface one has been shown to have the highest concentration of fluoride. In view of this rather low degree of substitution, the expression fluoride-substituted hydroxyapatite rather than fluorapatite should be used to refer to the product that results from fluoride substitution in biologic systems.

As shown in Table 4-2, chemical analyses of dental enamel indicate an average content of carbonate (expressed as carbon dioxide) of about 2.5 to 3.5 percent. Crystallographic inference and experimental evidence suggest that most of this carbonate is absorbed on the surface of the crystals and that very little is a part of the crystals themselves. The space positions occupied by the carbonate incorporated into the crystals, the atomic groups that are replaced, and even the true chemical nature of the $CO_2$ fraction (carbonate, bicarbonate?), are unknown.

The presence of carbonate in enamel has a detrimental effect on the crystallinity of the tissue, that is, on the degree of perfection of the crystal faces, the size of the crystals, and/or the existence of internal strains. Because their solubility in acids is greater than that of phosphates, the presence of carbonates in enamel also contributes to the susceptibility of the teeth to dental caries.

A second interesting fact of many biologic apatites concerns their stoichiometric deficiencies. When biologic or finely divided mineral or synthetic apatites are subjected to chemical analysis, it is frequently found that the Ca/P* ratio falls below the stoichiometric value of 1.67. Two conflicting explanations have been suggested. The first postulates that the excess phosphate is adsorbed on the high specific surface crystals. The second contends that there is statistical absence from the Ca I column, with provisions to maintain electrical balance by hydrogen bonds between oxygen atoms of neighboring phosphate tetrahedra. Both processes probably occur in biologic apatites; that is, they are calcium deficient lattices and they have phosphate, and other ions and groups as well, adsorbed on the surface of the crystals.

A second stoichiometric deficiency of biologic apatites has been mentioned by Kay and associates.[16] They reported that, in mineral hydroxyapatite, the hydroxyl rows are arranged in an orderly manner with the hydrogen ions consistently toward the same side of the oxygen ions and the hydroxyl axis almost superimposed with the direction of the c-axis. In biologic apatites, probably because of the speed of growth or because of the inavailability of enough energy during crystallization, a certain degree of internal disorder (higher entropy) is usually found in the hydroxyl rows, so that some hydrogen ions are located above the oxygen ions and some are below. Energy considerations prevent, however, that two consecutive hydroxyls in the same row could have their hydrogen ions facing one another. Consequently, each change in the orientation of the hydrogens on the hydroxyls of the same row results in the occurrence of a vacant place in that row, in order to separate the two approaching hydrogen ions. Fluoride ions, being of almost identical ionic radium and electrical charge as hydroxyls, fit perfectly in these lattice voids, thus contributing to perfect the crystalline structure of this deficient apatite. It is obvious that these more perfect lattices, with greater internal order (lesser entropy), may require more energy to be formed than the deficient more disordered specimens.

---

*It is customary to refer to the ratio $\dfrac{Ca + Mg}{P}$ as the corrected Ca/P ratio. This compensates for any degree of magnesium substitution.

Isometric substitutions produce changes in the unit cell dimensions of the apatite crystal, which, although minimal in magnitude, can be detected and can help in determining the nature and degree of a given substitution. Precise determination of the enamel apatite unit cell size yields values almost identical to those of precipitated hydroxyapatite. Since chemical data indicate that several components other than calcium, phosphorus, oxygen, and hydrogen are present in enamel, it follows that these other substances are foreign to the apatite itself, in which case they are not well enough crystallized, or they are present in very small amounts to record their own diffraction pattern, or their ions are substituting in the apatite in very small proportion, as is probably the case with magnesium (for calcium) and with fluoride (for hydroxyl).

Complete substitution of hydroxyl by fluoride results in a 0.5 percent contraction of the a-axis of the apatite crystal, with very little if any change in the a-axis dimension. Baud and associates,[17-19] working with bone apatite, found that the a-axis contraction from fluoride substitution is a linear function of the amount of fluoride incorporated into the apatite mass. This finding obviously permits an x-ray diffraction calculation of the amount of fluoride substituting for hydroxyl in a bone or tooth enamel specimen. The substitution of carbonate for some other component of the apatite, within the proportions common to biologic specimens, does not alter the linearity of the relationship between the a-axis contraction and the amount of fluoride substitution.

## THE STRUCTURE OF ENAMEL

Enamel consists of calcium phosphate (essentially hydroxyapatite) precipitated over a so-called organic matrix. The exact nature and structural characteristics of the organic matrix are not known.

The inorganic mass is formed by long rod-shaped crystal aggregates called enamel prisms, or rods. It was believed in the past that the rods were surrounded by a prism sheath and separated from and joined to one another by a so-called interprismatic substance. Both the prism sheaths and the interprismatic substance were believed to have a different composition from that of the rods themselves.

Modern electron microscopic observations disprove the existence of both the prism sheaths and interprismatic substance as definite chemical entities; similar to the prisms, the rods are composed of apatite crystals and organic matrix. The apatite crystals are bigger of enamel than those of dentin, cementum, and bone. They are ribbon-shaped or hexagonal prisms, measuring on the average 3,000 to 5,000 Å in length (range 250 to 10,000) and 500 Å in width (range 400 to 1,200). Their orientation within the prism changes from the center to the periphery of the prism. At the center the long axes of both crystals and prisms are parallel, while at the periphery they form an angle that may approach 90 degrees.

It is precisely this sudden change of orientation of the enamel crystals, which are anisotropically birefringent, that produces in the optical microscope the image of two separated structures surrounding and separating the prisms. Electron microscopy, obviously not subjected to optical birefringence, demonstrates that the only difference between the prisms, sheaths, and interprismatic substance is the change of direction of their component enamel crystals.

The change of orientation of the enamel crystals results in larger intercrystal spaces in the periphery than in the core of the prism. Since these spaces are occupied

66  *Improving dental practice through preventive measures*

**Table 4-4.** *Percentages of carbon dioxide and fluorine in enamel layers of teeth from areas with different levels of fluorine in the drinking water\**

| Fluorine (p.p.m.) in water supply | First layer Fluorine | First layer Carbon dioxide | Second layer Fluorine | Second layer Carbon dioxide | Third layer Fluorine | Third layer Carbon dioxide |
|---|---|---|---|---|---|---|
| 0.1 | 0.050 | 1.66 | 0.006 | 1.88 | 0.011 | 2.04 |
| 1.0 | 0.066 | 1.55 | 0.023 | 1.71 | 0.012 | 1.97 |
| 1.6 | 0.097 | 1.58 | 0.036 | 1.70 | 0.026 | 1.78 |
| 2.5 | 0.156 | 1.30 | 0.087 | 2.27 | 0.057 | 2.76 |
| 5.0 | 0.337 | 1.79 | 0.171 | 1.90 | 0.113 | 2.08 |

\*Data from McCann, H. G., Rasmussen, S., Brudevold, F., cited in Brudevold, F., McCann, H. G., and Gron, P.: Caries resistance as related to the chemistry of enamel. In Wolstenholme, G. E. W., and O'Connor, M., editors: Caries resistant teeth, London, 1965, J. & A. Churchill Ltd.

by organic substance, it follows that the concentration of organic substance is greater in the surface than in the interior of the enamel prisms. In addition to the periphery of the prisms, the so-called incremental striae of Retzius (which represent the periodicity of enamel opposition), as well as enamel defective cracks and, when present, the prism cross-striations, are sites of concentration of organic substance. The importance of these features in dental caries progression will be discussed later.

**Surface enamel**

The surface enamel, at least on smooth tooth surfaces, has a particular structure, which differs from deeper enamel in the following characteristics.
1. Morphologically it is interrupted by periodic depressions, the perykematas, which represent the external ending of the striae of Retzius.
2. Structurally the crystals are all parallel; that is, they do not form the characteristic prism arrangement. The crystals tend to be perpendicular to the enamel surface.
3. Chemically it is more mineralized and contains more fluoride, phosphate, and organic matter and less carbonate and water (Table 4-4).
4. It is covered by one or more organic films, the most superficial of them formed by the precipitation and denaturation of salivary proteins.

## PATHOGENESIS OF THE CARIOUS PROCESS

The elements of enamel that play a role in dental caries have been described; the means by which the process is initiated and progresses will now be discussed.

When the pathway of dental caries is followed on smooth surfaces of the teeth it can be observed that the first clinically visible alteration is not the formation of a cavity—in fact, the enamel surface appears to be intact—but a change of the luster and color of the enamel surface from the ivory, translucent, and lustrous aspect of sound enamel to a chalky whitish, opaque spot, the so-called white spot.

Instrumental observations such as x-ray densitometry, microscopic examination of stained ground sections, and other methods show that the white spot is the external manifestation of a process of enamel dissolution that has progressed underneath the surface of the enamel, while the surface layer remains practically untouched. The initiation of the lesion apparently occurs along the striae of Retzius.

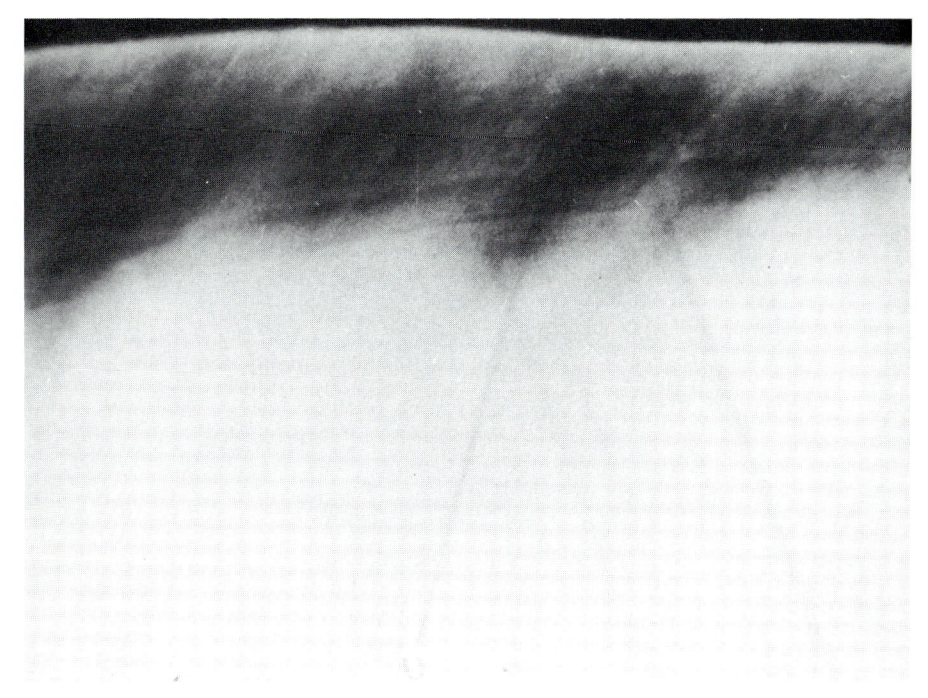

Fig. 4-2. Microradiograph of initial subsurface decalcification in dental caries. Notice the almost intact enamel surface, and how the dissolution progresses along the periphery of the enamel rods. (Courtesy Dr. John A. Gray.)

Further progression of the lesion results in the breakdown of the surface and deepening of the dissolution process. Microscopic examination shows that the progression of the lesion occurs chiefly through areas of concentration of organic substance, namely, the periphery of the enamel rods, the striae of Retzius, and enamel lamellae (defective enamel cracks filled with organic substance). In occlusal surfaces the carious lesion progresses through the rod's periphery after its initiation in (fissured?) pits and grooves. Fig. 4-2 shows the initial subsurface lesion.

The agents responsible for dental caries dissolve the prism substance but progress mainly through the organic components of enamel. In other words, the agents capable of producing dental caries have the ability to dissolve enamel prisms and to diffuse through the organic components that surround these prisms. Upon reaching the dentinoenamel junction, the carious lesion spreads laterally and progresses toward the pulp preferentially through the dentinal tubules. This gives dentinal caries its typical conic shape—base at the dentinoenamel junction and apex toward the pulp.

## POSSIBLE MECHANISMS OF CARIES FORMATION

As stated previously, enamel prisms are composed of apatite crystals separated by organic matrix. The initiation of enamel dissolution, then, can occur through one of the following processes.
1. The dissolution of the mineral components (acidogenesis)
2. The dissolution of the organic matrix (proteolysis)
3. The simultaneous dissolution of both organic and inorganic components

### The dissolution of the mineral components

Two types of chemical reactions may theoretically explain the dissolution of the mineral components: acid dissolution and chelation.

**Acid dissolution.** The theory of acid dissolution is the most widely accepted for the initiation and progression of dental caries. It is expressed by the equation

$$Ca_{10}(PO_4)_6(OH)_2 + 8H^+ \longrightarrow 10\ Ca^{++} + 6HPO_4^= + 2H_2O$$

Hydroxyapatite — Hydrogen ions — Free calcium ions — Hydrogen phosphate — Water

where the hydrogen ions (acid) react with the phosphate groups to form a soluble acid phosphate, thus breaking down the integrity of the tissue. The need for hydrogen ions implies the need for a low pH for this reaction to occur.

**Chelation.** A chelator, a compound with an affinity for metal ions (in this particular case, calcium), reacts with the tissue calcium ions to form a soluble calcium complex; this leads to the breakdown of the apatite crystals. Chelators operate over a wide range of pH values; therefore chelation can occur in the absence of acid conditions. In fact, the faster chelation rates generally occur in the presence of an alkaline pH.

There is a wealth of information which proves that acids in amounts and strength high enough to produce enamel dissolution do form in the tooth environment. Furthermore, the pH in carious cavities has been found to be consistently acid.

It has been possible to produce in the laboratory artificial carious lesions with the appearance of those naturally formed by exposing teeth in vitro to an acidic salivary-glucose-agar system. Time sequence studies of early lesions demonstrate that the first observable reactions are the presence of free minerals and a pH of 4.2 to 4.5 at the lesion. Free proteins are not observed until after decalcification has taken place.

There is general agreement that calcium chelators are present in the oral cavity; however, their concentration is so small that the participation of chelation in natural dental caries can be at best only minimal.

It is interesting to comment that acids and chelators appear to differ not only in the chemical but also in the morphologic pathway of enamel dissolution. Preliminary electron microscopic observations suggest that acids attack the enamel rod periphery and chelators attack the prism core.

### The dissolution of the organic matrix

It has been proposed that the initiation of the process of dental caries occurs because of the dissolution of the organic matrix by means of proteolytic enzymes produced by oral bacteria. Experimental evidence indicates, however, that the organic matrix of enamel is so petrified, that is, embedded in the mineral phase, that it is unavailable for enzymatic attack unless some decalcification initially has taken place. In addition, gnotobiotic studies have demonstrated that cariogenic bacteria are either nonproteolytic or at best only very slightly proteolytic. The first sign of free proteins in an in vitro lesion occurs after 10 days of exposure, that is, after acid decalcification has already been detected.

### The simultaneous dissolution of organic and inorganic matrices

The biochemical mechanisms responsible for the dissolution of the enamel will operate simultaneously on its organic and inorganic components. This type of process, for instance, is typical of bone resorption. The fact that the organic matrix of intact human enamel is not available for enzymatic destruction makes this conception of dental caries initiation untenable.

From a chemical viewpoint, then, the process of dental caries begins with the acid dissolution of the tooth (enamel) minerals. The breakdown of the organic matrix occurs by enzymatic and mechanical means once decalcification has occurred.

## THEORIES OF DENTAL CARIES

Through the years numerous theories have been proposed to explain the etiology of dental caries, taking into account the mechanisms of enamel dissolution. In general terms they can be classified as exogenous theories, which postulate that the origin of the lesion lies outside the teeth, and endogenous theories, which claim that caries is induced primarily by changes occurring inside the tooth.

### Exogenous theories

**The chemicoparasitic theory of Miller.** The most popular of all theories of caries etiology was formulated by W. D. Miller[20] in 1882. According to him, "dental caries is a chemico-parasitical disease consisting of two distinctly marked stages, decalcification or softening of the tissue and dissolution of the softened residue," produced by "all microorganisms of the mouth which possess the power of exciting an acid fermentation of foods," which thus "may and do take part in the first stage of dental caries," and "all [microorganisms] possessing a peptonizing or digestive action upon albuminaceous substances" which thus "may take in the second stage" (of proteolysis).

Modern refinements of this theory include the development of the concepts of dental plaque and its biochemical and bacteriologic dynamics, as well as the physiochemistry and chemistry of enamel dissolution.

**Proteolytic theories.** Gottlieb[21] proposed that carious lesions start in the organic matter occupying enamel cracks (lamellae) or in the prism sheaths, in areas not covered by the primary cuticle. Microbial enzymes dissolve the organic matrix and eventually the calcified enamel rod. However, only occasionally is the process totally proteolytic; most frequently a limited acid production accompanies the proteolysis. A yellow pigment is formed as a consequence of the enzymatic reaction, and Gottlieb[21] insists that this pigmentation is typical of true caries. In his opinion, the chalky enamel produced by acid alone is not carious.

According to Pincus[22] dental caries results from the action of a bacterial sulfatase on the sulfated mucopolysaccharides of enamel and dentin. The sulfuric acid removed from these compounds by the action of the sulfatase is in turn responsible for the dissolution of the tooth mineral. (The concentration of mucopolysaccharide in enamel is so low that it is difficult to conceive how caries can be produced by this mechanism.)

In Frisbie's[23] opinion the organic matrix of the tooth tissues is depolymerized by bacterial enzymes, following which acids released during the depolymerization or simply mechanical forces break down the inorganic components of the tooth.

**The proteolysis chelation theory.** Schatz and associates[24-26] proposed that the lesion results from the simultaneous degradation of the enamel organic matrix (particularly its keratin) by oral bacteria and of enamel minerals by chelators produced during the breakdown of the matrix, plus those present in dental bacteria, plaque, and food residues.

It has been not possible to demonstrate the availability of the organic matrix of intact enamel to bacterial enzymes. In addition, it is more likely that the small amount of chelators present in the dental plaque will complex free plaque calcium rather than the tightly bound enamel calcium.

**Endogenous theories**

Leimgruber[27] feels that the resistance of the teeth to dental caries depends on a posteruptive process of mineralization, which in turn is determined by a biologically active substance present in saliva, the so-called "maturation factor." This maturation factor chemically unites the protein and mineral components of enamel and dentin. Caries is interpreted as resulting from the rupture of the chemical bonds between organic and inorganic matrices.

Csernyei[28] visualizes dental caries as being determined by the plasma phosphatases, which dissolve the tooth apatites when the equilibrium fluoride-magnesium is altered by a deficiency of fluoride. Normally there is a physiologic equilibrium between phosphatase activators (magnesium) and phosphatase inhibitors (fluoride). When this equilibrium is altered in the dental pulp caries results through the effect of phosphoric acid released by the effect of pulp phosphatase.

Neuman and Di Salvo[29] have proposed a biophysical theory which postulates that the susceptibility to dental caries results from a lack of proper masticatory stress. Resistant teeth, they claim, result from a sclerosing effect produced by compressive forces originated from high chewing loads. It is said that the sclerosing effect consists of a loss of water plus an uncoiling of the polypeptide chains of the organic matrix, all of which produces a denser, more resistant tissue.

Only the theories of dental caries based on the initial acid dissolution of enamel have solid experimental support. The current interpretation of caries places the main etiologic role in the production of the so-called dental plaque (bacterial colonies) and of acids inside the plaque. Both acids and plaque are the result of metabolic processes of the cariogenic bacteria. The teeth themselves play in this this etiologic scheme only a secondary role, represented by their susceptibility—or resistance—to decay. In other words, the most important etiologic factors are those related to the production of cariogenic agents in the oral environment. When the cariogenic attack so originated is of sufficient intensity, very few teeth will escape its effect. The fact that 98 percent of Americans in an advanced and "sanitized" Western civilization suffer from dental caries is proof of this point.

This does not mean that nothing can be done to increase the resistance of the teeth to dental decay. Quite the contrary, this has so far been the most fruitful area of preventive dentistry.

## DENTAL FACTORS AFFECTING THE SUSCEPTIBILITY OF THE TEETH TO DECAY

There are a number of factors associated with the susceptibility or resistance of the teeth to dental caries. In general terms they can be classified as follows.
1. Anatomic factors, particularly the size and shape of the teeth, the depth of their grooves, fissures, and pits, and the dental arches' alignment
2. Chemical factors pertaining to the presence and anatomic distribution of certain elements

3. Structural factors, particularly the surface texture and internal arrangement
4. Crystallographic factors

**Anatomic factors**

The shape and size of a tooth, its alignment, and its particular type of surface texture determine to a certain degree the ability of the tooth to accumulate dental plaque and thus its resistance to dental caries. These three factors are themselves determined genetically but are also subjected to the influence of environmental variables, particularly nutrition.

The genetic template of tooth anatomy can be modified by nutritional manipulations during development, as shown by Paynter and Grainger,[30] and by Holloway and others.[31] However, none of the manifestations described has been unequivocally observed in humans; in fact, no evidence is available as to whether environmental factors can produce any significant change on the genetic makeup of human teeth.

**Chemical factors**

From the observation of Table 4-2, it is obvious that, as far as the most important components are concerned, there is no difference between carious enamel and sound enamel. There are, however, some interesting differences concerning the fluoride and carbonate content. Fluoride content is higher in carious enamel, possibly through a mechanism of concentration during reprecipitation; carbonate content is lower, probably through preferential (selective) solubility. However, sound enamel from sound teeth contains on the average more fluoride than sound enamel from carious teeth (Table 4-5).

It was mentioned previously that the surface enamel is almost intact in the early stages of dental caries formation. This represents a natural form of dental caries resistance, the study of which may offer clues for therapeutic caries prevention.

From a chemical viewpoint, surface enamel is more highly mineralized than subsurface enamel. It also contains more fluoride, phosphate, and organic substance, but less carbonate and water. To a certain degree the increased resistance to decay is attributed to these differences. Increased mineral and fluoride content increases enamel resistance, but the opposite is true for carbonate.

The contribution of fluoride to caries resistance is perhaps the most important single factor in this context and will therefore be discussed in greater detail.

**The reactions of enamel with fluoride.** It is universally accepted that, when fluoride is provided to humans or animals during periods of tooth formation, the

Table 4-5. *Enamel fluoride and dental caries experience*

| Fluoride in sound enamel | (p.p.m.) |
|---|---|
| Teeth from area of low dental caries experience* | 445 |
| Teeth from area of high dental caries experience* | 153 |
| Teeth from Aurora, Illinois; fluoride level of drinking water = 1.2 p.p.m.† | 133 |
| Teeth from control area; fluoride-free water† | 102 |

*Data from Ockerse, T.: The chemical composition of enamel and dentin in high and low caries areas in Africa, J. Dent. Res. 22:441, 1943.
†Data from McClure, F. J., and Likins, R. C.: Fluorine in human teeth studied in relation to fluorine in the drinking water, J. Dent. Res. 30:172, 1951.

precipitating apatites are partially fluoride-substituted. This is indicated from x-ray crystallography by a contraction of the a-axis dimension. The cariostatic effect of fluoridation of water supplies is attributed chiefly to this type of reaction. The fact that the surface layer of already calcified but unerupted teeth contains more fluoride than any other portion of the enamel points to a second pathway for fluoride incorporation into the apatite lattice, namely, ionic substitution of fluoride for hydroxyl ions. The fluoride must be derived (in this situation) from the tissue fluids bathing the teeth prior to eruption, that is, a very dilute fluoride solution. Chemically this reaction can be represented as follows

$$\underset{\text{Hydroxyapatite}}{Ca_{10}(PO_4)_6(OH)_2} + \underset{\text{Diluted fluoride}}{2F^-} \longrightarrow \underset{\text{Fluor-hydroxyapatite}}{Ca_{10}(PO_4)_6(OH)_{2-x}F_x}$$

where $x \leq 2$.

When the teeth have erupted, the application of a concentrated solution of fluoride—for example, sodium fluoride, potassium fluoride, or sodium fluosilicate—to the surface of the teeth the reaction, as observed by electron microscopy, electron diffraction, or x-ray diffraction, is the formation of calcium fluoride at the expense of the calcium ions of the enamel apatite. This reaction has been shown to be pH-dependent: at neutral or near neutral pH there is practically no observable reaction, while at pH 4.0 and below it proceeds rather rapidly, according to the following formula.

$$\underset{\text{Hydroxyapatite}}{Ca_{10}(PO_4)_6(OH)_2} + \underset{\substack{\text{Concentrated} \\ \text{fluoride}}}{20F\text{-}H^{+*}} \longrightarrow \underset{\substack{\text{Calcium} \\ \text{fluoride}}}{10\ CaF_2} + \underset{\substack{\text{Hydrogen} \\ \text{phosphate}}}{6HPO_4^=} + 2(OH)$$

This reaction occurs mainly on the surface of the enamel (or the enamel particles in experiments with powdered enamel) and is limited by the formation of the calcium fluoride precipitate.

Applications of stannous fluoride to the surface of the teeth and to powdered enamel have been shown to result in the formation of an amorphous precipitate on the surface of the enamel (or the enamel particles). The formation of this precipitate has been detected with electron diffraction and electron microscopy, but not with x-ray diffraction, thus indicating that the reaction is entirely superficial. It is generally accepted that the fluoride moiety of stannous fluoride reacts with enamel in much the same way as any other concentrated fluoride solution. The formation of the insoluble precipitate previously mentioned is, however, a limiting factor for the formation of calcium fluoride, and measurements of fluoride uptake by enamel after stannous fluoride topical treatment have consistently shown that tin reduces the amount of this uptake as compared, for example, to a sodium fluoride solution containing an equivalent amount of fluoride ions.

The reaction(s) of topical fluoride with enamel is greatly influenced by the crystallographic and chemical structural characteristics of the tissue. Enamel is composed of apatite crystals that have been shown by electron microscopy to be ribbon-

---

*It has been shown that this reaction may proceed also when an alkaline pH is present, provided that a mechanism for the release of calcium ions from the enamel is furnished to the system.

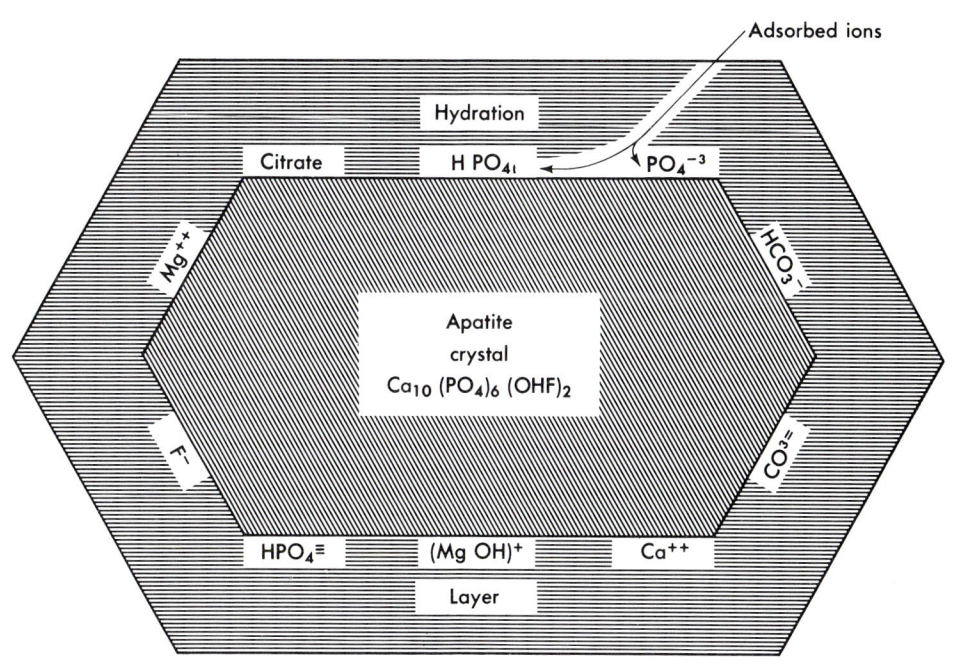

Fig. 4-3. Idealized view of the apatite crystal with its surrounding hydration layer and adsorbed ions.

shaped hexagonal prisms measuring, on the average, 3,000 to 5,000 Å in length (range 250 to 10,000 Å), and 500 Å in width (range from 400 to 1,200 Å). These crystals therefore have a rather large surface area, and there is evidence that electrical asymmetry on the crystal surface (which arises from the dissimilarity of the environment of internal and superficial atoms) sets up a powerful electric field, which pulls charged particles such as $Ca^{2+}$, $HPO_4^=$, $HCO_3^-$, $F^-$, $Mg^{2+}$, $CO_3^=$, citrate, and others and polarized water molecules toward the crystal surface. The apatite crystal can thus be visualized as a prism surrounded by a layer of absorbed ions and water, this last being called by most authors the hydration layer (Fig. 4-3).

The reaction(s) of enamel with elements or ions contained in solutions bathing the tissue can therefore involve: (1) the hydration layer; (2) the crystal surface; and (3) the interior of the crystal. Isotope studies suggest that, at least to a degree, this is the pattern with topical fluoride treatment. The reaction of enamel with fluoride solutions containing 100 μg or more of fluoride ions per milliliter can be visualized as follows. (1) Fluoride reacts with calcium ions removed (by hydrogen ions or any other mechanism) from the apatite lattice or dissolved in the hydration layer; calcium fluoride formed as a result of this reaction will deposit on the surface of the enamel crystals, from where most will be washed away shortly. (2) Some fluoride, from the treatment solution or from the calcium fluoride formed according to the process just described, will diffuse through the hydration layer to the surface of the crystals and eventually to their interior, forming a low concentration solution (less than 100 μg/ml.), and substituting them for hydroxyl ions. (3) Fluoride displaces carbonate (or bicarbonate) ions absorbed on the surface of the crystals.

From a mechanistical point of view the first and third processes are said to increase the resistance of enamel to acid dissolution because calcium carbonate is more soluble and calcium fluoride is less soluble than apatite. As far as the second process is concerned, there is no conclusive evidence in the literature of its occurrence as a result of a conventional topical fluoride treatment.

On the basis of the evidence reviewed so far, it would seem that the cariostatic ability of topical fluoride depends chiefly on the formation of calcium fluoride, and that of tin (II) on the formation of an insoluble layer of (probably) tin phosphate. The presence of fluoride, however, seems to be required in order to obtain cariostasis from tin, as tin (II) furnished to the enamel by compounds other than stannous fluoride has been shown to be effective to reduce the solubility rate of enamel against acetic acid, for instance, but not effective to reduce clinical dental caries.

Brudevold and his associates[32, 33] have postulated, however, that the anticaries efficacy of topical fluoride treatments depends mostly, if not exclusively, on the formation of fluorapatite, or, to be more accurate, on the substitution of fluoride for hydroxyl ions in the apatite lattice. Considering the basic chemical reactions concerning the interaction between enamel and fluoride, namely

$$Ca_{10}(PO_4)_6(OH)_2 + 2F^- \rightleftharpoons Ca_{10}(PO_4)_6 F_2 + 2(OH)^- \quad (1)$$
$$Ca_{10}(PO_4)_6(OH)_2 + 20F^- \rightleftharpoons 10\ CaF_2 + 6\ HPO_4^= + 2(OH)^- \quad (2)$$

and the reaction representing acid enamel dissolution,

$$Ca_{10}(PO_4)_6(OH)_2 + H^+ \rightleftharpoons Ca^{+2} + HPO^- + H_2O \quad (3)$$

they propose that there are two mechanisms to increase the rate of reaction (1), namely, increasing the concentration of fluoride, which in fact will displace the reaction toward reaction (2) and/or decreasing the pH, which in fact will promote reaction (3).

Observing that in both (2) and (3) one of the reaction products is phosphate, Brudevold and associates infer, applying the principal of LeChatelier, that the addition of phosphate to the reactants will displace the equilibrium in reactions (2) and (3) to the left, so that the treatment of enamel with rather concentrated fluoride solutions, at low pH levels, with the addition of phosphate, will result in fluoride substitution as indicated in reaction (1).

In testing this hypothesis, Brudevold and associates reported a substantial uptake of fluoride by enamel after what they called the acid phosphate-fluoride topical treatment, and, being unable to detect calcium fluoride formation, concluded that the fluoride taken up by the enamel had actually substituted for hydroxyl ions within the apatite lattice. This statement, based on negative inference, did not stand the proof of careful x-ray diffraction[34] and chemical studies,[35] which revealed the formation of calcium fluoride after acid phosphate-fluoride topical treatment. This outcome had been predicted by Brown and Wallace[36] on the basis of phase rule considerations.

Attempts to determine fluoride substitution reactions occurring after topical treatment by x-ray diffraction techniques, on the basis of the detection of fluorapatite formation, have consistently failed because in all probability no fluorapatite has been formed, but at best a solid solution of more or less fluoride-substituted hydroxyapatite. Even assuming that a small percentage of the hydroxyapatite crystals would have been transformed completely into fluorapatite, the similarity of the x-ray diffraction patterns of these two products is so marked that the detection of the reaction would have been impossible.

In a paper recently published, Frazier and associates[34] reported a contraction of the a-axis of powdered enamel treated for 62 hours with acid phosphate-fluoride, thus indicating incorporation of fluoride into the crystal lattice under *those experimental conditions*. No report has been published so far demonstrating conclusively the substitution of fluoride for hydroxyl ions in enamel apatite as a result of in vivo topical application of acid phosphate fluoride (or by any other topical treatment as well).

Concerning the mechanism of action of fluoride, theories have been proposed which claim that fluoride: (a) decreases oral bacteria growth, or acid formation; or (b) increases the resistance of the teeth to acid dissolution (intrinsic, dental effect).

The understanding of the true, intimate mechanism of fluoride uptake by enamel has academic as well as practical implications, if one wishes to attain the maximum protective results from a fluoride compound. Many authors claim that fluoride incorporated into the apatite lattice decreases the solubility of the enamel against acids. If this is actually the case, our efforts should be directed toward increasing the rate of the substitution reaction as much as possible. Among other things, this may require that the topical system provide energy in order to obtain the decrease in the enamel entropy which, according to modern ideas, characterizes the fluoride-substituted apatites.

Other studies affirm that the solubilities of both substituted and unsubstituted apatites, measured in terms of the amount dissolved at equilibrium in a given acid, are about the same, but that the presence of fluoride in the medium favors the reprecipitation of the dissolving or recently dissolved apatites. In this case the amount of apatite dissolved as a function of time, that is, the solubility rate, represented by the total amount of enamel dissolved minus the amount reprecipitated, at a given time will be less when fluoride is present in the medium than when it is not present. Inasmuch as fluoride-substituted apatites release fluoride to the medium when dissolving, they will decrease the solubility rate of the enamel of which they are a part. It is important to recognize, however, that what is required is the presence of fluoride in the medium, and not necessarily its presence in the crystal lattice. Fluoride present in the hydration layer, or absorbed on the surface of the crystal, or in any other enamel site (organic matrix?), from where it may gain access to the dissolving medium, will probably be as effective as fluoride incorporated into the crystals.

It is therefore obvious that both types of mechanisms depend on the amount of fluoride taken up by the enamel; and it is accepted that, other factors being equal, the resistance of dental enamel to acid dissolution increases with the increase of the fluoride of the enamel.

**Other chemical factors.** The situation with carbonate is opposite to that with fluoride. Since (calcium) carbonate is more soluble than (calcium) phosphate, then the less carbon dioxide present the more resistant the enamel would be. The lower concentration of carbonate in surface enamel is attributed to the selective (preferential) dissolution of carbon dioxide in weak mouth acids.

Some authors have postulated that there is a negative correlation between fluoride and carbonate concentration in hard tissues. While this has been proved in bone tissue, the situation is still controversial as far as enamel is concerned. In animal experiments Sobel[37] showed that the ingestion of a diet with (excessively) high phosphate-to-calcium ratio resulted in low carbonate content in the teeth and low caries experience in comparison to control animals. Conversely, a high calcium-to-phosphate ratio resulted in high enamel carbonate and high caries experience.

In addition to the concentration of minerals, surface enamel has also a higher concentration of organic substance (nonammoniacal nitrogen), probably derived from the saliva. The surface of enamel is covered by the so-called primary cuticle and on top of it, or on top of the enamel itself when the primary pellicle is worn out, by a second organic film, the so-called secondary pellicle or cuticle, which is probably formed by precipitated and denatured salivary proteins. The presence of this pellicle and the presence of salivary protein impregnating surface enamel are believed to play a role in caries resistance; these organic structures, while permeable to the hydrogen ions, do protect the enamel crystals against direct attack from the acid. Thus acid will progress below the surface, following organic pathways (striae of Retzius, lamellae) until it reaches enamel that: (a) is more susceptible on grounds of chemical composition (particularly less fluoride content); and (b) is less protected (not covered by the organic film described above).

In vitro dental caries tests have shown the need for a polymeric surface coating in order to produce white spot–like lesions.

Evidence has been accumulating which suggests that trace element imbalance plays a role in dental caries formation. Specific examples refer to differences in caries experience associated with geographic or geologic factors, which in turn can be traced to excess or deficiency of trace elements, as in Napier-Hastings (New Zealand), two populations with similar ethnic, socioeconomic, social and climatic characteristics but different molybdenum content in their soils and vegetables. Epidemiologic surveys indicate a greater caries experience in association with low molybdenum concentration and lesser caries experience with high molybdenum concentration.

Suggestions have been made that a trace amount of manganese in the water supply (approximately 0.3 p.p.m.) enhances the cariostatic effect of fluoride. On the other hand, it has been suggested that traces of selenium are conducive to higher caries susceptibility.

At present there is no clear picture of the type and direction of the relationship between most trace elements and dental caries, nor is there a clear understanding of the potential mechanisms involved.

**Crystallographic factors**

Since the enamel minerals, which are by weight close to 97 percent of mature enamel, are in a crystalline state, the possibility that the crystallographic characteristics of enamel play a role in caries initiation is worthy of consideration. Very little research, however, has been conducted in this connection.

In a study performed with enamel from a carious deciduous molar and a sound deciduous molar from the same child, it was found that the distances between the component atoms were smaller in the sound tooth than those in the affected tooth. This closer atomic packing has been interpreted as indicating a higher lattice energy content, and thus a greater resistance to breakdown in the sound tooth than in the carious tooth.

The very close atomic packing in enamel crystals is one of the reasons that so little fluoride reacts with intact enamel. In order to overcome this problem, experimental work is being conducted on how to "condition" the enamel surface in order to facilitate uptake of fluoride (and other ions).

The incorporation of fluoride into bone mineral improves the crystallinity of the tissue; that is, it produces larger, more regular apatite crystals (thus reducing their specific surface). The same has been proposed, though not proved, for enamel. Crystallographically, fluorapatite is almost identical to hydroxyapatite, so that it is very difficult to distinguish them from one another. With the small percentage of fluoride substitution usually found in enamel, the distinction is almost impossible.

**Structural factors**

According to Muhlemann,[38] "the morphogenesis, histodifferentiation, the appositional formation of enamel and dentin matrices and their consecutive mineralization are biological processes in need of nutritive energy, specific molecular tissue constituents and catalysts. Disturbances in energy transfer and deviations in the supply of nutrients during these stages of development may have repercussions on tooth morphology (size of the teeth), tissular topography (width and depth of occlusal fissures and pits), microscopic and molecular structure (surface texture of enamel, enamel prism harmony, apatite crystallinity), and chemical composition (organic, mineral and trace element content) of bone, enamel and dentin. In the case of teeth, disturbances during the development of the dental organ are unique since they are practically irreversible. Enamel can not be rebuilt like bone." It would appear, then, that nutritional conditions, which control the structural development of the teeth, should be of prime importance in determining their susceptibility or resistance to dental caries. There is no evidence, however, that differences in the structure of enamel produced by nutritional deficiencies increase or modify in any way the inherent susceptibility of the teeth to decay. In fact, teeth formed under extremely poor nutritional conditions have repeatedly been found to be exceptionally free of caries.

Several authors, including Lady Mellanby,[39] have reported, however, a greater incidence of caries in hypoplastic teeth. They attributed this effect to faulty enamel resulting from nutritional deficiencies, particularly vitamin D deficiency. Hypoplasia, however, results in rough tooth surfaces, which in turn favor the accumulation of plaque and food residues and thus caries attack. This effect is connected to the tooth environment rather than to the teeth themselves.

There is much evidence in man which suggests that the duration of food contact with the tooth surface is more important in caries causation than any nutritional factor operating during tooth formation or afterward.

## CONCLUSION

In the etiologic consideration of dental caries two types of factors must be considered: (a) those affecting the teeth themselves; and (b) those operating in the tooth environment.

Dental caries starts (in most instances) on the enamel surface; therefore this chapter presented modern concepts concerning the chemistry, crystallography, and structure of enamel and their relationships with dental caries. After explaining the mechanisms and theories of dental caries formation, the basic concepts referent to the reactions of fluoride with enamel were presented, along with other potential mechanisms for caries prevention.

On the basis of present knowledge it is possible to state that environmental factors play a bigger role in caries etiology and perhaps offer better hope of being controlled than factors related directly to the teeth.

**REFERENCES**

1. Hatchett, G.: Experiments and observations on shell and bone, Royal Soc. (London) Philosophical Transactions **89:**315, 1799.
2. Bassett, H.: The phosphates of calcium, IV, the basic phosphates, J. Biol. Chem. **11:**620, 1917.
3. Gassman, T. H.: Uber die kunstliche Darstellung des Haptbestandteiles der Knochen und der Zahne, Hoppe Seyler Z. Physiol. Chem. **178:**62, 1928.
4. Gross, R.: Die Kristalline Struktur von Dentin und Zahnschmeltz, Berlin, 1926, Festscr. Zahnaerztl. Inst. Univ. Greiswald.
5. De Jong, W. F.: La substance minerale dans les os, Rec. Trav. Chimiques Pays-bas **45:**445, 1926.
6. Mehmel, M.: The structure of apatite, Z. Krist. **75:**323, 1930.
7. Naray-Szabo, S.: Structure of fluorapatite, Z. Krist. **75:**387, 1930.
8. Gruner, J. W., McConnell, D., and Armstrong, W. D.: The relationships between crystal structure and chemical composition of enamel and dentin, J. Biol. Chem. **121:**771, 1939.
9. Klement, R.: Basiche zweiwertiger metalle, II, Bleihydroxylapatit, Z. Anorg. Allg. Chem **237:**161, 1938.
10. Lagergren, C., and Carlstrom, D.: Crystallographic studies of calcium and strontium hydroxyapatites, Acta Chem. Scan. **11:**545, 1957.
11. McDonald, N. S., Ezmirlian, F., Spain, P., and McArthur, C.: The ultimate site of skeletal deposition of strontium and lead, J. Biol. Chem. **189:**387, 1951.
12. McConnell, D.: The crystal chemistry of Frncolite and its relationship to calcified animal tissues. In: Metabolic interrelations (Trans. 4th Conference), New York, 1952, Josiah Macy Jr. Foundation.
13. Klement, R., and Hasselbach, H.: Uber Phosphate und Arsenate des zweiwertigen Zinns, Chem. Ber. **96:**1022, 1963.
14. McConnell, D., and Foreman, D. W.: The properties and structure of $Ca_{10}(PO_4)_6(OH)_2$; its relation to tin (II) apatite, Can. Miner **8:**431, 1966.
15. Trautz, O. R.: The use of x-ray diffraction in dental research, Ann. Dent. **12:**47, 1953.
16. Kay, M. I., Young, R. A., and Posner, A. S: Crystal structure of hydroxyapatite, Nature (London) **204:**1050, 1964.
17. Baud, C. A.: Etude biocristallographique des remaniements de la substance minerale osseuse in rapport avec son enrichissement en fluor, Compt. Rend. Soc. Biol. **150:**103, 1956.
18. Baud, C. A., and Slatkine, S.: Etude par diffraction des rayons x de la fixation in vivo du fluor dans la substance minerale des os, Advances Fluorine Res. **2:**107, 1964.
19. Baud, C. A., and Buchs, M.: Etude par des diffraction des rayons x de la substance minerale de l'os et de l'email dentaire. In: Stack, M. V., and Fearnhead, R. W., editors: Tooth enamel, Bristol, 1965, Wright.
20. Miller, W. D.: Microorganisms of the human mouth, Philadelphia, 1890, S. S. White.
21. Gottlieb, B.: Dental caries, Philadelphia, 1947, Lea & Febiger.
22. Pincus, P.: New hypothesis of dental caries, J. Canad. Dent. Assn. **26:**16, 1950.
23. Frisbie, H. H., and Nuckolls, J.: Caries of the enamel, J. Dent Res. **26:**181, 1947.
24. Martin, J. J., and others: Chelation or metal binding as a new approach to the problem of dental caries, Euclides (Madrid) **14:**311, 1954.
25. Schatz, A., and others: Some philosophical considerations on the proteolysis-chelation therapy of dental caries, Proc. Penn. Acad. Sci. **32:**20, 1958.
26. Schatz, A., and Martin, J. J.: Proteolysis-chelation theory of dental caries, J.A.D.A. **65:**368, 1962.
27. Leimgruber, C. H.: Le mechanism de la carie dentaire, Rev. Mens. Suisse. Odont. **66:**934, 1956.
28. Csernyei, J.: Dental caries—a biochemical process, New York D. J. **16:**241, 1950.

29. Neumann, H. H., and Di Salvo, N. A.: Does functional effort affect caries? J. Dent. Child. **22**:151, 1955.
30. Paynter, K. J., and Grainger, R. M.: Relation of nutrition to the morphology and size of rat molar teeth, J. Canad. Dent. Assn. **22**:519, 1956.
31. Holloway, P. J., Shaw, J. H., and Sweeney, E. A.: Nutritional influence on tooth size and morphology, J. Dent. Res. **39**:1108, 1960.
32. Brudevold, F: A study of acidulated fluoride solutions, I, in vitro effects on enamel, Arch. Oral Biol. **8**:167, 1963.
33. Wellock, W. D., and Brudevold, F.: A study of acidulated fluoride solutions, II, the caries inhibiting effect of single annual topical applications of an acidic fluoride and phosphate solution; a two year experience, Arch. Oral Biol. **8**:179, 1963.
34. Frazier, P. D., and Engen, D. W.: X-ray diffraction study of the reaction of acidulated fluoride with powdered enamel, J. Dent. Res. **45**:1144, 1966.
35. De Shazer, D. O., and Swartz, C. J.: The formation of calcium fluoride on the surface of hydroxyapatite after treatment with acidic phosphate-fluoride solutions, Arch. Oral Biol. **12**:1071, 1967.
36. Brown, W. E., and Wallace, B. M.: Phase rule considerations and the solubility of tooth enamel, Ann. N. Y. Acad. Sci. **131**:690, 1965.
37. Sobel, A. E., Shaw, J. H., Hanok, A., and Nobel, S.: Caries susceptibility in relation to composition of teeth and diet, J. Dent. Res. **39**:462, 1960.
38. Muhlemann, H. R.: Nutrition, tooth formation and caries susceptibility. In: Blix, G. M., editor: Nutrition and caries prevention, Symposium of the Swedish Nutrition, Uppsala, 1965, Almqvist & Wiksell.
39. Mellanby, M.: The effect of diet on the structure of teeth, Brit. D. J. **44**:1031, 1923.

# Chapter 5 Control of rampant dental caries

Russell W. Sumnicht

General discussion
    Definition, characteristics, and prevalence
    Cause
    Process
Control
    Considerations
    Treatment planning
    Individual control measures
        Initial caries removal
        Topical fluoride applications
        Patient counselling
        Dietary control
        Oral hygiene
        Caries activity tests
        Restorative procedures
        Recall
    Other factors
        Salivary factors
        Psychologic factors
        Systemic factors
        Familial factors
Conclusion

Dental caries, whether manifested by a single slowly developing lesion or by rapid destruction of multiple tooth surfaces, is initiated and sustained by acid demineralization of the inorganic content of susceptible tooth structure. The acids are formed as the result of bacterial enzyme fermentation of food debris under conditions conducive to such activity within the oral cavity. As with any disease, control of dental caries of any degree of severity is best achieved by eliminating the cause and establishing or reestablishing normal control mechanisms. Because of the fulminating nature of the disease, the control of rampant caries calls for a comprehensive effort and for special considerations relative to the timing, sequence, and extent of care.

## GENERAL DISCUSSION

**Definition, characteristics, and prevalence.** Massler defines rampant dental caries as "a suddenly appearing, widespread, rapidly burrowing type of caries resulting in early involvement of the pulp and affecting those teeth or dental surfaces usually regarded as immune to ordinary decay."[1]

In addition to rapidity of onset and progress and to indiscriminate involvement of tooth surfaces, rampant caries is characterized by lesions having very soft consistency and a light yellow or tan color. Because of the rapid rate of progress of these lesions, there is no time for dental pulps to form secondary dentin and therefore they are readily invaded. These developments, plus extensive involvement of lower anterior teeth and of lingual and cervical surfaces, indicate a serious breakdown of normal protective mechanisms.

Rampant dental caries can occur at any age but is found most commonly among children and young adults. Massler described it as affecting 5 to 8 percent of the population and as having a particularly high incidence among children between 4 and 8 years of age "ravishing the primary dentition," and among children and young adults between 11 and 19 years of age "in whom it mutilates the newly acquired dentition." There has been no significant change in these rates other than in areas where controlled fluoridation of water supplies has since been introduced and where substantial decreases in incidence of rampant caries can therefore be expected.[2]

Rampant caries has also been shown to be strongly influenced by familial factors. Klein[2-4] has reported extensive studies which indicate that children of caries-susceptible parents (particularly when both parents are caries susceptible) tend to have substantially more caries than do children of caries-immune parents and that siblings of caries-susceptible children tend to have substantially more than do siblings of caries-immune children. All authorities do not agree, but these tendencies are thought to be influenced more by diet, eating habits, oral hygiene practices, and other intra-family environmental factors than they are by heredity.[5]

**Cause.** It is generally accepted that acidogenic organisms, fermentable substrate (food or food debris), and tooth structure susceptible to dissolution by acids must be present in a mouth before teeth will decay. Dental plaque and saliva also play essential roles.

Classic studies by Orland and associates[6] and by Fitzgerald[7] show that teeth will not decay in the absence of bacterial organisms. Animals raised in germ-free conditions will not develop caries even though fed highly cariogenic diets. These animals and other caries-immune animals, when inoculated with organisms from caries-active animals and fed cariogenic diets, become caries-active. A number of investigators[8] have demonstrated the presence of acidogenic organisms at the forefront of carious lesions. A number of strains of streptococci have been shown to have etiologic roles in experimental animal caries.[9] In the presence of a caries-inducing diet, notably one containing high levels of sucrose, these organisms apparently induce plaque formation. The evidence suggests that cariogenic streptococci convert portions of sucrose to the polysaccharide dextran, a gummy and relatively inert and insoluble constituent of plaque. It causes plaque to adhere tightly to tooth structure and serves as a barrier to saliva and other outside influences that might otherwise interfere with intraplaque processes involved in dental caries.

Streptococci and sucrose have been similarly implicated as probable etiologic agents in dental caries in man. Streptococci isolated from plaque of patients with active caries have also been found to be geographically widespread in human populations, with prevalence of organisms tending to vary with prevalence of DMF teeth.[10]

The role of readily fermentable foods such as sucrose in active caries has been demonstrated by many investigators.[11, 12] The caries-reducing effectiveness of diets based on controlling consumption of carbohydrates has been well established.[13-15] Studies relating to the relationship between caries incidence and ingestion of sugar-containing foods leave little doubt that frequency of ingestion and the degree to which the foods adhere to tooth surfaces are critical factors. Stephan and Geis, in reporting a study on sixty cases of rampant caries, conclude that "frequent eating of carbohydrate foods and sweets between meals was the most common single factor associated with the development of rampant caries."[16] (See pp. 82-83.) There are a number of reports[17, 18] of destructive caries in young children associated with prolonged habitual use of nursing bottles, a condition that affords long and frequent exposure of teeth to milk sugars and often to added sweeteners as well. (See discussion of effect on malocclusions, p. 235.)

The vast evidence of protection against caries afforded by community fluoridated water and topically applied fluorides attests to the influence of tooth susceptibility on the carious process.

Bacterial plaque is believed to strongly influence caries activity by providing a means by which bacterial colonies live and function relatively undisturbed in intimate contact with tooth surfaces. Plaque consists largely of viable and nonviable bacteria mixed with mucin and possibly food debris and other materials and is found closely adherent to tooth surfaces in areas that are not easily reached for cleaning and where caries commonly occurs. The hydrogen ion concentration of inner layers of plaque substance in contact with the tooth surface has been demonstrated to fall to levels capable of demineralizing tooth structure within minutes following ingestion of fermentable carbohydrates.[19, 20]

Saliva has been described as the first line of defense against dental caries. Studies relative to the role played by saliva are concerned with its acid-buffering properties, chemical composition, possible antibacterial properties, rate of flow, and viscosity. High caries activity has definitely been shown to be associated with xerostomia.

**Process.** Any food, if retained in contact with tooth structure long enough, can be decomposed and can lead to caries production. However, most foods are cleared from the mouth before this degree of decomposition can take place. Dentistry's particular concern with sucrose and certain other carbohydrates is that breakdown and the formation of acids with resultant demineralization of susceptible tooth structure begin almost immediately with exposure of such foods to the action of acidogenic bacterial enzymes.

As has been mentioned, ingestion of cariogenic foods is accompanied by a lowering of the hydrogen ion concentration (pH) in the depths of dental plaque material. When the pH drops to 5.2 or lower, demineralization of susceptible tooth structure takes place. The frequency of such episodes depends on the frequency with which cariogenic foods are eaten, and the duration of activity depends on the rate at which the foods are cleared from the mouth. Thus unless the teeth are kept free of plaque or unless the food is removed as quickly as possible after eating frequent ingestion of cariogenic foods, particularly those that are not readily cleared from the mouth, is considered one of the most significant causative factors in high caries rates.

## CONTROL

**Considerations.** An essential step in the management of any disease is elimination or control of the cause. If caries activity depends on the simultaneous presence of appropriate bacterial organisms, fermentable substrate, and susceptible tooth structure, it appears logical that elimination or control of the cause of dental caries can be achieved by eliminating or controlling any one (preferably all) of these factors. Experience has shown that caries control can be achieved through dietary control or by increasing the caries resistance of tooth enamel through the use of fluorides. Evidence that caries incidence can be significantly lowered by means of oral hygiene or other mechanical means designed to reduce oral bacterial concentrations is meager. However, because of the implication of bacterial plaque in the caries process and because of the effects of food retention on prolonging this process, excellent oral hygiene practices are essential to a caries control program. It may be that the small volume of demonstrated success with oral hygiene as a means of inhibiting caries activity is the result of inadequate attention to oral hygiene instruction and to the effectitveness of measures used. Furthermore, proper oral hygiene practices are necessary for maintaining the health of periodontal tissues and thus are essential for comprehensive oral health care.

Oral health care should always be based on thorough examinations and sound treatment planning. In cases of lesser degrees of caries activity time is often not a critical factor—appointments may be arranged to suit the convenience of both doctor and patient and the sequence of procedures to be performed often is not an important determinant in the retention or loss of teeth. Furthermore, in many cases very little adjustment in self-care measures is necessary to establish effective caries control.

In cases of rampant caries, however, destruction progresses at such a pace that immediate attention and priority of attention to certain procedures are essential to minimize the destructive effects. An assumption should be made that there is a serious failure of all control mechanisms and that comprehensive efforts to restore them will be necessary. Early and frequent recall is needed to intercept the lesions of any continued caries activity and to make sure that the patient's home care is adequate. Of all measures, the importance of patient and parent cooperation to assure effective home care cannot be overstressed.

**Treatment planning.** Examination of the patient with rampant caries requires, among other procedures, obtaining radiographs adequate to determining the extent of tooth destruction, caries susceptibility tests as a basis for evaluating the effectiveness of subsequent corrective and control measures, determination of any use of drugs that may contribute to the condition, initiation of a diet record, and a physical examination to identify possible systemic etiologic factors.

Planning of care logically dictates giving priority consideration to those conditions causing pain or threatening imminent loss of teeth. If possible, this should be performed at the first appointment, even at the expense of completing the initial examination. Actively carious material should be removed from such teeth, and from as many other teeth as time will permit, with sufficient depth and extension of cavity preparations to permit placement and retention of sedative dressings.

Other measures to be given attention at the same or immediately succeeding appointments are removal and replacement with zinc oxide–eugenol cement of carious material in any remaining lesions, prophylaxis with the stannous fluoride–lava pumice, or zirconium silicate prophylaxis paste,[21] followed by topical application of a 10 percent stannous fluoride solution, and counselling of parents and patients with the objectives of establishing a caries-controlling diet and effective oral hygiene practices. Placement of permanent restorations and surgical procedures for other than emergency conditions are undertaken as early as possible, following initiation or accomplishment of the foregoing.

### Individual control measures

**Initial caries removal.** Removal of carious tooth material and replacement with zinc oxide–eugenol cement disrupts the caries process, protects the pulps of still vital teeth, and provides comfort for patients with early pulp involvement. In addition, ridding the mouth of all evidence of active caries is accompanied by a reduction in the oral *Lactobacillus* count, altering conditions in the mouth in such a way that involvement of additional tooth surfaces may be less likely to occur.[22]

All or most of the caries removal procedures can often be performed with the careful use of sharp chisels and excavators. Excavation of surface and soft material should be accomplished with sufficient extension and depth to retain the restorative material and assure isolation of the carious lesion. Care is taken to avoid exposure of vital dental pulps. A calcium hydroxide preparation is recommended for pulp capping. Use of crown forms or of orthodontic bands is often helpful in retaining the restorative cement on badly broken-down teeth.

**Topical fluoride applications.** Experience with the caries-inhibiting effects of topically applied fluoride preparations indicates such care to be of sufficient potential benefit to recommend their use as soon as practicable, following measures for the relief of pain and for the prevention of imminent loss of teeth.

A number of promising fluoride compounds and technics for applying fluorides to the teeth are under investigation. At the present time the procedure of choice in efforts to control rampant caries is the "triple" or "three-agent" approach in which a prophylaxis, using a prophylaxis paste containing stannous fluoride along with a fluoride-compatible polishing agent, is followed by a topical application of a 10 percent solution of stannous fluoride and home use of a stannous fluoride dentifrice. Such combined use of stannous fluoride preparations has been reported[23-29] as resulting in significant reductions in dental caries among both adults and children and as being effective in areas of both optimal and deficient levels of water fluoride.

**Patient counselling.** No measure is more important to the success of efforts to control rampant caries than the care a patient provides for himself. In essentially every case of rampant caries, effective home care requires a marked adjustment in diet and eating habits and the initiation or revision of oral hygiene practices. Very often the patient's condition has been complicated by a lack of knowledge of, or interest in, measures important to the preservation of oral health. Patient counselling must therefore not only provide the patient, and parents of the child patient, with instructions for home care, but it must also be planned and given in such a way as to motivate him (them) to desired action. The nature of the results appears to be determined largely by the placement of emphasis, with the extent of the effects determined by the quality, sincerity, and intensity of the effort. The importance of including parents in counselling of child patients cannot be overstressed. In discussing counselling, any use of the word *patient* should be read as including the words *and parent or parents* when the patient is a child.

The patient cannot be expected to make the difficult changes necessary to control his disease unless he realizes that failure to achieve control can have consequences of serious personal concern to him and that the disease and its effects can be intercepted or minimized through faithful observance of these changes.[31] Patient realization of these facts should be primary motivational objectives of counselling. Success will depend in large measure on the attention and preparation the dentist gives to this important aspect of oral health care.

**Dietary control.** The role of food in general, but of fermentable carbohydrates in particular, as a causative factor in rampant dental caries and the importance of establishing a corrective diet have been discussed. Diet evaluation and adjustment are essential to the successful control of the disease. A number of investigators[13-15] have reported reductions in caries activity as measured by caries activity tests, following abstinence from the eating of fermentable carbohydrates. Becks and associates reported restriction of carbohydrates as resulting in marked reductions of caries in 88.4 percent of a series of 655 cases of rampant caries and as causing complete elimination of caries activity in 62.3 percent of another series of 790 rampant caries cases.[13]

Diet-correcting measures should be initiated along with other interceptive procedures early[15] in the course of treatment. The procedures for performing such evaluations and the technics are described on p. 49.

The patient's diet record, his diet history, and, when available, the results of the salivary analysis are used as the basis for counselling the patient in home-care measures. This and subsequent salivary analyses are also used to evaluate the progress of the restriction of dietary carbohydrates.

When dietary requirements have been determined from an evaluation of the patient's diet record and diet history, they are discussed with the patient in such a way as to impress him with the importance to his future health of carefully following recommended changes. It is not easy to discontinue well-established dietary and eating habits abruptly; so much depends on the understanding and incentive imparted to the patient.

There are available a number of carefully developed dietary programs for control of caries,[14, 15] listing varieties and combinations of foods. Primary objectives of these programs include the restriction of fermentable carbohydrates,[14] the discontinuance of between-meal eating, and the assurance of adequate nutrition to meet daily recommendation of the Food and Nutrition Board of the National Academy of Sciences, National Research Council. (See p. 33.)

**Oral hygiene.** The role of bacterial plaque in providing foci for relatively undisturbed breakdown of fermentable foods to form acids on tooth surfaces and the rapidity with which fermentable foods are broken down following eating have been mentioned. Although evidence of reductions in dental caries attributable to maintenance of proper oral hygiene by the use of a toothbrush or other vehicle without a dentifrice is insufficient to be conclusive, deductive reasoning indicates that the teeth should be cleaned as soon as possible after eating and that instruction and motivation of the patient to good oral hygiene practices is an indispensable objective of patient counselling.[32]

Since the primary objective of brushing and related procedures is to clean the teeth, any method that will effectively reach and clean caries-susceptible areas is preferable. A technic in which disclosing materials are used enables the patient to evaluate the effectiveness of his efforts and to adjust his technics to reach areas that he has been missing. Use of disclosing materials is also helpful in pointing out to the patient inadequacies of measures he has been using, thus serving as an incentive for improvement. Following is a technic, using disclosing wafers, for patient instruction (again, it is important that parents of child patients be involved in these and other counselling procedures).

1. Materials
    a. Articulated models of the dental arches and a brush to demonstrate procedures.
    b. Hand and mouth mirrors.

c. Disclosing wafers.
   d. A soft to medium-textured multitufted nylon toothbrush (small for children and some adults—medium for most adults).
   e. A small tube of the stannous fluoride–calcium pyrophosphate dentifrice.
   f. Adjunctive aids for selected cases.
2. Procedures (accomplished with the patient, and parents as appropriate, standing before a mirror and wash basin as he would at home).
   a. Have the patient brush his teeth and rinse his mouth, using his usual technic.
   b. Have the patient use a disclosing wafer to stain remaining plaque and debris. (Apply petrolatum to prevent staining of the lips; have the patient chew a disclosing wafer for 30 seconds, swishing thoroughly to reach interproximal areas; and, finally, have him rinse to remove excess stain. Rinsing into a paper cup will prevent staining the sink—wafers are harmless if swallowed.)
   c. Point out areas the patient has missed (using hand and mouth mirrors as needed) and discuss inadequacies noted in his technic.
   d. Using models or other appropriate aids, demonstrate a toothbrushing method that provides a basic stroke suitable to the patient's needs. Point out how adjustments can be made to reach difficult areas. Then direct the patient in the application of these procedures in his own mouth. Holding the patient's hand and guiding it in performance of the procedures is often helpful. Adjunctive aids (dental floss, tape, balsa wood devices, etc.) may contribute to better results in some cases. In such cases the use of aids should be included in instructions and in supervised application.
   e. Have the patient brush his teeth under supervision. The objective is the removal of stain from all tooth surfaces. When the patient is too young to perform these procedures satisfactorily, a parent should do them for him.
   f. Have the patient restain his teeth and again check the results. Point out where improvements can be made.
   g. When satisfied with patient progress, provide him with disclosing wafers, instruct him to practice at home, and inform him that progress will be *reevaluated at the next and at succeeding appointments.* (Most patients should be able to remove most stained material in a single brushing after 1 week of conscientious practice.)
   h. At such time as the patient has demonstrated sufficient competence in his oral hygiene procedures, instruct him to check his effectiveness with disclosing wafers on a weekly basis until the technics become a matter of habit and then occasionally thereafter. Some dentists provide or have their patients obtain low-cost plastic-handled mouth mirrors for use in checking oral hygiene effectiveness at home.

**Caries activity tests.** A number of tests have been developed to evaluate oral conditions commonly associated with caries activity.[34, 35] These have been discussed in detail on pp. 8-11. Caries activity test results may be affected by any of a number of conditions, including such factors as the manner in which the saliva was collected, time between collection and testing, temperature, and test procedures. For this reason care and consistency in procedures are important. Also, for this reason some authorities advocate double checking with multiple tests to establish at least the initial base-line data.

**Restorative procedures.** Permanent restorations should be placed as soon as possible after establishment of all indicated control measures.[32] In some instances when retention of an initial zinc oxide–eugenol restoration cannot be satisfactorily achieved, a permanent restoration must be placed earlier to protect the tooth and its pulp.

Once control measures have been established, nothing is more important to the preservation of caries-affected teeth than carefully performed restorative procedures. The principles of good restorative care are generally known and are amply described in readily available literature, so they will not be discussed further. Meticulous attention to cavity preparation, use of pulp capping and pulpotomy technics, careful selection and use of restorative materials (including the use of supplemental expedients, such as cast gold or chrome steel crowns, orthodontic bands, and steel pins), and the polishing of restorations are all important.

**Recall.** When planned control and restorative measures have been accomplished, arrangements are made to recall the patient in 3 months. At that time a follow-up examination and radiographs are made; a prearranged salivary specimen is obtained for testing; a stannous fluoride prophylaxis and stannous fluoride topical application are given; oral hygiene is evaluated, using disclosing materials; counselling is given as needed; the nature of the patient's diet and dietary habits are determined, coordinated with the results of the salivary test, and corrected as required; and necessary restorative procedures are performed. Subsequent recall is made at 3-month intervals until it is apparent that longer intervals will suffice.

### Other factors

There is occasional evidence that a salivary inadequacy, psychologic or emotional problems, or systemic conditions may be playing a causative role in rampant caries. There is also strong evidence that familial factors influence caries activity. These factors should be considered in planning care for patients with rampant caries.

**Salivary factors.** Bibby has stated that, "When there is a close balance between carious breakdown or resistance of the enamel surface, the action of saliva can determine the outcome."[36] As has been mentioned, salivary factors that have been related to caries activity include rate of flow, viscosity, acid buffering properties, chemical composition, and possible antibacterial properties.

The one conclusion which appears to be definite is that at least a minimal volume of saliva is essential to caries control. Any condition, either permanent or temporary, whether pathologic or experimentally induced, that interferes seriously with salivary flow is almost invariably accompanied by high caries activity.[37, 38] There is also evidence[37] to suggest a tendency for higher caries rates to be associated with lower rates of salivary secretion, even when flow rates are considered to be within normal limits. When a patient with rampant caries fails to respond satisfactorily to other control measures, inadequate salivary flow rates should be suspected. McDonald[37] recommends that the stimulated flow rate be determined in every case of rampant caries. In case of deficiency, an attempt should be made to discover or correct the cause. Pathology or the results of surgery or irradiation affecting the salivary glands or their secretory nerve supplies may be involved, or the deficiency may be associated with emotional disturbances, the use of antihistaminic or tranquilizer drugs, vitamin B complex deficiency, habitual mouth breathing, changes occurring following menopause, or some other systemic condition.

Pilocarpine hydrochloride therapy has been suggested as a means of stimulating salivary flow in cases of xerostomia in which glands and nerve pathways are still functional.[37] The Council on Dental Therapeutics of the American Dental Association cautions that, "Cholinergic drugs such as pilocarpine and neostigmine (Prostigmin) bromide may be tried and may be beneficial, but their undesirable effects on other systems generally contradict their use for promoting salivation."[39] The patient's physician should be consulted in planning therapy in cases of dry mouth which are or appear to be related to systemic factors or to drug intake.

Other salivary factors have been mentioned as contributing to the complex role of saliva in the caries process. McDonald[37] reports indications of a direct relationship between salivary viscosity and the DMF index at all ages. He describes the patient with thick ropy saliva as invariably having "a dirty mouth, teeth covered with stain or materia alba, and greater-than-average to rampant caries," and relates viscosity to the type of saliva stimulated and to its mucin content. A buffering capacity imparted by such salivary ingredients as phosphates is believed to have a strong inhibiting effect on caries. The concentration of phosphate and calcium ions is also considered important in preventing dissolution of enamel.[35] Normal saliva is saturated with these ions—undersaturation may result in enamel dissolution while supersaturation may lead to precipitation of these salivary ingredients. Another of the many other possible involvements of saliva in the caries process is the suggestion that it may have antibacterial properties. Each of the foregoing possibilities can help explain the role of saliva in relation to caries activity.

**Psychologic factors.** There is considerable evidence that emotional factors may play a role in rampant caries. Sutton[40, 41] indicates a high correlation between severe mental stress and acute forms of the disease. In a series of 661 dentulous patients, 25 years of age or older, 169 were identified as having acute caries. Of these 169, 96 percent were reported as admitting recent mental stress—in contrast with only 2 percent of the others admitting such stress. The survey indicated that stress associated with acute caries was of several months' duration prior to diagnosis of the acute condition. Common causes of the reported stress were illness, either of the patient or of another member of his family, business conditions, or financial worries. In another study of 678 subjects the onset of caries and the beginning of stress were reported as being separated by a period of considerably less than a month.

Schwabacher[42] relates rampant caries to such interpersonal factors as repressed emotions, rebellion, dissatisfaction, and feelings of inferiority. He suggests that such mental states may induce bad eating habits or salivary flow deficiencies which in turn are conducive to caries activity.

**Systemic factors.** Burket[43] quotes a number of authorities as reporting marked increases in new carious lesions among adults with uncontrolled diabetes and with hypothyroid or hyperthyroid states. He cites conflicting evidence regarding caries experience among diabetics on low-refined carbohydrate diets but indicates that such diets are associated with lower caries attack rates. Explanations for increased caries activity among uncontrolled diabetics have suggested decreased salivary flow or the presence of an increased fermentable carbohydrate content in the saliva.

**Familial factors.** The dentist who sees a patient with rampant caries should make a point of investigating the possibility that others in the family may also be actual or potential victims of the disease. Early detection and interception are important to successful control and to preservation of the dentition.

Studies[2-4] referred to earlier show strong familial influences on caries experience. Children of caries-susceptible mothers are more likely to have a high caries rate than are children of caries-immune mothers; children of caries-susceptible fathers are more likely to have a high caries rate than are children of caries-immune fathers; and children whose parents are both caries susceptible are likely to have significantly higher rates than are children in any of the other groups. These relationships are shown to hold true even in areas with adjusted water-fluoride levels, where all child groups have less caries than corresponding groups in nonfluoride areas. The same familial influences are borne out in findings that siblings of children who are susceptible to caries are more likely to have high rates than are siblings of children who are immune to caries.

Whether these familial phenomena result more from hereditary or from other family-related factors is debatable. Most authorities believe that nonhereditary, environmental factors play the more influential role.

## CONCLUSION

The rapidly destructive nature of rampant dental caries suggests a serious breakdown of multiple protective mechanisms. Control of the disease and preservation of teeth depend on early interception of the destructive process, implementation of a comprehensive program to eliminate caries-conducive conditions and to establish a caries-resistant oral environment, and effective restoration of the damaged dentition. Success hinges as much on what the patient does to care for himself as it does on any other factor, so that special efforts in patient counselling are often necessary. Individual control measures are listed below in a typical procedural sequence. Results are most satisfactory when these procedures can be performed in a series of closely timed appointments.

1. Measures for relief of pain and discomfort
2. Removal of actively carious material from all lesions and careful replacement with an appropriate sedative dressing (zinc oxide–eugenol cement or calcium hydroxide first in deep lesions)
3. Stannous fluoride–lava pumice prophylaxis, followed by topical application of a 10 percent stannous fluoride solution
4. Diet record, diet history, and saliva tests (to be initiated at the first appointment)
5. Patient and parent counselling in diet, oral hygiene with the recommendation of use of the stannous fluoride–calcium pyrophosphate dentifrice, and other self-care measures (to be accomplished, as the need is indicated, throughout the entire course of care)
6. Establishment of a caries-controlling diet
7. Restoration of teeth with permanent restorative material
8. Periodic evaluation until satisfied with diet control and oral hygiene
9. Recall after 3 months

If response to the foregoing measures is not satisfactory, the possibility of inadequate salivary flow, mental stress, or a contributing systemic condition should be investigated.

## REFERENCES

1. Massler, M.: Teen-age caries, J. Dent. Child. 12: 57, 1945.
2. Klein, H.: The family and dental disease, V, caries experience among adults and offspring exposed to drinking water containing fluoride, Public Health Rep. 62:1247, 1947.

3. Klein, H., and Palmer, C. E.: Studies on dental caries, V, familial resemblance in siblings, Public Health Rep. **53**:1353, 1938.
4. Klein, H.: The family and dental disease, IV, dental disease (DMF) experience in parents and offspring, J.A.D.A. **33**:735, 1946.
5. Goodman, H. O.: Heredity factors in dental caries, Dent. Clin. N. Amer., September, 1968, p. 357.
6. Orland, F. J., and others: Experimental caries in germ-free rats inoculated with enterococci, J.A.D.A. **50**:259, 1955.
7. Fitzgerald, R. J.: Microbiological aspects of dental caries, J.A.D.A. **66**:597, 1963.
8. Canby, C. P., and Burnett, G. W.: Microorganisms of deep dental caries, J. Dent. Res. **39**:684, 1960.
9. Keyes, P. H.: Research in dental caries, J.A.D.A. **76**:1357, 1968.
10. Sumnicht, R. W.: Research in preventive dentistry, J.A.D.A. **79**:1193, 1962.
11. Gustafsson, B. E., and others: The Vipeholm dental caries study; the effect of different levels of carbohydrate intake on caries activity in 436 individuals observed for five years, Acta Odont. Scand. **22**:232, 1964.
12. Weiss, R. L.: Between-meal eating habits and dental caries experience in preschool children, Amer. J. Public Health **50**:1097, 1960.
13. Becks, H., Jensen, A. L., and Millarr, C. B.: Rampant dental caries; prevention and prognosis, J.A.D.A. **31**:1189, 1944.
14. Jay, P., Beeuwkes, A. M., and Husbands, J.: Dietary program for the control of dental caries, Ann Arbor, Michigan, 1964, The Overbeck Co., Publishers.
15. Nizel, A. E.: Food, nutrition and dental caries, Dent. Clin. N. Amer., July, 1962, p. 335.
16. Stephan, R. M., and Geis, S.: Comprehensive study of etiologic factors in rampant dental caries, 41st General Meeting, I.A.D.R. Abstract 132, 1963.
17. Fass, E. N.: Is bottle feeding a factor in dental caries? J. Dent. Child. **29**:245, 1962.
18. Winter, G. B.: Bottle feeding, sugar, and caries, Dent. Abstr. **10**:278, 1965.
19. Stephan, R. M.: The role of microbic dental plaque in the etiology of caries. In Muhler, J. C., and Hine, M. K., editors: A symposium on preventive dentistry, St. Louis, 1956, The C. V. Mosby Co.
20. Kleinberg, I., and Jenkins, G. N.: The pH of dental plaque before and after meals, Arch. Oral Biol. **9**: 493, 1964.
21. Dudding, N. J., and Muhler, J. C.: Technique of application of stannous fluoride in a compatible prophylactic paste and as a topical agent, J. Dent. Child. **29**:219, 1962.
22. Massler, M.: New concept for caries control, Your Child Patient **3**:2, 1964.
23. Protheroe, D. H.: Study to determine the effect of topical application of stannous fluoride on dental caries on young adults—preliminary report, Roy. Canad. D. Corps Quart. **3**:20, 1962.
24. Bixler, D., and Muhler, J. C.: Effect on dental caries in children in a nonfluoride area of combined use of three agents containing stannous fluoride; a prophylactic paste, a solution and a dentifrice, J.A.D.A. **68**:792, 1964.
25. Gish, C. W., and Muhler, J. C.: Effect on dental caries in children in a natural fluoride area of combined use of three agents containing stannous fluoride; a prophylactic paste, a solution and a dentifrice, J.A.D.A. **70**:914, 1965.
26. Scola, F. P., and Ostrom, C. A.: Clinical evaluation of stannous fluoride in naval personnel, 43rd General Meeting, I.A.D.R. Abstract 49, 1965.
27. Bixler, D., and Muhler, J. C.: Effect on dental caries in children in a nonfluoride area of combined use of three agents containing stannous fluoride; a prophylactic paste, a solution and a dentifrice, II, results at the end of 24 and 36 months, J.A.D.A. **72**:392, 1966.
28. Muhler, J. C., Spear, L. B., Jr., and Bixler, D.: The arrestment of incipient dental caries in adults after the use of three different forms of $SnF_2$ therapy; results after 30 months, J.A.D.A. **75**:1402, 1967.
29. Scola, F. P., and Ostrom, C. A.: Clinical evaluation of stannous fluoride when used as a constituent of compatible prophylactic paste, as a topical solution, and in a dentifrice in naval personnel, II, report of findings after two years, J.A.D.A. **77**:594, 1968.
30. Howard, R. L., and others: Motivation in prevention, I.A.D.R. Abstract 574, 1969.

31. Kegeles, S. S.: Some motives for seeking preventive dental care, J.A.D.A. **67:**90, 1963.
32. Brauer, J. C., and others: Dentistry for children, ed. 5, New York, 1964, McGraw-Hill Book Co.
33. Arnim, S. S.: The use of disclosing agents for measuring tooth cleanliness, J. Periodont. **34:**277, 1963.
34. Blechman, H.: Bacteria and dental caries, Dent. Clin. N. Amer., November, 1962, p. 321.
35. Alfonsky, D.: Saliva and its reaction to oral health, Birmingham, 1961, University of Alabama Press.
36. Bibby, B. G.: Prevention of dental caries, J. Prosth. Dent. **11:**1124, 1961.
37. McDonald, R. E.: Management of rampant caries, P.D.M., p. 3, 1961.
38. Aldous, J. A.: Induced xerostomia and its relation to dental caries, J. Dent. Child. **31:**160, 1964.
39. Council on Dental Therapeutics, American Dental Association: Accepted dental therapeutics 1969/1970, ed. 33, Chicago, 1968, The Association.
40. Sutton, P. R. N.: Mental stress and acute dental caries, Dent. Abstr. **8:**414, 1963.
41. Sutton, P. R. N.: The early onset of acute dental caries in adults following mental stress, New York Dent. J. **31:**387, 1965.
42. Schwabacher, E. D.: Interpersonal factors in rampant dental caries, J. Psychosom. Dent. Med. **5:**97, 1958.
43. Burket, L. W.: Oral medicine, ed. 4, Philadelphia, 1961, J. B. Lippincott Co.

# Chapter 6 Fluoride therapy

## George K. Stookey

Introduction
Systemic fluoridation
Alternative means of providing systemic fluoride therapy
    Fluoride tablets
    Vitamin-fluoride tablets
    Prenatal fluoride tablets
    Fluoridated salt
    Fluoridated milk
    Miscellaneous alternatives
Topical fluoride therapy
    Topical sodium fluoride therapy
    Topical stannous fluoride therapy
    Other fluorides as topical therapeutic agents
    Acid fluoride and acid fluoride–phosphate systems
    Fluoride mouthwashes
    Prophylactic pastes containing fluoride
Multiple fluoride therapy
Conclusion

## INTRODUCTION

This chapter is designed to summarize the current status of fluoride therapy. The first section is devoted to various types of systemic fluoride therapy that might be of value in the absence of communal fluoridation. The remainder of the material concerns the present status of topical fluoride therapy considering all major approaches or types of treatments with the exception of dentifrices, which will be considered in Chapter 7.

## SYSTEMIC FLUORIDATION

There is little doubt that the early finding of a relationship between the presence of fluoride in the drinking water and the prevalence of dental caries was one of the outstanding achievements of dental research during the past four decades. Following the discovery[1] of the presence of elevated levels of fluoride in the drinking waters of persons with "mottled enamel" (properly referred to as chronic endemic dental fluorosis),* a series of epidemiologic studies resulted in the statement that, for public health purposes, the minimal fluoride concentration in a domestic water supply is the highest concentration of fluoride incapable of producing a clinically recognizable degree of mottled enamel in as much as 10 percent of the population.[3] It was then

---

*There are a number of circumstances that result in enamel hypoplasia and "mottled enamel" is but one of the many forms of hypoplasia that is recognized. These causative circumstances include nutritional deficiencies, exanthematous diseases, congenital syphilis, hypocalcemia, birth injury, local infection or trauma, chemicals such as fluoride, and various idiopathic causes.[2]

shown that the concentration of fluoride in the water supply was inversely proportional to the prevalence of dental caries[4-7] and, further, that, although the concentration of fluoride added to the water was inversely related to the temperature of the area since differences in water consumption result from temperature differences, a maximal degree of protection against dental caries with minimal incidence of endemic dental fluorosis was obtained when drinking waters containing 0.8 to 1.2 p.p.m. fluoride were ingested during the first 12 years of life.[8] These early studies indicated that the amount of protection afforded the 6-year-old child by the presence of fluoride in the domestic water supply was about 60 percent. Numerous reports appearing in the literature in the past 30 years repeatedly confirmed these findings. No attempt will be made to review these works, since several reviews are presently available.[9-13]

There are, however, a number of aspects of communal fluoridation that warrant additional consideration, since only an appreciation of the mechanisms involved will allow the practitioner to intelligently discuss the subject with his patients and fellow associates.

Chronic endemic dental fluorosis has been shown to be a hypoplastic developmental defect, caused primarily by an inhibition in the normal metabolic activities of the ameloblast during the formative stage of tooth development. It has been suggested[14] that the ameloblast is the body cell most sensitive to the presence of fluoride and that, at levels of fluoride in the drinking water in excess of about 1.5 p.p.m., the ameloblasts form a defective enamel matrix that is unorganized and consists of an imperfect fusion of irregular and poorly staining enamel globules.[10] In addition, more elevated levels of fluoride have been shown to interfere with the calcification of the enamel matrix. In contrast, fluoride does not appear to exert any direct influence upon the odontoblasts although an indirect effect has been noted.

Clinically, chronic endemic dental fluorosis is found to have a wide range of manifestations directly dependent on the concentration of fluoride in the drinking water. These are characterized as ranging from questionable changes observed as an occasional white flecking or spotting of the enamel at fluoride concentrations approaching 1.5 p.p.m., to moderate and severe changes observed as a pitting and brownish staining of the enamel surface and even a corroded appearance of the teeth at fluoride concentrations in excess of 4 p.p.m.[15] Since chronic endemic dental fluorosis is a developmental defect, it cannot develop in mature enamel nor can it progress in the mature tooth with continued fluoride exposure regardless of the concentration of fluoride in the drinking water. Likewise, to answer a frequently asked question among practitioners, topical fluoride treatments, or any other type of fluoride therapy employed on erupted teeth, cannot result in the formation of chronic endemic dental fluorosis.

Although the exact mechanism or mechanisms involved in the influence of fluoride on dental caries has not yet been defined, most workers agree that only two concepts are of major concern. One concerns a bacteriostatic influence upon the oral flora, based primarily upon the well-known enzyme inhibition properties of fluoride, particularly certain glycolytic enzymes such as enolase or those enzymes requiring magnesium as a cofactor.[16] The early work of McClure, Bibby, and others concerning the influence of fluoride on the oral flora has been reviewed by Muhler and associates[10] and this work has indicated that salivary fluoride concentrations in excess of 250 p.p.m. are required to inhibit bacterial growth. However, more recent reports[17-22] have indicated that concentrations of fluoride as low as 0.5 p.p.m. have a detectable inhibitory influence upon the rate of acid production by the oral flora present in saliva and that concentrations approaching 10 p.p.m. have a pronounced inhibitory effect. These findings are of limited clinical significance since the concentration of fluoride in saliva is less than 0.25 p.p.m.[23, 24] Recent findings suggest that an accumulation of fluoride occurs within the dental plaque ranging in concentration from 6 to nearly 180 p.p.m.[25] and that the concentrations are significantly greater in subjects residing in an area where the water supply contains 2 p.p.m. fluoride as compared to a low-fluoride area. In these latter areas the fluoride concentrations of the plaque were 47 and 26 p.p.m., respectively. Concentrations of ionic fluoride in the plaque were subsequently reported[76] of 0.04 to 0.05 and 0.4 to 1.8 p.p.m. for the low and high fluoride areas, respectively. These later findings, coupled with the findings that the rate of acid production is markedly inhibited at these fluoride concentrations and the fact that at least a portion of the fluoride in the plaque is ionized and available to influence acid production,[27] suggest that this proposed mechanism may indeed play a role in the anticariogenic activity of fluoride ingested in drinking waters. However, additional research is needed to confirm these findings.

Most investigators, on the basis of a considerable accumulation of evidence, favor a second proposed mechanism to explain the anticariogenic properties of fluoride ingested as a constituent of the water supply. This theory is based on the observations that hydroxyapatite, the principal apatite structure of bone and tooth substance, when formed in vivo in the presence of fluoride in the circulating body fluids, as is true whenever one ingests drinking waters containing the optimal level of fluoride, is characterized by the conversion of a portion of the hydroxyl groups in hydroxyapatite to form fluoroapatite. This chemical transformation occurs during the period of calcification and results in an apatite crystal that is much less soluble in weak organic acids than is hydroxyapatite. This phenomenon then is used to explain the resistance of teeth calcified in the presence of fluoride against the subsequent development of dental caries. For this reason it is widely recommended[28] that, in order to receive the maximal amount of benefit from fluoridated communal water supplies, one must ingest these waters continuously during the period of enamel formation, namely, the first 8 years of life. In addition, it has been shown[6, 7] that the amount of fluoride in enamel and the resistance to dental caries increase with increasing concentrations of fluoride in the drinking water. Studies conducted to determine the concentration of fluoride in the outermost portion of enamel[29-31] indicate that the concentration of fluoride in enamel increases with duration of exposure; this latter finding has been used to explain the clinical observation of a lesser dental caries reduction of about 20 percent in children establishing residence in a fluoride area after the first 8 years of life. The mechanism of this latter reaction is thought to involve absorption of fluoride onto the enamel surface and a partial substitution of fluoride for the hydroxyl ions located in the surface of the enamel apatite crystals.

The information available in the literature is somewhat contradictory concerning changes in the concentration of fluoride in the blood following the ingestion of fluoride. Largent[32] reported variations in blood fluoride levels ranging from 0.009 to 6.9 p.p.m. in a subject ingesting 0.55 mg. fluoride and variations ranging from 0.55 to 7.7 p.p.m. in subjects ingesting 12 mg. fluoride as sodium fluoride daily. Smith and associates[33] examined the blood fluoride concentrations of residents of areas whose water supplies contained 0.06 and 1.36 p.p.m. fluoride and reported mean blood fluoride levels of 0.014 and 0.04 p.p.m. for the two groups, respectively. Singer and Armstrong[34] reported that residents of areas whose communal water supply contained 0.15 to 2.5 p.p.m. fluoride had comparable plasma fluoride levels, with mean values ranging from 0.14 to 0.16 p.p.m. for these concentrations, respectively. They reported an increased plasma fluoride level of 0.25 p.p.m. in residents of an area whose water supply contained 5.4 p.p.m. fluoride. Thus the relationship between the concentration of fluoride in the circulating body fluids, the concentration of fluoride in enamel, and the subsequent resistance to dental caries is not yet clear.

It is important to note that the supplementation of otherwise deficient communal water supplies with the optimal amount of fluoride is without question the most effective, practical, convenient, and economical means of providing the public a partial reduction in the incidence of dental caries. From a practical standpoint no other caries-preventive procedure is more convenient or requires less effort on the part of the recipient. The cost of fluoridation in communities with over 1,000 inhabitants is 5 to 15 cents per capita per year,[9] while in smaller communities[35] of less than 1,000 inhabitants it may be as low as $1.22 when economically oriented devices for installation and supervision of the addition of the fluoride compound are employed.

Nevertheless, it is apparent that the use of fluoridated communal water supplies provides dental health benefits to only a limited portion—in fact, only about forty percent of the population of the United States. At the present time about 74.5 million persons are receiving artificially fluoridated water while another 8.3 million are ingesting waters with naturally occurring fluoride. This fact becomes of even more concern when one finds that more than half of the communities in the United States have populations of less than 1,000 and that of these only 678, or about 6 percent, were fluoridating their water supply in the mid-1960's. In many of these small rural communities there is no immediately available dental service. Furthermore, a significant portion of our population resides in areas in which there is no communal water supply and still others reside in communities that oppose fluoridation for various reasons. Many children are presently beyond the age at which maximal benefits of communal fluoride may be derived.

Many facts are available that indicate the widespread prevalence of dental caries and the need for additional means of providing dental care, but suffice it to say that the mean dentist-population ratio is 1:1,900, nearly twice as great as the recommended value of 1:1,000, and that only slightly more than 40 percent of our populace visits a dentist once a year to receive minimal but scarcely adequate dental care, while nearly 60 percent need dental attention.[36] A recent survey on indigent families residing in three southern Indiana counties indicates that these figures may be relatively high for the number of patients seeing a dentist each year, particularly when the family income is low. In this study it was found that, in families with a mean income per year of $2,500, from 31 to 74 percent (dependent on age) of the persons had never visited a dentist. As a result of the deficiencies of communal fluoridation programs and the need for additional dental care, a number of alternative caries-preventive procedures have been suggested. These alternative methods for providing systemic fluoride therapy have included fluoride tablets and fluoride in table salt, in milk, in chewing gum, and in combination with various vitamins in either liquid or tablet preparations.

## ALTERNATIVE MEANS OF PROVIDING SYSTEMIC FLUORIDE THERAPY
### Fluoride tablets

In the past 20 years considerable attention has been given to the use of fluoride tablets since their use could conceivably represent a means by which individuals might derive the benefits of fluoride when a communal water supply is not available or when the available water supply is not fluoridated. Although only limited information is available in the literature concerning the metabolism of fluoride when provided in single daily dosages, as in a fluoride tablet, several clinical studies conducted almost entirely in Europe have been reported, in order to investigate the effectiveness of this procedure.

In considering those studies in which beneficial effects were obtained, Strean and Beaudet[37] reported in three separate studies the effectiveness of fluoride provided in tablets as calcium fluoride in both the presence and absence of vitamins C and D. The first two studies were conducted in an orphanage with supervised administration, while the third involved children who were private patients of dental practitioners. The fluoride tablet contained 3 mg. calcium fluoride (1.46 mg. fluoride), while the vitamin tablets contained 30 mg. ascorbic acid and 400 I.U. vitamin D (as calciferol) in addition to the fluoride. Strean and Beaudet reported that significant reductions ranging from 27.9 to 82 percent in dental caries were obtained in all subjects receiving the fluoride tablets regardless of vitamin content and further noted that the effect on dental caries was greater in those subjects provided the vitamin-fluoride tablets. A study in which 50,000 children, 6 to 8 years of age, in Hesse, Germany, received sodium fluoride tablets resulted in significant reductions in dental caries ranging from 22 to 40 percent.[38] In a short-term study Abary-Murillo[39] reported significant caries reductions with calcium fluoride troches. Held and Piguet[40] reported significant caries reductions after 3 years of ingestion of either a sodium fluoride tablet or a tablet containing bone meal in the permanent dentition of children 5 to 6 years of age at the initiation of the studies. Reductions in caries in the first permanent molars of 31.7 and 13.8 percent were noted in subjects provided the sodium fluoride and bone meal tablets, respectively, while reductions of 84.6 and 75.1 percent were reported in the incidence of caries in the remainder of the permanent dentition.

Bibby and associates[41] reported a 40.3 percent reduction in caries in a limited number of children ingesting a sodium fluoride lozenge, although no reduction was noted in subjects provided the fluoride in a pill formulation. Binder[42] reported a 35.1 percent reduction after 2 years in 565 children provided four sodium fluoride tablets daily, each of which contained 0.25 mg. fluoride. Kessler and Solth[43] similarly found a significant caries reduction of 33 percent in 602 preschool and school children following the use of sodium fluoride tablets. Schutzmannsky[44] reported on a study in which children 6 to 7 years of age were provided a single sodium fluoride tablet daily during the two-hundred-day school year only. In this study, conducted over a 4-year period, caries reductions of 9.2, 16.6, and 20.4 percent were noted after 2, 3, and 4 years with the latter two values being significant. No reductions in the incidence of caries in the first permanent molars were noted even after 3 years of use of the fluoride supplements. Arnold and associates[45] found that the daily use by 121 children, 4 to 15 years of age, of sodium fluoride tablets containing 1 mg. fluoride, provided by dissolving a tablet in one quart of water for use throughout the day, resulted in caries reductions comparable to those provided by fluoridated communal water supplies. In an extensive study involving more than 4,434 children 3 to 5 years of age, half of whom received sodium fluoride tablets, Ziemnowicz-Glowacka[46] reported a 38.5 percent reduction after 2 years and a comparable reduction of 42.4 percent after 3 years of ingestion of the tablets. Wrzodek[47] has reported a caries reduction of 25.5 percent following nearly 4 years of ingestion of sodium fluoride tablets by preschool and school children. Krusic[48] provided calcium fluoride tablets to 168 children 8 to 15 years of age and noted a significant reduction of 86.8 percent, while Pollak[49] reported caries reductions of about 38 percent after 3 years in 1,000 children 3 to 7 years of age provided a sodium fluoride tablet that also contained vitamins A, D, and E. Held and Dubois-Provost[50] reported a 50 percent reduction following the use of fluoride tablets, while Grissom and associates[51] reported a 34.1 percent reduction in caries in permanent teeth after 2 years of supervised ingestion of sodium fluoride tablets given during the school year only. In a 30-month study conducted at Indiana University,[52] the use of sodium fluoride tablets, containing 1 mg. fluoride, by children 3 to 6 years of age resulted in a reduction of 54.7 percent in the deciduous dentition but had no beneficial influence on the caries rate in the permanent teeth. A reverse finding of an effect in permanent but not in deciduous teeth has recently been reported by Kamocka and associates.[54]

More recent studies have tended to confirm that there is a beneficial influence of supplemental fluoride tablets on the prevention of dental caries in both the deciduous and permanent dentitions. Marthaler and Konig[55] observed a 46.6 percent reduction in the incidence of dental caries in the permanent dentition of children who had been ingesting fluoride tablets for 8 years. Similarly, Berner and others[56] reported a reduction of 84.1 percent in DMF teeth in children provided sodium fluoride tablets at school for 3 years and a 23.7 percent reduction after 4 additional years. DePaola and Lax[57] observed a reduction of 23.3 percent after providing sodium fluoride tablets for 2 years during the school year. Kailis and others[58] reported a 55.7 percent reduction in the incidence of dental caries in the deciduous dentition of kindergarten children who had ingested sodium fluoride tablets since birth.

Contradictory evidence relative to the use of fluoride tablets is also available in the literature. Stones and associates[60] provided sodium fluoride tablets containing 1.5 mg. fluoride to 250 institutionalized children 6 to 14 years of age with daily supervised administration for 2 years following a 2-year period in which the normal rate of caries development was determined. These investigators reported a reduction in caries in boys but not in the girls who participated in the study. Gustafsson and associates[61] provided sodium fluoride tablets in both the presence and absence of vitamins A, C, and D and calcium and failed to find any influence of the various supplements upon dental caries. Similarly, Bibby and associates[41] did not find a beneficial effect with sodium fluoride pills. In an extensive study involving some 7,200 children 7 to 11 years of age Jez[62] failed to find any beneficial influence from the daily use of calcium fluoride tablets for 30 months, while in a study involving 268 grammar school children Knychalska-Karwan and Laskowski[63] failed to find a significant reduction after 4 years of ingestion of sodium fluoride tablets. Similarly, in our own study[52] sodium fluoride tablets failed to provide any beneficial influence to the permanent dentition. These data are summarized in Table 6-1.

Of the twenty-seven literature reports of clinical studies pertaining to the use of fluoride tablets, five were either entirely or partially negative. Of the six studies conducted within the United States, four reported beneficial effects of fluoride tablets

**Table 6-1.** *Summary of clinical dental caries studies using various types of fluoride tablets and lozenges for systemic ingestion*

| Study | Fluoride compound | Daily dosage | Vehicle | Initial age of subjects (years) | Number of subjects | Duration | Reduction DMFS (defs) (percent) |
|---|---|---|---|---|---|---|---|
| Strean and Beaudet[37] | CaF$_2$ | 3 mg. | Tablet | 8-13 | 57 | 6 mo. | 27.9 |
| | CaF$_2$* | 3 mg.* | Tablet | 8-13 | 57 | 6 mo. | 39.5 |
| | CaF$_2$ | 3 mg. | Tablet | 8-13 | 68 | 8 mo. | 53.1 |
| | CaF$_2$* | 3 mg.* | Tablet | 8-13 | 73 | 8 mo. | 82.0 |
| Anonymous[38] | NaF | 1 mg. F | Tablet | 6-8 | 50,000 | 1 yr. | 22-40 |
| Abary-Murillo[39] | CaF$_2$ | 0.3 mg. | Troche | 8-15 | 20 | 6 mo. | 74.1 |
| Held and Piguet[40] | NaF | 1 mg. F | Tablet | 5-6 | 355 | 3 yr. | 31.7 (84.6)† |
| | CaF$_2$ | 1 mg. F | Tablet | 5-6 | 355 | 3 yr. | 13.8 (75.1)† |
| Bibby and others[41] | NaF | 1 mg. F | Pill | 5-14 | 133 | 12-14 mo. | 1.5 |
| | NaF | 1 mg. F | Lozenge | 5-14 | 119 | 12-14 mo. | 40.3 |
| Binder[42] | NaF | 1 mg. F‡ | Tablet | 6-9 | 565 | 2 yr. | 35.1 |
| Kessler and Solth[43] | NaF | 1 mg. F | Tablet | 4-8 | 602 | 1 yr. | 33.0 |
| Schutzmannsky[44] | NaF | 1 mg. F§ | Tablet | 6-7 | 400 | 2 yr. | 9.2 |
| | | | | | | 3 yr. | 16.6 |
| | | | | | | 4 yr. | 20.4 |
| Arnold and others[45] | NaF | 1 p.p.m. | Tablet‖ | 4-15 | 121 | 1-15 yr. | 60.0 |
| Ziemnowicz-Glowacka[46] | NaF | 1 mg. F | Tablet | 3-5 | 4,434 | 2 yr. | 38.5 |
| | | | | | | 3 yr. | 42.4 |
| Wrzodek[47] | NaF | 0.7-1 mg. F | Tablet | 6-9 | 13,585 | 4 yr. | 25.5 |
| Krusic[48] | CaF$_2$ | 1 mg. F | Tablet | 8-15 | 168 | 1 yr. | 86.8 |
| Pollak[49] | NaF | 1 mg. F¶ | Tablet | 3-7 | 1,000 | 1 yr. | 24.0 |
| | | | | — | | 3 yr. | 38.0 |
| Held and Dubois-Provost[50] | NaF | 1 mg. F | Tablet | 4-8 | — | — | 50.0 |
| Grissom and others[51] | NaF | 1 mg. F** | Tablet | 7-11 | 178 | 2 yr. | 34.1 |

\*Tablets also contained 30 mg. ascorbic acid and 400 I.U. vitamin D (calciferol).
†Reductions in first permanent molars and deciduous dentitions, respectively.
‡Ingested in four tablets daily, each of which contained 0.25 mg. F.
§Provided under supervision during two hundred–day school year.
‖One tablet containing 1 mg. F was dissolved in one quart of water daily.
¶Tablets contained vitamins A, D, and E in addition to fluoride.
\*\*Subjects provided tablets during school year (maximum of 180 tablets per year).
††Reductions in deciduous and permanent dentition, respectively.
‡‡Tablets also contained 2,500 I.U. vitamin A and 250 I.U. vitamin D.
§§Tablets also contained 70 mg. NaH$_2$PO$_4$ and were administered in schools (150 to 160 tablets per year).

Fluoride therapy 99

**Table 6-1.** *Summary of clinical dental caries studies using various types of fluoride tablets and lozenges for systemic ingestion—cont'd*

| Study | Fluoride compound | Daily dosage | Vehicle | Initial age of subjects (years) | Number of subjects | Duration | Reduction DMFS (defs) (percent) |
|---|---|---|---|---|---|---|---|
| Hennon and others[52] | NaF | 1 mg. F | Tablet | 3-6 | 50 | 30 mo. | 54.7 (0)†† |
| Minoguchi and others[53] | NaF | 0.5 mg. NaF | Tablet‡‡ | 6-12 | 75 | 6 yr. | 36.3 |
| Kamocka and others[54] | NaF | 1 mg. F | Tablet | 3-4 | — | 3 yr. | 0 (60)†† |
| Marthaler and König[55] | NaF | 0.5-1.0§ | Tablet | 1-7 | 995 | 8 yr. | 46.6 |
| Berner and others[56] | NaF | 1.0§ | Tablet | 5-7 | 210 | 3 yr. | 84.1 |
| Berner and others[56] | NaF | 1.0§ | Tablet | 5-7 | 1,000 | 7 yr. | 23.7 |
| DePaola and Lax[57] | NaF | 1.0§§ | Tablet | 6-9 | 327 | 2 yr. | 23.3 |
| Kailis and others[58] | NaF | 0.5-1.0 | Tablet | 4-6 | 234 | 6 yr. | (55.7) |
| Wigdorowixa[59] | NaF | 1.0 | Tablet | 4-7 | — | 3 yr. | 24.0 |
| Stones and others[60] | NaF | 1.5 mg. F | Tablet | 6-14 | 250 | 2 yr. | 0 |
| Gustafsson and others[61] | NaF | 1 mg. F | Tablet | 3-5 | 57 | 2 yr. | 0 |
| Jez[62] | $CaF_2$ | 1 mg. F | Tablet | 7-11 | 7,200 | 30 mo. | 0 |
| Knychalska-Karwan and Laskowska[63] | NaF | 1 mg. F | Tablet | 5-7 | 268 | 4 yr. | 4.5 |

upon dental caries. However, as a result of these collective positive findings, the Council on Dental Therapeutics[28] has classified fluoride tablets in Group B.

There are several reasons why additional research is needed prior to the generalized recommendation of the use of fluoride tablets. There is evidence available that suggests that the metabolism of fluoride, when ingested in a single dosage such as in a tablet, differs from that of persons residing in communal fluoride areas who ingest small quantities of fluoride in drinking water throughout the day and who eat food prepared with fluoride-containing water. Studies conducted in our own laboratories at Indiana University,[64, 65] as well as several other studies such as those by McClure[66] and by Machle and associates,[67] have indicated that over 95 percent of an ingested single dose of fluoride is rapidly excreted in the urine with only minor quantities retained by the body. While these studies have been conducted primarily in young adults, several additional studies involving both preschool and school children have shown that, even in young children, in whom skeletal and tooth tissue formation is occurring at a much more rapid rate than in young adults, the urinary

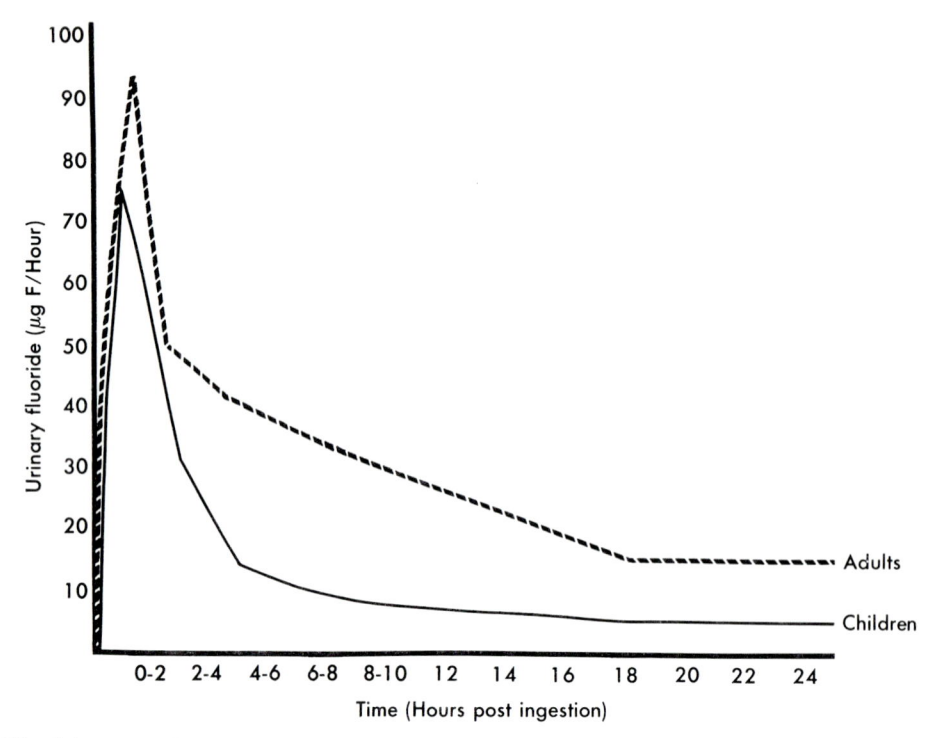

Fig. 6-1. Comparison of rate of urinary fluoride excretion in children and adults following the ingestion of 1 mg. fluoride as sodium fluoride in a tablet.

excretion pattern of the fluoride is such that a rapid rate of excretion occurs comparable to that observed in adults.

Typical findings relative to the rapid clearance of fluoride from the plasma are shown in Fig. 6-1. These data were obtained by providing 1 mg. fluoride in the form of a tablet to children 3 to 5 years of age and young adults 18 to 22 years of age with no appreciable previous exposure to fluoride. The appropriate fluoride excretion pattern was determined on the subjects prior to and immediately following the ingestion of the tablets, with urine specimens collected at predetermined intervals throughout a 24-hour period. These data indicate that in both groups of subjects the pattern of fluoride excretion in the urine was comparable.

The implication that the metabolism of fluoride ingested as a single dosage differs from that noted when fluoride is ingested more frequently is further supported by a recent study[65] in which young adults were provided 1.5 mg. fluoride (sodium fluoride) either as a single dose or in three doses of 0.5 mg. fluoride each. The data shown in Table 6-2 indicate that, of the total amount of fluoride ingested, 49.2 percent less fluoride was excreted in the urine when the ingestion of fluoride was in three doses as compared to a single dose.

Additional attempts have been made to investigate the metabolism of fluoride ingested in the form of a tablet. The results of a typical study are summarized in Fig. 6-2. In this study young adults with little or no previous exposure to fluoride were placed in a controlled dietary regimen with and without daily ingestion of a single fluoride tablet containing 1 mg. fluoride (sodium fluoride), and the concen-

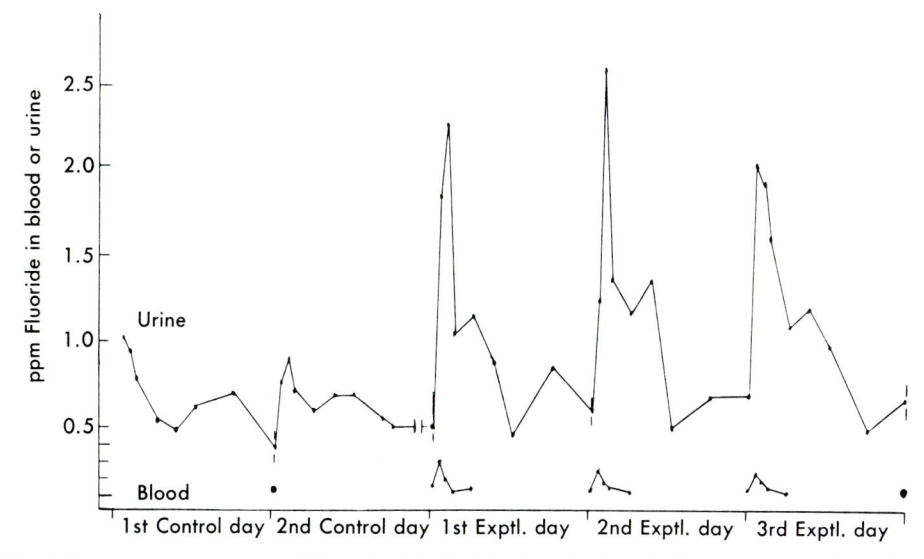

**Fig. 6-2.** Average parts per million fluoride in blood and urine of three young adult subjects ingesting a chewable vitamin tablet containing 1 mg. fluoride each morning at 8 A.M. for 3 days.

**Table 6-2.** *Urinary fluoride data in young adults ingesting equivalent amounts of aqueous fluoride as sodium fluoride in single or multiple dosages*

| Subject | Regimen | Number of days | p.p.m. | Urinary fluoride Total per day (mg.) | Average increase (mg.) |
|---------|---------|---------------|--------|-------------------------------------|-----------------------|
| H. L.   | Precontrol | 2 | 0.448 | 0.490 | — |
|         | 1.5 mg. F as NaF in single dose | 7 | 1.210 | 1.390 | 0.900 |
|         | Postcontrol | 7 | 0.557 | 0.498 | 0.008 |
| J. S.   | Precontrol | 2 | 0.322 | 0.568 | — |
|         | 0.5 mg. F as NaF, three doses | 7 | 0.490 | 1.025 | 0.457 |
|         | Postcontrol | 7 | 0.314 | 0.583 | 0.015 |

trations of fluoride in the blood and urine were noted at predetermined intervals of time. It was found that a slight increase in the blood-fluoride concentration followed the ingestion of a fluoride tablet, but that the concentration returned to the preexperimental level within 2 hours.

It appears that fluoride ingested in a tablet is rapidly absorbed and excreted. If the widely accepted conversion of hydroxyapatite of the developing tooth to fluoroapatite occurs in the presence of fluoride circulating in the body fluids and if this formation of fluoroapatite is at all related to an increased resistance to dental caries, it would appear that the rapid excretion of fluoride from the blood and circulating body fluids, as occurs following the ingestion of fluoride in single dosages, would not permit sufficient fluoride to be retained by the developing tooth tissue to be associated with a highly significant amount of caries resistance.

**Table 6-3.** *Recommended levels of supplemental fluoride therapy in children over 3 years of age**

| Fluoride concentration in drinking water (p.p.m.) | Recommended supplemental dosage level ||
|---|---|---|
| | NaF (mg. per day) | F- (mg. per day) |
| 0 | 2.2 | 1.0 |
| 0.2 | 1.8 | 0.8 |
| 0.4 | 1.3 | 0.6 |
| 0.6 | 0.9 | 0.4 |

*Data from Accepted Dental Remedies, ed. 33, Chicago, 1969, American Dental Association.

It has been recommended[28] that no supplemental fluoride be provided when the drinking water contains as much as or more than 0.7 p.p.m. fluoride. The recommended dosages are shown in Table 6-3 as a function of the inherent fluoride content of the drinking water for children over 3 years of age. The dosage should be reduced by half for children between 2 and 3 years of age, while no specific recommendations for children under 2 years of age have been made other than the use of artificially fluoridated water prepared by dissolving a tablet containing 1 mg. fluoride in a quart of water and using this water to prepare the formula and other foods for the children. In addition, as a precautionary measure against the storage of large quantities of sodium fluoride in the home, no more than 264 mg. should be dispensed at one time.[28]

A more practical disadvantage of the use of fluoride tablets involves the conscientiousness of both the parents and the children since this type of fluoride therapy requires consistent and continual daily ingestion of the tablets throughout the first 10 to 12 years of life in order to obtain maximal anticariogenic benefit. In a study conducted by Arnold and associates[45] it was found that only about half the subjects continued daily fluoride supplementation during the study in spite of the fact that these investigators used a very select group of children whose parents were dentists, physicians, or professional employees of the United States Public Health Service. In a study conducted in our clinic at Indiana University,[52] in which no attempt was made to select patients, it was found that 43 percent of the subjects had discontinued the regular ingestion of the tablets within the first 6 months of the program and that, after 3 years, 80 percent of the subjects had withdrawn from the program. Richardson has similarly reported on parental apathy in the administration of fluoride supplements with a discontinuation rate of 60 percent of 560 patients after 1 year.[68] It appears that the use of fluoride tablets as a means of supplemental fluoride therapy is fraught with several important limitations and that, although subsequent research may indicate that this type of therapy provides a significant degree of protection against dental caries, the practical aspects of using a sodium fluoride tablet may severely limit its role in preventive dentistry.

### Vitamin-fluoride tablets

In the past 5 years there has been a marked trend toward the use of sodium fluoride in combination with vitamins. Although there are numerous preparations available commercially, there is very little information available to support the use of these products. In addition, the Council on Dental Therapeutics[28] has been opposed to such combinations largely because of the problems involved in adjusting the fluoride dosage in accordance with the varying levels of fluoride in the water of some communities while maintaining the recommended level of vitamin supplementation.

Only limited information is available concerning the influence of various vitamins upon fluoride metabolism, or vice versa. Hennon and associates[69] have reported that a preparation containing vitamins A, C, and D, thiamine, riboflavin, pyridoxine, calcium pantothenate, cyanocobalamin, and biotin did not alter the metabolism of sodium fluoride in the rat. Showley and associates[70] similarly noted that vitamin A, thiamine, riboflavin, pyridoxine, and pantothenic acid did not markedly influence fluoride retention in the rat, although a greater retention of fluoride was noted at a reduced level of vitamin supplementation as compared to that noted when the minimal daily requirement of each vitamin was provided. Harkins and associates[71] have shown that relatively large doses of sodium fluoride added to a vitamin supplement had no effect on the growth rate or on food and vitamin utilization in the rat. With regard to the influence of individual vitamins Muhler[72] reported that elevated levels of ascorbic acid increased the retention of fluoride in the skeleton and soft tissues of guinea pigs. Suttie and Phillips[73] have reviewed the information available concerning vitamins and fluorosis and have suggested that elevated levels of vitamins A, C, and D tend to mitigate the symptoms of fluorosis, with ascorbic acid having the greatest effect. Stookey[74] similarly observed, in a series of controlled investigations in the rat and guinea pig in which a number of vitamins were individually evaluated for their influence upon fluoride metabolism, that optimal dosages of riboflavin, thiamine, pyridoxine, pantothenic acid, and vitamins A, C, and D did not significantly alter fluoride retention. Collectively, these limited studies suggest that the levels and types of vitamin supplementation provided in commercially available vitamin-fluoride preparations have no appreciable influence upon fluoride metabolism, although additional studies are needed concerning these relationships.

The first clinical dental caries study utilizing vitamin-fluoride supplements was conducted by Strean and Beaudet[37] and has been cited earlier. They concluded that the effectiveness of fluoride in reducing the incidence of dental caries was enhanced by the presence of vitamins. These workers found that the vitamin-fluoride combination tablets reduced caries by 39.5 and 82 percent in two studies, while the fluoride tablets alone provided reductions of 27.9 and 53.1 percent, respectively. Similar findings have been reported by Pollak,[49] who found a 38 percent reduction in dental caries in 2,000 children 3 to 5 years of age who had ingested a sodium fluoride tablet containing vitamins A, D, and E for 3 years. Gustafsson,[61] however, failed to find any anticariogenic effects associated with sodium fluoride tablets containing vitamins A, C, and D and calcium.

The results of a study conducted at Indiana University[75-77] suggest that the ingestion of chewable vitamin-fluoride tablets containing sodium fluoride and vitamins A, C, and D as well as certain members of the vitamin B complex may provide a substantial reduction in the prevalence of dental caries in the deciduous dentition. In this study children ranging in age from birth to 5 years were randomly divided into two groups and were provided either a vitamin-fluoride supplement or an identical vitamin supplement without added fluoride. The fluoride was provided as sodium fluoride at levels of 0.5 mg. fluoride per day for children less than 2 years

**Table 6-4.** *Caries prevalence in deciduous teeth of children according to length of time of product usage (Group I, vitamins only; Group II, vitamins and sodium fluoride)*

| Time period (months) | Group | Number of subjects | Deft (mean) | Percent difference | Defs (mean) | Percent difference |
|---|---|---|---|---|---|---|
| 0 ± 2 | I | 17 | 4.71 ± 1.33* | — | 9.71 ± 4.41 | — |
|  | II | 16 | 4.13 ± 1.17 | 12.3 | 6.38 ± 2.09 | 34.3 |
| 6 ± 2 | I | 34 | 4.50 ± 0.61 | — | 6.35 ± 1.18 | — |
|  | II | 34 | 3.50 ± 0.85 | 22.2 | 5.18 ± 1.46 | 19.8 |
| 11 ± 2 | I | 52 | 5.48 ± 0.69 | — | 8.25 ± 1.21 | — |
|  | II | 50 | 3.70 ± 0.69 | 32.5 | 5.42 ± 1.16 | 34.3 |
| 16 ± 2 | I | 49 | 5.94 ± 0.63 | — | 9.92 ± 1.35 | — |
|  | II | 50 | 3.72 ± 0.66 | 37.4‡ | 5.84 ± 1.18 | 41.1† |
| 22 ± 2 | I | 56 | 7.04 ± 0.70 | — | 12.75 ± 1.61 | — |
|  | II | 57 | 3.37 ± 0.56 | 52.1§ | 5.42 ± 1.12 | 57.5§ |
| 28 ± 3 | I | 90 | 6.38 ± 0.51 | — | 11.19 ± 1.21 | — |
|  | II | 99 | 3.03 ± 0.41 | 52.5§ | 4.55 ± 0.74 | 59.3§ |
| 35 ± 3 | I | 85 | 6.81 ± 0.54 | — | 12.38 ± 1.32 | — |
|  | II | 85 | 3.04 ± 0.40 | 55.1§ | 4.56 ± 0.77 | 63.2§ |
| 42 ± 1 | I | 73 | 7.32 ± 0.59 | — | 13.30 ± 1.44 | — |
|  | II | 66 | 3.18 ± 0.47 | 56.6§ | 5.05 ± 0.97 | 62.0§ |
| 48 ± 1 | I | 59 | 7.73 ± 0.62 | — | 14.25 ± 1.54 | — |
|  | II | 54 | 3.07 ± 0.48 | 60.3‡ | 4.61 ± 0.96 | 67.6§ |
| 54 ± 1 | I | 59 | 7.49 ± 0.50 | — | 14.14 ± 1.36 | — |
|  | II | 65 | 2.98 ± 0.45 | 60.2§ | 4.77 ± 0.94 | 66.3§ |
| 60 ± 1 | I | 44 | 8.02 ± 0.65 | — | 16.32 ± 1.53 | — |
|  | II | 58 | 2.64 ± 0.41 | 67.1§ | 4.21 ± 0.87 | 74.2§ |
| 66 ± 1 | I | 35 | 7.34 ± 0.65 | — | 14.00 ± 1.61 | — |
|  | II | 53 | 3.70 ± 0.55 | 49.6§ | 5.91 ± 1.13 | 57.8§ |

*Standard error of the mean.
†Probability < 0.05.
‡Probability < 0.02.
§Probability < 0.001.

of age and 1 mg. fluoride per day for children over 2 years of age. The results of this study are summarized in Tables 6-4 through 6-6. It is apparent (Table 6-4) that nearly 2 years of usage of the vitamin-fluoride product was required in order to obtain significant reductions in the prevalence of dental caries and that, after this period of ingestion of the vitamin-fluoride supplement, reductions of 52.1 and 57.5 percent in deft and defs, respectively, were noted. Slightly greater reductions of 55.1 and 63.2 percent in deft and defs, respectively, were noted after a 3-year use of the vitamin-fluoride supplement; this effect was maintained throughout the remainder of the 5½-year study period. Even greater caries reductions were noted (Table 6-5) when only those children who were less than 2 years of age at the initiation of the study were considered separately. In this instance reductions in caries

**Table 6-5.** *Caries prevalence in deciduous teeth of children 3 to 5 years of age, according to length of time of product usage (Group I, vitamins only; Group II, vitamins and sodium fluoride)*

| Length of use (months) | Group | Number of subjects | Deft (mean) | Percent difference | Defs (mean) | Percent difference |
|---|---|---|---|---|---|---|
| 0 ± 2 | I | 11 | 2.82 ± 0.81* | — | 3.82 ± 1.16 | — |
|  | II | 11 | 3.27 ± 1.31 | +16.8 | 5.18 ± 2.46 | +26.3 |
| 6 ± 2 | I | 25 | 4.20 ± 0.60 | — | 5.24 ± 0.93 | — |
|  | II | 23 | 2.91 ± 0.95 | 30.7 | 4.04 ± 1.56 | 22.9 |
| 11 ± 2 | I | 33 | 5.82 ± 0.97 | — | 8.58 ± 1.64 | — |
|  | II | 33 | 3.82 ± 0.87 | 34.4 | 5.45 ± 1.40 | 36.5 |
| 16 ± 2 | I | 37 | 5.92 ± 0.79 | — | 9.76 ± 1.66 | — |
|  | II | 35 | 3.06 ± 0.77 | 48.3† | 4.57 ± 1.28 | 53.2† |
| 22 ± 2 | I | 36 | 6.69 ± 0.89 | — | 11.81 ± 1.98 | — |
|  | II | 39 | 2.18 ± 0.42 | 67.4§ | 3.15 ± 0.78 | 73.3§ |
| 28 ± 3 | I | 52 | 5.58 ± 0.60 | — | 8.97 ± 1.25 | — |
|  | II | 47 | 2.23 ± 0.43 | 60.0§ | 3.02 ± 0.65 | 66.3§ |
| 35 ± 3 | I | 45 | 5.40 ± 0.64 | — | 8.38 ± 1.22 | — |
|  | II | 50 | 1.90 ± 0.43 | 64.6§ | 2.56 ± 0.71 | 69.5§ |
| 42 ± 1 | I | 29 | 5.72 ± 0.68 | — | 9.10 ± 1.36 | — |
|  | II | 25 | 1.76 ± 0.44 | 69.2§ | 2.12 ± 0.64 | 76.7§ |
| 48 ± 1 | I | 13 | 6.00 ± 0.93 | — | 9.85 ± 1.95 | — |
|  | II | 12 | 2.08 ± 0.76 | 65.3‡ | 2.83 ± 1.30 | 71.3‡ |

*Standard error of the mean.
†Probability < 0.02.
‡Probability < 0.01.
§Probability < 0.001.

**Table 6-6.** *Caries prevalence in permanent teeth of children according to length of time of product usage (Group I, vitamins only; Group II, vitamins and sodium fluoride)*

| Length of use (months) | Group | Number of subjects | DMFT (mean) | Percent difference | DMFS (mean) | Percent difference |
|---|---|---|---|---|---|---|
| 42 ± 1 | I | 23 | 2.39 ± 0.36* | — | 3.78 ± 0.67 | — |
|  | II | 12 | 1.83 ± 0.46 | 23.4 | 2.50 ± 0.74 | 33.9 |
| 48 ± 1 | I | 31 | 2.42 ± 0.32 | — | 4.06 ± 0.60 | — |
|  | II | 25 | 1.44 ± 0.35 | 40.5† | 2.20 ± 0.56 | 45.8† |
| 54 ± 1 | I | 40 | 2.40 ± 0.28 | — | 4.13 ± 0.55 | — |
|  | II | 40 | 1.35 ± 0.25 | 43.8§ | 1.73 ± 0.34 | 58.1‖ |
| 60 ± 1 | I | 30 | 2.73 ± 0.30 | — | 4.30 ± 0.47 | — |
|  | II | 42 | 1.60 ± 0.27 | 41.4§ | 2.19 ± 0.40 | 49.1§ |
| 66 ± 1 | I | 33 | 2.67 ± 0.37 | — | 4.67 ± 0.75 | — |
|  | II | 46 | 1.61 ± 0.26 | 39.7‡ | 2.26 ± 0.38 | 51.6§ |

*Standard error of the mean.
†Probability < 0.05.
‡Probability < 0.02.
§Probability < 0.01.
‖Probability < 0.001.

prevalence of 67.4 and 73.3 percent in deft and defs, respectively, were noted after a 2-year use of the vitamin-fluoride supplement, with comparable reductions being obtained in children who had ingested the fluoride preparation for about 3 years. This beneficial influence was maintained throughout the remainder of the 5-year study period. The use of a supplemental fluoride-vitamin preparation was also observed to have a significant beneficial influence on the permanent dentition (Table 6-6). In this particular study fluoride supplementation resulted in a reduction in dental caries prevalence of 39.7 and 51.6 percent in DMFT and DMFS, respectively, at the conclusion of the study period.

Comparable findings have been reported by Margolis and associates.[78] These investigators observed a mean deft prevalence in 535 children 3 to 5 years of age of 1.36 in the absence of fluoride-vitamin supplementation and a prevalence value of 0.62 in 686 children provided fluoride-vitamin supplementation representing a reduction of 54.4 percent.

An important practical consideration concerns the frequency of ingestion of the vitamin-fluoride supplement without supervision and the attitudes of the participants of the study. It was noted earlier that providing fluoride tablets without vitamins resulted in an 80 percent subject withdrawal in 3 years. In marked contrast, in the latter study involving vitamin-fluoride tablets, only 9.6 percent of the subjects withdrew from the program during a comparable period. These findings suggest that the combination of fluoride with vitamins for daily supplementation may represent a much more efficient and satisfactory means of providing daily fluoride supplementation in the absence of communal fluoridation than the use of fluoride tablets alone. Nevertheless, additional research is needed to confirm the few reported clinical trials with vitamin-fluoride supplements.

**Prenatal fluoride tablets**

Since the mechanism of action of systemic fluoride involves the conversion of hydroxyapatite to fluoroapatite during tooth formation and since the deciduous dentition and the first permanent molars undergo complete or partial calcification in utero, it has been suggested that fluoride must be provided prenatally in order to achieve maximal protection against dental caries.

However, some major conflicts are apparent in the literature regarding the ability of fluoride to pass the placenta. These conflicts stem from the consistent finding in laboratory studies, involving various animal species and different technics, that low levels of fluoride, comparable to the level obtained in fluoridated drinking water, do not pass the placental tissues in significant amounts to become incorporated in the skeletal hard tissues of the fetus in sufficient amounts to reduce dental caries. These studies have been the subject of a recent review,[79] and no attempt will be made here to reconsider these numerous (nearly 100) studies. Another recent report[80] has suggested that low levels of fluoride pass the placenta of the guinea pig and that this species, which has not heretofore been evaluated in the laboratory, may represent an exception to the results reported previously in other animal species.

A number of attempts have been made to investigate the prenatal metabolism of fluoride in the human by determining the concentration of fluoride in the maternal and fetal circulation simultaneously and the amount of fluoride retained in the fetal hard tissues. The results of these studies are summarized in Table 6-7 and indicate that, in general, increasing amounts of fluoride provided in the drinking water

**Table 6-7.** *Summary of studies concerning concentration of fluoride in maternal and fetal soft and hard tissues*

| Study | Prenatal dietary regimen | Vehicle | Maternal blood | Placenta | Fetal blood | Femur | Mandible and/or maxilla | Teeth |
|---|---|---|---|---|---|---|---|---|
| Martin[81] | 0.1 p.p.m. F | Drinking water | — | — | — | 19.6 | 19.0 | 12.2 |
| Blayney and Hill[82] | 1.0 p.p.m. F | Drinking water | — | — | — | 96.2 | 106.1 | 67.5 |
| Gardner and others[83] | 0.06 p.p.m. F | Drinking water | — | 0.74 | — | — | — | — |
|  | 1.0 p.p.m. F | Drinking water | — | 2.09 | — | — | — | — |
| Feltman and Kosel[84] | 0.0 p.p.m. F | Drinking water | — | 0.68 | 0.22 | — | — | — |
|  | 1.0 p.p.m. F | Drinking water | — | 0.85 | 0.38 | — | — | — |
| Gedalia and others[85, 86] | 0.05 p.p.m. F | Drinking water | — | — | — | 43.8 | 46.9 | 40.8 |
|  | 0.55 p.p.m. F* | Drinking water | 0.18 | — | — | — | — | — |
|  | 0.55 p.p.m. F | Drinking water | 0.09 | 0.15 | 0.11 | 130.0 | — | — |
|  | 0.55 p.p.m. F | Drinking water | — | — | — | 92.5 | 78.8 | 69.7 |
|  | 1.1-1.2 p.p.m. F | Drinking water | — | — | — | 114.8 | 105.3 | 63.0 |
| Feltman and Kosel[87] | Control | Drinking water | — | 0.76 | 0.25 | — | — | — |
|  | 1 p.p.m. F | Drinking water | — | 0.91 | 0.34 | — | — | — |
| Ziegler[88] | Control | Milk | 0.15 | 0.36 | 0.13 | — | — | — |
|  | 1 p.p.m. F | Milk | 0.28 | 0.68 | 0.15 | — | — | — |
| Held[89] | 5 mg. F/day (5 days) | Tea | 0.28 | — | 0.27 | — | — | — |
| Held[90] | 25 mg. F/day (21 days) + 1.5 mg. F/day (45 days) | Pill | 0.24 | — | 0.21 | — | — | — |
| Feltman and Kosel[91] | Control | Tablet | — | 1.01 | 0.17 | — | — | — |
|  | 1 mg. F (NaF, Na$_2$PO$_3$F, or CaF$_2$ for 7 years) | Tablet | — | 1.11 | 0.41 | — | — | — |
| Feltman and Kosel[91] | 1 mg. F (NaF, Na$_2$PO$_3$F, or CaF$_2$ for 8 years) | Tablet | — | 0.90 | 0.22 | — | — | — |
| Feltman and Kosel[91] | Control | Tablet | — | 1.06 | 0.13 | — | — | — |
|  | 1 mg. F (NaF, Na$_2$PO$_3$F, or CaF$_2$ for 13 years) | Tablet | — | 1.26 | 0.36 | — | — | — |

*Nonpregnant women.

during pregnancy resulted in increasing amounts of fluoride in the maternal blood, placenta, and fetal blood, suggesting that fluoride may pass the human placenta. In addition, analyses conducted on various fetal hard tissues indicate that similar increases in the fluoride content of these tissues occur with increasing concentrations of fluoride in the drinking water. The data also suggest that the use of prenatal fluoride tablets may result in concentrations of fluoride in the placenta and fetal blood comparable to that noted in the presence of fluoridated drinking water, although this relationship has not been examined simultaneously in the same study.

Little information has been offered to suggest an influence of prenatal fluoride upon the subsequent development of dental caries. The first report of this nature

Table 6-8. *Mean number of DMF and def teeth of children who ingested NaF tablets and data reported from other studies, after 10 years of fluoridation and after use of a natural fluoride water**

| Age group (years) | NaF tablets deft ± SE§ | NaF tablets DMFT ± SE | Aurora, Illinois† deft | Aurora, Illinois† DMFT | Grand Rapids, Mich.‡ Base line deft | Grand Rapids, Mich.‡ Base line DMFT | Grand Rapids, Mich.‡ 10 years of F deft | Grand Rapids, Mich.‡ 10 years of F DMFT | Brantford, Ontario‡ deft | Brantford, Ontario‡ DMFT |
|---|---|---|---|---|---|---|---|---|---|---|
| 4-5 | 1.2 ± 0.6 | — | 2.7 | — | 5.2 | — | 2.5 | — | 2.6 | — |
| 6-9 | 1.8 ± 0.4 | 0.6 ± 0.2 | 3.4 | 0.8 | 5.8 | 2.3 | 3.1 | 1.0 | 3.4 | 0.9 |
| 10-12 | 0.9 ± 0.3 | 2.2 ± 0.3 | 1.3 | 2.5 | 1.5 | 6.5 | 1.6 | 2.9 | 1.4 | 2.8 |
| 13-15 | — | 4.5 ± 0.9 | — | 3.8 | — | 11.0 | — | 6.7 | — | 5.0 |

*From Feltman, R., and Kosel, G.: J. Dent. Med. 16:190, 1961.
†Aurora—a natural fluoride water.
‡Grand Rapids and Brantford—fluoridated water.
§SE—standard error.

Table 6-9. *Dental caries data in deciduous teeth after 13 years of fluoridation at Evanston, Illinois**

| Year | Number of years of fluoridation | Six: Age at time of first exposure (years) | Six: deft rate | Six: Change from 1946 (percent) | Seven: Age at time of first exposure (years) | Seven: deft rate | Seven: Change from 1946 (percent) | Eight: Age at time of first exposure (years) | Eight: deft rate | Eight: Change from 1946 (percent) |
|---|---|---|---|---|---|---|---|---|---|---|
| 1946 | None | | 4.83 | | | 5.50 | | | 5.77 | |
| 1948 | 1 | 5 | 5.08 | + 5.16 | 6 | 5.41 | – 1.64 | 7 | 6.20 | +74.58 |
| 1950 | 3 | 3 | 4.78 | – 0.93 | 4 | 6.68 | + 2.14 | 5 | 6.54 | +13.22 |
| 1951 | 4 | 2 | 5.00 | – 6.00 | 3 | 5.50 | + 1.49 | 4 | 6.75 | +16.87 |
| 1953 | 6 | Birth | 4.33 | –10.37 | 1 | 5.18 | – 5.86 | 2 | 5.99 | + 3.71 |
| 1955 | 8 | Preconception | 3.09 | –35.91 | In utero | 4.04 | –26.64 | Birth | 4.78 | –17.21 |
| 1958 | 11 | Preconception | 3.36 | –30.32 | Preconception | 3.78 | –31.24 | Preconception | 3.83 | –33.62 |
| 1960 | 13 | Preconception | 3.30 | –31.74 | Preconception | 3.64 | –33.85 | Preconception | 4.11 | –28.80 |

*From Blayney, J. R., and Hill, I. N.: J.A.D.A. 69:291, 1964. Copyright by the American Dental Association. Reprinted by permission.

was made by Feltman and Kosel[87]; their data are summarized in Table 6-8. These investigators found that the use of prenatal sodium fluoride tablets resulted in a significant decrease in the incidence of dental caries in the deciduous dentition comparable to that observed in areas of natural and artificially fluoridated water supplies such as in Aurora, Illinois, Grand Rapids, Michigan, and Brantford, Ontario. Blayney and Hill[82] have reported similar findings after 13 years of fluoridation in the dental caries study at Evanston, Illinois; these data are presented in Table 6-9. A rearrangement of the dental caries data, reported from other classic artificial communal fluoridation studies such as the study given in Table 6-10, support these findings. The results of a survey conducted by Katz and Muhler[92] are summarized in Table 6-11 and indicate similar conclusions, namely, that the presence of fluoride in the drinking water for 8 years or longer results in significant reductions in the prevalence of dental caries in the deciduous dentition. However, Carlos and associates[93] failed to find any influence of communal fluoride on dental caries in deciduous teeth after 2 years of fluoridation. Likewise, Horowitz and Heifetz[94] failed to observe any added beneficial influence on dental caries in the deciduous dentition of fluoridation initiated up to 1 year prior to the birth of children. Other reports[82] have noted that a signficant effect on the deciduous dentition is apparent only after several years of fluoridation; this factor may well explain the negative findings of Carlos and associates and those of Horowitz and Heifetz.

The only reported study investigating the influence of prenatal fluoride tablets upon dental caries involved tablets containing only the fluoride compound and inert fillers. Unfortunately the prenatal preparations now commercially available and commonly prescribed contain a variety of vitamins and minerals, and many of these minerals, particularly calcium, have been shown[96] to significantly reduce the metabolic availability of the fluoride. The results of a study[97] conducted to determine

Table 6-10. *Effectiveness of fluoridation on caries experience in deciduous teeth in relation to the age at which children (or their mothers) began to be exposed to fluoride**

| Study | Age (years) | \-2 | \-1 | 0 | 1 | 2 | 3 | 4 | 5 | 6 | 7 | 8 | 9 | 10 |
|---|---|---|---|---|---|---|---|---|---|---|---|---|---|---|
| Grand Rapid, Michigan | 4 | 2.5 | 2.7 | 3.0 | 3.2 | 3.4 | 5.4 | 4.2 | | | | | | |
| | 5 | 2.3 | 2.5 | 3.3 | 4.0 | 3.9 | 5.1 | 6.1 | 5.4 | | | | | |
| | 6 | 2.9 | 3.8 | 4.0 | 4.6 | 4.8 | 5.4 | 5.7 | 7.0 | 6.4 | | | | |
| | 7 | 3.1 | 3.5 | 3.9 | 4.1 | 4.8 | 5.2 | 5.8 | 6.1 | 7.7 | 6.3 | | | |
| | 8 | 3.3 | 3.5 | 3.3 | 4.1 | 4.9 | 4.7 | 5.1 | 5.1 | 5.1 | 8.0 | 5.8 | | |
| | 9 | | 3.0 | 2.3 | 3.7 | 3.9 | 4.2 | 4.4 | 4.1 | 4.1 | 4.4 | — | 4.6 | |
| | 10 | | | | 2.4 | 2.6 | 2.4 | 2.4 | 2.9 | 3.2 | 3.2 | 2.8 | — | 2.9 |
| Brantford, Ontario | 5 | 2.7 | 3.0 | 2.6 | 3.1 | 3.0 | 4.1 | 4.1 | 5.4 | | | | | |
| | 6 | 3.2 | 3.2 | 3.4 | 3.9 | 3.6 | 4.7 | 4.9 | 5.7 | 6.5 | | | | |
| | 7 | 3.5 | 3.7 | 3.8 | 4.4 | 4.1 | 5.1 | 5.2 | 6.1 | 6.4 | 6.7 | | | |
| | 8 | | 4.0 | 3.7 | 4.6 | 4.2 | 5.3 | 5.3 | 5.9 | 6.4 | 6.5 | 6.5 | | |
| | 9 | | | 3.3 | 4.2 | 3.9 | 4.9 | 4.7 | 5.1 | 5.1 | 5.4 | 5.7 | 6.0 | |
| | 10 | | | | 2.9 | 2.8 | 3.4 | 3.2 | 4.5 | 3.9 | 3.6 | 3.8 | 4.1 | 4.0 |

*Data from Arnold, F. A., Jr., and others: Public Health Rep. 71:652, 1956, and the Ontario Department of Health.

**Table 6-11.** *Influence of fluoride ingested prenatally in drinking water on prevalence of dental caries in children**

|  | Deciduous teeth ||||  Permanent teeth ||||
|---|---|---|---|---|---|---|---|---|
| Study | Mean age (years) | Number of subjects | Mean deft | Mean defs | Mean age (years) | Number of subjects | Mean DMFT | Mean DMFS |
| Bloomington, Indiana† | 4.5 | 14 | 4.1 | 5.9 | 5.6 | 70 | 0.2 | 0.2 |
|  | 5.6 | 70 | 3.9 | 7.1 | 6.6 | 91 | 1.0 | 1.2 |
|  | 6.6 | 91 | 5.5 | 11.7 | 7.4 | 16 | 2.0 | 3.0 |
|  | 7.4 | 16 | 5.2 | 11.5 | 8.6 | 15 | 3.3 | 5.4 |
| Muncie, Indiana‡ | 5.7 | 86 | 2.3 | 4.5 | 5.7 | 86 | 0.07 | 0.09 |
|  | 6.5 | 118 | 3.7 | 7.9 | 6.5 | 118 | 0.7 | 0.9 |
|  | 7.2 | 37 | 3.3 | 7.9 | 7.2 | 37 | 1.2 | 1.5 |
| West Lafayette, Indiana§ | 4.6 | 13 | 1.3 | 2.2 | 5.5 | 24 | — | — |
|  | 5.5 | 24 | 1.5 | 1.9 | 6.6 | 16 | 0.3 | 0.3 |
|  | 6.6 | 16 | 3.4 | 6.1 | 7.2 | 7 | 0.6 | 0.6 |
|  | 7.2 | 7 | 2.3 | 4.4 |  |  |  |  |
| Indianapolis, Indiana‖ | 4.5 | 10 | 0.8 | 1.4 | 5.6 | 45 | 0.1 | 0.15 |
|  | 5.6 | 45 | 2.1 | 3.3 | 6.6 | 112 | 0.6 | 0.8 |
|  | 6.6 | 112 | 2.1 | 3.9 | 7.4 | 83 | 1.1 | 1.5 |
|  | 7.4 | 83 | 2.3 | 4.8 |  |  |  |  |
| Frankfort, Indiana¶ | 4.6 | 20 | 1.0 | 1.6 | 5.8 | 70 | 0.04 | 0.04 |
|  | 5.8 | 70 | 2.6 | 4.7 | 6.6 | 170 | 0.4 | 0.4 |
|  | 6.6 | 170 | 2.9 | 6.1 | 7.3 | 68 | 0.7 | 1.0 |
|  | 7.3 | 68 | 3.5 | 7.6 | 8.3 | 16 | 0.9 | 1.7 |

*From Katz, S., and Muhler, J. C.: Prenatal fluoride and dental caries experience in deciduous teeth, J.A.D.A. 76:305, 1968.
†Nonfluoride area.
‡Survey conducted after 8 years of artificial fluoridation.
§Survey conducted after 9 years of artificial fluoridation.
‖Survey conducted after 12 years of artificial fluoridation.
¶Natural fluoride area (1 p.p.m. F).

the metabolic availability of the fluoride in a typical commercial prenatal tablet preparation as evaluated by skeletal fluoride retention in the rat are summarized in Table 6-12. These data indicate that the presence of the minerals in the prenatal supplement reduced the utilization of the fluoride by about 40 percent. Thus while the available data suggest a prenatal influence of fluoride upon dental caries in the deciduous dentition after several years of maternal fluoride exposure no evidence is available to support the usefulness of presently available prenatal preparations containing vitamins and minerals. Until such information is available one cannot recommend such preparations as a substitute for communal fluoridation.

**Fluoridated salt**

The use of table salt containing fluoride, either added intentionally or present as a natural constituent, such as in sea salt, has been suggested as an alternative means of providing fluoride to the developing dentition. It has been suggested[98] that, since the average daily per capita consumption of salt is 9 Gm., the addition of

Table 6-12. *Fluoride content of carcasses and femurs of rats provided fluoride either alone or in a typical commercially available prenatal supplement*[97]

| Group | Number of animals | Regimen | Carcass Ash weight (Gm.) | Carcass p.p.m. F | Carcass Total μg F | Femur Ash weight (mg.) | Femur p.p.m. F | Femur Total μg F | Net retention (percent) |
|---|---|---|---|---|---|---|---|---|---|
| A | 11 | Control diet | 5.27 ±0.38* | 261 ± 41 | 1,377 ± 246 | 363 ±32 | 343 ± 57 | 125 ± 27 | — |
| B | 13 | Control diet + fluoride | 5.18 ±0.37 | 3,558 ±410 | 18,335 ±1,931 | 376 ±29 | 5,112 ±552 | 1,919 ±276 | 62.5 |
| C | 12 | Prenatal supplement diet | 5.32 ±0.60 | 219 ± 76 | 1,177 ± 449 | 356 ±41 | 284 ± 90 | 103 ± 37 | — |
| D | 13 | Prenatal supplement diet + fluoride | 5.27 ±0.40 | 2,256 ±424 | 11,827 ±2,037 | 372 ±39 | 2,788 ±279 | 1,039 ±125 | 38.6 |

*Standard error of the mean.

200 mg. sodium fluoride per kilogram of salt would provide an equivalent amount of fluoride to that received by ingesting drinking water containing 0.7 to 0.9 p.p.m. fluoride. Although a slight reduction in the incidence of dental caries was noted when a slightly greater level of fluoride (280 mg. sodium fluoride per kilogram sodium chloride) was employed by Marthaler[99] in a 5-year clinical study involving 662 children 8 to 14 years of age, he concluded that the failure of the fluoride supplementation to provide the expected results was due primarily to the fact that the amount of fluoride ingested in the salt was only about half the optimal level. Similarly, since sea salt normally contains about 40 p.p.m. fluoride, the use of this material would require a daily consumption of about 25 Gm. to provide 1 mg. fluoride. Although certain people, particularly in the Far East, ingest these quantities daily,[100] very little is known concerning the influence on dental caries of fluoride ingested in this manner. Very little data are available concerning this method as an alternative means of providing fluoride therapy, and until much additional information is provided, particularly with regard to the regulation of fluoride consumption and clinical effectiveness, such a procedure should not be recommended.

**Fluoridated milk**

The use of fluoridated milk has been suggested[88] as a substitute for communal fluoridation but has received only limited support. Muhler and Weddle[101] noted that, in the rat, less fluoride was metabolically available when ingested in milk as compared to water. Muhler and associates[65] reported similar findings in human beings, while Ericsson[102] noted that, although the absorption of fluoride from milk was less complete than that observed from water, the elevated level of fluoride in the blood remained for a longer period of time when the fluoride was ingested in milk. Light and others[103] have suggested that the use of fluoridated milk resulted in complete caries prevention in a study involving a single family. Kopel[104] has reported that the provision of children 6 to 10 years of age with 1 mg. fluoride added to a half pint of milk provided with the school lunch resulted in an 80 percent reduction in the incidence of dental caries. Rusoff and associates[105] have similarly reported a marked reduction in the incidence of caries in children, associated with the ingestion of fluoride in milk. Nevertheless, much additional information is needed regarding the variation in the amount of ingestion of milk; further evidence of efficacy prior to the establishment of this procedure as a substitute for communal fluoridation is also necessary.

### Miscellaneous alternatives

A variety of additional alternative procedures have been suggested as a substitute for communal fluoridation, but little or no information is available to support these suggestions. For example, Ege[106] has suggested that the addition of 3.5 mg. fluoride per kilogram of breakfast cereal would be a convenient and efficient means of providing fluoride in Denmark since 98 percent of the population of that country regularly ingests cereals; this level of fluoride fortification would provide 0.6 to 1.5 mg. fluoride daily, depending on the amount of cereal ingested. Emslie and associates[107] have suggested the possibility of fluoride-enriched chewing gum and have reported that 80 to 90 percent of fluoride, added to chewing gum as either radioactive sodium fluoride or stannous fluoride, was released within 15 minutes of chewing. Lind and others[108] employed a gum containing 25.5 mg. potassium fluoride in a clinical study involving 229 11-year-old children. Under supervision, the children chewed the gum five times during a 6-month period; the investigators reported a caries reduction of about 15 percent, a value that was not statistically significant. Still other suggested means have been offered; however, none of these procedures has undergone enough investigation to be considered further as alternative means of providing systemic fluoride therapy at the present time.

## TOPICAL FLUORIDE THERAPY

It is apparent that not only is systemic fluoride, as provided from communal fluoridation, only partially effective in controlling dental caries, but it further requires the presence of a communal water supply and ingestion during the first 10 to 12 years of life to achieve the maximal degree of caries protection of about 60 percent of the population. It has further been shown that, at the present time, only a maximum of one-third of the population receives the benefits of either naturally or artificially fluoridated drinking water and that, even today, additional methods of controlling dental caries are needed.

Since the discovery of the anticariogenic properties of fluoride, one of the most significant advances has been the development of various means of applying fluorides to the erupted dentition to partially prevent the subsequent development of dental caries. In the past 30 years the use of topical fluoride applications, fluoride-containing dentifrices, prophylactic pastes, mouthwashes, and multiple combinations of treatments have been proposed and evaluated. With the exception of dentifrices, which will be described in Chapter 7, all of the various approaches to topical fluoride therapy will be considered.

### Topical sodium fluoride therapy

The clinical studies utilizing topical applications of sodium fluoride are summarized in Tables 6-13 to 6-15. The first clinical study with sodium fluoride was reported by Bibby[109] in 1942 and indicated that the use of the half-mouth technic in which two quadrants of each mouth served as control for the two treated quadrants and a series of three applications of 0.1 percent sodium fluoride in children resulted in caries reductions of about 31 percent after one year. Bibby and Turesky[110] subsequently reported reductions of 27.6 and 29.8 percent after 2 and 5 years, respectively. Knutson and Armstrong[111-113] employed a similar technic except that the number of initial fluoride applications was increased and the concentration of the sodium fluoride solution was 2 percent. These investigators reported reductions in DFT of 39.7, 41.4, and 36.7 percent, and in DFS of 23.4, 34.6, and 32.8 percent after 1, 2, and 3 years, respectively. Within the next decade numerous studies were reported (as shown in Table 6-13), and a variety of factors were investigated clinically. For example, it was reported by Knutson and associates[117] that four applications were required for maximal effectiveness and that a thorough prophylaxis prior to the topical applications was essential. It was further noted that repeated applications at yearly intervals were necessary to maintain a beneficial effect. A review of the literature indicates that, while a wide range of degrees of effectiveness have been reported, the majority of reported results have indicated that the use of four applications of sodium fluoride, applied according to the technic of Knutson,[118] results in caries reductions of 30 to 40 percent in the permanent teeth of children residing in an area where the water supply is fluoride deficient.

Only two reports[155, 156] have appeared regarding the efficacy of topically applied sodium fluoride in children reared in an optimal fluoride area. As shown in Table 6-13, both of these reports were essentially negative and indicate that this means of caries prevention is of little value in an optimal fluoride area.

The results reported following topical applications of sodium fluoride on deciduous teeth are summarized in Table 6-14. The results obtained in nonfluoride areas are less than those found in the permanent dentition, and one might conclude that this procedure results in about 25 to 30 percent fewer carious lesions. Only one study[161] has been reported pertaining to the use of this technic in a fluoride area, and these investigators found reductions of 21 and 12 percent in deft and defs, respectively. These latter data suggest that this procedure may be of only limited value in an optimal fluoride area.

The clinical dental caries studies concerning the use of sodium fluoride in adults are summarized in Table 6-15. It may be seen that five of the seven studies have been negative, although two studies[164, 166] suggested significant benefit. No studies have been reported utilizing this procedure in adults residing in an optimal fluoride area. As a result it has been generally concluded that sodium fluoride applied topically is of little value for adults.

**Topical stannous fluoride therapy**

Following the early findings that topical applications of sodium fluoride were beneficial in partially preventing the subsequent development of dental caries, an attempt was made to find related agents that might be of even greater value in controlling dental caries. While a variety of compounds were suggested from various laboratory evaluation procedures (and will be subsequently discussed), the agent that drew major attention was stannous fluoride.

Thus stannous fluoride, following its critical evaluation in the laboratory, was employed in a considerable number of clinical studies. The studies that evaluate the influence of topically applied stannous fluoride in the permanent dentition of

*Text continued on p. 124.*

**114**  *Improving dental practice through preventive measures*

**Table 6-13.** *A review of clinical dental caries studies using topically applied sodium areas*

| Study | Number of subjects | Technic | Initial age of subjects (years) | Prophylaxis |
|---|---|---|---|---|
| *Nonfluoride area* | | | | |
| Bibby[109] | 90 | Half-mouth | 10-12 | Yes |
| | 80 | | | |
| Bibby and Turesky[110] | 39 | Half-mouth | 10-12 | Yes |
| Knutson and Armstrong[111-113] | 289 | Half-mouth | 7-15 | Yes |
| | 270 | | | |
| | 242 | | | |
| McCauley and Dale[114] | 21 | Half-mouth | 2-13 | No |
| Jordan and others[115] | 241 | Half-mouth | 6-12 | Yes |
| | 575 | | | |
| | 161 | | | |
| Fulton and Tracy[116] | 69 | Whole-mouth | | Yes |
| Knutson and others[117] | 472 | Half-mouth | 7-15 | No |
| | 504 | | | |
| | 482 | | | |
| Galagan and Knutson[119] | 301 | Half-mouth | 7-15 | Yes |
| | 247 | | | |
| | 249 | | | |
| Galagan and Knutson[120] | 304 | Half-mouth | 6-16 | Yes |
| | 362 | | | Yes |
| | 335 | | | Yes |
| | 276 | | | Yes |
| | 208 | | | No |
| | 371 | | | Yes |
| | 272 | | | Yes |
| Tschappat[121] | 213 | Half-mouth | 12-14 | |
| Hewat and Rice[122] | 97 | Half-mouth | 5-13 | Yes |
| Syrrist[123] | 116 | Half-mouth | 12 | Yes |
| Miller[124] | 73 | Whole-mouth | 6-14 | Yes |
| Davies[125] | 146 | Whole-mouth | 9-12 | Yes |
| Floren[126] | 94 | Half-mouth | | Yes |

\*Applications spaced at 3-month intervals.
†Applications spaced at 6-month intervals.
‡Applications of NaF followed by single application of 5 percent CaCl₂.
§Used 2 weeks of supervised toothbrushing in place of prophylaxis.
‖Applications made at 3- to 4-month intervals.
¶Treated at 6-month intervals over 3-year period.
\*\*Reapplications made at 6-month intervals.
††Reported as DPT and DFS.

*fluoride evaluated in permanent teeth of children residing in nonfluoride and fluoride*

| Fluoride concentration (percent) | Number of applications | Length of application (minutes) | Years after initial application | Reduction (percent) DMFT | DMFS |
|---|---|---|---|---|---|
| 0.1 | 3 | 4 | 1 | — | 45.9 |
|  | 6 | 4 | 2 | — | 27.6 |
| 0.1 | 6 | 4 | 5 | — | 29.8 |
| 2 | 7-15 | 3 | 1 | 39.7†† | 23.4 |
|  | 7-15 | 3 | 2 | 41.4 | 34.6 |
|  | 7-15 | 3 | 3 | 36.7 | 32.8 |
| 0.1 | 3-11 | 1 | 1 | 0 | 0 |
| 2 | 1 | 1-2 | 1 | 4.9 | 8.3 |
|  | 2 | 1-2 | 1 | 10.0 | 17.0 |
|  | 3 | 1-2 | 1 | 21.0 | 16.4 |
| 2 | 2 | 1-2 | 1 |  | 53.0 |
| 2 | 2 | 4 | 2 | 9.3 | 11.7 |
|  | 4 | 4 | 2 | 20.1 | 15.6 |
|  | 6 | 4 | 2 | 21.3 | 21.2 |
| 2 | 2 | 4 | 1 | 21.7 | 13.5 |
|  | 4 | 4 | 1 | 40.7 | 33.7 |
|  | 6 | 4 | 1 | 41.0 | 28.3 |
| 2 | 3* | 3-4 | 1 | 26.7 | 24.1 |
| 2 | 2† | 3-4 | 1 | 14.6 | 13.1 |
| 1 | 2 | 3-4 | 1 | 14.7 | 12.1 |
| 1 | 4 | 3-4 | 1 | 39.2 | 32.0 |
| 2‡ | 2 | 3-4 | 1 | +10.3 | + 8.7 |
| 2 | 2 | 3-4 | 1 | 20.3 | 13.3 |
| 2 | 4 | 3-4 | 1 | 32.4 | 27.0 |
| 1 | 1 | 4 | 1 |  | 5.0 |
| 1 | 2 | 4 | 1 |  | 22.0 |
| 2 | 12 | 4 | 1 | 18.8 | 36.4 |
| 2 | 7 | 7-8 | 2 | 8.4 | 3.2 |
| 1 | 4† | 2 | 2 | 0 | 0 |
| 2 | 4 | 3-4 | 1 |  | 58.3 |
| 4 | 3 | 4 | 2 |  | 0 |

**Table 6-13.** *A review of clinical dental caries studies using topically applied sodium areas—cont'd*

| Study | Number of subjects | Technic | Initial age of subjects (years) | Prophylaxis |
|---|---|---|---|---|
| *Nonfluoride area—cont'd* | | | | |
| Chrietzenberg[127] | 234 | Whole-mouth | 6-12 | Yes§ |
| | 230 | Whole-mouth | 6-12 | Yes |
| Hewat and others[128] | 111 | Half-mouth | 13-14 | Yes |
| Marshall-Day[129] | 100 | Half-mouth | 14-15 | |
| Abary-Murillo[39] | 20 | Whole-mouth | 10-16 | Yes |
| Adler[130] | 400 | Half-mouth | 7-12 | Yes |
| Adler[131] | 4,621 | Half-mouth | 8-14 | Yes |
| Walton[132] | 80 | Whole-mouth | 8-12 | Yes |
| Bergman[133] | 114 | Half-mouth | 11-12 | Yes |
| Cohen and Schiffrin[134] | 95 | Whole-mouth | 6-16 | Yes |
| | 87 | | | |
| Sarkany[135] | 447 | Half-mouth | 7-14 | Yes |
| Hawes and others[136] | 46 | Half-mouth | | Yes |
| Syrrist and Karlsen[137] | 91 | Half-mouth | 12 | Yes |
| University of Toronto[138] | 238 | Whole-mouth | | Yes |
| Howell and others[139] | 92 | Whole-mouth | 6-16 | Yes |
| McLaren and Brown[140] | 483 | Half-mouth | 6-11 | Yes |
| | 405 | | | |
| Schutzmannsky[141] | 418 | Half-mouth | 7-13 | Yes |
| Kimmelman[142] | 89 | Half-mouth | 5-16 | Yes |
| Dominick and Wodniecki[143] | 566 | Whole-mouth | 7-16 | Yes |
| | 233 | Half-mouth | | |
| Nevitt and others[144] | 298 | Half-mouth | 9-14 | Yes |
| Czarnocka and others[145] | 312 | Whole-mouth | 7-13 | Yes |
| Harris[146] | 429 | Whole-mouth | 6-11 | Yes |
| Miller and Hobson[147] | 12 | Whole-mouth | 3-6 | Yes |
| | 44 | Whole-mouth | | |
| Berggren and Welander[148] | 568 | Whole-mouth | 7-14 | Yes |
| Mercer and Muhler[149] | 151 | Whole-mouth | 6-14 | Yes |

Fluoride therapy 117

fluoride evaluated in permanent teeth of children residing in nonfluoride and fluoride

| Fluoride concentration (percent) | Number of applications | Length of application (minutes) | Years after initial application | Reduction (percent) DMFT | Reduction (percent) DMFS |
|---|---|---|---|---|---|
| 2 | 4 | 3-4 | 1 | 49.3 | |
| 2 | 4 | 3-4 | 1 | 46.5 | |
| 2 | 4 | 3 | 1 | | 17.8 |
| 2 | 4 | 3-4 | 1 | 11.2 | 9.5 |
| 2 | 5 | 3-4 | 0.5 | | 92.9 |
| 2 | 4 | 4 | 1 | 0 | 0 |
| 2 | 4 | 4 | 1 | 0 | 0 |
| 2 | 4 | 3-4 | 2 | 43.0 | |
| 2 | 4 | 5 | 3 | | 54.0 |
| 2 | 4 | 3-4 | 1 | | 42.6 |
| 2 | 4 | 3-4 | 2 | | 43.8 |
| 2 | 4 | 4 | 1 | 0 | 0 |
| 1 | 4.9 | | 3 | | 30.0 |
| 2 | 7¶ | 7-8 | 2 | 48.5 | 47.0 |
|  |  |  | 5 | 13.2 | 21.0 |
| 2 | 2 | 4 | 2 | | 30.0 |
| 2 | 4 | 4 | 2 | 23.6 | 36.3 |
| 2 | 4 | 3-4 | 1 | | 38.6 |
|  |  |  | 2 | | 17.6 |
| 2 | 1 | 4 | 1 | | 36.4 |
|  | 1 |  | 2 | | 20.0 |
|  | 2 |  | 3 | | 38.5 |
|  | 2 |  | 4 | | 22.2 |
|  | 3 |  | 5 | | 28.6 |
| 2 | 1 | 7-12 | 1 | | |
| 2 | 6¶ | 4 | 5 | | 35.5 |
|  |  |  | 5 | | |
| 2 | 4 | 4 | 1.33 | 35.9 | 22.6 |
| 2 | 9** | 2-5 | 5 | | 33.4 |
| 2 | 4 | 3 | 5 | 44.3 | |
| 1 | 12 | 2 | 2 | 73.3 | |
|  | 12 | 2 | 2 | 0 | |
| 1 | 9 | 4 | 2 | 25-30 | 25-30 |
| 2 | 1 | 4 | 1 | 0 | 0 |

**118** *Improving dental practice through preventive measures*

**Table 6-13.** *A review of clinical dental caries studies using topically applied sodium areas—cont'd*

| Study | Number of subjects | Technic | Initial age of subjects (years) | Prophylaxis |
|---|---|---|---|---|
| *Nonfluoride area—cont'd* | | | | |
| Law and others[150] | 269 | Half-mouth | 7-13 | Yes |
| Torell and Ericsson[151] | 159 | Whole-mouth | 10 | Yes |
| Badzian-Kobos[152] | 50 | Half-mouth | 6-8 | Yes |
| Averill and others[153] | 242 | Whole-mouth | 7-11 | Yes |
| Cons and Janerich[154] | 270 | Whole-mouth | 6-11 | Yes |
| *Fluoride area* | | | | |
| Downs and Pelton[155] | 600 | Half-mouth | 6-18 | Yes |
| Galagan and Vermillion[156] | 282 | Half-mouth | 7-16 | Yes |

**Table 6-14.** *Review of clinical dental caries using topically applied sodium fluoride on*

| Study | Number of subjects | Technic | Initial age of subjects (years) | Prophylaxis |
|---|---|---|---|---|
| *Nonfluoride area* | | | | |
| Jordan and others[115] | 241 | Half-mouth | 6-12 | Yes |
| | 575 | Half-mouth | 6-12 | Yes |
| | 161 | Half-mouth | 6-12 | Yes |
| Ast[157] | 260 | Half-mouth | 2-7 | Yes |
| Jordan[158] | 152 | Whole-mouth | 4-6 | Yes |
| Wittich[159] | 40 | Half-mouth | 3-6 | Yes |
| Sarkany[135] | 447 | Half-mouth | 7-14 | Yes |
| Sundvall-Hagland[160] | 107 | Half-mouth | 3-5 | Yes |
| *Fluoride area* | | | | |
| McDonald and Muhler[161] | 76 | Whole-mouth | 3-12 | Yes |

*Reductions based upon comparison to comparable group of children.

**Table 6-15.** *Review of clinical dental caries studies using topically applied sodium fluoride*

| Study | Number of subjects | Technic | Fluoride water supply | Initial age of subjects (years) |
|---|---|---|---|---|
| Arnold and others[162] | 94 | Whole-mouth | No | 17-23 |
| Frank[163] | 35 | Half-mouth | No | 20-25 |
| Klinkenberg and Bibby[164] | 139 | Half-mouth | No | 18-40 |
| Driak[165] | 72 | Half-mouth | No | 24-29 |
| Rickles and Becks[166] | 47 | Half-mouth | No | 22-34 |
| Kutler and Ireland[167] | 147 | Half-mouth | No | 20-42 |
| Carter and others[168] | 60 | Whole-mouth | No | 19-39 |

*fluoride evaluated in permanent teeth of children residing in nonfluoride and fluoride*

| Fluoride concentration (percent) | Number of applications | Length of application (minutes) | Years after initial application | Reduction (percent) DMFT | DMFS |
|---|---|---|---|---|---|
| 2 | 4 | 4 | 1 | 35.0 | 35.3 |
| 2 | 4 | 3-4 | 2 |  | 19.8 |
| 2 | 24 | 4 | 2 | 62.8 |  |
| 2 | 4 | 1-2 | 2 | 16.0 | 11.4 |
| 2 | 4 | 4 | 3 | 17.2 | 11.2 |
| 2 | 4 | 3-4 | 1 | 0.4 | 0 |
| 2 | 4 | 3-4 | 1 | 8.9 |  |

*deciduous teeth of children residing in nonfluoride and fluoride areas*

| Fluoride concentration (percent) | Number of applications | Length of application (minutes) | Years after initial application | Reduction (percent) deft | defs |
|---|---|---|---|---|---|
| 2 | 1 | 3-4 | 1 | 4.9 | + 3.1 |
| 2 | 2 | 3-4 | 1 | 14.5 | 10.1 |
| 2 | 3 | 3-4 | 1 | 40.0 | 16.7 |
| 2 | 4 | 3-4 | 1 |  | 22.0 |
| 2 | 3-4 | 3-4 | 3 | 33.6 |  |
| 2 | 4 | 3-4 | 2 |  | 22.2 |
| 2 | 4 | 3-4 | 1 |  | 32.0 |
| 2 | 4 |  | 1 |  | 19 (34)* |
|   |   |   | 2 |  | 14 (23) |
|   |   |   | 3 |  | 77 (12) |
| 2 | 4 | 4 | 1 | 21.0 | 12.0 |

*in adults*

| Prophylaxis | Fluoride concentration (percent) | Number of applications | Length of application (minutes) | Years after initial application | Reduction (percent) DMFT | DMFS |
|---|---|---|---|---|---|---|
| Yes | 1 | 1 | 5 | 1 | 0 | 0 |
| Yes | 2 | 1 |  | 0.5 | 0 | 0 |
| Yes | 1 | 5 | 4 | 1 | 47.3 | 44.5 |
| Yes | 2 | 1 |  | 3 | 0 | 0 |
| Yes | 2 | 4 | 4 | 2 | 18.8 | 36.8 |
| Yes | 2 | 4 | 4 | 1 | 0 | 0 |
| Yes | 2 | 4 | 4 | 1 | 12.0 |  |

120  *Improving dental practice through preventive measures*

**Table 6-16.** *Review of clinical dental caries studies using topically applied stannous*

| Study | Number of subjects | Technic | Initial age of subjects (years) | Prophylaxis |
|---|---|---|---|---|
| *Nonfluoride area* | | | | |
| Howell and others[139] | 194<br>195 | Whole-mouth | 6-16 | Yes |
| McLaren and Brown[140] | 483<br>405 | Whole-mouth | 6-11<br>6-11 | Yes |
| Slack[169] | 328 | Half-mouth | | Yes |
| Slack[170] | 299 | Half-mouth | 6 | Yes |
| Muhler[171] | 45 | Whole-mouth | 6-15 | Yes |
| Jordan and others[172] | 234 | Whole-mouth | 12-13 | Yes |
| Jordan and others[173] | 209 | | | |
| Abdul-Ghaffar and Muhler[174] | 185<br>182 | Whole-mouth | 6-15 | Yes |
| Nevitt and others[144] | 290 | Half-mouth | 9-14 | Yes |
| Rothhaar[175] | 350 | Whole-mouth | 3-15 | Yes |
| Law and others[150] | 273<br>281 | Half-mouth | 7-13 | Yes |
| Mercer and Muhler[149] | 154<br>152 | Whole-mouth | 6-14 | Yes |
| Gish and others[176] | 157<br>170<br>188<br>201<br>192<br>216<br>204<br>203 | Whole-mouth | 6-8 | Yes |
| Salter and others[177] | | Whole-mouth | 6-7 | Yes |
| Thomsen[178] | 51 | Whole-mouth | 8-9 | Yes |
| Peterson and Williamson[179] | 111 | Whole-mouth | 9-13 | Yes |
| Harris[180] | 212 | Half-mouth | 7-12 | Yes |

\*Applied as a spray.
†SnF$_2$ treatment preceded by single application of 4 percent NaF.
‡Applications given at 6-month intervals.
§Variable response according to caries activity before initial treatment.
∥Results obtained on different subjects by second examiner.
¶Reapplication given at end of first year.
\*\*Reductions calculated from comparison of data of children treated with NaF.
††SnF$_2$ topical applications given at 6-month intervals.

## Fluoride therapy

fluoride on permanent teeth of children residing in nonfluoride and fluoride areas

| Fluoride concentration (percent) | Number of applications | Length of application (minutes) | Years after initial application | Reduction (percent) DMFT | Reduction (percent) DMFS |
|---|---|---|---|---|---|
| 2 | 4 | 4 | 2 | 83.1 | 58.8 |
| 2 | 4* | 4 | 2 | 60.9 | 65.5 |
| 2 | 4 | 3-4 | 1 | | 46.3 |
|   | 4 | 3-4 | 2 | | 18.9 |
| 2 | 3 | | 1 | | 24.9 |
| 2 | 3 | 3-4 | 1 | 31.7 | 33.2 |
|   |   |     | 2 | 5.9  | 29.2 |
| 8 | 1 | 4 | 0.25 | 45.0 | 48.0 |
| 8 | 1 | 4 | 1 | 20.0 | 14.4 |
| 8 | 1 | 4 | 2 | 37.9 | 38.3 |
| 8 | 2 | 4 | 1 | 100.0 | 78.2 |
| 8† | 1 | 4 | 1 | 100.0 | 60.6 |
| 2 | 4 | 3-4 | 1.25 | 44.4 | 29.0 |
| 8 | 1‡ | 4 | 3 | | 60-100§ |
|   |    |   | 5 | | 60-100§ |
| 2 | 4 | 3-4 | 1 | 33.8 | 31.6 |
| 8 | 1 | 3-4 | 1 | 18.8 | 24.9 |
| 8 | 1 | 4 | 1 | 50.0 | 51.3 |
| 8 | 2 | 4 | 1 | 53.2 | 53.3 |
| 8 | 1 | 4 | 5 | 30.0** | 35.0 |
| 2 | 4 | 3-4 | 4 | 20.0 | 25.0 |
|   |   |     | 3 | 30.0 | 23.0 |
|   |   |     | 2 | 28.0 | 26.0 |
| 8 | 1 | 4 | 1 | 64.7 | 55.8 |
|   | 2 | 4 | 1 | 29.4 | 29.5 |
| 10 | 1 | 4 | 0.5 | 65.0 | 67.0 |
| 8 | 1¶ | 4 | 2 | 26.2 | 24.2 |
| 8 | 1 | 4 | 3 | 23.6 | |

**Table 6-16.** *Review of clinical dental caries studies using topically applied stannous*

| Study | Number of subjects | Technic | Initial age of subjects (years) | Prophylaxis |
|---|---|---|---|---|
| *Nonfluoride area—cont'd* | | | | |
| Mercer and Muhler[181] | 80 (115)‖ | Whole-mouth | 5-15 | Yes |
| | 82 (117)‖ | | | |
| | 69 ( 96) | | | |
| | 76 (106) | | | |
| | 60 ( 72) | | | |
| | 53 ( 82) | | | |
| Torell and Ericsson[151] | 141 | Whole-mouth | 10 | Yes |
| | 162 | | | |
| Hoskova and Komarek[182] | 235 | Half-mouth | 6 | Yes |
| Wellock and others[183] | 211 | Whole-mouth | 8-12 | Yes |
| Muhler and others[184] | 109 | Whole-mouth | 12-14 | Yes |
| | 103 | | | |
| | 100 | | | |
| Muhler[185] | 250 | Whole-mouth | 6-13 | Yes |
| Hass[186] | 245 | Whole-mouth | 6-12 | No |
| Averill and others[153] | 241 | Whole-mouth | 7-11 | Yes |
| Horowitz and Lucye[187] | 259 | Whole-mouth | 8-10 | Yes |
| | 223 | Whole-mouth | 8-10 | Yes |
| Caprioglio and others[188, 189] | 489 | Whole-mouth | 4-14 | Yes |
| | 489 | Whole-mouth | 4-14 | Yes |
| Cartwright and others[190] | 172 | Whole-mouth | 6-19 | Yes |
| Bordoni and others[191] | 132 | Whole-mouth | 6-12 | Yes |
| Cons and Janerich[154] | 579 | Whole-mouth | 6-11 | Yes |
| *Fluoride area* | | | | |
| Muhler[185] | 232 | Whole-mouth | 6-17 | Yes |
| | 199 | | | |
| Muhler[192] | 176 | Whole-mouth | 6-17 | Yes |
| | 134 | | | |
| | 78 | | | |
| Horowitz and Heifetz[193] | 346 | Whole-mouth | 7-11 | Yes |
| | 306 | Whole-mouth | 7-11 | Yes |
| | 283 | Whole-mouth | 7-11 | Yes |
| | 327 | Whole-mouth | 7-11 | Yes |
| | 289 | Whole-mouth | 7-11 | Yes |
| | 249 | Whole-mouth | 7-11 | Yes |
| Ship and others[194] | 897 | Whole-mouth | 11-14 | Yes |

*fluoride on permanent teeth of children residing in nonfluoride and fluoride areas—cont'd*

| Fluoride concentration (percent) | Number of applications | Length of application (minutes) | Years after initial application | Reduction (percent) DMFT | Reduction (percent) DMFS |
|---|---|---|---|---|---|
| 10 | 1‡ | 0.5 | 0.5 | 84.3 (51.6)‖ | 77.2 (46.2)‖ |
| 8 | 1‡ | 4 | | 84.3 (50.5) | 81.1 (42.8) |
| 10 | | | 1 | 82.0 (47.8) | 77.1 (48.5) |
| 8 | | | | 80.5 (38.0) | 78.3 (39.8) |
| 10 | | | 2 | 66.7 (51.0) | 61.2 (47.6) |
| 8 | | | | 67.8 (44.0) | 69.3 (47.0) |
| 10 | 1 | 4 | 2 | | 3.5 |
| 8 | 1 | 4 | 1 | | 63.0 |
| | | | 2 | | 33.0 |
| 8 | 1 | 4 | 1 | −9.0 | 0 |
| 8 | 1‡ | 4 | 0.25 | 55.0 | 44.0 |
| | | | 0.5 | 52.0 | 53.0 |
| | | | 0.75 | 48.9 | 54.8 |
| 8 | 1‡ | 1 | 0.5 | 51.2 | 52.2 |
| | | | 1 | 54.8 | 51.9 |
| 8 | 1 | 4 | 1 | 30.1 | 21.1 |
| 4 | 4 | 1-2 | 2 | 8.0 | 6.8 |
| 8 | 1 | 4 | 1 | +27.4 | +28.2 |
| 8 | 2 | 4 | 2 | + 2.7 | + 8.3 |
| 8 | 2 | 4 | 2 | 47.5 | 38.5 |
| 8 | 3 | 4 | 3 | 39.5 | 40.2 |
| 8 | 4 | 4 | 2 | 37.5 | |
| 8 | 2-7 | 4 | 3 | | 57-90* |
| 8 | 3 | 4 | 3 | 7.5 | 7.2 |
| 8 | 1†† | 4 | 0.5 | 35.2 | 35.9 |
| 8 | | | 1 | 34.9 | 31.1 |
| 8 | | | 1.5 | 35.6 | 36.1 |
| 8 | | | 2 | 46.4 | 35.3 |
| 8 | | | 2.5 | 54.3 | 49.2 |
| 8 | 1 | 1 | 1 | 16.9 | 10.0 |
| 8 | 2 | | 2 | 20.4 | 12.7 |
| 8 | 3 | | 3 | 20.9 (56.0)* | 21.1 (61.3)* |
| 10 | 1 | 0.5 | 1 | 0.0 | 0.0 |
| 10 | 2 | | 2 | 2.2 | 5.1 |
| 10 | 3 | | 3 | 13.5 (56.0)* | 3.8 (51.6)* |
| 8 | 1 | 4 | 1 | 0.0 | |

children reared in the presence and absence of a fluoridated water supply are summarized in Table 6-16. It may be seen that 24 of the 29 studies have been positive, with five recent studies indicating a failure to find any significant beneficial effect of topically applied stannous fluoride. The remaining studies have shown generally greater reductions than were noted with sodium fluoride. Since it has been shown[195] that the half-mouth experimental technic is not valid because of the intra-oral transfer of fluoride and tin to the untreated quadrant particularly in lower quadrants, the reductions obtained with this experimental procedure may be somewhat lower than the actual value. For the most part these suggestions are borne out from the data reported in Table 6-16. When one considers the studies using the whole-mouth technic and comparable groups for the control values it is apparent that the beneficial influence of topical applications of stannous fluoride, as measured by reductions in subsequent caries development, is of the magnitude of 40 to 60 percent. Only three studies have been reported concerning the effect of topically applied stannous fluoride on permanent teeth developed in the presence of an optimal fluoride water supply. In one study,[192] as shown in Table 6-16, caries reductions of about 50 percent were reported after 2½ years. However, both of the more recent studies failed to indicate a beneficial influence of this treatment procedure.[193, 194]

Table 6-17. *Review of clinical dental caries studies using topically applied stannous*

| Study | Number of subjects | Technic | Initial age of subjects (years) | Prophylaxis |
|---|---|---|---|---|
| *Nonfluoride area* | | | | |
| Compton and others[196] | 112 | Whole-mouth | 2-4 | Yes |
| Salter and others[177] | 92 | Whole-mouth | 6-7 | Yes |
| | | Whole-mouth | 6-7 | Yes |
| Burgess and others[197] | 150 | Whole-mouth | 2-5 | Yes |
| | 121 | | | |
| *Fluoride area* | | | | |
| McDonald and Muhler[161] | 86 | Whole-mouth | 3-12 | Yes |

*Treatments given at yearly intervals.

Table 6-18. *Review of clinical dental caries studies using topically applied stannous*

| Study | Number of subjects | Technic | Initial age of subjects (years) | Prophylaxis |
|---|---|---|---|---|
| Protheroe[198] | 80 | Half-mouth | 17-21 | Yes |
| | 79 | Half-mouth | 17-21 | Yes |
| Muhler[171] | 37 | Whole-mouth | 17-34 | Yes |
| Muhler[199] | 228 | Whole-mouth | 17-38 | Yes |
| Harris and others[200] | 280 (303)† | Whole-mouth | 30.1‡ | Yes |

*Single topical applications made at 6-month intervals.
†Independent data for second examiner.
‡Mean age.

The results obtained when stannous fluoride was applied to the deciduous dentition in the presence and absence of an optimal fluoride water supply are summarized in Table 6-17. It may be seen that the beneficial influence of stannous fluoride approaches a 40 percent reduction in the development of dental caries and, further, that this degree of protection is not influenced by and exists in addition to the beneficial influence of communal fluoridation.

The results obtained in the four studies in which the influence of topically applied stannous fluoride was evaluated in adults are summarized in Table 6-18. All the studies reported a beneficial effect, three reported reductions of 15 to 16 percent in surfaces and 24 to 39 percent in teeth, while a fourth reported about a 45.3 to 54 percent reduction in surfaces. These data indicate that topically applied stannous fluoride, in contrast to sodium fluoride, provides significant benefits to adults.

On numerous occasions in the past several years, discussions have arisen relative to the agent of choice for topical application, particularly with regard to the use of sodium or stannous fluoride. Reviews of this subject have either criticized the studies comparing the efficacy of these agents on a variety of grounds[201] or have left the matter up to the clinician.[202] The results of the studies that directly compare these two compounds are summarized in Table 6-19. While it is true that some criticisms of each study may be offered, there are likewise a number of factors that

*fluoride on deciduous teeth of children residing in nonfluoride and fluoride areas*

| Fluoride concentration (percent) | Number of applications | Length of application (minutes) | Years after initial application | Reduction (percent) deft | Reduction (percent) defs |
|---|---|---|---|---|---|
| 8 | 1 | 4 | 1 |  | 28.0 |
| 8 | 1 | 4 | 1 | 45.2 | 42.4 |
| 8 | 2 | 4 | 1 | 35.6 | 42.8 |
| 8* | 1 | 4 | 1 |  | 14.8 |
|  |  |  | 2 |  | 25.1 |
| 4 | 4 | 4 | 1 | 57.1 | 37.0 |

*fluoride on adults*

| Fluoride concentration (percent) | Number of applications | Length of application (minutes) | Years after initial application | Reduction (percent) DMFT | Reduction (percent) DMFS |
|---|---|---|---|---|---|
| 10 | 1 | 4 | 1 |  | 54.0 |
| 10 | 1 | 4 | 2 |  | 45.3 |
| 10 | 1* | 4 | 1 | 39.0 | 15.0 |
| 10 | 1 | 4 | 1 | 24.0 | 16.0 |
| 10 | 1 | 4 | 1 |  | 15.0 (7.4)† |

**Table 6-19.** *Review of clinical dental caries studies directly comparing the effectiveness of*

| Study | Technic | Initial age of subjects (years) | Fluoride in water supply | Number of subjects | Fluoride compound |
|---|---|---|---|---|---|
| McDonald and Muhler[161] | Whole-mouth | 3-12 | Yes | 86 | $SnF_2$ |
|  | Whole-mouth | 3-12 | Yes | 76 | NaF |
| Mercer and Muhler[149] | Whole-mouth | 6-14 | No | 154 | $SnF_2$ |
|  |  |  |  | 152 | $SnF_2$ |
|  |  |  |  | 151 | NaF |
| McLaren and Brown[140] | Half-mouth | 6-11 | No | 483 | $SnF_2$ |
|  |  |  |  |  | NaF |
|  |  |  |  | 405 | $SnF_2$ |
|  |  |  |  |  | NaF |
| Nevitt and others[144] | Half-mouth | 9-14 | No | 290 | $SnF_2$ |
|  |  |  |  | 298 | NaF |
| Law and others[150] | Half-mouth | 7-13 | No | 273 | $SnF_2$ |
|  |  |  |  | 281 | $SnF_2$ |
|  |  |  |  | 269 | NaF |
| Howell and others[139] | Whole-mouth | 6-16 | No | 194 | $SnF_2$ |
|  |  |  |  | 195 | $SnF_2$ |
|  |  |  |  | 192 | NaF |
| Torell and Ericsson[151] | Whole-mouth | 10 | No | 141 | $SnF_2$ |
|  |  |  |  | 159 | NaF |
| Gish and others[176] | Whole-mouth | 6-8 | No | 157 | $SnF_2$ |
|  |  |  |  | 170 | NaF |
|  |  |  |  | 188 | $SnF_2$ |
|  |  |  |  | 201 | NaF |
|  |  |  |  | 192 | $SnF_2$ |
|  |  |  |  | 216 | NaF |
|  |  |  |  | 204 | $SnF_2$ |
|  |  |  |  | 203 | NaF |
| Averill and others[153] | Whole-mouth | 7-11 | No | 125 | NaF |
|  |  |  |  | 124 | $SnF_2$ |
| Cons and Janerich[154] | Whole-mouth | 6-11 | No | 270 | NaF |
|  |  |  |  | 270 | $SnF_2$ |

\*Applied as a spray.
†These values indicate superiority over NaF since the latter served as the control.

may be offered in defense of the various studies. For example, a considerable amount of laboratory and clinical research resulted in the establishment of a recommended procedure of application as described for each agent by Knutson[118] and by Dudding and Muhler.[203] It would then seem only logical to compare these agents when each is employed in the recommended manner as was performed in certain comparable studies.[150, 154, 176] Similarly, one might suggest that each compound be evaluated at identical concentrations and with identical methods of application. This approach was also employed in four studies.[139, 140, 144, 150] Regardless of the criticisms of design, one cannot ignore the findings of the ten studies reported to date, comparing *topical applications of sodium fluoride and stannous fluoride*

| Fluoride concentration (percent) | Prophy-laxis | Number of applications | Length of applications (minutes) | Years after initial application | Reduction (percent) DMFT | Reduction (percent) DMFS |
|---|---|---|---|---|---|---|
| 4 | Yes | 4 | 4 | 1 | 57.0 | 37.0 |
| 2 | Yes | 4 | 4 | 1 | 21.0 | 12.0 |
| 8 | Yes | 1 | 4 | 1 | 50.0 | 51.3 |
| 8 |  | 2 | 4 | 1 | 53.2 | 53.3 |
| 2 |  | 1 | 4 | 1 | 0 | 0 |
| 2 | Yes | 4 | 3-4 | 1 |  | 46.3 |
| 2 | Yes | 4 | 3-4 | 1 |  | 38.6 |
| 2 | Yes | 4 | 3-4 | 2 |  | 18.9 |
| 2 | Yes | 4 | 3-4 | 2 |  | 17.6 |
| 2 | Yes | 4 | 3-4 | 1.25 | 44.4 | 29.0 |
| 2 | Yes | 4 | 4 | 1.25 | 35.9 | 22.6 |
| 2 | Yes | 4 | 3-4 | 1 | 33.8 | 31.6 |
| 8 | Yes | 1 | 3-4 | 1 | 18.8 | 24.9 |
| 2 | Yes | 4 | 4 | 1 | 35.0 | 35.3 |
| 2 | Yes | 4 | 4 | 2 | 83.1 | 58.8 |
| 2 | Yes | 4 | 4* | 2 | 60.9 | 65.5 |
| 2 | Yes | 4 | 4 | 2 | 23.6 | 36.3 |
| 8 | Yes | 1 | 4 | 2 |  | 3.5 |
| 2 | Yes | 4 | 3-4 | 2 |  | 19.8 |
| 8 | Yes | 1 | 4 | 5 | 30.0† | 35.0† |
| 2 | Yes | 4 | 3-4 |  |  |  |
| 8 | Yes | 1 | 4 | 4 | 20.0 | 25.0 |
| 2 | Yes | 4 | 3-4 |  |  |  |
| 8 | Yes | 1 | 4 | 3 | 30.0 | 23.0 |
| 2 | Yes | 4 | 3-4 |  |  |  |
| 8 | Yes | 1 | 4 | 2 | 28.0 | 26.0 |
| 2 | Yes | 4 | 3-4 |  |  |  |
| 2 | Yes | 4 | 1-2 | 2 | 16.0 | 11.4 |
| 4 | Yes | 4 | 1-2 | 2 | 8.0 | 6.8 |
| 2 | Yes | 4 | 4 | 3 | 17.2 | 11.2 |
| 8 | Yes | 3 | 4 | 3 | 7.5 | 7.2 |

these two anticariogenic agents. Half of the studies have indicated a very pronounced superiority of the stannous salt, while lesser degrees of superiority were noted in two additional studies. However, two studies reported that sodium fluoride was superior to stannous fluoride. Unfortunately, the two most recent attempts[153, 154] to resolve this matter failed to find a significant benefit from either treatment procedure in spite of the magnitude of information to the contrary. By far the majority of the clinical investigations conducted to date indicate that stannous fluoride is more effective in children. One might proceed a bit further and point out that, in establishing the merits of these two compounds, one must recall that topically applied

128 *Improving dental practice through preventive measures*

**Table 6-20.** *Review of clinical dental caries studies utilizing topical applications of various*

| Study | Fluoride compound | Technic | Fluoride in water supply | Initial age of subjects (years) | Number of subjects |
|---|---|---|---|---|---|
| Howell and Muhler[210] | SnClF | Whole-mouth | No | 6-15 | 394 |
| | NaF | Whole-mouth | No | 6-15 | 397 |
| Howell and Muhler[211] | SnClF | Whole-mouth | No | 6-15 | 357 |
| | NaF | Whole-mouth | No | 6-15 | 363 |
| Gish and others[212] | KSnF$_3$ | Whole-mouth | No | 6-15 | 390 |
| | H$_2$O | Whole-mouth | No | 6-15 | 411 |
| Gish and others[213] | KSnF$_3$ | Whole-mouth | No | 6-15 | 319 |
| | H$_2$O | Whole-mouth | No | 6-15 | 364 |
| Gish and others[214] | KSnF$_3$ | Whole-mouth | No | 6-15 | 294 |
| | H$_2$O | Whole-mouth | No | 6-15 | 342 |
| Muhler[171] | SnClF | Whole-mouth | No | 6-15 | 101 |
| | H$_2$O | Whole-mouth | No | 6-15 | 107 |
| Muhler[215] | SnClF | Whole-mouth | No | 6-15 | 220 |
| | SnClF | Whole-mouth | No | 6-15 | 188 |
| Hawes and others[136] | Na$_2$PO$_3$F | Half-mouth | No | 12† | 150 |
| | KF | Half-mouth | No | 12 | |
| Bibby and others[216] | PbF$_2$ | Half-mouth | No | 11-13 | 120 |
| Klinkenberg and Bibby[164] | PbF$_2$ | Half-mouth | No | 18-40 | 139 |
| Galagan and Knutson[119] | PbF$_2$ | Half-mouth | No | 7-15 | 272 |
| | | | | | 214 |
| | | | | | 262 |
| Cheyne[209] | KF | Whole-mouth | No | 4-6 | 27§ |
| East and others[217] | KF | Half-mouth | No | — | 48 |
| Stones and others[60] | KF | Whole-mouth | No | 6-14 | 65 |
| Peterson and Jordan[218] | Na$_2$SiF$_6$ | Half-mouth | No | 8-14 | 133 |
| | NaF | Half-mouth | | | |
| | Na$_2$SiF$_6$ | Half-mouth | No | 8-14 | 199 |
| | Na$_2$SiF$_6$ | Half-mouth | No | 8-14 | 156 |
| | NaF | Half-mouth | | | |
| Berggren and Welander[219] | NaF | Whole-mouth | No | 10 | 177 |
| | ZrF$_4$ | | | | 176 |
| | FeF$_3$ | | | | 167 |
| Muhler and others[220] | SnZrF$_6$ | Whole-mouth | No | 5-15 | 66 |
| Muhler and others[220] | SnZrF$_6$ | Whole-mouth | No | 6-14 | 233 |
| | SnZrF$_6$ | Whole-mouth | No | 6-14 | 245 |

\*Results obtained in children treated with NaF served as controls.
†Mean age.
‡pH 4.0.
§No control group; "control" data obtained on each subject prior to initiating study.

## fluoride solutions

| Prophy-laxis | Fluoride concentration (percent) | Number of applications | Length of application (minutes) | Years after initial application | Reduction (percent) DMFT | DMFS |
|---|---|---|---|---|---|---|
| Yes | 4 | 4 | 4 | 1 | 86.9* | 83.5* |
| Yes | 1 | 4 | 4 | 1 | | |
| Yes | 4 | 4 | 4 | 2 | 33.0 | 23.5 |
| Yes | 1 | 4 | 4 | 2 | | |
| Yes | 4 | 4 | 4 | 0.83 | 53.7 | 39.2 |
| Yes | | | | | | |
| Yes | | | | 2 | 47.5 | 38.5 |
| Yes | | | | | | |
| Yes | 4 | 4 | 4 | 3 | 39.5 | 40.2 |
| Yes | | | | | | |
| Yes | 4 | 4 | 4 | 1 | 42.9 | 36.5 |
| Yes | | | | | | |
| Yes | 4 | 4 | 4 | 0.5 | 46.9 | 32.5 |
| Yes | 4 | 4 | 4 | 1 | 51.9 | 36.5 |
| Yes | 15 | 4 | | 1 | | 20.0 |
| | 10 | | | | | Positive |
| Yes | 0.01 | 3 | 5 | 1 | 0 | 0 |
| Yes | 0.06 | 4 | 5 | 1 | 39.6 | 27.5 |
| Yes | 0.06 | 2 | 3-4 | 1 | | 2.4 |
| | | 4 | 3-4 | 1 | | 6.7 |
| | | 6 | 3-4 | 1 | | 3.2 |
| Yes | 0.15 | 2 | 2 | 1 | | 48.8 |
| Yes | 0.15 | 4 | 6 | 1 | 0 | |
| Yes | 2.6‡ | 8 | 7 | 3 | 0 | 0 |
| Yes | 0.9 | 4 | 4 | 2 | +21.4 | +11.7 |
| | 2 | 4 | 4 | 2 | | |
| Yes | 0.9 | 2 | 4 | 2 | 15.7 | 12.8 |
| Yes | 0.9 | 1 | 4 | 2 | 0 | 0 |
| | 2 | 4 | 4 | 2 | | |
| No | 0.5 | 5 | 3 | 2 | 29 | |
| | 0.25 | 5 | 3 | 2 | 17 | |
| | 0.56 | 5 | 3 | 2 | 33 | |
| Yes | 16 | 2 | 1 | 0.75 | 93.2 | 95.5 |
| Yes | 24 | 2 | 1 | 1 | 80.9 | 75.8 |
| Yes | 24 | 1 | 1 | 1 | 64.6 | 65.1 |

stannous fluoride has been shown to be of significant value in adults and in residents of areas already enjoying the benefits of a fluoridated water supply, whereas the use of sodium fluoride has not been shown to be of any significant value in either of these situations.

The discussions in the literature relative to the value of these two anticariogenic agents have also pointed out that there are additional disadvantages to the use of stannous fluoride, such as taste, gingival blanching, the instability of aqueous solutions, and the unesthetic pigmentation, all of which are absent when sodium fluoride is employed. Considerations of taste have little scientific merit, since therapeutic agents are not selected on the basis of taste but rather upon efficacy. The influence of stannous fluoride upon the gingiva has been repeatedly investigated[171, 204, 205] and shown to be of little consequence. The requirement of preparing fresh solutions has not detracted to any great degree from the acceptance of the agent. The presence of pigmentation following the use of stannous fluoride has been pointed out repeatedly[206, 207] and has been suggested as being caused by the formation of a tin phosphate at the site of either active or incipient carious lesions. Moreover, this pigmentation has been shown repeatedly to be associated with caries arrestment. These latter studies have been quite dramatic and have noted still another advantage of stannous fluoride. A recent study in adults[208] has indicated very dramatically the role of stannous fluoride in arresting presently carious lesions. While several studies have indicated that sodium fluoride is of little value in arresting carious lesions or in preventing the subsequent development of additional carious lesions on an already carious tooth, stannous fluoride has been found to be equally effective in preventing new lesions in both previously sound and previously carious teeth. Two recent studies[181, 208] have indicated that not only is a single application sufficient to obtain significant caries reductions but, further, that the length of application may be reduced to as little as 15 seconds in contrast to the 4-minute applications recommended for sodium fluoride application. It appears that there are many scientific reasons upon which to base one's recommendations for the use of stannous fluoride as the topical agent of choice at the present time.

Table 6-21. *Review of clinical dental caries studies using topically applied acidulated*

| Study | Initial age of subjects (years) | Fluoride in water supply | Technic | Prophy-laxis | Number of subjects | Fluoride concen-tration (percent) |
|---|---|---|---|---|---|---|
| Bibby and others[222] | Young adults | No | Whole-mouth | No | 31 | 0.1 |
|  |  |  |  |  | 15 | 0 |
| Roberts and others[223] | 11-13 | No | Whole-mouth | No | 187 | 0.01 |
|  |  |  |  |  | 169 | — |
| Tempestini[224] | 6-10 | No | Half-mouth | No | 89 | 2 |
| Rickles and Becks[166] | 22-34 | No | Half-mouth | Yes | 22 | 2 |

*Reductions noted when questionable lesions are excluded.

## Other fluorides as topical therapeutic agents

In the course of the development of new compounds for use in the control of dental caries, a variety of agents have been considered and, on the basis of laboratory studies, some of these materials have been evaluated clinically. The results of these studies are summarized in Table 6-20. While Cheyne[209] reported significant caries reductions with potassium fluoride in the first topical fluoride study reported in the literature, subsequent studies with this compound were of little success. Similar findings were noted with lead fluoride. While all of the studies with stannous chlorofluoride and potassium fluorostannite were positive, these compounds offer few advantages over stannous fluoride and are certainly lacking in investigative evidence. Sodium silicofluoride, sodium monofluorophosphate, zirconium fluoride, and ferric fluoride are likewise lacking in effectiveness. A recent report[220] indicates that stannous hexafluorozirconate is highly effective in the control of dental caries; this compound warrants additional investigation. It thus appears that to date only stannous fluoride has been sufficiently evaluated to warrant recommendation as a successor to sodium fluoride.

## Acid fluoride and acid fluoride–phosphate systems

A recent development in topical fluoride therapy that has received considerable attention in spite of limited clinical evaluation is the use of acidulated fluoride-phosphate. The concept of acidulated sodium fluoride is not new and was suggested for clinical study by Bibby more than 20 years ago. The results of the studies using acidulated sodium fluoride are summarized in Table 6-21. It is apparent that, while slight reductions were noted in two of the four studies, the treatment actually increased the incidence of dental caries in the other two studies. In view of these findings this approach to caries control was abandoned, at least temporarily.

Recently this concept was again brought into focus when Brudevold and associates[221] noted an increased uptake of fluoride in enamel following the topical application of acidulated sodium fluoride–phosphate mixtures and suggested an improved efficacy of sodium fluoride in preventing dental caries in human beings when used

*sodium fluoride*

| pH | Number of applications | Length of application (minutes) | Frequency of application | Years after initial application | Reduction (percent) DMFT | DMFS |
|---|---|---|---|---|---|---|
| 4.0 | 150+ | — | 3 times a week | 1 | | +35.7 (21.9)* |
| 4.0 | | — | | | | +31.4 (+6.6)* |
| 4.0 | 100+ | | 2 times a week | 1 | +30.5 | +24.8 |
| 4.0 | | | | | | |
| | 4 | 3-4 | | 1 | | 19.0 |
| 3.5 | 4 | 4 | 1 every 3 months | 2 | 0 | 12.7 |

132  *Improving dental practice through preventive measures*

**Table 6-22.** *Review of clinical dental caries studies using topically applied acidulated*

| Study | Initial age of subjects (years) | Fluoride in water supply | Technic | Prophylaxis | Number of subjects | Fluoride concentration (percent) |
|---|---|---|---|---|---|---|
| Wellock and Brudevold[225] | 8-11 | No | Whole-mouth | Yes | 115 | 1.23 F (NaF + HF) |
|  |  |  |  |  | 115 | 1.23 F (NaF + HF) |
| Pameijer and others[226] | 4-10 | No | Half-mouth | Yes | 77 | 2 NaF (0.9 F) |
| Wellock and others[183] | 8-12 | No | Whole-mouth | Yes | 220 | 1.23 F (NaF + HF) |
|  |  |  |  |  | 195 | 1.23 F (NaF + HF) |
| Muhler and others[184] | 12-14 | No | Whole-mouth | Yes | 101 | 8 $SnF_2$‡ |
|  |  |  |  |  | 92 | 8 $SnF_2$ |
|  |  |  |  |  | 94 | 8 $SnF_2$ |
| Muhler and others[184] | 6-13 | No | Whole-mouth | Yes | 250 | 3.6 NaF |
|  |  |  |  |  | 250 | 8 $SnF_2$ |
|  |  |  |  |  | 249 | 3.6 NaF |
|  |  |  |  |  | 239 | 8 $SnF_2$ |
| Averill and others[153] | 7-11 | No | Whole-mouth | Yes | 234 | 2 |
| Szwejda and others[227] | 7-8 | No | Whole-mouth | Yes | 182 | 1.23 F (NaF + HF) |
| DePaola[228] | 7-11 | No | Whole-mouth | Yes‖ | 201 | 0.25 |
| Cartwright and others[190] | 6-19 | No | Whole-mouth | Yes | 172 | 1.23 F (NaF + HF) |
| Horowitz[229-231] | 9-12 | No | Whole-mouth | Yes | 214 | 1.23 F (NaF + HF) |
|  |  |  |  |  | 187 |  |
|  |  |  |  |  | 167 |  |
|  |  |  |  |  | 205 | 1.23 F (NaF + HF) |
|  |  |  |  |  | 191 |  |
|  |  |  |  |  | 162 |  |
|  |  |  |  |  | 209 | 1.23 F (NaF + HF) |
|  |  |  |  |  | 196 |  |
|  |  |  |  |  | 182 |  |

\*Reapplications made at early intervals.
†Reduction obtained by comparison to other quadrants treated with 2 percent NaF.
‡Single applications of $NaH_2PO_4$ followed by $SnF_2$ were given at 6-month intervals.
§Single applications given at 6-month intervals.
‖Utilized 3.3 percent $NaF$-$HF$-$NaH_2PO_4$ (3 percent) prophylaxis paste (pH 5.0).

*phosphate-fluoride systems*

| Phosphate concentration (percent) | pH | Number of applications | Length of application | Years after initial application | Reduction (percent) DMFT | DMFS |
|---|---|---|---|---|---|---|
| 0.1 M H₃PO₄ | 2.8 | 1* | 4 | 1 | 55.0 | 71.0 |
| 0.1 M H₃PO₄ | 2.8 | 2 | 4 | 2 | 67.0 | 70.0 |
| 0.15 M H₃PO₄ | 3.6 | 4 | 3 | 0.25-1.25 |  | 51.0† |
| 0.1 M H₃PO₄ | 3-3.5 | 1* | 4 | 1 | 44.0 | 46.0 |
| 0.1 M H₃PO₄ | 3-3.5 | 2 | 4 | 2 | 44.0 | 52.0 |
| 10  NaH₂PO₄ | 2.8, 4.5 | 1 | 4 | 0.25 | 68.0 | 74.0 |
| 10  NaH₂PO₄ | 2.8, 4.5 | 1 | 4 | 0.5 | 69.0 | 71.0 |
| 10  NaH₂PO₄ | 2.8, 4.5 | 2 | 4 | 0.75 | 62.0 | 75.0 |
| 1.8 (K₂HPO₄ + H₃PO₄) | 6.0 | 1§ | 1 | 0.5 | 52.3 | 50.3 |
| 8  NaH₂PO₄ | 3.0 | 1§ | 1 | 0.5 | 84.9 | 80.1 |
| 1.8 (K₂HPO₄ + H₃PO₄) | 6.0 | 2 | 1 | 1 | 51.2 | 51.5 |
| 8  NaH₂PO₄ | 3.0 | 2 | 1 | 1 | 65.5 | 67.0 |
| 0.3 NaH₂PO₄ + H₃PO₄ | 4.43 | 4 | 1-2 | 2 | 12.0 | +2.3 |
| 0.1 M H₃PO₄ | 3.5 | 1 | 1 | 1 | +0.3 | +0.5 |
| 0.3 NaH₂PO₄ | 3.77 | 2 | 1 | 1 | 37.5 | 31.0 |
| 0.1 M H₃PO₄ | 2.8 | 4 | 4 | 2 | 49.2 |  |
| 0.1 M H₃PO₄ | 3-3.5 | 1 | 4 | 1 | 17.0 | 22.4 |
|  |  | 2 | 4 | 2 | 25.7 | 33.0 |
|  |  | 3 | 4 | 3 | 26.0 | 28.0 |
| 0.1 M H₃PO₄ | 3-3.5 | 2 | 4 | 1 | 28.3 | 27.1 |
|  |  | 4 | 4 | 2 | 32.9 | 35.9 |
|  |  | 6 | 4 | 3 | 38.1 | 41.3 |
| 0.1 M H₃PO₄ | 3-3.5 | 1 | 4 | 1 | 11.9 | 13.7 |
|  |  | 2 | 4 | 2 | 12.2 | 21.6 |
|  |  | 3 | 4 | 3 | 15.5 | 24.4 |

**Table 6-22.** *Review of clinical dental caries studies using topically applied acidulated*

| Study | Initial age of subjects (years) | Fluoride in water supply | Technic | Prophy-laxis | Number of subjects | Fluoride concentration (percent) |
|---|---|---|---|---|---|---|
| Selvig[232] | 8-11 | No | Whole-mouth | Yes | 115 | 1.23 F (NaF + HF) |
|  |  |  |  |  | 132 |  |
| Gray and others[233] | 3-4 | No | Whole-mouth | Yes | 128 | 1.23 F (NaF + HF) |
| Jordan and others[234] | 6-12 | No | Whole-mouth | Yes | 428 | 1.23 F (NaF + HF) |
| DePaola and others[235] | 6-8 | No | Whole-mouth | No | 245 | 1.0 NaF |
|  |  |  |  |  | 216 | 0.25 NaF |
|  |  |  |  |  | 205 | 0.25 NaF |
| Cons and Janerich[154] | 6-11 | No | Whole-mouth | Yes | 277 | 1.23 F (NaF + HF) |
|  |  |  |  |  | 277 | 1.23 F (NaF + HF) |

in this manner. An improved fluoride uptake in enamel was noted 20 years earlier with acidulated sodium fluoride, and this latter type of therapy was selected for clinical investigation on this basis only to be subsequently found to be of no clinical value.

To date fifteen studies have been reported using acidulated fluoride–phosphate systems. The findings are summarized in Table 6-22. These studies considered collectively suggest that the acidulated sodium fluoride–phosphate mixture may be significantly more effective than sodium fluoride alone when used in children reared in the absence of communal fluoridation. While Wellock and associates[183] reported this type of therapy to be more effective than stannous fluoride under these experimental conditions, Muhler and associates[184] reported comparable findings for the two treatment procedures. More recent studies utilizing topically applied acidulated sodium fluoride–phosphate systems have failed to confirm the early expectations of a high degree of efficacy. In fact, of the last ten studies, three failed to find a significant effect with this treatment procedure and only one reported a caries reduction greater than 41 percent. It is interesting to note that the two studies[184] conducted using stannous fluoride–phosphate systems suggest that this system may be considerably more effective than either stannous fluoride alone or the acidulated sodium fluoride–phosphate mixture.

It has been suggested[225] that the acidulated sodium fluoride–phosphate mixture is not only a marked improvement in terms of efficacy of fluoride therapy but is not accompanied by the suggested disadvantages of taste, stability, gingival tissue blanching, and pigmentation associated with the use of stannous fluoride.

*phosphate-fluoride systems—cont'd*

| Phosphate concentration (percent) | pH | Number of applications | Length of application | Years after initial application | Reduction (percent) DMFT | DMFS |
|---|---|---|---|---|---|---|
| 0.1 M H₃PO₄ | 3-3.5 | 2 | 4 | 1 | 55 | |
| | | 4 | 4 | 2 | 67 | |
| 0.1 M H₃PO₄ | 3-3.5 | 2 | 4 | 2 | 32.8 | |
| 0.1 M H₃PO₄ | 3-3.5 | 1 | 4 | 1 | 26.1 | 34.7 |
| 0.1 M H₃PO₄ | 3.8 | 3 | 1-2 | 1 | 23.4 | 20.6 |
| 0.03 M H₃PO₄ | 3.8 | 6 | 1-2 | 2 | 5.6 | 11.1 |
| 0.03 M H₃PO₄ | 3.8 | 9 | 1-2 | 3 | 1.4 | 12.8 |
| 0.1 M H₃PO₄ | 3 | 3 | 4 | 3 | 16.0 | +2.1 |
| 0.1 M H₃PO₄ | 3 | 3 | 4 | 3 | 25.0 | 18.0 |

**Table 6-23.** *Summary of enamel decalcification data with various fluoride systems*

| Treatment system | Fluoride concentration | Enamel decalcification (µg Ca) pH 1.5 | pH 3.0 | pH 4.5 |
|---|---|---|---|---|
| NaF | 1,000 p.p.m. F | 37,608 | 1,056 | 137 |
| NaF + H₃PO₄ | 1,000 p.p.m. F | 69,300 | 38,030 | 292 |
| SnF₂ | 1,000 p.p.m. F | 1,515 | 186 | 175 |
| NaF | 1.8% F | 155,504 | 57,892 | 137 |
| NaF + H₃PO₄ | 1.8% F | 108,050 | 12,513 | 182 |
| SnF₂ | 1.8% F | 25,409 | 1,583 | 148 |

Recent studies[236] have suggested, however, that serious decalcification may result from the use of the acidulated sodium fluoride–phosphate systems at a pH of 3.0 or less as was used in at least two of the clinical studies. A portion of these data are shown in Table 6-23, and it may be seen that, at both fluoride concentrations examined, markedly greater amounts of enamel decalcification were apparent with the nontin-containing systems. At a pH of about 3.0, the amount of calcium leached from the enamel surface with the sodium fluoride–phosphate system was from eight to two hundred times greater than that noted with stannous fluoride. Before one can justify a recommendation of this recently suggested means of controlling dental caries, much additional work is needed not only to confirm the present evidence but also to determine if this treatment is of any value in adults or in persons reared in the presence of fluoride. While a discussion of fluoride mechanisms is

136  *Improving dental practice through preventive measures*

Table 6-24. *Summary of clinical dental caries studies employing fluoride rinses*

| Study | Fluoride source and concentration (percent) | Frequency of rinses | Length of rinse (minutes) | Number of subjects | Initial age of subjects (years) | Years of observation | Reduction (percent) DMFT | Reduction (percent) DMFS |
|---|---|---|---|---|---|---|---|---|
| Bibby and others[222] | NaF (0.01; pH 4.0) | 3/week | | 31 | 20-24 | 1 | | +108 |
| Roberts and others[223] | NaF (0.01; pH 4.0) | 2/week | 1 | 187 | 11-13 | 1 | +34 | +21 |
| Weisz[237, 238] | NaF (0.25) | 2/day | | 74 | 5-6 | 10 | | 89 |
| Fjaestad-Seger and others[239] | NaF (0.2) | 1/2 weeks | 3 | | | 1 | | |
| Berggren and Welander[148] | NaF (1.0) | 9/2 years | 4 | 568 | 7-14 | 2 | 11 | 25-39 |
| Torell and Siberg[240] | NaF (0.2) | 1/month | 3 | 912 | 8-9 | 1 | | 21 |
| Goaz and others[241] | Na₂PO₃F (6.0)* | 1/day | 1-2 | 129 | 7-14 | 1.2 | | 42 |
| Berggen and Welander[219] | NaF (0.5) ZrF₄ (0.25) FeF₃ (0.56) | 5/2 years 5/2 years 5/2 years | 3 3 3 | 177 176 167 | 10 10 10 | 2 2 2 | 19 17 33 | |
| Forsman[242] | NaF (0.2) | 1/2 weeks | | 526 | 10-12 | 1 2 | | 50 80 |
| Torell and Ericsson[151] | NaF (0.05) NaF (0.2) | 1/day 1/2 weeks | | 190 211 | 10 10 | 2 2 | | 50 25 |

| | | | | | | |
|---|---|---|---|---|---|---|
| Torell and Ericsson[243] | NaF (0.2) | 1/2 weeks | 40,000 | 6-15 | 5 | 51 |
| Ollinen[244] | NaF (0.5) | 1/month | | | 3.5 | 64 |
| Kasakura[245] | NaF (0.1) | 1/day | 41 | 10-11 | 2 | 60 | 92 |
| Hundstadbraaten[246] | NaF (1.0) | 1/3 months | 803 | 7-13 | 3 | | 43 |
| Kann[247] | NaF (0.2) | 1/2 weeks | 18,250 | | | | |
| Englander and other[248] | NaF (1.1) + 0.1 M PO$_4$ (pH 4.5) | 1/day | 154 | 11-14 | 1.75 | 64 | 75 |
| | NaF (1.1) | 1/day | 151 | 11-14 | 1.75 | 67 | 80 |
| Swerdloff and Shannon[249] | SnF$_2$ (0.1) | 1/day | 83 | 11-15 | 0.5 | 33 | 31 |
| Bullen and others[250, 251] | NaF (1.2) + PO$_4$ (pH 3) | 5/year | 331 235 | 6 6 | 1 2 | | 39 15 |
| Conchie and others[252] | NaF (1.2) + PO$_4$ (pH 3) | 9/2 years | 567 494 444 | 12-13 12-13 12-13 | 1 2 3 | 18 23 24 | 17 24 25 |
| Koch[253] | NaF (0.5) | 1/2 weeks/ 3 years | 85 | 10 | 3 5 | | 25 0 |
| Horowitz and others[254, 255] | NaF (0.6) + PO$_4$ (pH 3) | 5/year | 130 | 11-14 | 2 | 8 | 8 |
| | NaF (0.6) + PO$_4$ (pH 3) | 5/year | 144 | 11-14 | 2 | +9 | 2 |
| | NaF (1.2 F) + PO$_4$ (pH 3) | 5/year | 168 | 11-14 | 2 | 9 | 5 |

*Subjects resided in communal fluoride area.

beyond the scope of this text, it may be stated that, if the mechanism suggested for the acidulated sodium fluoride–phosphate systems is valid, one would not expect additional benefit from the treatment in persons reared in the presence of optimal fluoride in the drinking water. Additional studies are also needed to determine if this system has any influence on caries arrestment; again, on a purely theoretical basis one would not predict a pronounced influence of this treatment on already existing lesions. Likewise the safety of such treatments warrants further investigation. In short, while this means of therapy may truly represent an additional means of providing fluoride therapy, much additional information is needed.

**Fluoride mouthwashes**

An additional concept that has received a limited amount of interest is the use of mouthwashes containing fluoride. The first clinical study utilizing this concept was reported by Bibby and associates.[222] These investigators employed a 0.1 percent acidulated sodium fluoride (pH 4.0) mouthwash three times weekly in young adults and failed to find any beneficial effect attributable to the treatment. Weisz[237, 238] reported that the use of a 0.25 percent sodium fluoride mouthwash twice daily in children 5 to 9 years of age resulted in caries reductions of 80 to 90 percent after 2 to 10 years of regular usage.

A more recent approach has been the use of fluoride solutions applied either with a toothbrush or as a mouthwash under supervision; these studies are summarized in Table 6-24. Berggren and Welander[148] reported on the use of a 1 percent sodium fluoride solution applied with a toothbrush nine times during two consecutive school years for 4 minutes each time. These investigators reported caries reductions of 25 to 39 percent at the end of the study period, although it was noted that the reductions occurred largely in the maxillary teeth. Torell and Siberg[240] reported caries reductions of 21.3 percent in school children after 1 year's use of a mouthwash containing 0.2 percent sodium fluoride. The mouthwash was used once each month for a 3-minute period under supervision. These investigators failed to find any beneficial effect from the use of a 0.2 percent potassium fluoride mouthwash in the same study. Goaz and associates[241] noted about a 40 percent reduction in dental caries in children residing in a fluoride area following the daily application with a toothbrush of a 6 percent sodium monofluorophosphate solution throughout a 14-month study period. Berggren and Welander[219] employed the supervised toothbrushing procedure at about 2-month intervals and reported reductions of 29 percent with 0.5 percent sodium fluoride, 17 percent with a 0.25 percent solution of zirconium fluoride, and 33 percent with a 0.56 percent ferric fluoride solution. Forsman[242] reported reductions in caries of 50 and 80 percent in children using a 0.2 percent sodium fluoride solution once each 2 weeks for 1 and 2 years, respectively. Torell and Ericsson[151] reported a 50 percent reduction in caries in a 2-year study in children following the daily use of a 0.05 percent sodium fluoride mouthwash, but only a 25 percent reduction when a 0.2 percent sodium fluoride mouthwash was used at 2-week intervals. As shown in Table 6-24, a number of more recent studies have tended to confirm the efficacy of this approach to the control of dental caries. A total of twenty-one studies have been reported; only the two initial studies, which utilized acidulated sodium fluoride,[222, 223] and the recent report by Horowitz and others[254, 255] have failed to demonstrate a beneficial effect.

It appears that mouthwashes are valuable in the control of dental caries. One should note, however, that the presence of such mouthwashes containing relatively high concentrations of fluoride in the home may represent a potential health hazard from a toxicity viewpoint. The use of these mouthwashes must be accompanied by the proper precautionary measures and their indiscriminate use should be avoided.

**Prophylactic pastes containing fluoride**

Early in the history of topical fluoride therapy Bibby and associates[222] suggested that the use of sodium fluoride in a prophylactic paste might be of significant value. As summarized in Table 6-25, these investigators reported on two pilot studies utilizing prophylactic pastes containing sodium fluoride, acidulated to pH 4.0 with hydrogen peroxide and found only a limited degree of success, considerably less than these same investigators noted with topical applications of sodium fluoride. No additional studies have been reported in the United States with sodium fluoride in prophylactic pastes since this early report. Several Russian investigators[143, 256, 257] have reported on the use of a prophylactic paste containing 75 percent sodium fluoride, but the results reported to date are too inconsistent to receive much support at this time. Peterson and associates[258] recently reported a very modest effect with an acidulated fluoride–phosphate paste containing potassium fluoride.

To date, eight studies have been conducted using stannous fluoride in a prophylactic paste, and these findings are also summarized in Table 6-25. These studies, with one exception,[187] have been consistently positive with caries reductions largely between 30 and 40 percent. Interestingly, these studies indicated a comparable degree of effectiveness in both children and in adults reared in both the presence and absence of communal fluoridation. It is apparent that the use of a prophylactic paste containing stannous fluoride will afford a significant degree of protection against the subsequent development of dental caries and warrants consideration as a means of effectively providing fluoride therapy in a caries-preventive program.

A recent development has been the use of a zirconium silicate paste containing 9 percent stannous fluoride as a patient-applied treatment procedure. This approach has been employed as a potential means of providing dental health benefits to a greater segment of the population than can be reached through operator-applied topical treatment procedures in the dental office. The practical value of this technic is readily apparent when one realizes that treatments are performed annually or semiannually generally in groups of thirty to forty subjects, although several hundred may be treated simultaneously, with a total time requirement of less than half an hour.

Table 6-26 summarizes the results that have been obtained by various investigators employing this approach in the control of dental caries. It is apparent from the ten studies reported that this procedure results in a significant reduction in the incidence of dental caries of about 50 percent. Moreover, these data indicate that this procedure is of added value in the prevention of dental caries in children residing in an area already deriving the benefits of communal fluoridation. In view of the dental health benefits associated with this procedure and the manpower problem currently facing the dental profession, this procedure should have considerable application in the future.

**MULTIPLE FLUORIDE THERAPY**

Throughout the foregoing review regarding available means of providing fluoride therapy it is apparent that none of the procedures in themselves is able to completely prevent the subsequent development of dental caries. It has been shown that various

140  Improving dental practice through preventive measures

**Table 6-25.** *Summary of clinical dental caries using prophylactic pastes containing either*

| Study | Initial age of subjects (years) | Fluoride in water supply | Technic | Treatment concentration (percent) |
|---|---|---|---|---|
| *Sodium fluoride* | | | | |
| Bibby and others[222] | 6-14 | No | Half-mouth | 1 NaF + pumice + $H_2O_2$ (pH 4.0) |
|  | 6-15 | No | Half-mouth | 1 NaF + pumice + $H_2O_2$ (pH 4.0) |
| Tusnova[256] | 7-14 | No | Half-mouth | 75 NaF + pumice |
| Diminick and Wodniecki[143] | 7-14 | No | Half-mouth | 75 NaF + pumice |
| Kiseleva and others[257] | 6-14 | No | Whole-mouth | 75 NaF + pumice |
| Peterson and others[258] | 10-13 | No | Whole-mouth | 2.1(F)KF·$2H_2O$ – $PO_4$ – lava pumice |
|  | 11-13 | Yes | Whole-mouth | 2.1(F)KF·$2H_2O$ – $PO_4$ – lava pumice |
| *Stannous fluoride* | | | | |
| Peterson and others[259] | 10-13 | No | Whole-mouth | 17.5 $SnF_2$ + silex |
| Bixler and Muhler[260] | 5-18 | No | Whole-mouth | 8.9 $SnF_2$ + lava pumice |
| Gish and Muhler[261] | 6-14 | Yes | Whole-mouth | 8.9 $SnF_2$ + lava pumice |
| Muhler and Bixler[262] | 17-59 | No | Whole-mouth | 50 $SnF_2$ + silex |
| Bixler and Muhler[263] | 17-36 | No | Whole-mouth | 15 $SnF_2$ + silex |
| Muhler[264] | 6-15 | No | Whole-mouth | 50 $SnF_2$ + lava pumice |
| Gish and Muhler[265] | 6-15 | No | Whole-mouth | 8.9 $SnF_2$ + lava pumice |
| Horowitz and Lucye[187] | 8-10 | No | Whole-mouth | $P_F$ 8.9 $SnF_2$ + lava pumice |

*Results obtained when questionable lesions are excluded.
†Independent data from second examiner with second group of children.

types of therapy represent only a contribution to a fluoride therapy program and that each procedure in itself may play a significant but limited role in caries prevention but frequently only under specific experimental conditions.

Following the clinical findings of a great degree of versatility with stannous fluoride, that is, the ability of this agent to provide anticariogenic benefits in both children and adults in both the presence and absence of communal fluoride, it was suggested by Muhler and associates[260] that the use of multiple stannous fluoride treatments might more nearly achieve the goal of complete caries protection. As a

## Fluoride therapy

*sodium fluoride or stannous fluoride*

| Number of subjects | Number of applications | Frequency of applications | Years after initial application | Reduction (percent) DMFT | Reduction (percent) DMFS |
|---|---|---|---|---|---|
| 47 | 3 | 4 mo. | 1 | | 21.0 (42)* |
| 95 | 2 | 6 mo. | 1 | | 12.0 (25)* |
| 869 | 1 | 6 mo. | 1 | | 50.0 |
| 233 | 6 | 6 mo. | 5 | | Positive |
| 942 | 3 | 3 mo. | 1 | | 0.0 |
| 256 | 2 | 12 mo. | 2 | 13.5 (12.2) | 15.7 (15.3) |
| 202 | 2 | 12 mo. | 2 | 19.0 ( 7.8) | 15.1 (12.3) |
| 121 | 1 | 6 mo. | 2 | 35.1 | 41.9 |
| 141 | 1 | None | 2 | 27.9 | 34.2 |
| 109 (114)† | 1 | 6 mo. | 6 mo. | 12.9 (38.7)† | 17.5 (40.2)† |
| 99 (106) | | | 1 | 30.6 (38.8) | 34.6 (34.2) |
| 81 ( 85) | | | 18 mo. | 23.6 (35.5) | 31.4 (37.2) |
| 71 ( 82) | | | 2 | 29.1 (35.6) | 29.1 (37.8) |
| 111 (104)† | 1 | 6 mo. | 6 mo. | 37.6 (56.2)† | 46.6 (60.4)† |
| 107 ( 99) | | | 1 | 29.3 (45.1) | 39.6 (41.7) |
| 71 ( 89) | | | 3 | 33.3 (24.5) | 39.2 (30) |
| 108 | 1 | 6 mo. | 6 mo. | | 24.5 |
| 82 | | | 1 | | 36.6 |
| 159 | 1 | 6 mo. | 6 mo. | 31.5 | 27.2 |
| | | | 1 | 41.0 | 30.5 |
| 230 | 1 | 6 mo. | 6 mo. | 59.7 | 62.0 |
| 194 | | | 1 | 45.7 | 49.7 |
| 160 | 1 | 6 mo. | 6 mo. | 33.7 | 32.6 |
| 227 | 1 | 12 mo. | 2 | +5 | +6 |

result, a series of independent studies was initiated. The results of these studies are summarized in Table 6-27. These studies included the evaluation of stannous fluoride in an area of communal fluoridation using a compatible lava pumice–stannous fluoride prophylactic paste, an aqueous solution of stannous fluoride for topical application, and a stannous fluoride–calcium pyrophosphate dentifrice for home use. As shown in Table 6-27, it is apparent that, while some anticariogenic benefits were derived from each portion of the multiple treatment program, by far the most benefits were obtained when the greatest number of treatments were employed.

142  *Improving dental practice through preventive measures*

Table 6-26. *Summary of clinical caries studies utilizing self-application of a stannous fluoride–zirconium silicate prophylactic paste*

| Study | Fluoride in water supply | Initial age of subjects (years) | Treatment | Number of applications | Frequency of applications (months) | Number of subjects | Years after initial application | Reduction (percent) DMFT | Reduction (percent) DMFS |
|---|---|---|---|---|---|---|---|---|---|
| Muhler and Kelley[266] | No | 10-13 | P_F + D_F | 2 | 6 | 38 | 0.5 | 76 (29)* | 80 (36) |
|  |  |  |  |  |  | 28 | 1 | 66 (66) | 63 (69) |
| Gish and Mercer[267] | Yes | 6-14 | P_F | 2 | 6 | 108 | 1 | 22 | 51 |
|  |  |  |  | 4 | 6 | 110 | 2 | 17 | 14 |
|  |  |  |  | 6 | 6 | 105 | 3 | 30 | 25 |
| Gish and Mercer[268] | No | 6-14 | P_F | 2 | 6 | 201 | 1 | 34 | 42 |
|  |  |  |  | 4 | 6 | 175 | 2 | 39 | 43 |
|  |  |  |  | 6 | 6 | 162 | 3 | 32 | 37 |
| Christman[266] | No | 11-13 | P_F + D_F | 2 | 6 | 139 | 1 | 97 | 77 |
| Barnes and Nazhat[266] | No | 11-13 | P_F | 2 | 6 | 12 | 1 | 73 (31) | 59 (12) |
|  |  |  | P_F + D_F | 2 | 6 | 19 | 1 | 59 (64) | 69 (68) |
| Lang and others[269] | Yes | 6-10 | P_F | 1 | 6 | 70 | 0.5 | 56 (29; 47) | 65 (33; 48) |
|  |  |  | P_F | 2 | 6 | 67 | 1 | 67 (39; 53) | 70 (45; 56) |
|  |  |  | P_F | 3 | 6 | 42 | 1.5 | 41 (27; 41) | 42 (38; 42) |
|  |  |  | P_F + D_F | 1 | 6 | 79 | 0.5 | 61 (34; 50) | 65 (38; 51) |
|  |  |  | P_F + D_F | 2 | 6 | 78 | 1 | 58 (50; 62) | 57 (51; 57) |
|  |  |  | P_F + D_F | 3 | 6 | 46 | 1.5 | 54 (33; 44) | 53 (39; 46) |
| Jordan and others[270] | No | 9-12 | P_F | 1 | 6 | 362 | 0.5 | 25 | 28 |
|  |  |  |  | 2 | 6 | 320 | 1 | 12 | 16 |
|  |  |  |  | 3 | 6 | 296 | 1.5 | 20 | 23 |
|  |  |  |  | 4 | 6 | 243 | 2 | 15 | 19 |
| Gish and others[268] | No | 6-14 | P_F + R_F + E | 2 | 6 | 223 | 1 | 21 | 21 |
|  |  |  | P_F + R_F + E | 4 | 6 | 194 | 2 | 20 | 28 |
|  |  |  | P_F + R_F + D_F + E | 2 | 6 | 212 | 1 | 35 | 30 |
|  |  |  | P_F + R_F + D_F + E | 4 | 6 | 178 | 2 | 39 | 34 |
|  |  |  | P_F + R_F | 2 | 6 | 354 | 1 | 22 | 14 |
|  |  |  | P_F + R_F | 4 | 6 | 311 | 2 | 26 | 25 |
|  |  |  | P_F + R_F + D_F | 2 | 6 | 339 | 1 | 33 | 29 |
|  |  |  | P_F + R_F + D_F | 4 | 6 | 287 | 2 | 28 | 30 |
| Oshiro[271] | Yes | 8-11 | P_F | 1 | 12 | 249 | 1 | 100 | 100 |
|  |  |  |  | 2 | 12 | 238 | 2 | 69 | 100 |
| Kelley and others[272] | No | 6-14 | P_F | 1 | 12 | 81 | 1 | 41 | 64 |

*Value in parentheses represent results for independent examiner(s) for same children

Fluoride therapy 143

**Table 6-27.** *Summary of clinical dental caries studies utilizing multiple stannous fluoride therapy in a solution, prophylactic paste, and $Ca_2P_2O_7$ dentifrice*

| Study | Initial age of subjects (years) | Fluoride in water supply | Technic | Treatment | Number of subjects | Years after initial application | Reduction (percent) DMFT | DMFS |
|---|---|---|---|---|---|---|---|---|
| Bixler and Muhler[260] | 5-18 | No | Whole-mouth | $P_F$* | 109 (114)† | 0.5 | 12.9 (38.7)† | 17.5 (40.2)† |
| | | | | $P_F + D_F$* | 115 (110) | | 33.6 (31.1) | 47.2 (37.4) |
| | | | | $P_F + T_F$* | 108 (120) | | 34.5 (52.8) | 46.5 (59.8) |
| | | | | $P_F + T_F + D_F$* | 113 (129) | | 88.8 (76.4) | 97.4 (77.1) |
| | | | | $P_F$ | 99 (106)† | 1 | 30.6 (38.8)† | 34.6 (34.2)† |
| | | | | $P_F + D_F$ | 109 (110) | | 31.4 (27.2) | 37.3 (32.4) |
| | | | | $P_F + T_F$ | 103 (108) | | 46.1 (40.1) | 47.6 (41.9) |
| | | | | $P_F + T_F + D_F$ | 108 (122) | | 72.5 (54.7) | 74.6 (58.4) |
| Bixler and Muhler[263] | 5-18 | No | Whole-mouth | $P_F$* | 81 (85)† | 2 | 23.6 (35.5)† | 31.4 (37.2)† |
| | | | | $P_F + D_F$* | 89 (86) | | 29.2 (24.5) | 36.9 (31.7) |
| | | | | $P_F + T_F$* | 84 (74) | | 35.3 (46) | 38.5 (43.1) |
| | | | | $P_F + T_F + D_F$* | 83 (97) | | 66.1 (50.2) | 70.3 (55.4) |
| | | | | $P_F$* | 71 (82) | | 29.1 (35.6) | 29.1 (37.8) |
| | | | | $P_F + D_F$* | 82 (82) | | 34.9 (32.8) | 38.7 (36.1) |
| | | | | $P_F + T_F$* | 86 (68) | | 39.2 (58.2) | 39.7 (55.6) |
| | | | | $P_F + T_F + D_F$* | 69 (74) | | 63.5 (48.9) | 66.8 (49.9) |
| Gish and Muhler[261] | 6-14 | Yes | Whole-mouth | $P_F$* | 111 (104)† | 0.5 | 37.6 (56.2)† | 46.6 (60.4)† |
| | | | | $P_F + T_F$* | 117 (97) | | 83.5 (62.9) | 89.9 (59.7) |
| | | | | $P_F + T_F + D_F$* | 110 (104) | | 83.5 (77.5) | 89.2 (77.1) |
| | | | | $P_F$ | 107 (99) | 1 | 29.3 (45.1) | 39.6 (41.7) |
| | | | | $P_F + T_F$ | 113 (95) | | 68.4 (57.9) | 75.4 (57.6) |
| | | | | $P_F + T_F + D_F$ | 108 (98) | | 62.4 (76) | 69.6 (73.3) |
| Gish and Muhler[265] | 6-14 | Yes | Whole-mouth | $P_F$ | 71 (89) | 3 | 33.3 (24.5) | 39.2 (30) |
| | | | | $P_F + T_F$ | 65 (82) | | 53.5 (39) | 60.4 (43.8) |
| | | | | $P_F + T_F + D_F$ | 68 (92) | | 53.5 (48.4) | 54.3 (55.7) |
| Peterson and others[259] | 10-13 | No | Whole-mouth | $P_F$† | 141 | 2 | 27.9 | 34.2 |
| | | | | $P_F$‡ | 121 | | 35.1 | 41.9 |
| | | | | $P_F + T_F$† | 163 | | 29.3 | 32.2 |
| Muhler and others[273] | 20-26 | Yes | Whole-mouth | $P_F + T_F + D_F$§ | 100 | 0.5 | 98 | 92 |
| | | | | | 83 | 1 | 77 | 69 |
| | | | | | 83 | 1.5 | 72 | 68 |

*Treatments were made at 6-month intervals; $SnF_2$ when used, was applied as an 8 percent topical solution, a prophylactic paste ($P_F$) containing 8.9 percent $SnF_2$ and/or an $SnF_2$-$Ca_2P_2O_7$ dentifrice ($D_F$) containing 0.4 percent $SnF_2$.
†Data obtained independently by a second examiner on different subjects.
‡Single treatments given only initially; topical application consisted of 8 percent $SnF_2$.
§Treatments given at 6-month intervals.
‖Incomplete report.
¶Length of time of $SnF_2$ topical application decreased to 15 seconds.

*Continued.*

**Table 6-27.** Summary of clinical dental caries studies utilizing multiple stannous fluoride therapy in a solution, prophylactic paste, and $Ca_2P_2O_7$ dentifrice—cont'd

| Study | Initial age of subjects (years) | Fluoride in water supply | Technic | Treatment | Number of subjects | Years after initial application | Reduction (percent) DMFT | DMFS |
|---|---|---|---|---|---|---|---|---|
| | | | | | 45 | 2 | 70 | 68 |
| | | | | | 44 | 2.5 | 68 | 59 |
| Scola and others[274, 275] | 17-24 | No | Whole-mouth | $P_F$§ | 177 | 0.5 | 9 | 11 |
| | | | | $P_F + T_F$ | 181 | | 26 | 35 |
| | | | | $P_F + D_F$ | 171 | | 33 | 54 |
| | | | | $P_F + T_F + D_F$ | 165 | | 53 | 40 |
| | | | | $P_F + T_F + D_F$¶ | 160 | | 63 | 59 |
| | | | | $P_F$ | 157 | 1 | 12 | 12 |
| | | | | $P_F + T_F$ | 153 | | 47 | 43 |
| | | | | $P_F + D_F$ | 139 | | 29 | 48 |
| | | | | $P_F + T_F + D_F$ | 142 | | 51 | 45 |
| | | | | $P_F + T_F + D_F$¶ | 138 | | 73 | 54 |
| | | | | $P_F$ | 106 | 2 | 26 | 12 |
| | | | | $P_F + T_F$ | 107 | | 34 | 27 |
| | | | | $P_F + D_F$ | 102 | | 47 | 42 |
| | | | | $P_F + T_F + D_F$ | 108 | | 50 | 48 |
| | | | | $P_F + T_F + D_F$¶ | 105 | | 77 | 61 |
| Muhler and Bixler[262] | 17-59 | No | Whole-mouth | $P_F$ | 108 | 0.5 | | 24.5 |
| | | | | $P_F + D_F$ | 111 | | | 42.2 |
| | | | | $P_F + T_F$ | 106 | | | 40.1 |
| | | | | $P_F + T_F + D_F$ | 110 | | | 89.0 |
| | | | | $P_F$ | 82 | 1 | | 36.6 |
| | | | | $P_F + D_F$ | 77 | | | 30.1 |
| | | | | $P_F + T_F$ | 81 | | | 44.8 |
| | | | | $P_F + T_F + D_F$ | 71 | | | 73.3 |
| Bixler and Muhler[263] | 17-36 | No | Whole-mouth | $P_F$ | 159 | 0.5 | 31.5 | 27.2 |
| | | | | $P_F + T_F$ | 155 | | 48.3 | 44.2 |
| | | | | $P_F + T_F + D_F$ | 146 | | 64.0 | 56.1 |
| | | | | $P_F$ | 101 | 1 | 41.0 | 30.5 |
| | | | | $P_F + T_F$ | 102 | | 61.2 | 55.4 |
| | | | | $P_F + T_F + D_F$ | 98 | | 56.7 | 51.5 |
| Gish[276] | 6-15 | No | Whole-mouth | $P_F + T_F$ | 148 | 0.5 | 60.9 | 61.7 |
| Horowitz and Lucye[187] | 8-10 | No | Whole-mouth | $P_F$ | 227 | 2 | +5 | +6 |
| | | | | $T_F$ | 223 | 2 | +3 | +8 |
| | | | | $P_F + T_F$ | 225 | 2 | +3 | 1 |

In a nonfluoride area Bixler and Muhler[260] noted an 80 to 90 percent reduction in dental caries in children 6 months after a treatment in which stannous fluoride was employed in a prophylactic paste, a topical solution, and in a dentifrice. After 1 and 2 years, these reductions decreased to about 60 to 70 percent. Comparable findings were reported by Gish and Muhler[261] when this same series of treatments was employed in children born and raised in an optimal fluoride area. Similar findings have been obtained recently in adults residing in a fluoride area[273] and in a nonfluoride area.[208] Equally dramatic findings are those of Scola and Ostrom,[274, 275] which indicate that, in a military population after 2 years of investigations, caries protections of more than 60 percent were afforded those persons who received the multiple stannous fluoride treatments. Conversely, Horowitz and Lucye[187] failed to find any beneficial influence from this treatment procedure.

Collectively, these findings indicate that, while the goal of complete prevention of dental caries has not yet been realized with fluoride therapy, by far the closest approximation to this goal may be achieved through the regular use of a stannous fluoride multiple treatment program in an area with optimal fluoride in the communal water supply.

## CONCLUSION

The evidence available in the literature regarding the role of various types of fluoride therapy in the prevention of dental caries has been reviewed. It has been shown that, with regard to systemic fluoride therapy, no substitute for the use of a water supply containing the optimal amount of fluoride may be recommended at this time, although subsequent research may confirm the limited information available that indicates vitamin-fluoride tablets have significant value. A consideration of the suggested means of providing topical fluoride therapy to the erupted dentition indicates that (1) sodium fluoride is of value as a caries preventive agent, but only in children reared in the absence of communal fluoride, (2) stannous fluoride provides significant benefits to all aspects of our population, (3) certain other fluorides, including fluoride-phosphate systems, presently indicate promise as anticariogenic agents but require much additional independent clinical evaluation before their role in a caries-prevention program may be determined and their use indiscriminantly recommended, and (4) by far the greatest contribution toward the complete control of dental caries may be obtained through a multiple treatment stannous fluoride program that includes the use of stannous fluoride in a compatible prophylactic paste, a solution for topical application, and in a calcium pyrophosphate dentifrice for home use in an area with optimal fluoride in the communal water supply.

## REFERENCES

1. McKay, F.: Mottled enamel: early history and its unique features. In Moulton, F. R., editor: Fluorine and dental health, Washington, D. C., 1942, Pub. 19, American Association for the Advancement of Science.
2. Shafer, W. G., Hine, M. K., and Levy, B. M.: A textbook of oral pathology, Philadelphia, 1958, W. B. Saunders Co.
3. Dean, H. T., and Elvove, E.: Studies on the minimal threshold of the dental signs of chronic endemic fluorosis (mottled enamel), Public Health Rep. 50:1719, 1935.
4. Dean, H. T.: Endemic fluorosis and its relation to dental caries, Public Health Rep. 53: 1443, 1938.
5. Dean, H. T., and others: Domestic water and dental caries, including certain epidemiological aspects of oral L. acidophilus, Public Health Rep. 54:862, 1939.

6. Dean, H. T., and others: Domestic water and dental caries, II, a study of 2,832 white children aged 12-14 years, of eight suburban Chicago communities, including L. acidophilus studies, of 1,761 children, Public Health Rep. 56:761, 1941.
7. Dean, H. T., Arnold, F. A., Jr., and Elvove, E.: Domestic water and dental caries, V, additional studies of the relation of fluoride domestic waters to dental caries experience in 4,425 white children, aged 12 to 14 years, of 13 cities in 4 states, Public Health Rep. 57:1155, 1942.
8. Arnold, F. A., Jr.: Fluorine in drinking water: its effect on dental caries, J.A.D.A. 36:28, 1948.
9. Cox, G. J.: Fluorine and dental caries. In Jeans, P. C., Elvehjem, C. A., and King, C. G., editors: Survey of the literature of dental caries, Pub. 225, Washington, D. C., 1952, National Academy of Sciences, National Research Council.
10. Muhler, J. C., Hine, M. K., and Day, H. G.: Preventive dentistry, St. Louis, 1954, The C. V. Mosby Co.
11. Muhler, J. C., and Hine, M. K.: Fluorine and dental health: the pharmacology and toxicology of fluorine, Bloomington, 1959, Indiana University Press.
12. McClure, F. J.: Fluoride drinking waters: a selection of Public Health Service papers on dental fluorosis and dental caries: physiological effects, analysis, and chemistry of fluoride, Pub. 825, Washington, D. C., 1962, United States Public Health Service.
13. Campbell, I. R.: The role of fluorine in public health: the soundness of fluoridation of communal water supplies, Cincinnati, Ohio, 1963, University of Cincinnati Press.
14. Smith, F. A., and Hodge, H. C.: Fluoride toxicity. In Muhler, J. C., and Hine, M. K., editors: Fluorine and dental health, Bloomington, 1959, Indiana University Press.
15. Dean, H. T., and Elvove, E.: Further studies on the minimal threshold of chronic endemic dental fluorosis, Public Health Rep. 52:1249, 1937.
16. Frajola, W. J.: Fluoride and enzyme inhibition. In Muhler, J. C., and Hine, M. K., editors: Fluorine and dental health, Bloomington, 1959, Indiana University Press.
17. Wright, D. E., and Jenkins, G. N.: The effect of fluoride on acid production of saliva-glucose mixtures, Brit. D. J. 96:30, 1954.
18. Bramstedt, F., Kroncke, A., and Naujoks, R.: Experimentelle Untersuchungen zur Fluorwirkung im Speichel, Schweiz. Mschr. Zahnheilk. 65:770, 1955.
19. Lilienthal, B.: The effect of fluoride on acid formation by salivary sediment, J. Dent. Res. 35:197, 1956.
20. Lilienthal, B., and Martin, W. D.: Investigation of the anti-enzymatic action of fluoride at the enamel surface, J. Dent. Res. 35:189, 1956.
21. Jenkins, G. N.: The effect of pH on the fluoride inhibition of salivary acid production, Arch. Oral Biol. 1:33, 1959.
22. Jenkins, G. N.: Some effects of fluoride on the metabolism of salivary bacteria, J. Dent. Res. 39:684, 1960.
23. McClure, F. J.: Domestic water and dental caries, III, fluorine in human saliva, Amer. J. Dis. Child. 62:512, 1941.
24. Martin, D. J., and Hill, I. N.: The Evanston dental caries study, V, the fluorine content of saliva and its relationship to (A) oral *Lactobacillus* counts and (B) the prevalence of dental caries, J. Dent. Res. 29:291, 1950.
25. Hardwick, J. L., and Leach, S. A., editors: The fluoride content of the dental plaque, Proceedings of the Ninth Congress of ORCA, Oxford, England, 1963, Pergamon Press.
26. Jenkins, G. N., Ferguson, D. B., and Edgar, W. M.: Bound and ionised fluoride in plaque, Abst. 488, San Francisco, March, 1968, Int. Ass. Dent. Res.
27. Dawes, C., and others: The relation between the fluoride concentrations in the dental plaque and in drinking water, Brit. D. J. 119:164, 1965.
28. American Dental Association: Council on Dental Therapeutics, Accepted dental therapeutics, 1969/1970, ed. 33, Chicago, 1969, The Association.
29. Isaac, S., and others: The relation of fluoride in the drinking water to the distribution of fluoride in enamel, J. Dent. Res. 37:318, 1958.
30. Yoon, S. H., and others: Distribution of fluoride in teeth from areas with different levels of fluoride in the water supply, J. Dent. Res. 39:845, 1960.

31. Jackson, D., and Weidmann, S. M.: The relationship between age and fluorine content of human dentine and enamel: a regional survey, Brit. D. J. 107:303, 1959.
32. Largent, E. J.: Metabolism of inorganic fluorides. In Shaw, J. H., editor: Fluoridation as a public health measure, Washington, D. C., 1954, American Association for the Advancement of Science.
33. Smith, F. A., Gardner, D. E., and Hodge, H. C.: Investigations on the metabolism of fluoride, II, fluoride content of blood and urine as a function of the fluorine in drinking water, J. Dent. Res. 29:596, 1950.
34. Singer, L., and Armstrong, W. D.: Regulation of human plasma fluoride concentration, J. Appl. Physiol. 15:508, 1960.
35. Striffler, D. F., and others: Fluoridation of water supplies in small rural communities, Public Health Rep. 80:25, 1965.
36. Dentistry in the United States, summary report of the Commission on the Survey of Dentistry in the United States, Washington, D. C., 1960, American Council on Education.
37. Strean, L. P., and Beaudet, J. P.: Inhibition of dental caries by ingestion of fluoride-vitamin tablets, New York J. Med. 45:2183, 1945.
38. Anonymous: Fluor-Grossaktion im Land Hessen, Deutsches Zahnh. Ztschr. 6:543, 1951.
39. Abary-Murillo, J.: Fluoride therapy, J. Philippine D. A. 5:19, 1952.
40. Held, A. J., and Piguet, F.: Kariesprophylaxe mit Fluortabletten, Stoma 7:213, 1954.
41. Bibby, B. G., Wilkins, E., and Witol, E.: A preliminary study of the effects of fluoride lozenges and pills on dental caries, Oral Surg. 8:213, 1955.
42. Binder, K.: Vorlaufiger Bericht uber die bisherigen Erfahrungen und Resultate der Fluortablettenverabfolgung an Wiener Schulkinder, Oester. Ztschr. Stomat. 55:653, 1958.
43. Kessler, W., and Solth, K.: Ergebnisse der Zahnkariesprophylaxe durch interne Fluor-Gaben, Stoma 11:14, 1958.
44. Schutzmannsky, G.: Kariesprophylaxe durch Fluortablettengabe, Deutsches Zahnh. Ztsch. 14:1713, 1959.
45. Arnold, F. A., Jr., McClure, F. J., and White, C. L.: Sodium fluoride tablets for children, D. Progress 1:8, 1960.
46. Ziemnowicz-Glowacka, W.: Sodium fluoride tablets as a means to reduce the incidence of caries in kindergarten pupils, Czas. Stomat. 13:719, 1960; Dent. Abstr. 6:397, 1961.
47. Wrzodek, G.: Ueber die Kariesprophylaxe mit Fluor in Hessen, Zahnh. Welt Reform 61:136, 1960; Dent. Abstr. 5:716, 1960.
48. Krusic, V.: Caries-reducing effects of tablets containing $CaF_2$ in Slovenian school children, Zobozdrov. vest. 15:27, 1960; Dent. Abstr. 6:243, 1961.
49. Pollak, H.: Caries prevention by administration of mulgatum fluoride tablets, Deutsches Zahnh. Ztschr. 14:363, 1960; Dent. Abstr. 6:119, 1961.
50. Held, A. J., and Dubois-Prevost, R.: Fluorides for dental prophylaxis, Ann. Biol. Clin. 19:497, 1961.
51. Grissom, D. K., and others: A comparative study of systemic sodium fluoride and topical stannous fluoride applications in preventive dentistry, J. Dent. Child. 31:314, 1964.
52. Hennon, D. K., Stookey, G. K., and Muhler, J. C.: A clinical study concerning the systemic ingestion of fluoride tablets in children, J. Dent. Child. (In press.)
53. Minoguchi, G., Ono, T., and Tamai, S.: Prophylactic application of fluoride for dental caries in Japan, Int. Dent. J. 13:510, 1963.
54. Kamocka, D., Sebastyanska, Z., and Spychalska, M.: Effect of fluoride tablets on caries in Polish preschool children, Czas. Stomat. 17:299, 1964; Dent. Abstr. 9:682, 1964.
55. Marthaler, T. M., and Konig, K. G.: The effect of fluoride tablet administration in schools on the caries incidence in 6- to 15-year-old children, Schweiz. Mschr. Zahnheilk. 77:539, 1967.
56. Berner, L., Fernex, F., and Held, A. J.: A study on the cariostatic effect of sodium fluoride (Zymafluor) tablets; results of thirteen year observations, Schweiz. Mschr. Zahnheilk. 77:528, 1967.
57. DePaola, P. F., and Lax, M.: The caries-inhibiting effect of acidulated phosphate–fluoride chewable tablets: a two-year double-blind study, J.A.D.A. 76:554, 1968.
58. Kailis, D. G., and others: Fluoride and caries: observations on the effects of prenatal

and postnatal fluoride on some Perth pre-school children, Med. J. Austral. 2:1037-40, 1968.
59. Wigdorwixa-Makowerowa, N.: Wroclaw investigations into fluorine prophylaxis of dental caries, Postery Hig. Med. Dosw. 21:287, 1967.
60. Stones, H. H., and others: The effect of topical applications of potassium fluoride and of the ingestion of tablets containing sodium fluoride on the incidence of dental caries, Brit. D. J. 86:263, 1949.
61. Gustafsson, B. E., and others: The Vipeholm dental caries study; the effect of different levels of carbohydrate intake on caries activity in 436 individuals observed for five years, Acta Odont. Scand. 2:232, 1954.
62. Jez, M.: Izledki mnoziene fluorizacije zobovja solske mladine, Zobozdrav. vest. 17:113, 1962; Dent. Abstr. 8:298, 1963.
63. Knychalska-Karwan, Z., and Laskowska, L.: Use of fluoride tablets in Polish children, Dent. Abstr. 9:53, 1964.
64. Bixler, D.: Blood and urinary studies using fluoride tablets, J. Dent. Res. 39:1119, 1960.
65. Muhler, J. C., and others: Blood and urinary fluoride studies following the ingestion of single dosages of fluoride, J. Oral Ther. 2:241, 1966.
66. McClure, F. J.: Nondental physiological effects of trace quantities of fluoride. In Moulton, F. R., editor: Dental caries and fluorine, Washington, D. C., 1946, American Association for the Advancement of Science.
67. Machle, W., Scott, E. W., and Largent, E. C.: The absorption and excretion of fluorides; the normal fluoride balance, J. Indust. Hyg. 24:199, 1942.
68. Richardson, A. S.: Parental participation in the administration of fluoride supplements, Canad. J. Pub. Health 58:508-13, 1967.
69. Hennon, D. K., Stookey, G. K., and Muhler, J. C.: Fluoride retention in rats receiving various vitamin-sodium fluoride preparations, J. Pediat. 64:272, 1964.
70. Showley, J. E., and others: The influence of vitamin supplementation on fluoride retention in animals fed a synthetic or stock corn diet, J. Oral Ther. 2:346, 1966.
71. Harkins, R. W., Longnecker, J. B., and Sarett, H. P.: The effect of NaF on the growth of rats with varying vitamin and calcium intakes, J. Nutrition 81:81, 1963.
72. Muhler, J. C.: Effect of vitamin C on skeletal fluoride storage in the guinea pig, J.A.D.A. 56:335, 1958.
73. Suttie, J. W., and Phillips, P. H.: Fluoride ingestion and vitamin metabolism. In Muhler, J. C., and Hine, M. K., editors: Fluorine and dental health, Bloomington, 1959, Indiana University Press.
74. Stookey, G. K.: Factors influencing fluoride metabolism, Indiana University, 1970 (doctoral dissertation).
75. Hennon, D. K., Stookey, G. K., and Muhler, J. C.: The clinical anticariogenic effectiveness of supplementary fluoride–vitamin preparations: results at the end of three years, J. Dent. Child. 33:3, 1966.
76. Hennon, D. K., Stookey, G. K., and Muhler, J. C.: The clinical anticariogenic effectiveness of supplementary fluoride–vitamin preparations: results at the end of four years, J. Dent. Child. 34:439, 1967.
77. Hennon, D. K., Stookey, G. K., and Muhler, J. C.: The clinical anticariogenic effectiveness of supplementary fluoride–vitamin preparations: results after five and a half years. (Unpublished report, 1969.)
78. Margolis, F. J., Macauley, J., and Freshman, E.: The effects of measured doses of fluoride—a five-year preliminary report, Amer. J. Dis. Child. 113:670-2, 1967.
79. Zipkin, I., and Babeaux, W. L.: Maternal transfer of fluoride, J. Oral Ther. 1:652, 1965.
80. Hudson, J. T., and Stookey, G. K.: Studies on the placental transfer of fluoride in the guinea pig, I.A.D.R. Abstract 46, 1965.
81. Martin, D. J.: The Evanston dental caries study, I, determination of fluorine in foods, bones, and teeth, J. Dent. Res. 27:27, 1948.
82. Blayney, J. R., and Hill, I. N.: Evanston dental caries study, XXIV, prenatal fluorides—value of water-borne fluorides during pregnancy, J.A.D.A. 69:291, 1964.
83. Gardner, D. E., and others: Fluoride content of placental tissue as related to fluoride content of drinking water, Science 115:208, 1952.

84. Feltman, R., and Kosel, G.: Prenatal ingestion of fluorides and their transfer to the fetus, Science 122:560, 1955.
85. Gedalia, I., and others: Placental transfer of fluorine in the human fetus, Proc. Soc. Exp. Biol. Med. 106:147, 1961.
86. Brzezinski, A., Bercovici, B., and Gedalia, I.: Fluorine in the human fetus, Obstet. Gynec. 15:329, 1960.
87. Feltman, R., and Kosel, G.: Prenatal and postnatal ingestion of fluorides—14 years of investigation—final report, J. Dent. Med. 16:190, 1961.
88. Ziegler, E.: Untersuchungen uber die Fluorierung der Milch zur Cariesprophylaxe, Mitt. Gesch. Med. Naturwiss. 28:13, 1956.
89. Held, H. R.: Der Durchtritt des Fluors durch die Placenta und sein Uebertritt in die Milch, Schweiz. med. Wschr. 82:297, 1952.
90. Held, H. R.: Fluormedikation und Blutluor, Schweiz. med. Wschr. 84:251, 1954.
91. Feltman, R.: Prenatal and postnatal ingestion of fluorides—a progress report, Dent. Dig. 62:353, 1956.
92. Katz, S., and Muhler, J. C.: Prenatal fluoride and dental caries experience in deciduous teeth, J.A.D.A. 76:305, 1968.
93. Carlos, J. P., Gittelsohn, A.M., and Haddon, W., Jr.: Caries in deciduous teeth in relation to maternal ingestion of fluoride, Public Health Rep. 77:658, 1962.
94. Horowitz, H. S., and Heifetz, S. B.: Effects of prenatal exposure to fluoridation on dental caries, Public Health Rep. 82:297-303, 1967.
95. Arnold, F. A., Jr., and others: Effect of fluoridated public water supplies on dental caries prevalence; tenth year of the Grand Rapids-Muskegon Study, Public Health Rep. 71:652, 1956.
96. Weddle, D. A., and Muhler, J. C.: The effects of inorganic salts on fluorine storage in the rat, J. Nutrition 54:437, 1954.
97. Stookey, G. K., Hennon, D. K., and Muhler, J. C.: The skeletal retention and anticariogenic efficacy of fluoride when administered in the presence of a prenatal vitamin-mineral supplement, J. Dent. Res. 48:1224-30, 1969.
98. Bohne, C.: Fluoridated NaCl: large scale tests in Switzerland, Zahnarztl. Praxis 7:8, 1956.
99. Marthaler, T. M.: Zur Frage des Fluorvollsalzes lerstklinische Resultate (fluoride addition to table salt; first clinical results), Schweiz. Mschr. Zahnh. 71:671, 1961; Dent. Abstr. 7:55, 1962.
100. Hadjimarkos, D. M.: Sea salt and dental caries, Nature 195:392, 1962.
101. Muhler, J. C., and Weddle, D. A.: Utilizability of fluorine storage in the rat when administered in milk, J. Nutrition 55:347, 1955.
102. Ericsson, Y.: The state of fluorine in milk and its absorption and retention when administered in milk, investigations with radioactive fluorine, Acta Odont. Scand. 16:51, 1958.
103. Light, A. E., and others: Effect of fluoridated milk on deciduous teeth, J.A.D.A. 56:249, 1958.
104. Kopel, H.: Fluoridated milk of value in preventing dental cavities in children, J. Dent. Child. 28:334, 1961.
105. Rusoff, L. L., and others: Fluoride addition to milk and its effect on dental caries in school children, Amer. J. Clin. Nutrition 11:94, 1962.
106. Ege, R.: Berigelse af dem Danske kost Med Fluorid, Tandlaegebladet 65:445, 1961; Dent. Abstr. 7:93, 1962.
107. Emslie, R. D., Veall, N., and Duckworth, R.: Chewing gum as a vehicle for the administration of fluoride: studies with $F^{18}$, Brit. D. J. 110:121, 1961.
108. Lind, V., Stelling, E., and Nystrom, S.: Fluorhaltigt Tuggummi som Kariesprofylaktikum, Odont. Revy 12:341, 1961; Dent. Abstr. 7:456, 1962.
109. Bibby, B. G.: Use of fluorine in the prevention of dental caries, II, effects of sodium fluoride applications, J.A.D.A. 31:317, 1944.
110. Bibby, B. G., and Turesky, S. S.: A note on the duration of caries inhibition produced by fluoride applications, J. Dent. Res. 26:105, 1947.

111. Knutson, J. W., and Armstrong, W. D.: Effect of topically applied sodium fluoride on dental caries experience, Public Health Rep. 58:1701, 1943.
112. Knutson, J. W., and Armstrong, W. D.: Effect of topically applied sodium fluoride on dental caries experience, II, report of findings of second year, Public Health Rep. 60: 1085, 1945.
113. Knutson, J. W., and Armstrong, W. D.: Effect of topically applied sodium fluoride on dental caries experience, III, report of findings for the third study year, Public Health Rep. 61:1683, 1946.
114. McCauley, H. B., and Dale, P. P.: Observation of increased caries activity following interruption of topical fluorine applications, J. Dent. Res. 24:305, 1945.
115. Jordan, W. A., and others: The effects of various numbers of topical applications of sodium fluoride, J.A.D.A. 33:1385, 1946.
116. Fulton, J. T., and Tracy, E. T.: Use of topical fluorine on school age children and its effect on dental caries, Connecticut Health Bull. 60:55, 1946.
117. Knutson, J. W., Armstrong, W. D., and Feldman, F. M.: Effect of topically applied sodium fluoride on dental caries experience, IV, report of findings with two, four, and six applications, Public Health Rep. 62:425, 1947.
118. Knutson, J. W.: Sodium fluoride solution: technic for applications to the teeth, J.A.D.A. 36:37, 1948.
119. Galagan, D. J., and Knutson, J. W.: Effect of topically applied sodium fluoride on dental caries experience, V, report of findings with two, four, and six applications of sodium fluoride and of lead fluoride, Public Health Rep. 62:1477, 1947.
120. Galagan, D. J., and Knutson, J. W.: Effect of topically applied sodium fluoride on dental caries experience, VI, experiments with sodium fluoride and calcium chloride; widely spaced applications; use of different solution concentrations, Public Health Rep. 63:1215, 1948.
121. Tschappat, K.: Uber die lokale Fluorapplikation zur Kariesprophylaxe und ihre statistische Answertung mit dem "Berner Kariesindex," Schweiz. Mschr. Zahnh. 58:961, 1948.
122. Hewat, R. E. T., and Rice, F. B.: Control of dental caries by topical applications of sodium fluoride: experimental study on 97 children in Wellington, New Zealand D. J. 45:215, 1949.
123. Syrrist, A.: Experimental studies on the effect of sodium fluoride on human dental enamel; investigations into the potentialities of topical application of sodium fluoride to teeth as a means of caries control, Odont. Tskr. 57:447, 1949.
124. Miller, J.: Clinical investigations in preventive dentistry, Brit. D. J. 91:92, 1951; D. Pract. 1:66, 1950.
125. Davies, G. N.: Dental caries control and the general practitioner, New Zealand D. J. 46:25, 1950.
126. Floren, I.: Experiments with fluoride applications on school children in Goteborg, Odont. Tskr. 58:66, 1950.
127. Chrietzenberg, J. E.: Toothbrushing as a substitute for quick cleaning in the topical fluoride technic, J.A.D.A. 42:435, 1951.
128. Hewat, R. E. T., Eastcott, D. F., and Leslie, G. H.: Control of dental caries by topical applications of sodium fluoride; second experimental study in Wellington, New Zealand D. J. 47:123, 1951.
129. Marshall-Day, C. D.: Effect of topical sodium fluoride on dental caries during adolescence, J. Dent. Res. 30:514, 1951.
130. Adler, P.: Collective and cooperative caries prophylaxis with fluoride, Zahnh. Praxis 3:26, 1952.
131. Adler, P.: Kariesschutz durch Fluor (caries protection by fluoride), Oester. Ztschr. Stomat. 49:247, 1952.
132. Walton, W. E.: Topical sodium fluoride, Pennsylvania D. J. 19:23, 1952.
133. Bergman, G.: The caries inhibiting action of sodium fluoride; experimental studies, Acta Odont. Scand. 11:112, 1953.
134. Cohen, A., and Schiffrin, L.: Dental caries in handicapped children after topical sodium fluoride, Oral Surg. 6:562, 1953.

135. Sarkany, I.: A helyi fluorkezeles hatekonysage (the effectiveness of local fluoride applications), Orv. hetil. **94:**321, 1953.
136. Hawes, R. R., Sannes, S., and Brudevold, F.: Pilot studies of three topical fluoride application procedures, J. Dent. Res. **33:**661, 1954.
137. Syrrist, A., and Karlsen, K.: A five-year report on the effect of topical applications of sodium fluoride on dental caries experience, Brit. D. J. **97:**1, 1954.
138. University of Toronto, Division of Dental Research, Faculty of Dentistry: Topical application of sodium fluoride, J. Ontario D. A. **31:**326, 1954.
139. Howell, C. L., and others: Effect of topically applied stannous fluoride on dental caries experience in children, J.A.D.A. **50:**14, 1955.
140. McLaren, H. R., and Brown, H. K.: A study of the use of topically applied stannous fluoride solution in prevention of dental caries, Canad. J. Pub. Health **46:**387, 1955.
141. Schutzmannsky, G.: 5-Jahres-Ergebnisse lokaler Fluorapplikation, Deutsches Zahn. Heilk. **22:**166, 1955.
142. Kimmelman, B. B.: Clinical caries control: effectiveness of 2% sodium fluoride cream, I.A.D.R. Abstract 34, 1956.
143. Dominick, K., and Wodniecki, J.: Die lokale Fluorapplikation bei Schulkindern in Olkusz (Polen), Odont. Revy **8:**335, 1957.
144. Nevitt, G. A., Witter, D. H., and Bowman, W. D.: Topical applications of sodium fluoride and stannous fluoride, Public Health Rep. **73:**847, 1958.
145. Czarnocka, K., and others: Topical fluoridation of teeth in children, Czas. Stomat. **12:** 699, 1959.
146. Harris, R.: Observations on the effect of topical sodium fluoride on caries incidence in children, Australian D. J. **4:**257, 1959.
147. Miller, J., and Hobson, P.: Silver nitrate and sodium fluoride on enamel caries, Brit. D. J. **106:**246, 1959.
148. Berggren, H., and Welander, E.: Supervised tooth brushing with a sodium fluoride solution in 5,000 Swedish school children, Acta Odont. Scand. **18:**209, 1960.
149. Mercer, V. H., and Muhler, J. C.: Comparison of a single application of stannous fluoride with a single application of sodium fluoride or two applications of stannous fluoride, J. Dent. Child. **28:**84, 1961.
150. Law, F. E., Jeffreys, M. H., and Sheary, H. C.: Topical applications of fluoride solutions in dental caries control, Public Health Rep. **76:**287, 1961.
151. Torell, P., and Ericsson, Y.: Two-year clinical tests with different methods of local caries-preventive fluorine application in Swedish school children, Acta Odont. Scand. **23:**287, 1965.
152. Badzian-Kobos, K., and Pankiewicz, H.: Beitrag zur anwendung der fluorideirung der kauflache der durchbrechenden ersten bleibenden molaren, Deutsch Stomat. **17:**337, 1967.
153. Averill, H. M., Averill, J. E., and Ritz, A. G.: A 2-year comparison of three topical fluoride agents, J.A.D.A. **74:**996-1001, 1967.
154. Cons, N. C., and Janerich, D. T.: Albany topical fluoride study—2 year preliminary report, I.A.D.R. Abstract 545, 1969.
155. Downs, R. A., and Pelton, W. J.: The effect of topically applied fluorides in dental caries experience on children residing in fluoride areas, J. Colorado State D.A. **29:**7, 1950.
156. Galagan, D. J., and Vermillion, J. R.: Effect of topical fluoride on teeth matured on fluoride bearing water, Public Health Rep. **70:**1114, 1955.
157. Ast, D. B.: Sodium fluoride dental caries prophylaxis, New York Dent. J. **16:**441, 1950.
158. Jordan, W. A.: A three-year study on the effects of a 2% topical sodium fluoride on deciduous molars, North-West Den. **29:**265, 1950.
159. Wittich, H. C.: The effect of topical application of sodium fluoride upon deciduous teeth, North-West Den. **29:**113, 1950.
160. Sundvall-Hagland, I.: Sodium fluoride application to the deciduous dentition; a clinical study, Acta Odont. Scand. **13:**5, 1955.
161. McDonald, R. E., and Muhler, J. C.: The superiority of topical application of stannous fluoride on primary teeth, J. Dent. Child. **24:**84, 1957.

162. Arnold, F. A., Jr., Dean, H. T., and Singleton, D. C., Jr.: The effect of caries incidence of a single topical application of fluoride solution to the teeth of young adult males of a military population, J. Dent. Res. **23:**155, 1944.
163. Frank, R.: Research and clinical evaluation of local applications of sodium fluorides, Schweiz. Mschr. Zahnh. **60:**283, 1950.
164. Klinkenberg, E., and Bibby, B. G.: Effect of topical applications of fluorides on dental caries in young adults, J. Dent. Res. **29:**4, 1950.
165. Driak, F.: Kariesprophylaxe mit besonderer Berucksichtigung der Impragnierungsmethoden, Oester. Ztschr. Stomat. **48:**153, 1951.
166. Rickles, N. H., and Becks, H.: The effects of an acid and a neutral solution of sodium fluoride on the incidence of dental caries in young adults, J. Dent. Res. **30:**757, 1951.
167. Kutler, B., and Ireland, R. L.: The effect of sodium fluoride application on dental caries experience in adults, J. Dent. Res. **32:**458, 1953.
168. Carter, W. J., and others: The effect of topical fluoride on dental caries experience in adult females of a military population, J. Dent. Res. **34:**73, 1955.
169. Slack, G. L.: The effect of topical application of stannous fluoride solution in the prevention of dental caries, J. Dent. Res. **34:**785, 1955.
170. Slack, G. L.: The effect of topical application of stannous fluoride on the incidence of dental caries in 6-year-old children, Brit. D. J. **101:**7, 1956.
171. Muhler, J. C.: Effect on gingiva and occurrence of pigmentation on teeth following the topical application of stannous fluoride or stannous chlorofluoride, J. Periodont. **28:** 281, 1957.
172. Jordan, W. A., Snyder, J. R., and Wilson, V.: Stannous fluoride clinical study in Olmsted County, Minnesota, Public Health Rep. **73:**1010, 1958.
173. Jordan, W. A., Snyder, J. R., and Wilson, V.: A study of a single application of eight per cent stannous fluoride, J. Dent. Child. **26:**355, 1959.
174. Abdul-Ghaffar, H., and Muhler, J. C.: Pretreatment of teeth with sodium fluoride prior to stannous fluoride application in children, J. Dent. Res. **38:**901, 1959.
175. Rothhaar, R. E.: Topical stannous fluoride in a pedodontic practice, J. Dent. Child. **27:**140, 1960.
176. Gish, C. W., Muhler, J. C., and Howell, C. L.: A new approach to the topical application of fluorides for the reduction of dental caries in children; results at the end of five years, J. Dent. Child. **29:**65, 1962.
177. Salter, W. A. T., McCombie, F., and Hole, L. W.: The anticariogenic effects of one and two applications of stannous fluoride on the deciduous and permanent teeth of children age 6 and 7, J. Canad. D. A. **28:**363, 1962.
178. Thomsen, C.: Om anvendelse of tinfluoridi caries profylaksen, Tandlaegebladet **66:**1, 1962; Dent. Abstr. **7:**338, 1962.
179. Peterson, J. K., and Williamson, L.: Effectiveness of topical application of eight percent stannous fluoride, Public Health Rep. **77:**39, 1962.
180. Harris, R.: Observations on the effect of eight per cent stannous fluoride on dental caries in children, Australian D. J. **8:**335, 1963.
181. Mercer, V. H., and Muhler, J. C.: The effect of a 30-second topical $SnF_2$ treatment on dental caries reductions in children, J. Oral Ther. **1:**141, 1964.
182. Hoskova, M., and Komarek, K.: Effect of topical use of stannous fluoride, Cesk. Stomat. **64:**390, 1964.
183. Wellock, W. D., Maitland, A., and Brudevold, F.: Caries increments, tooth discoloration, and state of oral hygiene in children given single annual applications of acid phosphate–fluoride and stannous fluoride, Arch. Oral Biol. **10:**453, 1965.
184. Muhler, J. C., Stookey, G. K., and Bixler, D.: Evaluation of the anticariogenic effect of mixtures of stannous fluoride and soluble phosphates, J. Dent. Child. **32:**154, 1965.
185. Muhler, J. C.: The anticariogenic effectiveness of a single application of stannous fluoride in children residing in an optimal communal fluoride area, J. Dent. Child. **27:** 51, 1960.
186. Hass, R. L.: Effectiveness of a single application of stannous fluoride after toothbrushing, J.A.D.A. **71:**1391, 1965.

187. Horowitz, H. S., and Lucye, H. S.: A clinical study of stannous fluoride in a prophylaxis paste and as a solution, J. Oral Ther. 3:17-25, 1967.
188. Caprioglio, D., and Resta, C.: The value of topical applications of eight percent stannous fluoride in the reduction of dental caries in children—a 2-year study, Dent. Cosmos 35:1543, 1967.
189. Caprioglio, D., Carlino, W., and Resta, C.: Effetti di applicazioni topiche con fluoruro stannoso (8%) sulla riduzione della carie dentale nei bambini, II, risultati dopo tre anni, Riv. Ital. Stomat. 22:1274, 1967.
190. Cartwright, H. V., Lindahl, R. L., and Bawden, J. W.: Clinical findings on the effectiveness of stannous fluoride and acid phosphate fluoride as caries reducing agents in children, J. Dent. Child. 35:36-40, 1968.
191. Bordoni, N., and others: Topical application of stannous fluoride—its statistical evaluation, Rev. Assoc. Odont. Argent. 56:155, 1968.
192. Muhler, J. C.: The anticariogenic effectiveness of a single application of stannous fluoride in children residing in an optimal fluoride area, II, results at the end of 30 months, J.A.D.A. 61:431, 1960.
193. Horowitz, H. S., and Heifetz, S. B.: Evaluation of topical applications of stannous fluoride to teeth of children born and reared in a fluoridated community: final report, J. Dent. Child. 36:355, 1969.
194. Ship, I., Cohen, A., and Laster, L.: The effects of acidulated fluorophosphate and stannous fluoride topical applications on DMFT in adolescents in a fluoridated community, I.A.D.R. Abstract 278, 1967.
195. Meckel, A. H., and Francis, M. D.: Intraoral transfer of stannous fluoride, J. Dent. Res. 43:81, 1964.
196. Compton, F. H., and others: The Riverdale preschool project, J. Canad. D.A. 25:478, 1959.
197. Burgess, R., and others: Topical stannous fluoride for preschool children, J. Dent. Res. 40:712, 1961.
198. Protheroe, D. H.: A study to determine the effect of topical application of stannous fluoride on dental caries in young adults, Roy. Canad. D. Corps Quart. 3:18, 1962.
199. Muhler, J. C.: The effect of a single topical application of stannous fluoride on the incidence of dental caries in adults, J. Dent. Res. 37:415, 1958.
200. Harris, N. O., and others: Stannous fluoride topically applied in aqueous solution in caries prevention in a military population, SAM-TDR-64-26, Brooks Air Force Base, Texas, 1964, United States Air Force School of Aerospace Medicine.
201. Weisz, W. S.: A comparison of the relative effects of sodium and stannous fluoride when applied topically, J. Dent. Child. 29:65, 1962.
202. Mandel, I. D., and Cagan, R.: Pharmaceutical agents for preventing caries—a review, II, topical application procedures, J. Oral Ther. 2:128, 1965.
203. Dudding, N. J., and Muhler, J. C.: Technique of application of stannous fluoride in a compatible paste and as a topical agent, J. Dent. Child. 29:219, 1962.
204. Swieterman, R. P., Muhler, J. C., and Swenson, H. M.: The effect of highly concentrated solutions of stannous fluoride on human gingival tissues, J. Periodont. 32:131, 1961.
205. Higgason, J. C., Swenson, H. M., and Muhler, J. C.: Effect on gingival tissues of albino rats of concentrated solutions of topically applied sodium or stannous fluoride, J. Periodont. 34:357, 1963.
206. Muhler, J. C.: Stannous fluoride enamel pigmentation—evidence of caries arrestment, J. Dent. Child. 27:157, 1960.
207. Mercer, V., and Muhler, J. C.: The clinical demonstration of caries arrestment following topical stannous fluoride treatments, J. Dent. Child. 32:65, 1965.
208. Scola, F. P., and Ostrom, C. A.: Clinical evaluation of stannous fluoride in naval personnel, I.A.D.R. Abstract 49, 1965.
209. Cheyne, V. D.: Human dental caries and topically applied fluorine; a preliminary report, J.A.D.A. 29:804, 1942.
210. Howell, C. L., and Muhler, J. C.: The effect of topically applied stannous chlorofluoride on the dental caries experience in children, Science 120:316, 1954.

154 *Improving dental practice through preventive measures*

211. Howell, C. L., and Muhler, J. C.: The effect of topically applied stannous chlorofluoride on the dental caries experience in children, II, results two years after initial treatment, J.A.D.A. **55**:493, 1957.
212. Gish, C. W., Muhler, J. C., and Howell, C. L.: The effect of topically applied potassium fluorostannite on the dental caries experience in children, J. Dent. Res. **36**:780, 1957.
213. Gish, C. W., Muhler, J. C., and Howell, C. L.: The effect of topically applied potassium fluorostannite on the dental caries experience in children, II, results at the end of two years, J. Dent. Res. **37**:417, 1958.
214. Gish, C. W., Muhler, J. C., and Howell, C. L.: The effect of topically applied potassium fluorostannite on the dental caries experience in children, III, results at the end of three years, J. Dent. Res. **38**:881, 1959.
215. Muhler, J. C.: Effects of fluoride and non-fluoride containing tin salt on the dental caries experience in children, J. Dent. Res. **37**:422, 1958.
216. Bibby, B. G., DeRoche, E., and Wilkins, E.: The effect of topical applications of lead fluoride on dental caries, J. Dent. Res. **26**:446, 1947.
217. East, B. R., and others: A study of the topical application of potassium fluoride in caries prevention, J. Dent. Res. **24**:267, 1945.
218. Peterson, J. K., and Jordan, W. A.: Relative caries-inhibiting value of topically applied sodium silicofluoride and sodium fluoride: final report of a two yaer study at Mound, Minnesota, J. Dent. Res. **36**:124, 1957.
219. Berggren, H., and Welander, E.: The caries-inhibiting effect of sodium, ferric and zirconium fluorides, Acta Odont. Scand. **22**:401, 1964.
220. Muhler, J. C., Bixler, D., and Stookey, G. K.: The clinical effectivness of stannous hexafluorozirconate as an anticariogenic agent, J.A.D.A. **76**:558, 1968.
221. Brudevold, F., and others: A study of acidulated fluoride solutions, I, in vitro effects on enamel, Arch. Oral Biol. **8**:167, 1963.
222. Bibby, B. G., and others: Preliminary reports on the effect on dental caries of the use of sodium fluoride in a prophylactic cleaning mixture and in a mouthwash, J. Dent. Res. **25**:207, 1946.
223. Roberts, J. F., Bibby, B. G., and Wellock, W. D.: The effect of an acidulated fluoride mouthwash on dental caries, J. Dent. Res. **27**:497, 1948.
224. Tempestini, O.: Problems of fluoride in individuals and public health control of caries, Riv. Ital. Stomat. **4**:323, 1949.
225. Wellock, W. D., and Brudevold, F.: A study of acidulated fluoride solutions, II, the caries inhibiting effect of single annual topical applications of an acidic fluoride and phosphate solution; a two year experience, Arch. Oral Biol. **8**:179, 1963.
226. Pameijer, J. H. N., Brudevold, F., and Hunt, E. E., Jr.: A study of acidulated fluoride solutions, III, the cariostatic effect of repeated topical sodium fluoride applications with and without phosphate: a pilot study, Arch. Oral Biol. **8**:183, 1963.
227. Szwejda, L. F., Tossy, C. V., and Below, D. M.: Fluorides in community programs; results from a fluoride gel applied topically, J. Public Health Dent. **27**:192, 1967.
228. DePaola, P. F.: Combined use of a sodium fluoride prophylaxis paste and a spray containing acidulated sodium fluoride solution, J.A.D.A. **75**:1407-11, 1967.
229. Horowitz, H. S.: The effect on dental caries of topically applied acidulated phosphate-fluoride: results after one year, J. Oral Ther. **4**:286, 1968.
230. Horowitz, H. S.: Effect on dental caries of topically applied acidulated phosphate-fluoride: results after two years, J.A.D.A. **78**:568, 1969.
231. Horowitz, H. S.: Effect of topically applied acidulated phosphate-fluoride on dental caries in Hawaiian school children, I.A.D.R. Abstract 549, 1969.
232. Selvig, K. A.: Local application of acidulated phosphate-fluoride in school children, Norske Tannlaegeforen Tid. **78**:483, 1968.
233. Gray, A. S., Hawk, D. R., and Jordan, I. I.: Pilot dental program for Penticon school children, J. Canad. D. A. **35**:316, 1969.
234. Jordan, W. A., Pugnier, V. A., and McKee, D. P.: Evaluating acidulated phosphate fluoride solution as a caries inhibitor, North-West Den. **48**:207-10, 1969.
235. DePaola, P. F., and others: The relationship of cariostasis, oral hygiene, and past caries experience in children receiving three sprays annually with acidulated phosphate-fluoride: three-year results, J.A.D.A. **77**:91, 1968.

236. Stookey, G. K., Hudson, J. T., and Muhler, J. C.: Laboratory studies concerning the effectiveness and safety of various fluoride and fluoride–phosphate systems, J. Dent. Res. **46:**503, 1967.
237. Weisz, W. S.: Two year study of efficacy of sodium fluoride mouth wash, Pennsylvania D. J. **15:**36, 1947.
238. Weisz, W. S.: The reduction of dental caries through use of a sodium fluoride mouthwash, J.A.D.A. **60:**438, 1960.
239. Fjaestad-Seger, M., Norstedt-Larsson, K., and Torell, P.: Forsok med enkla metoder for klinisk fluorapplikation. Sverig. Tandlak-Farb. Tidn. **53:**169, 1961.
240. Torell, P., and Siberg, A.: Mouthwash with sodium fluoride and potassium fluoride, Odont. Revy **13:**62, 1962.
241. Goaz, P. W., and others: Effect of daily applications of sodium monofluorophosphate solutions on caries rate in children, J. Dent. Res. **42:**965, 1963.
242. Forsman, B.: Effect of mouth rinses with sodium fluoride in schools at Vixjo, Sverig. Tandlak.-Forb. Tidn. **57:**705, 1965.
243. Torell, P., and Ericsson, Y.: The value in caries prevention of methods for applying fluorides topically to the teeth, Int. Dent. J. **17:**564, 1967.
244. Ollinen, P.: Munskoljning eller borstning med olika fluoridlosningar, Sverig. Tandlak.-Forb. Tidn. **58:**913, 1966.
245. Kasakura, T.: Dental observation on school feeding, part 3, effect of the dental caries prevention by oral rinsing with sodium fluoride solution after school feeding, Odontology **54:**22-32, 1966.
246. Hundstadbraaten, K.: Effect on dental caries in children of supervised toothbrushing with a sodium fluoride; results after three years, Norske. Tannlaegefor. T. **76:**164, 1966.
247. Kann, J.: Systematic controlled use of mouth rinses with fluoride, Tandlaegebladet **69:** 838, 1965.
248. Englander, H. R., and others: Clinical anticaries effect of repeated topical sodium fluoride applications by mouthpieces, J.A.D.A. **75:**638, 1967.
249. Swerdloff, G., and Shannon, I. L.: Feasibility of the use of stannous fluoride mouthwash in a school system, J. Dent. Child. **36:**363, 1969.
250. Bullen, D. C. T., McCombie, F., and Hole, L. W.: One year effect of supervised toothbrushing with an acidulated fluoride-phosphate solution, J. Canad. D.A. **31:**231, 1965.
251. Bullen, D. C. T., McCombie, F., and Hole, L. W.: Two year effect of supervised toothbrushing with an acidulated fluoride-phosphate solution, J. Canad. D. A. **32:**89-93, 1966.
252. Conchie, J. M., McCombie, F., and Hole, L. W.: Three years of supervised toothbrushing with a fluoride-phosphate solution, J. Public Health Dent. **29:**11-18, 1969.
253. Koch, G.: Caries increment in school children during and two years after end of supervised rinsing of the mouth with sodium fluoride solution, Odont. Revy **20:**323, 1969.
254. Horowitz, H. S., and Heifetz, S. B.: A review of studies on the self-administration of topical fluorides, Canad. J. Pub. Health **59:**393, 1968.
255. Heifetz, S. B., Horowitz, H. S., and Driscoll, W. S.: Evaluation of a self-administered procedure for the topical application of acidulated phosphate-fluoride: results after two years, I.A.D.R. Abstract 544, 1969.
256. Tusnova, M. N.: Fluoridation of teeth for prophylactic purposes against caries, Stomatologiia **2:**11, 1950.
257. Kiseleva, M. M., Reusova, E. P., and Sofronova, A. F.: Data on the effectiveness of local fluoridation, Stomatologiia **38:**10, 1959.
258. Peterson, J. K., and others: Effectiveness of an acidulated phosphate fluoride-pumice prophylactic paste: a two-year report, J. Dent. Res. **48:**346, 1969.
259. Peterson, J. K., Jordan, W. A., and Snyder, J. R.: Effectiveness of stannous fluoride-silex-silicone prophylaxis paste, North-West Den. **42:**276, 1963.
260. Bixler, D., and Muhler, J. C.: Combined use of three agents containing stannous fluoride: a prophylactic paste, a solution, and a dentifrice, J.A.D.A. **68:**792, 1964.
261. Gish, G. W., and Muhler, J. C.: Effect on dental caries in children in a natural fluoride area of combined use of three agents containing stannous fluoride: a prophylactic paste, a solution, and a dentifrice, J.A.D.A. **70:**914, 1965.
262. Muhler, J. C., and Bixler, D.: Clinical evaluation of multiple stannous fluoride therapy in adults. (Unpublished report, 1962.)

263. Bixler, D., and Muhler, J. C.: Clinical evaluation of multiple stannous fluoride therapy in adults. (Unpublished report, 1963.)
264. Muhler, J. C.: Unpublished data.
265. Gish, C. W., and Muhler, J. C.: Unpublished data.
266. Muhler, J. C.: Mass treatment of children with a stannous fluoride zirconium silicate self-administered prophylactic paste for partial control of dental caries, J. Amer. Coll. Dent. **35:**45, 1968.
267. Gish, C. W., and Mercer, V. H.: Child self-application of a zirconium silicate-stannous fluoride anticariogenic paste—clinical results after 1 and 2 years, I.A.D.R. Abstract 552, 1969.
268. Gish, C. W., Mercer, V. H., and Smith, C. E.: Unpublished reports, 1969.
269. Lang, L. A., and others: The clinical efficacy of a self-applied stannous fluoride prophylactic paste; results after eighteen months, J. Dent. Child. **37:**27, 1970.
270. Jordan, W. A., Pugnier, V. A., and McKee, D. P.: Unpublished report, 1969.
271. Oshiro, R. S.: Unpublished report, 1969.
272. Kelley, G. E., and others: The clinical evaluation of a patient administered $SnF_2$-$ZrSiO_4$ prophylactic paste in children, I, results after one year in the Virgin Islands, J.A.D.A. **81:**142, 1970.
273. Muhler, J. C., and others: Arrestment of incipient dental caries in adults following three different forms of $SnF_2$ therapy, J.A.D.A. **75:**1406, 1967.
274. Scola, F. P., Nielsen, A. G., and Ostrom, C. A.: Clinical evaluation of stannous fluoride, progress report, I.A.D.R. Abstract 41, 1963.
275. Scola, F. P., and Ostrom, C. A.: Clinical evaluation of stannous fluoride when used as a constituent of a compatible prophylactic paste, as a topical solution, and in a dentifrice in naval personnel, II, report of findings after two years, J.A.D.A. **77:**594, 1968.
276. Gish, C. W.: Personal communication.

## Chapter 7 Dentifrices and oral hygiene

### Joseph C. Muhler

Historical aspects
Dentifrice composition and function of component parts
Subjects' reaction to brushing with and without a dentifrice
Dentifrice stomatitis
What dentifrice should your patients use?
    Stannous fluoride–calcium pyrophosphate dentifrices
    Sodium monofluorophosphate dentifrices
    Chlorophyll dentifrices
    Ammoniated dentifrices
    Antibiotic dentifrices
    Antienzyme dentifrices
    Neutral dentifrices
Brushing after meals
    Anticalculus dentifrices
What type of toothbrush should your patients use?
    Electric toothbrushes
What is the best way to brush one's teeth?
Conclusion

## HISTORICAL ASPECTS

In the past decade there has been more interest in the use of dentifrices than at any other time in dental history. A number of factors account for this, most of which are important not only to one's personal dental health today but also to the future dental health of our children. On August 1, 1960, the Council on Dental Therapeutics of the American Dental Association placed a stannous fluoride calcium pyrophosphate dentifrice* into a "B" classification. This in itself was an epic step forward in dental health in that it was the first time the American Dental Association ever formally recognized a commercial dentifrice advertised to the public as having "therapeutic" value against tooth decay. Subsequently, in 1964 this classification was changed to "A"—recognition of complete acceptance by the Council on Dental Therapeutics. Subsequently three other stannous fluoride dentifrices (Cue, Fact, and Super Stripe) received the "B" classification, and in 1969 the first non-stannous fluoride dentifrice† was placed in the "A" classification.

The function of a dentifrice is not limited to providing an agent useful for reducing tooth decay, however. Historically, a dentifrice is a substance whose primary function is to clean the accessible surfaces of the teeth when used with a toothbrush and whose secondary functions are to polish the teeth, to improve gingival health, and to help reduce mouth odors. Hopefully, it may someday be possible to have an effective dentifrice for controlling, or preventing, salivary calculus.

---
*Crest brand dentifrice, manufactured by The Procter and Gamble Co., Cincinnati, Ohio.
†Colgate-MFP brand dentifrice. This product contains 2.0 percent sodium N-lauroyl sarcosinate and 0.76 percent sodium monofluorophosphate as the active agents.

The history of dentifrices is, in a sense, the history of dentistry. Probably the control of pain and the desire for clean teeth more closely parallel the development of dentistry as we know it today than any one factor or combination of factors. It is paradoxical that these two different factors are related to each other in any way. However, if one could and would clean his teeth properly every day in the manner required to eliminate the dental plaque he would in fact probably suffer no dental pain from tooth decay. The old adage "A clean tooth never decays" is widely accepted, the critical problem being that it is extremely difficult to clean properly the areas of the tooth that decay most readily.

Dental caries is not a disease of civilized man as some would want you to believe. Without any doubt, primitive man suffered from tooth decay. In fact, archeologists have found evidence both in skeletons and written manuscripts indicating that prehistoric man even attempted primitive forms of dentistry to help restore teeth affected by tooth decay. Such records are available as far back in history as 3700 B.C. As history developed, so did superstitions and magic, the latter being used to ward off evil spirits believed to cause the toothache.

If one lived in the fifth century, a common "prescription" for halitosis was to use the ashes of the heads of a rabbit and three mice mixed with an equal amount of marble dust, all of which were mixed with water. The Romans may have been the first to use a combination of different substances especially formulated to be used as a dentifrice, which consisted of flour of pumice, burned egg shells, stag's horns, mice, and lizards. The historical saying that "The battle against cavities and bad breath has been waged for more than 5,000 years" has in fact considerable documentary evidence to support it.

Similarly, the history of the use of a toothbrush is as old as any form of health history since man has attempted to find a cure for dental pain, which results in most instances from tooth decay, as long as history has been recorded. The need for the use of a toothbrush is not limited to human needs; the crocodile, for example, after a meal stretches out on the river bank and opens his mouth, and then the small zick-zack bird enters to pick out with his beak the small impacted food particles in and about the crocodile's teeth. Not having access to such forms of oral hygiene, man developed the toothbrush some 300 years ago.

The toothbrush probably had its beginning from the toothpick. It was the custom of the Neanderthal man to remove food particles from his teeth with the aid of a plain twig of a tree, while natives of Africa and Asia used bamboo twigs. Later as civilization progressed silver or gold toothpicks became the mark of a wealthy, cultured, and important man. Toothpicks were eventually broadened at one end so as to have a larger area with which to clean more of the teeth and mouth. The early history of the Arabians and Persians contained references to such items. Definite times during the day were set aside by the Greeks in order that all could clean their teeth. Their toothbrushes were known as siwaks. The modern patrician family employed slaves to clean their teeth with small sticks of evergreen. These slaves were known as mastickes (the evergreen tree was known as mastic wood) and may be considered as the forerunners of our modern dental hygienists.

The modern toothbrush and dentifrice are a far cry from these early concoctions. Today's dentifrice is especially formulated from chemically pure substances in scrupulously clean laboratories and factories only after years of exacting testing and research for safety and effectiveness on every ingredient used. There are three forms

**Table 7-1.** *Comparison of different constituents of various physical forms of dentifrices and their percentage composition*

| Dentifrice ingredient | Paste | Powder | Liquid |
|---|---|---|---|
| Abrasive | Calcium pyrophosphate (40%) | Dicalcium phosphate dihydrate (94.2%) Sodium tripolyphosphate (3%) | None |
| Foaming agent | Synthetic detergent (1.5%) | Sodium lauryl sulfate (0.25%) | Alkyl sulfate (1%) |
| Humectant(s) | Glycerol (25%) | None | Glycerol (10%) |
| Binding agent(s) | Gum tragacanth (1.4%) | None | Gum tragacanth (0.75%) |
| Water | 28.8% | None | 63.3% |
| Flavoring agent | 0.9% | 2% | 0.82% |
| Sweetening agent | Trace | Saccharin (0.25%) | 0.03% |
| Alcohol | None | None | (24%) |
| Miscellaneous ingredients (therapeutic agents) | | | |
| Stannous fluoride | 0.4% | None | None |
| Sodium fluoride | None | 0.1% | 0.1% |
| Sodium copper chlorophyllin | None | 0.2% | None |

of dentifrices—liquid, powder, and paste. In some European countries one can still purchase "block" or solid dentifrice (essentially, flavored soap), but this form of dentifrice is not used in the United States. While by far the greatest volume of dentifrice manufactured and sold is of the paste variety, each form has specific dental applications and all are valuable for meeting different dental needs under special circumstances. A typical composition of each of the three forms of dentifrice is shown in Table 7-1.

## DENTIFRICE COMPOSITION AND FUNCTION OF COMPONENT PARTS

Basically, all pastes and powders contain an agent to clean as well as to polish teeth. This is the abrasive, or the "polishing agent"; it is a misnomer since many substances will clean teeth but will not polish them. Dentifrice manufacturers spend millions of dollars each year in an attempt to find effective agents for both cleaning and polishing teeth with the minimum amount of damage to the teeth and their supporting structures. The need for a dentifrice containing an abrasive is important in that about 85 to 90 percent of the population of the United States need to use an abrasive to effectively remove the stained deposits on their teeth. These stains form rapidly (within a few days); most people are required to brush more than once a day to prevent rapid re-formation of the deposits. A dentifrice that has good cleaning properties and produces a high polish is desirable because a highly polished tooth surface will stain less readily and will remain clean longer.

As stated previously, it is possible either to remove the stained deposits on teeth and not polish the teeth satisfactorily or to clean the teeth and actually damage enamel and dentin by using a polishing agent that is too abrasive. Cleaning and polishing may or may not be related to each other. The obvious goal of the dentifrice manufacturer is to produce a dentifrice containing a polishing agent that will clean very well with no damage to the teeth and that will provide a high polish. A number of different polishing agents along with their abrasiveness are shown in Table 7-2. Levigated alumina, for example, produces a very smooth and shiny surface but is too abrasive to use daily in a dentifrice. The calcium phosphates used in dentifrices today produce excellent smoothness and, in addition, are good cleaners. Chalk, on the other hand, produces a rough appearance of the tooth but does clean fairly well. The technics used to evaluate abrasiveness as reported in Table 7-2 are extremely sensitive and accurate in that they evaluate abrasiveness by measuring the tooth loss in terms of radioactivity of dentin (in terms of radiophosphorus). Such data suggest that several commercial products are extremely abrasive. Serious questions can be raised as to the need for such products if such data represent tooth damage. If there is evidence that a commercial product can produce a significant benefit to oral health, there may well be reason to have a moderately increased level in abrasiveness over other nontherapeutic products since the benefit produced far outweighs any potential damage. No such reasoning justifies the use of commercial products with high levels of dentin abrasiveness and no therapeutic benefits.

**Table 7-2.** *Comparison of a number of different polishing agents used as constituents of commercial dentifrices and their abrasiveness to dentin*

| Abrasive | Dentifrice brand name | Dentin abrasion ($P^{32}$) |
|---|---|---|
| Levigated alumina | None | 748 ± 30 |
| $(NaPO_3)_x$ | Pepsodent with $SnF_2$ | 194 ± 2 |
| $(NaPO_3)_x + CaHPO_4$ | Colgate MFP | 336 ± 24 |
| $CaCO_3$ | Iodent No. 2 | 321 ± 12 |
| | Thermodent | 58 ± 3 |
| | Phillips | 347 ± 9 |
| | Detoxol | 128 ± 11 |
| | Macleans | 433 ± 16 |
| | Caroid (powder) | 610 ± 16 |
| | Dr. Lyon's Powder | 807 ± 32 |
| | Dr. Forhan's | 179 ± 4 |
| $CaHPO_4$ | Plus White | 406 ± 24 |
| $Ca_2P_2O_7$ | Crest | 217 ± 9 |
| $Ca_2P_2O_7$, high $\beta$-phase | Gleem | 246 ± 12 |
| $CaHPO_4 \cdot 2H_2O$ | Kolynos Super-White | 162 ± 7 |
| | Kolynos with NaF | 219 ± 3 |
| | Listerine | 77 ± 4 |
| | Rexall with NaF | 78 ± 11 |
| | Iodent Junior with $SnF_2$ | 199 ± 8 |
| | Amm-i-dent | 83 ± 2 |
| | Amm-i-dent with NaF | 120 ± 4 |
| $Ca_{10}(PO_4)_6F_2$ | Amurol | 64 ± 3 |
| $CaHPO_4 \cdot 2H_2O + CaHPO_4 + CaCO_3$ | Ultra Brite | 457 ± 28 |
| $CaHPO_4 \cdot 2H_2O + CaCO_3 + ZrSiO_4$ | Pepsodent | 220 ± 10 |
| $SiO_2 \cdot nH_2O + Al\ PO_4$ | Vote | 441 ± 24 |

Almost all dentifrices contain a foaming agent to aid in the cleaning ability of the abrasive. In the early 1930's and until the mid 1940's, soap was used as the foaming agent in over half of all dentifrices; others used no foaming agent. The soap was added, according to the manufacturer, to lower the surface tension and, as a result, to increase the cleaning ability of the dentifrice. However, other disadvantages were produced by adding soap that limited the composition of the dentifrice. For example, soap is an effective detergent only when used in an alkaline solution, and, as a result, the dentifrice was often so alkaline as to cause damage to the oral mucous membrane. Similarly, soap is not compatible with many of the calcium salts used as polishing agents in the dentifrice. The restriction of using only a limited number of flavoring agents in the presence of soap was a considerable disadvantage also. As a result, many dentifrices containing soap did not have the best consumer properties from a taste viewpoint. Dentifrice manufacturers began to look for foaming agents that did not have the disadvantage of soap. It was discovered that several different synthetic detergents could be substituted for soap, eliminating many of soap's disadvantages but still possessing the foaming qualities of soap. Essentially all dentifrice manufacturers are using synthetic detergents today. These chemicals have the same action as soap in lowering the surface tension, loosening surface stains, and making surface stains more easily removed with the toothbrush. As a class, detergents are neutral in reaction but can be used in either acid or alkaline solutions; they do not react with the saliva, are not injurious to gingival tissues, are not inactivated by calcium salts used as abrasives, and do not adversely affect the taste qualities of the dentifrice.

The other major ingredients are agents that give the dentifrice its body—the binding agent—and substances that keep the product from drying out—the humectant. Minor amounts of flavoring and sweetening agents are also added.

Liquid dentifrices differ from pastes and powders essentially in that they contain no abrasive. As stated previously, most people require some abrasive in order to satisfactorily remove the stain and food debris from the teeth. As a result, liquid dentifrices did not enjoy a successful commercial market, although the stain that accumulates on the teeth of people who used them could easily be removed by using a paste or powder dentifrice once or twice every other week. Their loss to the consumer is unfortunate since there are certain specific cases in which liquid dentifrices are indicated in clinical practice. For example, for those patients who have considerable gingival recession, liquid dentifrices are useful since they will not damage the dentin as would a product containing an abrasive. For patients having a considerable amount of dentin or cementum abrasion, such products are useful for the same reason.

Some dentists continue to recommend salt and soda for their patients as a dentifrice. While baking soda is a fair agent to remove stain from the teeth, those dental scientists who have spent many years studying the use of dentifrices and the public's reaction to them know that such a combination is not used for more than a few days, or weeks at the most, by the majority of the people who need a dentifrice. This is because it is not only too messy to use and handle, but also because it does not have the necessary properties the public has come to want and expect of a dentifrice. Furthermore, its taste is unpleasant, and one of the major contributions that the dentifrice manufacturer has made in helping the masses of people brush their teeth more frequently is to make dentifrices pleasant to use. Since most dentists feel that one needs to brush his teeth more than once a day, it is a severe handicap to a product if it does not have highly acceptable taste qualities. Similarly, salt and soda contain no detergent or soap, and such substances are quite important not only in increasing the cleaning ability of a dentifrice, but also in acting as a foaming agent to help dislodge particles from between the teeth.

## SUBJECTS' REACTION TO BRUSHING WITH AND WITHOUT A DENTIFRICE

A group of fifty college students participated in a study in order to determine their reactions to brushing their teeth without a dentifrice, with a paste dentifrice, and with salt and soda (powder dentifrice). The general reaction of the participants who used no dentifrice was most unfavorable. This is indicated by the fact that 46 percent of the subjects withdrew from the study and only 4 percent stated that they liked to brush without a dentifrice (Table 7-3).

Table 7-3. *Comparison of the ability of three different types of dentifrices to prevent pellicle formation*

| Group | Time (weeks) | Number of subjects | Number of subjects with pellicle formation (percent) |
|---|---|---|---|
| No dentifrice | 2 | 31 | 12 (61) |
|  | 5 | 27 | 25 (93) |
| Dentifrice | 2 | 47 | 3 (6) |
|  | 5 | 47 | 4 (9) |
| Salt and soda (powder) | 2 | 40 | 4 (10) |

Table 7-4. *Patient preference of three different types of dentifrices and their reasons for being motivated to brush their teeth*

| Question: List in order of your preference: No dentifrice, paste dentifrice, and powder dentifrices | | | | |
|---|---|---|---|---|
| Paste-powder-water | | | 59% | |
| Paste-water-powder | | | 13% | |
| Powder-paste-water | | | 5% | |
| Undecided | | | 3% | |
| Withdrew | | | 20% | |

| Question: List three things, in order of importance, that motivate you to brush your teeth | | | | |
|---|---|---|---|---|
|  | Total | I | II | III |
| Cleanliness | 18% | 25% | 23% | 6% |
| Breath | 14% | 6% | 31% | 3% |
| Habit | 12% | 6% | 12% | 17% |
| Appearance | 7% | 6% | 6% | 10% |
| Taste | 17% | 23% | 6% | 23% |
| Health of teeth | 20% | 28% | 16% | 16% |
| Social pressure | 5% | 3% | 6% | 6% |
| Obligation to study | 2% | 3% | 0% | 3% |
| Didn't know | 5% | 0% | 0% | 16% |

By contrast, in the group using a paste dentifrice, 88 percent of the participants stated that they preferred this procedure and only 5 percent withdrew. When the participants were given a salt and soda powder, 20 percent withdrew and 8 percent said that they liked using the powder. Pellicle formation was found in 61 percent of the subjects using no dentifrice, in contrast to only 6 percent using a paste dentifrice and 10 percent using a powder dentifrice after a 2-week evaluation period.

The replies given when the participants were asked to list their motivations for toothbrushing are shown in Table 7-4. Of the total answers, most frequently listed (20 percent) was health of teeth as their motivation for brushing their teeth. It is encouraging to find that the efforts of the dental profession are making an impression in educating the public to the need for maintaining good oral hygiene and its relation to mouth health. Habit was given by 12 percent as their reason for brushing; this shows the importance of teaching regular brushing habits at an early age. Only 7 percent listed appearance as the motivating power for brushing.

Little is known about the effectiveness of various methods advocated for maintaining oral hygiene. One would be hard pressed to find scientific support, for instance, for the commonly heard statement to the effect that rinsing your mouth following the ingestion of food is associated with better oral health. In order to ascertain some relative comparison of different technics, a 1-month study was designed by the United States Army Dental Corps to compare the results of two commonly advocated field expedients—vigorous rinsing with water and the use of a stick or twig—and the use of a toothbrush and dentifrice. A total of 156 recently commissioned Medical Service Corps officers attending a basic orientation course at the Army's Medical Field Service School were examined and periodontal, calculus, debris, and oral hygiene scores recorded. Most of these officers were recent college graduates and eager to cooperate. The examining officer had no idea of the nature of the study or in which group any officer belonged.

The study population was divided into three groups as nearly alike as possible on the basis of initial examination findings. The oral hygiene method to be followed by each group was determined by tossing a coin. One group was supplied with toothbrushes and dentifrices and asked to brush their teeth as frequently as possible and after each meal. The second group was given a supply of wooden Stim-U-Dents to simulate twigs or sticks and asked to limit oral hygiene to the use of this technic after each meal. They were instructed to use the point of the stick to clean interproximally and to chew the blunt end carefully to form a brush for use on the re-

Table 7-5. *Comparison of three oral hygiene methods (periodontal index data)*

| Group | Number of subjects | Mean score Initial | Mean score Final | Mean change | Change (percent) | Same | Number plus | Number minus |
|---|---|---|---|---|---|---|---|---|
| Brush | 52 | .33 | .353 | +.023 | + 6.9 | 14 | 20 | 18 |
| Stick | 51 | .28 | .247 | −.033 | −11.7 | 13 | 19 | 19 |
| Rinse | 50 | .28 | .376 | +.096 | +34.0 | 20 | 21 | 9 |
| Rinse* | 32 | .29 | .453 | +.163 | +56.2 | 12 | 17 | 3 |
| All | 153 | .31 | .329 | +.019 | + 6.1 | 59 | 77 | 49 |

*Those reported brushing five times or less in month.

**Table 7-6.** *Comparison of three oral hygiene methods (debris index data)*

| Group | Number of subjects | Mean score Initial | Mean score Final | Mean change | Change (percent) | Same | Number plus | Number minus |
|---|---|---|---|---|---|---|---|---|
| Brush | 52 | .60 | .74 | +.14 | + 22.5 | 11 | 26 | 15 |
| Stick | 51 | .62 | .79 | +.16 | + 25.6 | 11 | 28 | 12 |
| Rinse | 50 | .57 | 1.25 | +.68 | +120.5 | 3 | 41 | 6 |
| Rinse* | 32 | .64 | 1.51 | +.87 | +136.9 | 2 | 30 | 0 |
| All | 153 | .60 | .92 | +.32 | + 54.1 | 25 | 95 | 33 |

*Those reported brushing five times or less in month.

**Table 7-7.** *Comparison of three oral hygiene methods (calculus index data)*

| Group | Number of subjects | Mean score Initial | Mean score Final | Mean change | Change (percent) | Same | Number plus | Number minus |
|---|---|---|---|---|---|---|---|---|
| Brush | 52 | .17 | .197 | +.027 | +16.3 | 43 | 7 | 2 |
| Stick | 51 | .19 | .157 | −.033 | −17.1 | 38 | 3 | 10 |
| Rinse | 50 | .16 | .180 | +.020 | +12.7 | 40 | 5 | 5 |
| Rinse* | 32 | .20 | .238 | +.038 | +18.8 | 25 | 3 | 3 |
| All | 153 | .17 | .199 | +.005 | + 2.9 | 121 | 15 | 17 |

*Those reported brushing five times or less in month.

maining surfaces. The third group was asked to limit cleaning procedures to vigorous rinsing with water, coffee, or mouthwash after meals.

A second examination was performed at the end of 1 month. Three of those examined initially were not available. Mean initial and final scores and numerical and percentage changes in scores are shown in Tables 7-5 to 7-9. Each of the tables is devoted to a separate index, giving mean initial and final scores, numerical and percentage changes in scores, the number of scores remaining the same, the number increasing, and the number decreasing. A separate grouping of rinsers, those who reported brushing five times or less during the month, is also shown.

Table 7-5 presents the periodontal findings. Stick users had a decrease in periodontal index of 11.7 percent, with all others having increases from 6.9 percent for brushers to as high as 56.2 percent among the special rinser group. Differences between brushers and stick users do not appear as evident if the number of scores remaining the same, going up, or going down are compared.

The results for the debris findings are given in Table 7-6. Where brushers and stick users had increases of 22.5 percent and 25.6 percent, the rinser group went up 120.5 percent, and the special rinser group went up 136.9 percent.

The calculus findings are shown in Table 7-7. Again, the stick users seem to have an advantage, showing a reduction of 17.1 percent as compared to increases of 16.3 percent for brushers, 12.7 percent for rinsers, and 18.8 percent for the special rinser group.

After the final examination each study participant was interviewed for information not obtained from the clinical examinations. Questions were asked in such a way as to encourage honest answers. Each was asked the following questions.

**Table 7-8.** *Results of comparing three oral hygiene methods (extent to which instructions followed)*

| Group | Completely | Most of time | Part of time | None | Total |
|---|---|---|---|---|---|
| Brush | 15 | 21 | 16 | 0 | 52 |
| Stick | 15 | 18 | 15 | 3 | 51 |
| Rinse | 11 | 24 | 10 | 5 | 50 |

**Table 7-9.** *Results of comparing three oral hygiene methods (opinion of assigned method)*

| Group | Good | Some good | Not good | No opinion | Total |
|---|---|---|---|---|---|
| Brush | 49 | 0 | 0 | 2 | 51* |
| Stick | 24 | 21 | 6 | 0 | 51 |
| Rinse | 2 | 16 | 30 | 2 | 50 |

*One not present for interview.

1. Were you able to follow instructions for a whole month?
2. To what extent did you follow them?
3. What do you think of the method your group followed as a means of maintaining oral hygiene?
4. If the method was unsatisfactory, in what way was it inadequate?

The extent to which each procedure was followed is shown in Table 7-8. Answers demonstrated that class scheduling and relocation of billets early in the month made it difficult to brush after each meal. This was particularly true during a 2-week period ending about 4 days prior to the final examination during which the class underwent field training. The degree of participation reported was classified as complete, most of the time, part of the time, and none. From the lack of enthusiasm for rinsing as a brushing substitute it was surprising that so many stayed with this procedure for the entire period. Many stated that they brushed only on weekends, before social engagements, or before going to church, others that they kept from brushing for as long as they could but finally gave it up and resumed brushing.

Opinions as to the acceptability of the self-care measure followed are summarized in Table 7-9. All the brushers indicated satisfaction. Among those who used the sticks, opinion was divided, some even expressing the belief that this method was better in some ways than brushing. Some stated that the sticks presented an advantage in being convenient to carry. Others listed such disadvantages as unfamiliarity and awkwardness of use; also, they break easily. Some felt that the sticks cleaned well, but they missed the taste and freshness left in the mouth following use of a dentifrice. Others complained of halitosis or of a bad taste in the mouth. Rinsing was generally unpopular. Members of the rinsing group complained of inadequate cleaning, of grimy, gritty, or dirty-feeling teeth, and also of halitosis or bad oral taste.

## DENTIFRICE STOMATITIS

There has been during recent years an unmeasurable undercurrent of opinion among dentists to the effect that 7 to 10 percent of the population develops stomatitis by using commercially available dentifrices. However, no data appear in the literature to support or define these conclusions. In questioning oral pathologists or dentists who have observed such oral inflammation and who associate the changes with the use of dentifrices, one concludes that the inflammation disappears if the patient discontinues using his present dentifrice. Unrelated pieces of data suggest that, if in fact such changes are associated with dentifrices, no one particular dentifrice is more prone to produce these effects than any other. Most workers feel that the essential oils used in dentifrices can produce oral inflammation in susceptible patients but that the magnitude of the population affected must be almost insignificant.

The only clinical evaluation that has compared different dentifrices for their

**Table 7-10.** *Relationship of dentifrices to idiopathic gingival reaction*

|  | Total subjects | Subjects with no idiopathic gingival reaction | Subjects with idiopathic gingival reaction | Percentage of subjects with idiopathic gingival reaction |
|---|---|---|---|---|
| I. Dentifrice | | | | |
| Crest | 494 | 475 | 19 | 3.8 |
| Ultra Brite | 128 | 88 | 40 | 31.3 |
| Macleans | 88 | 55 | 33 | 37.5 |
| Vote | 32 | 25 | 7 | 21.9 |
| Plus White | 40 | 30 | 10 | 25.0 |
| Colgate* | 147 | 123 | 24 | 16.3 |
| Total | 929 | 796 | 133 | 14.3 (Mean) |

| II. Gingival reactions | Number of reactions |
|---|---|
| Crest | |
| Slough | 1 |
| Redness | 18 |
| Ultra Brite | |
| Slough | 5 |
| Redness | 28 |
| Swelling | 5 |
| Sensitivity | 2 |
| Macleans | |
| Slough | 9 |
| Redness | 22 |
| Sensitivity | 2 |
| Vote | |
| Slough | 1 |
| Redness | 6 |
| Plus White | |
| Redness | 10 |
| Colgate | |
| Slough | 14 |
| Redness | 9 |
| Swelling | 1 |

*Not Colgate-MFP.

effect on oral stomatitis has been conducted by Hutchins and Barnes.[1] During a 3-month period all patients presenting themselves to four military dental clinics for dental examinations were questioned as to which dentifrice (by brand name) they used. This question was asked and recorded by auxiliary dental personnel in the absence of the dentists, who subsequently examined each subject's oral condition. If the patient routinely used either of the following dentifrices, he was included in the study: Crest, Colgate, Ultra Brite, Macleans, Vote, or Plus White. If the patient did not use one of these dentifrices he was excluded from the study. A total of 929 patients served as subjects in the study, which used these criteria. All subjects were unaware of the design and purpose of the study.

After the dentifrice data had been recorded the patients were examined by one of four dentists. If the examiner noted any evidence of idiopathic gingival reactions, this information was recorded on the patient's dental chart. Examiners were extremely careful to record only idiopathic gingival reactions. Extreme effort was made in order to rule out every possible known local and/or systemic cause for the gingival reaction noted. Among the idiopathic gingival reactions noted were gingival slough, gingival swelling, and areas of bright red coloration that were incompatible with the color of the adjacent gingival tissue. In some instances the subjects complained of "unnatural" gingival sensitivity. When no etiologic factor could be found these instances were recorded as being idiopathic gingival reactions.

All examiners were unaware of the dentifrices used by the subjects and were also unaware of which patients were included as subjects in the study. All examinations were performed using mouth mirrors and reflective illuminating light.

Following the examinations the auxiliary personnel who had recorded the dentifrice information provided by the subjects extracted the idiopathic gingival reaction notations from the dental charts and entered this information on the data sheets.

The subjects in this study were military personnel and civilian dependents of military personnel. Approximately 20 percent of the subjects were female. The subjects ranged in age from 18 to 38 years, with a mean age of 21 years. The data obtained in this study are found in Table 7-10. From these data it is impossible to associate any dentifrice constituent with the observed clinical findings. Both Ultra Brite and Macleans contain chloroform and both produce a high incidence of gingival reactions. However, Vote and Plus White do not contain chloroform yet produce a high degree of idiopathic gingival changes. This entire area of dentifrice research needs further study before any definite conclusion can be made.

## WHAT DENTIFRICE SHOULD YOUR PATIENTS USE?

Not only are there different physical types of dentifrices, but also there are dentifrices that are used for different purposes, although the claims for many of these have never been substantiated either in the laboratory or by clinical trials. For example, some dentifrices are claimed to reduce the sensitivity of the teeth, others to improve specifically one's breath, some to reduce tartar, and others to reduce dental caries. Almost any dentifrice that contains a flavoring agent will improve one's breath—temporarily. There are no reports which show that any of the other claims made for dentifrices can be substantiated other than for those dentifrices that contain stannous fluoride or sodium monofluorophosphate.

The type of dentifrice a person needs to use depends in great measure on his particular state of oral health. The dentist, of course, is the only counsel in such matters and should advise the patient only after he has thoroughly examined the oral soft and hard tissues and becomes acquainted with each patient's particular clinical case. For example, if the patient is elderly and has had a severe amount of gingival damage, resulting in a considerable amount of exposed dentin or cementum, the dentist may suggest a liquid dentifrice for the majority of the time the patient brushes his teeth. Almost every dentifrice available today that contains an abrasive is safe for routine use, with the exception of one or two more recently introduced brands. There are, however, differences in their cleaning and polishing ability because of differences in the abrasive used. While minor exceptions to the rule exist, powder dentifrices as a class are more abrasive than paste dentifrices, and similar differences exist between the paste dentifrices.

It is not possible to formulate a rule applicable to every patient in regard to which dentifrice has the best cleaning and polishing properties and still produces minimum abrasiveness for the simple reason that all patients do not have similar stains and films on their teeth. For example, a heavy cigar or cigarette smoker may require a different type dentifrice to properly clean and polish his teeth from that required by a nonsmoker.

In the last few years patients have been selecting dentifrices not solely on their taste or cleaning ability, although admittedly both are important, but more so on the basis of their therapeutic claims. By far the greatest attention given to the therapeutic dentifrices, both by the profession and by the patient, has been directed toward a dentifrice containing stannous fluoride as the active ingredient and calcium pyrophosphate as the compatible polishing agent.*

### Stannous fluoride–calcium pyrophosphate dentifrices

Two important developments have made it possible to formulate truly effective anti–tooth decay dentifrices. The first was the discovery by a group of research scientists at Indiana University that stannous fluoride appeared to be more active than sodium fluoride. However, it was still another thing to capture the effectiveness of this compound in a dentifrice, since the use of all conventional abrasives would not only inactivate the fluoride but also the stannous ion. So, in a sense, two problems had to be solved in formulating the new dentifrice containing stannous fluoride. As in the case in many scientific advancements, the answer to the problem came not through great genius, but through very hard work. This group of dental scientists assisted by others from the company manufacturing the dentifrice were working on this problem when it was found that dicalcium phosphate, the most common abrasive in use at that time, could be made relatively compatible with stannous fluoride through heat treatment. The new product formed was calcium pyrophosphate, whose properties are such that it permits both the tin (II) and fluoride ions to remain active in the dentifrice.

Even after this important discovery, it remained for the manufacturer to devote many additional years of work and study to improve the dentifrice so as to maintain the activity of the stannous fluoride and so that it would, in addition, have good consumer properties. One of the major problems to be evaluated was how long it could remain on the shelf and still retain its activity. It was known that, when the active tin (II) loses its effectiveness to combine with the tooth, the effectiveness

---

*Crest brand dentifrice, manufactured by the Procter and Gamble Co., Cincinnati, Ohio.

of the dentifrice decreases. In order to stabilize the dentifrice a reservoir of active tin (II) ions was placed in the dentifrice in addition to the stannous fluoride, so that when some of the active tin (II) ions in the stannous fluoride would react with water or air and become inactive, the reservoir of tin (II) ions would take their place. Such a development has led to the present formulation, which has an excellent stability for long periods of time.

In order to obtain professional acceptance of the stannous fluoride–calcium pyrophosphate dentifrice, an extensive clinical testing program was undertaken. The clinical tests that have been conducted using the stannous fluoride–calcium pyrophosphate dentifrice that contains the final product formulation are summarized in Table 7-11. These data show repeated positive clinical tests using the stannous fluoride–calcium pyrophosphate dentifrice by not only several different independent investigators, but also in several different experiment sites. Of real value to preventive dentistry, since it is the object of preventive dentistry to eliminate dental caries as far as possible, is that added benefit is derived from topical applications of stannous fluoride when the stannous fluoride–calcium pyrophosphate dentifrice is used. Furthermore, these clinical data show among both children and adults, in both fluoride and nonfluoride areas, that the maximum clinical effectiveness of stannous fluoride is obtained when used as a constituent of a compatible prophylactic paste (lava pumice), followed by topical applications of stannous fluoride followed by the routine use of the stannous fluoride–calcium pyrophosphate dentifrice. Such a program has several advantages for dentistry: it provides an effective caries-control program for all members of the population, whether they are young or old or reside in an urban or rural community. Such accomplishments aid substantially in dentistry's goal to eliminate dental caries for all people. No added benefits have been demonstrated for any other dentifrice when used in such a preventive program.

Besides the stannous fluoride–calcium pyrophosphate dentifrice, a wide variety of other dentifrices for which therapeutic claims have been made have at one time or another appeared on the commercial market. Some of these are still available,

**Table 7-11.** *A comparison of the clinical effectiveness of the $SnF_2$-$Ca_2P_2O_7$ dentifrice when evaluated under different clinical conditions in both children and adults*

| Clinical conditions | Length of study (years) | Reduction in dental caries (percent DMFS) |
|---|---|---|
| Fluoride area[2] | 2 | 32 |
| Supervised brushing | | |
|   Three times a day[3] | 2 | 46 |
|   Three times a day[4] | 1 | 52 |
|   One time a day[5] | 2 | 21 |
| In conjunction with $SnF_2$ topical[6] | 3 | 63 |
| In conjunction with $SnF_2$ topical and $SnF_2$ prophylaxis | | |
|   Children*[7, 8] | 1 | 71 |
| | 3 | 58 |
|   Adults[9, 10] | 1 | 54 |
| | 2½ | 64 |

*In natural fluoride area.

170  *Improving dental practice through preventive measures*

**Table 7-12.** *A comparison of clinical effectiveness of a sodium monofluorophosphate dentifrice under different clinical conditions**

| Clinical condition | Length of study (years) | Percentage reduction in dental caries |
|---|---|---|
| Fluoride area[11] | 3 | 17 |
| Unsupervised brushing[12, 13] | 2 | 20 |
|  | 3 | 18 |
| Brushing supervised |  |  |
| One time a day[14] | 2½ | 19 |
| Two times a day[15] | 2 | 34 |
| Three times a day[16] | 1.8 | 21 |

*Colgate-MFP brand dentifrice.

and it is with some difficulty that the consumer knows which of these is really as effective as the advertisements claim. In general, three different forms of therapeutic dentifrices are presently available for use.

1. The suggested control of dental caries
2. The suggested control of dental calculus (tartar)
3. The suggested control of sensitive teeth

Some dentifrices, of course, make no therapeutic claims, resting simply on the ability of the product to have a pleasant taste and to effectively clean the teeth.

### Sodium monofluorophosphate dentifrices

A dentifrice containing insoluble metaphosphate and anhydrous dicalcium phosphate as the polishing agent and 0.76 percent sodium monofluorophosphate and 2.0 percent sodium N-lauroyl sarcosinate has received the "A" classification by the American Dental Association. The studies concerning its clinical effectiveness, which have been published and which were conducted with an appropriate control group, are found in Table 7-12 arranged in a manner similar to the studies reported for the $SnF_2$-$Ca_2P_2O_7$ dentifrice clinical data found in Table 7-11. While the product is clinically effective as an anticariogenic dentifrice, additional work is required to demonstrate its effectiveness when used with other anticariogenic agents (such as fluoride topicals and fluoride containing prophylactic pastes) and when used by adults.

### Chlorophyll dentifrices

The beginning of the therapeutic dentifrice era in regard to the control of tooth decay began on a major scale with the introduction on the market of the chlorophyll dentifrices. These dentifrices claimed to reduce tooth decay, based on the known properties of chlorophyll to reduce bacterial growth, and to reduce the acid formed within the dental plaque. No clinical studies were ever published to support these claims. Today, a few dentifrices still contain chlorophyll, but their claims are limited to helping improve the breath. Adequate proof for this claim still awaits experimental clinical verification.

### Ammoniated dentifrices

The next therapeutic dentifrices to appear were the ammoniated dentifrices. These contain chemicals that have either active ammonia compounds or compounds that are converted to active ammonia in the mouth, resulting in less acid being formed in the dental plaque. A considerable number of clinical trials have been conducted with a wide variety of different ammoniated dentifrices with varying results. One such product has shown some effectiveness in reducing tooth decay, although as yet sufficient clinical evidence is not available for the Council of Dental Therapeutics to place it in an approved category.

**Antibiotic dentifrices**

Following in order were the antibiotic dentifrices. The most frequently discussed were those containing penicillin as the active ingredient. These products were based on the premise that the antibiotic would destroy the bacteria thought responsible for producing acid within the dental plaque, and in experimental animal studies they looked quite promising. Clinical results were inconclusive, however, one study showing some effectiveness and others no effectiveness. These products are not commercially available today since it has been shown that some people may become sensitized by the small amount of penicillin in the dentifrice, making it dangerous to use the drug when critically needed.

The only other antibiotic dentifrice receiving clinical investigation in human beings is tyrothricin, even though many others have been studied extensively in animals. A single and as yet unsubstantiated clinical study showed a 25 percent reduction in dental caries at the end of 2 years.

**Antienzyme dentifrices**

Next were the antienzyme dentifrices, the most popular of which is the dentifrice containing a detergent with sodium N-lauroyl sarcosinate. This is the active ingredient called Gardol. These dentifrices are thought to act in a manner similar to the antibiotic dentifrices in principle, but instead of interfering with bacterial growth they are thought to effect the enzyme systems required for the breakdown of foods by bacteria to form acids. The Council of Dental Therapeutics of the American Dental Association has stated that there is not sufficient clinical evidence available upon which to make an adequate evaluation of these dentifrices.

Sodium dehydroacetate, another suggested antienzyme, has so little clinical evidence supporting its use that no evaluation of it is possible.

**Neutral dentifrices**

A number of dentifrices claim reductions in tooth decay and a reduction in mouth odors simply on the basis that when used with the toothbrush they reduce the bacterial content of the oral cavity. It is a well-established fact that the bacterial count of the mouth can be drastically reduced after brushing one's teeth and tongue. The question that remains unanswered is whether or not the simple reduction in bacteria count for only a short period of time following toothbrushing will reduce dental caries. This should not be interpreted to mean that frequency and thoroughness of toothbrushing itself is not related to reduction in tooth decay, since this is not the case. Consider, for example, the clinical studies that have been conducted with the stannous fluoride–calcium pyrophosphate dentifrice in terms of frequency of brushing each day. Table 7-13 suggests that the clinical effectiveness is directly related to the frequency of toothbrushing, that is, the more times each day you brush with this dentifrice the greater its effectiveness (see also Table 7-11). Clinical studies

**Table 7-13.** *Comparison of the increased anticariogenic benefit of the $SnF_2$-$Ca_2P_2O_7$ dentifrice when used as an unsupervised product once or three times a day*

| Brushing regimen | Reduction in one-year increments (DMF surfaces) (percent) |
|---|---|
| Unsupervised | 23 |
| Supervision one time a day | 34 |
| Supervision three times a day | 57 |

are available to show a positive relationship of toothbrushing to gingival health. It certainly follows that by brushing more than once a day one should expect less dental caries and calculus as well as better gingival health.

## BRUSHING AFTER MEALS

While conclusive clinical evidence is not available to support after-meal brushing as an effective anticariogenic technic, scientific evidence suggests that such a procedure would be effective. Fosdick,[17] for example, in the only study so far reported, observed a reduction in dental caries of 50 percent by after-meal brushing using a nontherapeutic product (calcium phosphate polishing agent) when compared to another group not practicing similar brushing habits.

### Anticalculus dentifrices

There are no clinical studies that show that any of the dentifrices available today significantly reduce calculus.

## WHAT TYPE OF TOOTHBRUSH SHOULD YOUR PATIENTS USE?

For all practical purposes there are two kinds of toothbrushes, those with natural bristles and those with synthetic (nylon) bristles. While the type of brush a particular patient should use from the standpoint of bristles is an individual matter of preference, most people will prefer a brush with a synthetic bristle because it will not wear out as soon as most natural bristle brushes, and it will dry out much faster after use. The idea that many people are sensitive to synthetic bristles is not based upon experimental fact.

Beside the type of bristle, the number of rows and the number of tufts in each row of bristles are worthy of comment. In general, only the dentist can advise a patient of what brush is best for his personal use since the arrangement of the teeth, their relationship to the cheeks and lips, and the presence or absence of extracted teeth all influence the number of bristles best required to clean a particular patient's mouth. In advising a patient as to what type of brush to use, the dentist should evaluate if a straight-handle brush or one with a bent head is best suited to clean the patient's mouth. Generally speaking, a straight-handled brush with synthetic fibers and a small head is best for most patients.

Should the bristles be soft or hard? Again, this is a matter that only the dentist can decide after examining the state of the patient's oral health. Most dentists are beginning to recommend a multitufted medium hard bristled brush, which is necessary to allow patients to do a thorough cleaning of the hard-to-get-at areas. If the patient has a considerable amount of gingival irritation, a soft toothbrush must be used initially so as to permit the gingival tissue to heal. Similarly, young children during the period of the mixed dentition may have considerable pain and gingival irritation, and frequently they will not brush their teeth at all, or else not thoroughly enough, unless they use a soft bristle brush. If the gingival tissues are in a good state of health and if the patient is practicing careful toothbrushing, a hard bristle brush is more effective for brushing the occlusal surfaces. However, research may ultimately show that a softer brush may be more helpful in cleaning thoroughly the spaces in the gingival crevice. Dental floss is necessary to clean thoroughly between the teeth.

**Electric toothbrushes**

The use of electric toothbrushes has increased greatly in the past several years. One is impressed with the fact that patients brush more frequently—at least initially—after purchasing such products. There is some evidence to suggest that those patients who do not have good toothbrushing habits may benefit by using an electric toothbrush since it does a good portion of the labor for them.

Numerous articles have appeared in the literature concerning the comparative effectiveness of mechanical and manual toothbrushes, particularly with regard to their influence on oral hygiene and periodontal health. The majority of these reports have suggested that a mechanical toothbrush is superior to a manual toothbrush with regard to the removal of dental plaque.[18-25] However, a number of reports[26-33] failed to indicate a significant superiority of either of these types of toothbrushes. The use of a mechanical toothbrush has been shown to be superior to a manual toothbrush with regard to the inhibition of pellicle formation.[34] Investigations concerning dentin abrasion have generally concluded that the mechanical toothbrushes are less abrasive than manual toothbrushes,[35-39] although one group of investigators failed to find any difference between the two types of brushes.[40] Considerable attention has been directed toward the possible advantageous use of mechanical toothbrushes for handicapped patients[41-47] and for children receiving orthodontic treatment.[48, 49]

The two types of toothbrushes also have been investigated with regard to their comparative influence on calculus formation and gingival health. These studies have generally shown that the mechanical toothbrush is superior to the manual toothbrush with regard to the removal and prevention of calculus deposition,[50, 51] although this observation was not confirmed in at least one study.[31] Numerous studies have also reported a superiority of mechanical toothbrushes with regard to their ability to promote gingival health[52-56] although, again, some reports* have failed to confirm such findings.

**WHAT IS THE BEST WAY TO BRUSH ONE'S TEETH?**

A considerable number of different technics have been suggested for use in cleaning one's teeth. The best one for a particular patient must be determined by the dentist only after a complete oral examination. A number of factors must be considered in making this decision, among which are the arrangement of the teeth, whether or not there are missing teeth and where they are in the mouth, the state of the gingival health, the presence or absence of exposed dentin or cementum, and the

---

*See references 26, 30, 31, and 57-60.

cooperation of the patient. Regardless of what particular technic is recommended, certain general principles apply to all cases. The main purpose of the toothbrush is to remove dental plaque from between the teeth and in the free gingival crevice with the minimum amount of damage to the teeth and their surrounding soft tissues. In principle, one can do this by brushing the teeth with the technic that most effectively gets the bristles in between each tooth, down into the pits and fissures of the molars and bicuspid teeth, and into the gingival crevice and effectively massages the gingival tissues. A definite pattern of brushing one's teeth is oftentimes found very helpful.

In order to aid one's ability to clean the teeth properly, many dentists recommend the use of disclosing tablets. These disclosing solutions are highly colored and are useful in picturing in color the areas on the teeth where plaque accumulates, so that one may learn to brush such areas more carefully.

## CONCLUSION

In this chapter the historical developments of concepts leading to current methods of controlling dental caries through the use of a toothbrush and a dentifrice were discussed. The composition of a modern dentifrice was presented and the function of each of the individual constituents of the dentifrice was shown. The effects that different commercial dentifrices have in the partial control of dental caries were compared and the clinical data supporting the effectiveness were shown. Based upon available clinical data, the stannous fluoride–calcium pyrophosphate dentifrice is the only product that has been shown to be effective in children and adults and when used by children whose teeth calcified and maturated in an optimal fluoride area. For optimal use of this dentifrice, I suggest that it be used in an optimal fluoride area, preceded by a prophylaxis with lava pumice and stannous fluoride and a topical application of stannous fluoride.

## REFERENCES

1. Hutchins, D. W., and Barnes, G. P.: Relationship of dentifrices to idiopathic gingival reactions. Personal communication.
2. Gish, C. W., and Muhler, J. C.: Effectiveness of a $SnF_2$-$Ca_2P_2O_7$ dentifrice on dental caries in children whose teeth calcified in a natural fluoride area, II, results at the end of 24 months, J.A.D.A. 73:853, 1966.
3. Muhler, J. C.: Effect of a stannous fluoride dentifrice on caries reduction in children during a three-year study period, J.A.D.A. 64:216, 1962.
4. Bixler, D., and Muhler, J. C.: Experimental clinical human caries test; design and interpretation, J.A.D.A. 65:482, 1962.
5. Jordon, W. A., and Peterson, J. K.: Caries inhibiting value of a dentifrice containing stannous fluoride, final report of a two year study, J.A.D.A. 58:42, 1959.
6. Muhler, J. C.: A practical method for reducing dental caries in children not receiving the established benefits of communal fluoridation, J. Dent. Child. 28:5, 1961.
7. Gish, C. W., and Muhler, J. C.: Effect on dental caries in children in a natural fluoride area of combined use of three agents containing stannous fluoride: a prophylactic paste, a solution and a dentifrice, J.A.D.A. 70:914, 1965.
8. Bixler, D., and Muhler, J. C.: Effect on dental caries in children in a nonfluoride area of combined use of three agents containing stannous fluoride: a prophylactic paste, a solution and a dentifrice, II, results at the end of 24 and 36 months, J.A.D.A. 72:392, 1966.
9. Scola, F. P., and Ostrom, C. A.: Clinical evaluation of stannous fluoride when used as a constituent of a compatible prophylactic paste, as a topical solution, and in a dentifrice in naval personnel, J.A.D.A. 73:1306, 1966.

10. Muhler, J. C., and others: The arrestment of incipient dental caries in adults after the use of three different forms of SnF₂ therapy: results after 30 months, J.A.D.A. **75**:1402, 1967.
11. Mergele, M. E.: Report II, an unsupervised brushing study on subjects residing in a community with fluoride in the water, Bull. Acad. Med. New Jersey **14**:251, 1968.
12. Fanning, E. A., Gotjamanos, T., and Vowles, N. J.: The use of fluoride dentifrices in the control of dental caries: methodology and results of a clinical trial, Aust. Dent. J. **13**: 201, 1968.
13. Naylor, M. N., and Emslie, R. D.: Clinical testing of stannous fluoride and sodium monofluorophosphate dentifrices in London school children, Brit. D. J. **123**: 17, 1967.
14. Moller, I. J., Holst, J. J., and Sorensen, E.: Caries reducing effect of a sodium monofluorophosphate dentifrice, Brit. D. J. **124**:209, 1968.
15. Thomas, A. E., and Jamison, H. C.: Effect of a combination of two cariostatic agents on caries in children: two year clinical study of supervised brushing in children's homes, Bull. Acad. Med. New Jersey **14**:241, 1968.
16. Mergele, M. E.: Report I, a supervised brushing study in state institutional schools, Bull. Acad. Med. New Jersey **14**:247, 1968.
17. Fosdick, L. S.: The clinical effectiveness of a neutral dentifrice in reducing dental caries, J.A.D.A. **50**:761, 1950.
18. Cross, W. G., Forrest, J. O., and Wade, A. B.: A comparative study of tooth cleansing using conventional and electrically operated toothbrushes, Brit. D. J. **113**:19, 1962.
19. Lefkowitz, W., and Robinson, H. B. G.: Effectiveness of automatic and hand brushes in removing dental plaque and debris, J.A.D.A. **65**:651, 1962.
20. Hoover, D. R., and Robinson, H. B. G.: Effect of automatic and hand toothbrushing on gingivitis, J.A.D.A. **65**:361, 1962.
21. Parfitt, G. J.: Cleansing the subgingival space, J. Periodont. **34**:13, 1963.
22. Conroy, C. W.: Comparison of automatic and hand toothbrushes, J.A.D.A. **70**:921, 1965.
23. Goldman, H. M., and others: Comparative cleansing efficiency of power-driven and conventional toothbrushes, I, effect of uninstructed patients, Periodontics **3**:200, 1965.
24. Ritsert, E. F., and Binns, W. H., Jr.: Adolescents brush better with an electric toothbrush, J. Dent. Child. **34**:354, 1967.
25. Powers, G. K.: A comparison of effectiveness in interproximal plaque removal of an electric toothbrush and a hand toothbrush, Periodontics **5**:37, 1967.
26. Chilton, N. W., DiDio, A., and Rothner, J. T.: Comparison of the clinical effectiveness of an electric and a standard toothbrush in normal individuals, J.A.D.A. **64**:777, 1962.
27. Quigley, G. A., and Hein, G. W.: Comparative cleansing efficiency of manual and power brushing, J.A.D.A. **65**:26, 1962.
28. Eliott, J. R.: A comparison of the effectiveness of a standard and an electric toothbrush, J. Periodont. **34**:375, 1963.
29. Beube, F. E., Schwartz, M., and Thompson, R. H.: A comparison of effectiveness of plaque removal of an electric toothbrush and a conventional hand toothbrush, Periodontics **2**:71, 1964.
30. Smith, W. A.: A clinical evaluation of an electric toothbrush, J. Periodont. **35**:127, 1964.
31. Rainey, B. L., and Ash, M. M.: A clinical study of a short stroke reciprocating action electric toothbrush, J. Periodont. **35**:455, 1964.
32. Ash, M. M., Rainey, B. L., and Smith, W. A.: Evaluation of manual and motor-driven toothbrushes, J.A.D.A. **69**:321, 1964.
33. Glass, R. L.: A clinical study of hand and electric toothbrushing, J. Periodont. **36**:322, 1965.
34. Iwerson, A. E., and Werking, D. H.: Hand and automatic toothbrushing effectiveness of inhibiting brown pellicle, J.A.D.A. **68**:178, 1964.
35. Phaneuf, E. A., and others: Automatic toothbrush: a new reciprocating action, J.A.D.A. **65**:12, 1962.
36. Terry, I. A., and Harrington, J. H.: Abrasive tests on acrylics, J.A.D.A. **65**:377, 1962.
37. Harrington, J. H., and Terry, I. A.: Automatic and hand toothbrushing abrasion studies, J.A.D.A. **68**:343, 1964.

38. Manly, R. S., and others: A method for measurement of abrasion of dentin by toothbrush and dentifrice, J. Dent. Res. **44**:533, 1965.
39. McConnell, D., and Conroy, C. W.: Comparison of abrasion produced by a simulated manual vs. a mechanical toothbrush, J. Dent. Res. **46**:1002, 1967.
40. Hein, J. W., Quigley, G. A., and Soparkar, P. M.: Comparable clinical abrasion of electric and hand toothbrushes, I.A.D.R. Abstract 492, 1966.
41. Chilton, N. W., and Kutscher, A. H.: Use of an electric toothbrush by a severely handicapped man, J. New Jersey D. Soc. **33**:20, 1961.
42. Kelner, M.: The use of an electrically powered toothbrush in the home dental care of handicapped children, Penn. D. J. **28**:3, 1961.
43. Greene, A., and others: The electric toothbrush as an adjunct in maintaining oral hygiene in handicapped patients, J. Dent. Child. **29**:169, 1962.
44. Vowles, J. K.: Assessment of an automatic action toothbrush (Broxident) in spastic children, Brit. D. J. **115**:327, 1963.
45. Copestoke, E.: Electrically operated toothbrushes, Brit. D. J. **114**:83, 1963.
46. Cohen, M. M., and Winer, R. A.: Comparative effectiveness of manually and power operated toothbrushing on tooth deposits, Periodontics **2**:122, 1964.
47. Smith, J. F., and Blankenship, J.: Improving oral hygiene in handicapped children by the use of an electric toothbrush, J. Dent. Child. **31**:198, 1964.
48. Kobayashi, L. Y., and Ash, M. M.: A clinical evaluation of an electrical toothbrush used by orthodontic patients, Angle Orthodont. **34**:209, 1964.
49. Womack, W. R., and Gray, A. H.: Comparative cleansing efficiency of an electric and a manual toothbrush in orthodontic patients, Angle Orthodont. **38**:256, 1968.
50. Sanders, W. E., and Robinson, H. B. G.: Effect of toothbrushing on deposition of calculus, J. Periodont. **33**:386, 1962.
51. Manhold, J. H., Jr.: Gingival tissue health with hand and power brushing: a retrospective with corroborative studies, J. Periodont. **38**:23, 1967.
52. Berman, C. L., and others: Observations of the effect of an electric toothbrush, J. Periodont. **33**:195, 1962.
53. Derbyshire, T. C., and Mankodi, S. M.: Gingival keratinization with hand and electric toothbrushes: a cytological comparison, J.A.D.A. **68**:255, 1964.
54. Lobene, R. R.: Evaluation of altered gingival health from permissive powered toothbrushing, J.A.D.A. **69**:585, 1964.
55. Lobene, R. R.: The effect of an automatic toothbrush on gingival health, J. Periodont. **35**:137, 1964.
56. Fraleigh, C. M.: Tissue changes with manual and electric brushes, J.A.D.A. **70**:380, 1965.
57. Toto, P. D., and Farchione, A.: Clinical evaluation of an electrically powered toothbrush in home periodontal therapy, J. Periodont. **32**:249, 1961.
58. Manhold, J. H., Jr., Franzetti, J., and Fitzsimmons, L.: Effect of the electric toothbrush on human gingiva: histologic and microrespirometer evaluation, J. Periodont. **36**:135, 1965.
59. Bechlem, D. N., Saxe, S. R., and Stern, L. B.: A histologic study of the effect upon the gingivae of using toothbrush in the presence of marginal periodontitis, Periodontics **3**:90, 1965.
60. Glickman, I., Petralis, R., and Marks, K. M.: The effect of powered toothbrushing and interdental stimulation upon microscopic inflammation and surface keratinization of the interdental gingiva, J. Periodont. **36**:108, 1965.

Chapter 8 Preventive pedodontics

James R. Roche

> Objectives of pedodontic care
> Early diagnosis
>     Technic for examining a child under 2 years of age
>     Oral findings
>     Nursing bottle caries
> Preventive behavior management
> Dental caries—prevention and control
>     Examination procedures
>     Preventing initiation of new carious lesions
>     Operative dentistry
> Dental aberrations affecting the developing occlusion
>     Ankylosis of teeth
>     Ectopic eruption of first permanent molar
>     Local factors affecting delayed eruption
>     Premature loss of primary molars and cuspids
>     Anterior crossbite
> Recall evaluation

## OBJECTIVES OF PEDODONTIC CARE

Historically, dental care for children has been designed primarily to prevent oral pain and infection, the occurrence and progress of dental caries, premature loss of primary teeth, loss in arch length, and the association between fear and dental care. During the progress of the pedodontic service the dentist continues to be responsible for guiding the child and parent, intercepting the effects of oral disorders on health and dental alignment, and preventing oral disease.[1]

Current surveys[2] demonstrate that dental caries and gingivitis are major oral health problems for children of low-income families in the United States. Among children 5 to 9 years of age who were examined without the aid of dental radiographs 87 percent required restorations and 35 percent were in need of extractions. Restorations were necessary for 91 percent of the adolescents, ages 10 to 16, and extractions were needed for at least 25 percent of this age group. Children under 10 years of age demonstrated a 9 percent prevalence of mild gingivitis or inflamed gingiva that completely circumscribed the tooth without pocket formation. Gingivitis was present in 35 percent of the adolescents, with 1 percent of the affected group revealing evidence of a definite breakdown in the epithelial attachment.

Rayner[3] has indicated that the socioeconomic status of families, as might be expected, has an influence on the mother's attitude on the value of oral health and the preventive use of the dentist for children 11 to 14 years of age.

A study by Moore[4] of 1,123 children aged 7 to 13 years, using the papillary-marginal-attached index, indicated that 93 percent of the children demonstrated evidence of gingivitis. Neglected gingivitis in children has been suggested as a predisposing factor in advanced periodontal disease among adults.

**178** *Improving dental practice through preventive measures*

The prevention of dental caries in children is a persistent problem. Hennon[5] recently published a report on the prevalence of dental caries in preschool children. Of the children 18 to 23 months old 8.3 percent demonstrated dental caries, and the children in this group affected with decay had an average defs of 1.75. Of the study group between 24 and 36 months of age 35.3 percent demonstrated dental caries with an average of 5.13 defs. Presently the number of rampant caries cases of the primary dentition observed in the dental practice may be markedly reduced, as a result of the fluoridation of communal water supplies. In comparing the prevalence of dental caries for 5-year-old children from fluoride and nonfluoride communities, Murray[6] reported that the children from fluoride areas demonstrated a 63.6 percent lower caries experience than the children from a low fluoride region.

Intensified oral health education programs by elementary and high schools and dental societies and more effective methods of prevention and control in the dental office are believed to have decreased the dental caries experience in the mixed and permanent dentitions. Community dental health education projects and dental care programs are alerting parents to the importance of pedodontic care.

Recent surveys[7] among members of the Association of Pedodontic Diplomates and the Academy of Pedodontics indicate that approximately 30 percent of pedodontic services were for recall patients receiving preventive services, that is, prophylaxis, examination, and topical application of fluoride, and 40 percent of the pedodontists' patients received restorations. Certainly after emergency oral care the appropriate priority of services should be directed toward preventing dental caries and periodontal disease. Comprehensive dental treatment is a form of prevention and includes intercepting the progress of diseases of the soft and hard tissues of the mouth and alleviating oral disorders.

Currently both the family dentist and the pedodontist need to promote orderly and energetic preventive programs for all child patients if prevention is to continue as the keystone of pedodontic care.

## EARLY DIAGNOSIS

Examination of the child's oral structures from the age of 16 to 22 months provides an opportunity for diagnosing early dental caries, recording abnormal erup-

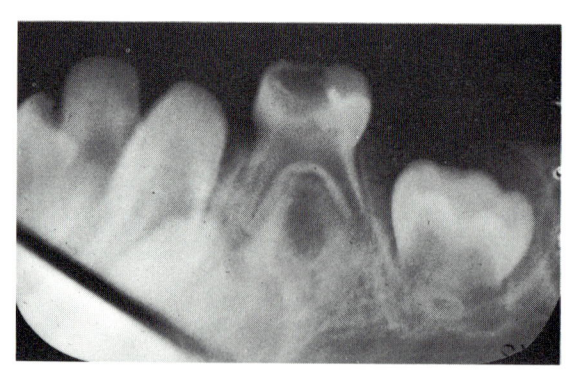

Fig. 8-1. Periapical radiograph of a 14-month-old child demonstrating a mandibular right first primary molar with extensive dental caries involving the pulp; emphasizes the uncommon extensive dental caries at a very young age.

tion, and establishing a preventive oral health plan. Home preventive measures may be emphasized to the parents during the child's teething period so as to influence his future oral health. Clinical experience in several pedodontic practices indicates that parents are most receptive to learning about home preventive dental care during the teething period.

Detection of decay near the child's eighteenth month may prevent the progress of incipient carious lesions. Dental caries may occur to an alarming degree in children under 2 years of age (Fig. 8-1).

It is beneficial to oral health if a carious lesion is diagnosed during the incipient form, and it is much easier to perform a very small restoration on a young child than to provide an extensive restoration when the child is only a few months older.

## Technic for examining a child under 2 years of age

Unlike the child of 2 years of age or more, who may accompany the dental assistant into the treatment room, the child under 2 years of age usually responds best when he is transferred from the reception area to the treatment room in the company of his parent.

Fig. 8-2 illustrates the treatment room scene, in which the chairside assistant has placed the parent in a reclined and comfortable position in the dental chair. The child is seated on the mother's lap, his head resting against her shoulder and upper arm. The mother is in a position to restrain the child by placing her arms around his

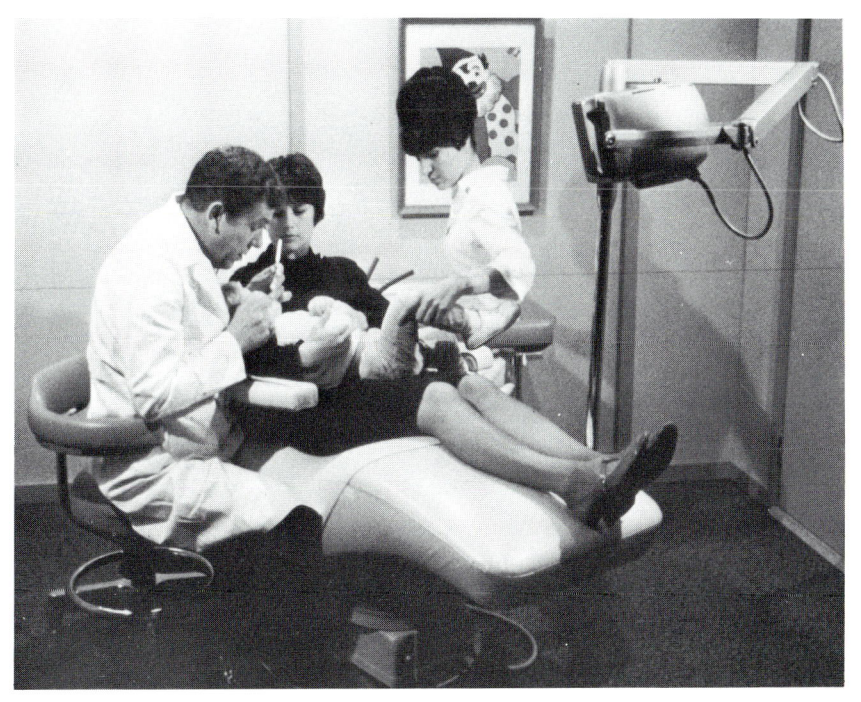

**Fig. 8-2.** The child under 2 years of age is positioned across his mother's lap and his head is supported by his mother's arm. The dentist firmly cradles the young patient's head to prohibit irrational head movements. The chairside assistant applies light hand contact to the child's legs to provide restraint if needed.

**180** *Improving dental practice through preventive measures*

arms and chest. The chairside assistant is seated higher than the dentist so that she can hand him the required instruments safely and effectively. She is also ready to grasp the child's feet or possibly his arms if the mother loses her hold. The dentist should cradle the child's head in his arm to prohibit irrational head movements of the child.

The examination procedure begins with a slow digital inspection of the child's soft tissues. A sharp explorer, an unmarred front-surface mirror, and adequate light are aids for detecting incipient carious lesions in the examination. Breaks in the continuity of the enamel surface that feel soft under firm palpation with the explorer may be considered as carious lesions. The chairside assistant may pass a dry cotton roll to the dentist for use in drying the occlusal fissures of the primary molars or the labial surfaces of the incisors. Usually only light "on guard" restraint of the patient's feet is required by the chairside assistant's left hand, which permits her to efficiently record the dentist's dictation of the examination of the soft tissues and the dentition.

**Oral findings**

Aberrations in the number or form of primary teeth may be signs of anomalies within the mandible that should receive early treatment planning (Fig. 8-3). Detection of dental caries in the crevice of fused or geminated primary crowns may prevent extensive and rapid tooth loss (Fig. 8-4).

Another disorder that may be present during the teething period is eruptive hematoma (Fig. 8-5). Shafer[8] has reported that eruptive hematoma appears a few weeks before the eruption as blood-filled "eruptive cysts" overlying unerupted teeth. Eruptive hematoma may be observed more frequently in the tissues covering the primary second molars or first permanent molars and is classified as a particular type of dentigerous cyst. The normal follicular space surrounding the erupting tooth is enlarged with the tissue fluid or blood. No treatment is indicated, and usually the

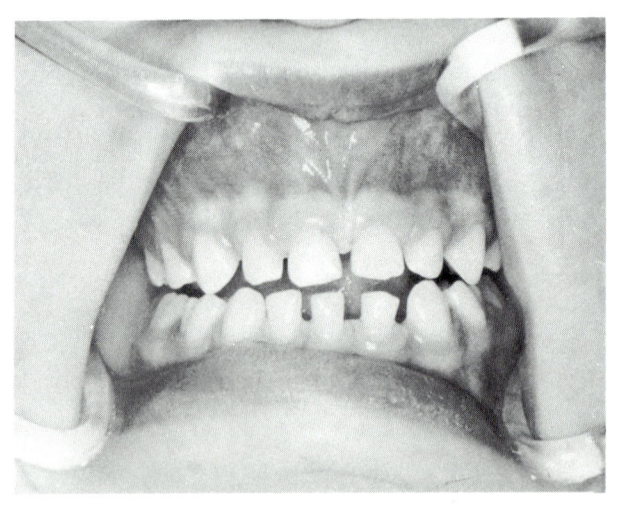

Fig. 8-3. The mandibular left primary lateral incisor is congenitally missing or delayed in eruption, or anomalies are present within the mandible.

tooth will emerge through the tissue without delay and the hematoma will be reduced.

Tasanen[9] recently reported a comprehensive study including a control group on the age-old controversy of the effects of teething as related to oral and systemic symptoms. The study group consisted of 192 tooth eruptions in 126 children with 107 controls. The results indicated that teething did not increase the incidence of infection, did not cause a rise in temperature, erythrocyte sedimentation rate, or white cell count, and did not cause diarrhea, cough, or sleep disturbance. This impressive study demonstrated an increase in daytime restlessness, finger sucking or rubbing of the gingiva, and drooling, along with some possible influence on a decrease in appetite. One-third of the study group demonstrated no change in the color of the mucosa overlying the erupting tooth, one-third of the babies had a slight increase in the redness of tissue overlying the erupting tooth, and the other one-third demonstrated a marked redness of the gingival tissue overlying the erupting tooth.

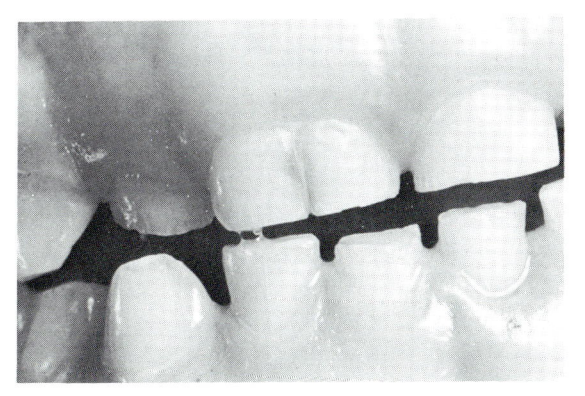

Fig. 8-4. Crowns of fused or geminated primary incisors may demonstrate a significant labial crevice, which is a predisposing area for the initiation of decay.

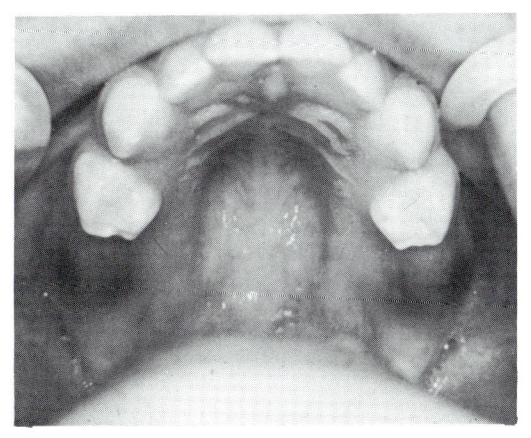

Fig. 8-5. Eruptive hematomas are represented as elevated portions of gingival tissue appearing bluish in color and overlying the eruptive maxillary right and left secondary primary molars. No treatment is indicated.

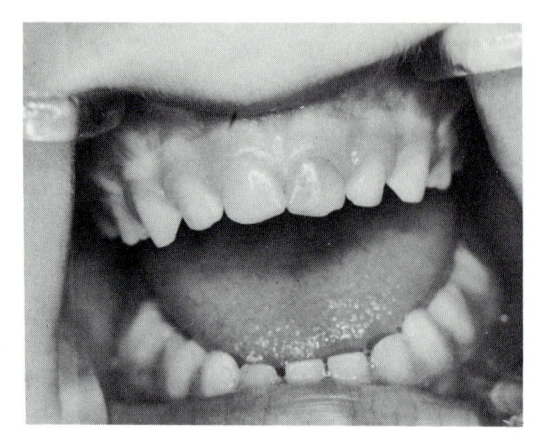

Fig. 8-6. The preschool child is particularly vulnerable to traumatic injury of the dentition. The maxillary left primary central and lateral incisors demonstrate Class I fractures, and the left central incisor is discolored as a result of a blow to the primary teeth.

Tasanen's findings obviously indicate that young children who are awake at night or who have elevated temperatures during the teething period should be referred to a physician for a physical examination in consideration of a possible coincidental infection such as otitis media or bronchitis. Thus a systemic disturbance can perhaps be intercepted because the dentist did not try to relate the symptoms to the process of erupting primary teeth.

Fractured and discolored primary incisors may be present during the teething period (Fig. 8-6). A study by Ravn[10] indicates that children in the age range of $1\frac{1}{2}$ to $2\frac{1}{2}$ years are most vulnerable to blows of the primary dentition. Preventive pedodontics should include the identification of primary teeth that have been traumatized; the affected teeth should be evaluated periodically. Although subsequent findings may indicate a marked constriction of the pulpal canals, the injured primary incisors will often remain free of apical pathology and normal exfoliation will follow. In other cases the discolored or fractured primary incisors will demonstrate delayed root resorption and prolonged retention, thereby causing the deflection of the permanent tooth. Periapical pathology may result from traumatized incisors, and periodic oral and radiographic examinations are indicated until the traumatized primary teeth have exfoliated.

**Nursing bottle caries**

Occasionally, children beyond the age of 1 year continue to receive a nursing bottle filled with milk or sugary fluids during naptime and bedtime. During the receptionist's recording of the child's preliminary medical history, the parent may indicate that the child beyond the weaning period has received the nursing bottle to pacify his behavior or to aid with his sleep. Intercepting this parental habit of prolonged bottle feeding may prevent the occurrence or progression of the rampant pattern of decay known as nursing bottle caries.

The carbohydrate contents of the nursing bottle becomes pooled around the maxillary anterior teeth and provides a culture medium for acid-forming microorganisms. During sleep the salivary flow is diminished and clearance of liquids from

*Preventive pedodontics* 183

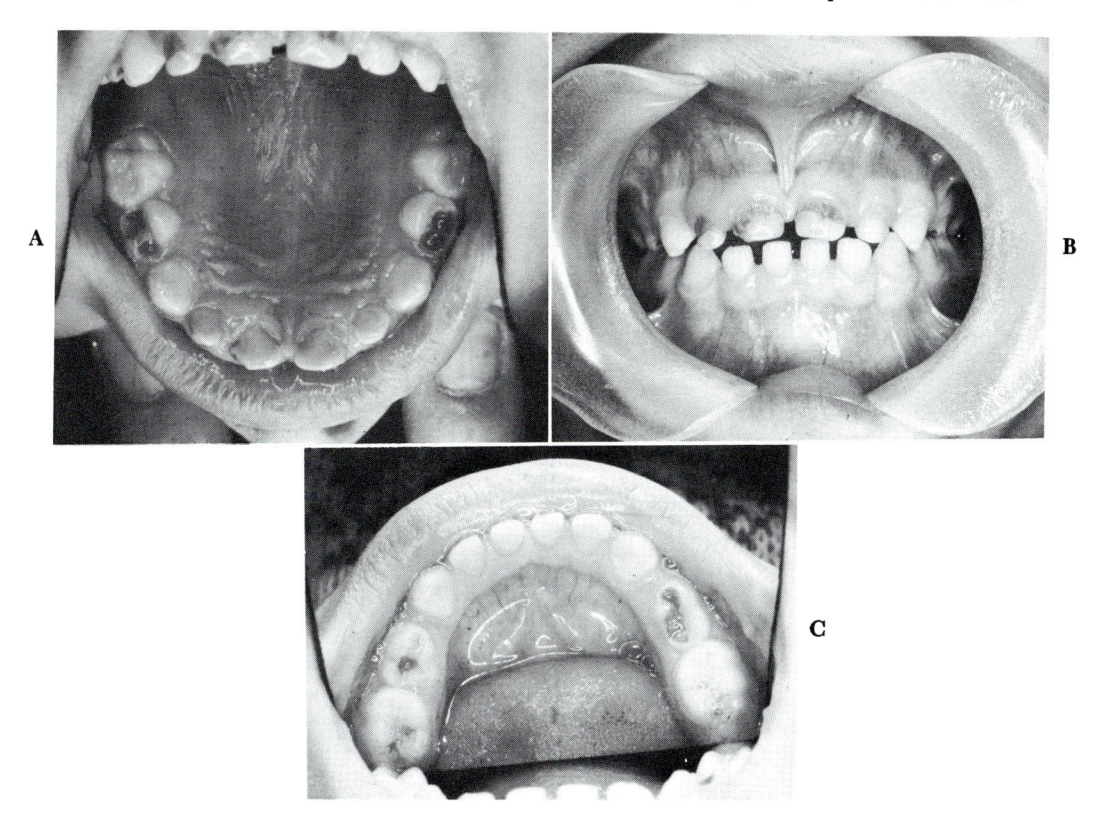

Fig. 8-7. A, Nursing bottle caries, an extensive type of tooth decay involving the maxillary anterior teeth; may occur from the pooling of milk or sugary fluids around these teeth. B, Occlusal view of maxillary primary teeth demonstrating circumvential carious lesions of the incisors and the extensively decayed occlusal areas of the first primary molar. C, Occlusal view of mandibular primary teeth demonstrating the first primary molars markedly involved by the decay process. The unaffected mandibular primary incisors have been protected by the position of the tongue during bottle feeding.

the mouth is slowed. Typically, these circumvential carious lesions begin at the cervical third on the labial surface of the maxillary anterior teeth; they may extend onto the proximal and lingual areas (Fig. 8-7). These lesions progress rapidly and may contribute to the fracturing away of the incisal portions of the maxillary primary incisors with resulting pulpal necrosis and periapical abscess formation. Within a few months the occlusal areas of all the first primary molars may be involved extensively with this rapidly advancing decay. The mandibular primary incisors are usually unaffected by bottle feeding, since the child's tongue is positioned over these teeth while the nipple is held in his mouth.

Several studies[11-13] have indicated the relationship between prolonged nursing bottle feeding and the formation of this typical pattern of decay, particularly if the nursing bottle contains a sweetened liquid or if sugars are added to the milk.

The etiology of nursing bottle caries remains controversial. Finn[14] presented a critical literature review of the possible relationship between plain milk and nursing bottle caries. He concluded that questionable evidence was available to demonstrate that bottle feeding of plain milk without added sugars causes this peculiar pattern

184 *Improving dental practice through preventive measures*

of decay formation. Michal[15] surveyed parents of children with nursing bottle caries, and he reported case histories of prolonged bottle feeding of only plain milk.

Although nursing bottle caries may be more prevalent in families of a low socioeconomic level, Michal has reported an increased number of cases from educated, middle-income parents.

Consultation with parents may also reveal that the child has been receiving frequent administrations of sugary-flavored medicines. This history would indicate the need for more frequent recall examinations.

Early examination of the child between the ages of 16 and 22 months may prevent or intercept the possible ill effects of prolonged nursing bottle feeding. During consultation with the child's physician it would be appropriate for the dentist to recommend that bottle feeding be discontinued to reduce the risk of dental caries.

## PREVENTIVE BEHAVIOR MANAGEMENT

Proper guidance of the child patient toward the acceptance of dental procedures helps to prevent behavior problems. Because of the limited experience of young patients, each of their dental visits contains an element of stress.

Planned management of the child's first visit can cultivate good rapport between the parents and the office staff. While the parent and the receptionist are seated comfortably in the business office, the receptionist can obtain the child's medical and dental history and make friends with him. In addition, a preliminary evaluation can be recorded of the parent's anxiety over the child's dental visit. Identifying the degree of parental fear toward dentistry may assist in preparing the dentist and staff for the child's reactions to the dental procedures. The receptionist's sincere interest in the child and the parent projects a similar feeling on the part of the entire staff, and potential problems of child management related to fear or defiance can be alleviated greatly by the receptionist's effective management of the parent during their first conversation.

At the time the child is to receive care the receptionist can improve communication with the young patient in the reception area by speaking to the child at eye level and in a relaxed manner (Fig. 8-8).

Unlike the child under 2 years of age, the older patient is taken to the treatment room while the parent remains in the reception area. This separation gives the child encouragement for the visit by exemplifying the parent's confidence in the dentist. It also enables the dentist to give undivided attention to the child patient and makes it easier for him to hold the child's attention. Accompanying the child from the reception area to the treatment room is usually uneventful. Misunderstandings on the part of the child can be prevented at this point, if the receptionist remembers to maintain a positive attitude toward the child's dental needs and the value of good dental health.

The dentist and his office staff can often identify the child's overt or disguised feelings of anxiety. Acclimating the child to the dental instruments, initial procedures, and anticipated sensation is an important step in controlling anxiety. If members of the dental team show interest in the child by determining his feelings and concerns, they can more effectively condition his attitude toward the immediate procedure and future treatment.

The defiant child requires an unemotional approach, a positive procedural plan, and firm and modulated voice control. Children want to know the rules, and the

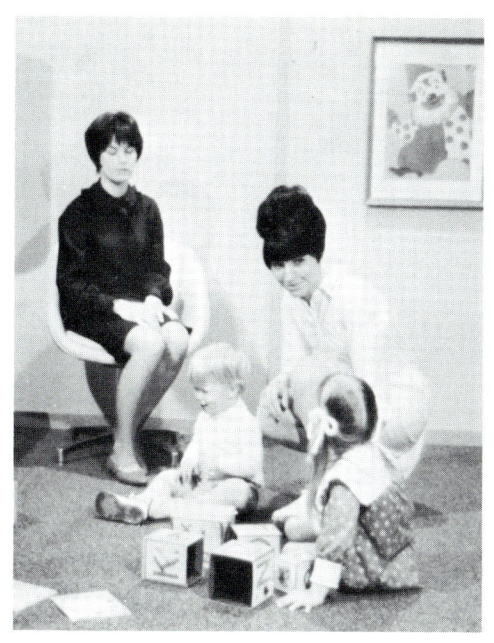

**Fig. 8-8.** The receptionist communicates a friendly interest in the child at eye level, while explaining that the dentist will look at the child's teeth in the next room.

defiant child in particular needs to understand limitations to resistive habits. The entire dental staff can render calm guidance if they adopt a mature emotional attitude that respects children and if they interpret the child's occasional insulting remarks as reactions to the situation rather than something personal.

The fearful child needs understanding and gradual reconditioning with repeated explanation of the proposed procedure, demonstration of the technic, and a positive progression of the plan. Attempting to talk a patient out of fear is usually ineffective. Discriminating between fear and defiance in a continuously crying child of 2 to 4 years of age may not be easy. A repetition of "tell and show" may subsequently require an immediate "go ahead" to accomplish the technic and reinforce the ease of the procedure.

Each member of the staff should speak so that the child can understand. Instructions should be consistent with the child's limited vocabulary and experience. All staff members should refrain from embarrassing the child by making fun of his transitory speech imperfections or by laughing at his limited ability to express himself. To develop an effective dialogue, the dentist should listen carefully to the child patient so that he can discover the best avenue of communication.

Time invested in acclimating the child to the dental procedures and attempting to understand his actions may prevent uncooperative behavior and provide increased efficiency during the subsequent procedures.

## DENTAL CARIES—PREVENTION AND CONTROL
### Examination procedures

Pedodontic services are based on a thorough examination of the oral tissues, occlusion, and all surfaces of the erupted teeth. A prophylaxis is an essential pre-

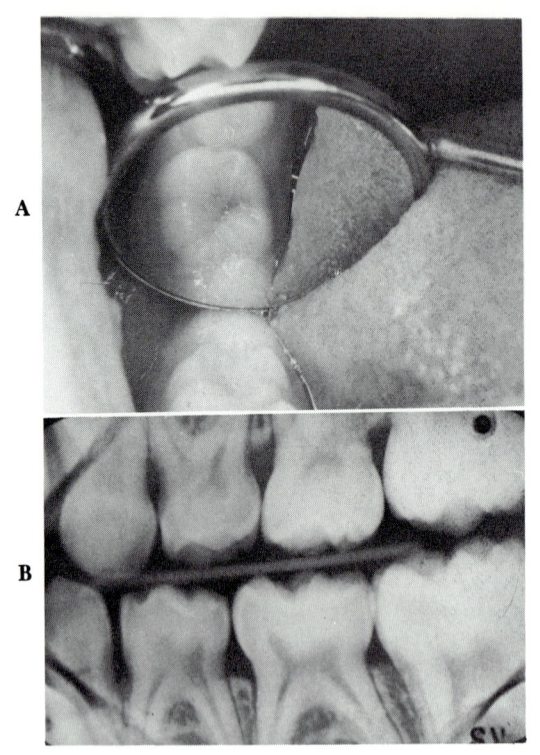

Fig. 8-9. **A,** Mirror view of a mandibular right first permanent molar demonstrating discoloration in the occlusal fissures. A sharp explorer was unable to demonstrate a softness. **B,** Posterior bite-wing radiograph demonstrating an extensive rarefied area in the mesial portion of the occlusal just beneath the enamel surface of the mandibular right first permanent molar. An extensive carious lesion was present that could have been prevented by careful evaluation of earlier radiographs.

liminary to an efficient examination. A laboratory study by Kelley[16] using zirconium silicate–stannous flouride prophylaxis paste* demonstrated that zirconium silicate is a better cleaning agent than lava pumice, silex, or flour of pumice. The study further indicated that the paste is an effective means of providing a topical application of stannous fluoride with a beneficial enamel antisolubility effect. In addition, a dental prophylaxis may be an important step in conditioning or reconditioning the child to oral health procedures.

Posterior bite-wing radiographs for children whose primary molars have proximal contact are essential in determining the number and extent of decayed areas. Hennon's study demonstrated that 76 percent of interproximal dental caries in the primary dentition of patients between 24 and 39 months of age would not have been diagnosed without radiographs.

The young patient's lack of understanding, fear of discomfort, gagging, or other impediments to adequate radiographs may be dealt with by presenting the procedure confidently and performing one or more "fake-take" exercises.

Dental caries can be correctly diagnosed by correlating the oral findings with the

---

*Zircate Treatment Paste, L. D. Calk Company, Milford, Delaware.

radiographic evaluation. Extensive tooth destruction may be prevented by analyzing the posterior bite-wing radiographs in the occlusal region at the dentinoenamel junction. Occasionally discolored occlusal pit and fissures may present maximum resistance to a sharp explorer; yet the radiograph may reveal evidence of a hemisphere of decay beneath the enamel surface (Fig. 8-9).

## Preventing initiation of new carious lesions

During the consultation period with the child's parents, it is essential that they be informed of the oral findings, recommended treatment, and estimated expense. The control of dental caries is approached by investigating causes, correcting improper habits, and providing proper restorations. Unhurried and private consultation with parents may reveal anxieties or possible family conflicts that are contributing to improper eating habits or diminished salivary flow. Fear of dental procedures acquired from their own experiences may have influenced the parents to neglect the dental needs of their child.

If the child's dentition shows evidence of a high caries susceptibility, examining the parents and other siblings may provide insight for motivating the parents to preventive measures.

Home preventive measures need enthusiastic presentation. Motivating the child to use adequate toothbrushing habits and the parents to exert supervision should be a continuous teaching process. Oral hygiene for the child is important since the presence of oral debris is related to the degree of gingivitis. Proper toothbrushing immediately after each meal removes gross amounts of food debris and bacterial plaque and helps to correct gingivitis resulting from poor oral hygiene. By using a large model of the dentition and an oversized brush, the hygienist or assistant can demonstrate the proper toothbrushing method and explain to the parents the style of junior brush recommended by the dentist. She can also emphasize the benefits of brushing the teeth or rinsing the mouth immediately after eating.

The use of disclosing dye tablets containing erythrosine (F.D.C. Red No. 3) has been recommended by Arnim[17] as an educational aid. On subsequent visits the disclosing dye will help the staff to show the young patient and his parent the areas of oral debris that have been missed by ineffective positioning of the toothbrush. The gift of a 2-minute timer can encourage the child to take the proper time for the toothbrushing exercise at home. The parents may be instructed in the use of dental floss for removing oral debris. The floss is passed between the proximal contacts and drawn occlusally.

The dentist may instruct the office staff to recommend to parents a medium nylon bristle junior brush with a straight trim for the child's primary or mixed dentition. A study by Kimmelman and Tassman[18] indicated that medium bristle toothbrushes remove stains from the child's teeth more effectively than hard or soft bristle brushes. Starkey[19] also recommends the straight form medium brush and the scrub-brush method for brushing the primary dentition. It would be better for the parents of a preschool child to brush their child's teeth than to relinquish this important health measure to the child. McClure[20] compared various methods of brushing the teeth of preschoolers. His results demonstrated that parents were able to clean the child's teeth better than the child. Also, parents who had been instructed in the scrub-brush method performed better than parents using other methods. During the eruption of the permanent incisors the roll method of brushing can be demonstrated to the parent and the child; however, the child may be 9 years old before he can wield the brush properly. Therefore the parent should supervise the roll method during the early years of the mixed dentition.

Studies[21, 22] have demonstrated that electric toothbrushing can be significantly superior to the use of manual brushes in removing debris for the primary and mixed dentitions. A study of preschool children by Hall[23] demonstrated that an electric toothbrush removes significantly more debris than a manual brush. Even with a preschool group practicing self-brushing, the electric toothbrush was more effective in removing material from the teeth. Irrespective of whether an electric or manual toothbrush is used, the instructed parent can perform this task more effectively than the preschool child. A study by Ritsert[24] revealed that adolescents preferred an electrically operated toothbrush to the use of a manual brush. Also, the automatic brush proved to be 23 percent more effective than manual brushing for removing debris. The electric toothbrush has been recognized as beneficial for use by the parents of handicapped children in improving oral hygiene and decreasing gingivitis in their children.

An important responsibility of the dentist is the surveillance of oral hygiene and gingival health for his patient during the period that his orthodontic colleague is providing corrective treatment. It would be appropriate for the dentist to recommend the use of an electric toothbrush during home care for the adolescent patient who is wearing banded appliances. Womack[25] has reported on the effectiveness of an electric toothbrush* for patients 10 to 17 years of age who were wearing multi-banded appliances. The study group using the electric toothbrush maintained superior dental cleanliness to that of the group of orthodontic patients using the manual toothbrush. Neither the electric nor manual toothbrush damaged the appliances or gingival tissues.

It would be appropriate to recommend to parents the daily use by their children of a stannous fluoride–calcium pyrophosphate dentifrice for reducing the dental caries experience.

The topical application of 10 percent stannous fluoride is effective in reducing the number of new carious lesions. During the prophylaxis with the Zircate Treatment Paste, unwaxed dental floss is drawn between the teeth, carrying the stannous fluoride into the interproximal areas. At this time the one-application technic of applying 10 percent aqueous solution of stannous fluoride for a 30-second tooth-contact period may be given. Maximum benefit from stannous fluoride in the reduction in dental caries experience is obtained when the child receives a prophylaxis with the Zircate Treatment Paste and a topical application of stannous fluoride in the office, followed by daily home use of a stannous fluoride–calcium pyrophosphate dentifrice.

Diet surveys help to establish a baseline reference for diet discussions with parents.[26, 27] Better cooperation will be obtained from the parents in completing an accurate diet survey if the objective of the survey is explained to them beforehand. The parents should understand that the dentist is concerned with the child's eating habits and the types of food he eats as they relate to the decay process. If the parents believe that their ability to manage their child's diet is being questioned, they may be reluctant to provide a reliable survey and may develop a barrier against subse-

---

*Broxodent, E. R. Squibb and Sons, Inc., New Brunswick, New Jersey.

quent dietary recommendations. The dentist must be convinced of the value of using the diet record as an educational measure before the parents are asked to take time to complete the forms. The hygienist can assist in providing a diet consultation with the parents who have completed the diet record of their child's 7-day food intake. In a quiet and private environment the hygienist can explain the relationship between diet and dental caries and can give the parents the American Dental Association Booklet, *Diet and Dental Health*. The calculated quantity of refined carbohydrate from the child's diet record will provide a substantial basis for the consultation. The quantity of refined carbohydrates in the child's sample diet can be illustrated, the frequency of fermentable carbohydrate intake reviewed, and the importance of selecting foods from the four basic food groups stressed.

The hygienist maintains control of the printed material used in acquainting the parents with the important effects of diet on oral health and marks topics of interest. This procedure encourages the parents to refer to the selected information after they return home. During the child's teething period the parents are usually eager for dental health education; they can be very receptive to information on how foods and fluids may promote decay.

Recommendations to parents should depict the child's mealtime experience as an enjoyable time of day. Rust[28] indicated the importance of avoiding forced feeding of children, which may result in the development of strong dislike for certain foods.

Advising parents to completely restrict the child's between-meal snack habit may result in a better mealtime diet; however, society has placed an obvious emphasis on the between-meal snack. Educating parents on special snacks of a nonrefined carbohydrate nature—such as open-faced meat sandwiches, cheese and meat cubes, and fresh fruit—may be the recommendation of choice.

## Operative dentistry

Restorative dentistry is valuable in controlling dental caries in children. Restoration of carious lesions prevents the loss of teeth from the progression of decay into the pulp with resulting pulpal necrosis and possible alveolar abscess. Furthermore, complete restorative procedures have the potential of reducing the number of oral microorganisms involved in the formation of dental caries.

The presence of multiple and extensive carious lesions may require the expeditious removal of gross layers of caries and the arresting of the decay process by temporarily sealing all lesions with zinc oxide–eugenol dressings.

If the radiographs demonstrate that the carious lesion is close to the pulp, indirect pulp treatment may be the procedure of choice to maintain pulpal vitality. The superficial layers of decay are removed with the use of a No. 4 round bur at low speed. The bur is directed laterally at the level of the dentinoenamel junction and a layer of caries is permitted to remain over the deepest area of potential pulpal exposure. A sedative dressing composed of an accelerated-setting zinc oxide–eugenol mixture (such as Temrex*) is placed in the cavity and contoured properly to avoid displacement by occlusion. Extensive destruction requires cementing a band around the treated tooth to prevent displacement of the dressing. After a convalescent period of 8 weeks or longer the tooth is anesthetized and isolated with a rubber dam.

---

*Temrex Cement, Interstate Dental Company, Inc., New York, New York.

The zinc oxide–eugenol is removed, and the remaining caries is carefully excavated to a sound dentin base.

Because of the deposit of secondary dentin, an entry into the pulp usually will not be evident after the convalescent period. If an entry is present into the pulp, pulpotomy or pulpectomy treatment should be considered. The cavity preparation should be completed, a cavity liner or base placed, and the tooth restored.

## DENTAL ABERRATIONS AFFECTING THE DEVELOPING OCCLUSION

Early, thorough, and periodic examination procedures can assist in identifying oral abnormalities and can provide the basis for intercepting and possibly aborting a permanent defect in alignment.

Radiographic findings should be correlated with visual and tactile evaluations in diagnosing aberrant dental development. Panoramic radiographs can be helpful in determining the presence of all unerupted tooth masses in patients older than 4 years. When properly instructed by trained assistants, young patients and their parents have accepted panoramic radiography with cooperation. If panoramic equipment is not available, a preschool radiographic survey as described by Matlock[29] can be used for children between the ages of 3 and 6 years. This survey consists of a maxillary and a mandibular anterior occlusal film, a maxillary right and left posterior occlusal film, and a right and left lateral jaw film.

Brown[30] stated that an adequate radiographic technic for children should detect anomalies of number, shape, position, and texture. MacRae[31] compared three dental radiographic views with an eight-film survey for children 6 to 9 years old. This study demonstrated that right and left posterior bite-wing radiographs and a maxillary incisor view failed to reveal 22 percent of the anomalies detected by additional views of the maxillary and mandibular molars and the mandibular incisors.

### Ankylosis of teeth

During the period of resorption for the primary molar roots, a solid union may occur between the osseous tissue and the root surface. The firm attachment between the primary root and the bone results in the following: depression of the primary tooth inferior to the plane of occlusion, atypical contacts with adjacent normal teeth, a solid sound to percussion, lack of mobility, and a disruption in the image of the periodontal membrane space radiographically (Fig. 8-10). Lamb[32] reported that the prevalence of ankylosed primary molars in a study group of 2,105 children, ages 8 to 12, was 3.2 percent. Ankylosis occurred much more often in the mandible than in the maxilla, and the mandibular second primary molars were most frequently involved.

Diagnosis of an ankylosed primary molar requires periodic evaluation of the proximal contacts. Occasionally primary molars diagnosed as being ankylosed will subsequently demonstrate root resorption and will exfoliate normally. If marked atypical proximal contact occurs definitive treatment consists of extracting the ankylosed pirmary molar and placing an immediate space management appliance to prevent proximal tipping of adjacent teeth with resultant loss of arch length. Ankylosis of the primary molar may result in prolonged retention of the primary tooth.

The delayed eruption of a permanent tooth depressed inferior to the plane of occlusion may indicate that it is ankylosed. The diagnosis of an ankylosed permanent molar presents the opportunity to intercept the hindered eruption. "Rocking" the

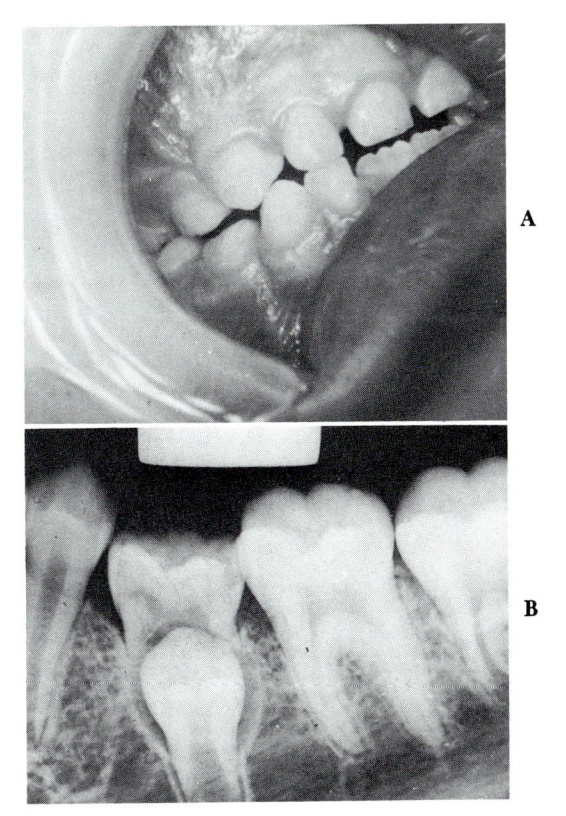

Fig. 8-10. **A,** The mandibular right first primary molar demonstrates a depressed position in the arch and can be easily detected during the evaluation of the occlusion. **B,** The radiographic appearance of an ankylosed primary molar may demonstrate a partial or complete absence of the periodontal membrane space.

anesthetized permanent molar with extraction forceps may break the osteoid bridge between the root and the bone and permit continued eruption of the tooth. Occasionally orthodontic consultation with consideration for multibanded anchorage may be required to provide a force occlusally to encourage movement of the loosened ankylosed molar.

### Ectopic eruption of first permanent molar

Preventive measures include the diagnosis and treatment of ectopic eruption of the first permanent molar. The abnormal mesioangular positioning of the first permanent molar prior to complete emergence into the mouth may compel the permanent molar to become impacted beneath the distal portion of the primary second molar crown.

Pulver[33] studied the problem of ectopic eruption of the maxillary first permanent molar and concluded that this aberration may result from a combination of the following circumstances.
1. Larger than normal mean sizes of all maxillary primary and permanent teeth
2. Larger affected first permanent molars and second primary molars
3. Smaller maxillae

**192** *Improving dental practice through preventive measures*

4. Posterior position of the maxillae in relation to cranial base
5. Abnormal angulation of eruption of the maxillary first permanent molar
6. Delayed calcification of some affected first permanent molars

Although ectopic eruption of the first permanent molar has been suspected of signaling an arch length inadequacy, this is not always the case.

Studies[34, 35] have indicated that the prevalence of ectopic first permanent molar eruption is between 2 and 3 percent. Carr[36] reported an increased prevalence of the ectopic first permanent molar eruption among children with cleft lip and cleft palate. The study group received palate closure at 24 months of age, and 29 percent of the girls and 22.9 percent of the boys demonstrated ectopic eruption.

Early diagnosis of the aberrant position of the first permanent molar from radiographs will indicate the need either to provide close surveillance of the eruptive pattern for this tooth or to intercept the severe mesial inclination of the malposed permanent molar with appliance therapy.

The dentist should be alert to the possible ectopic eruption of the first permanent molar. The permanent molar may produce severe resorption of the distal root and a portion of the crown of the second primary molar. Young[35] reported that 66 percent of the ectopic erupted first permanent molars were self-correcting without interceptive appliances; however, the displaced permanent molar may remain locked and may contribute to premature loss of the second primary molar (Fig. 8-11). The early loss of the second primary molar and the severe mesioangular positioning

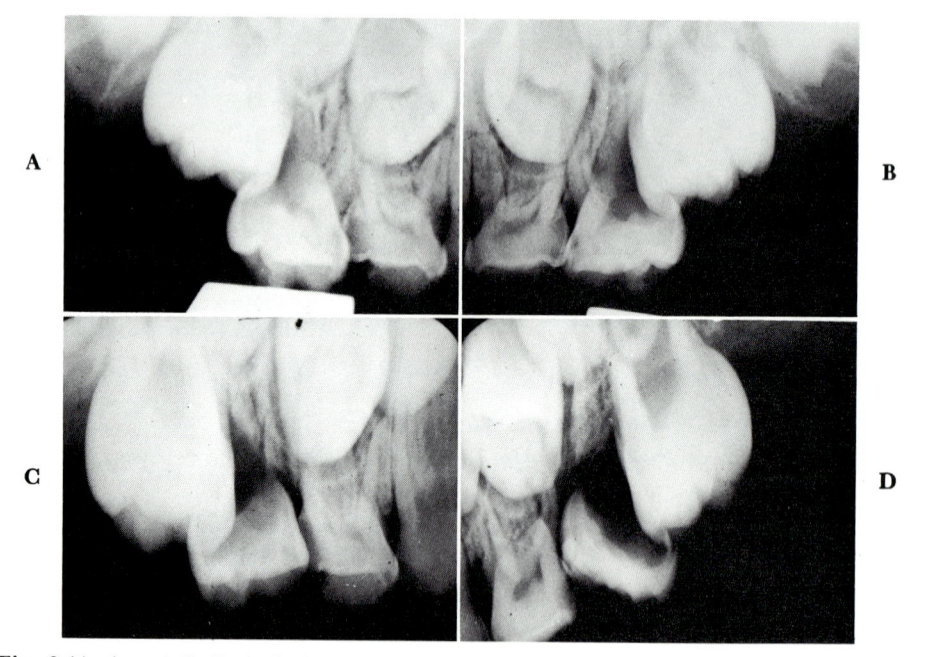

**Fig. 8-11. A** and **B**, Periapical radiographs demonstrating ectopic eruption of the maxillary right and left first permanent molars, with destruction of the distal portion of the second primary molars. **C** and **D**, Periapical radiographs 10 months later, demonstrating the continued ectopic eruption of the maxillary right and left first permanent molars with the continued extensive destruction and displacement of the second primary molars.

*Preventive pedodontics* 193

of the ectopic permanent molar result in significant loss of arch length. It may be possible to prevent premature loss of the second primary molar, or at least to prevent loss in arch length.

Occasionally, if the partially impacted permanent molar is only slightly locked inferior to the distal convexity of the second primary molar, the impacted tooth may be influenced to tip distally and become unlocked by inserting a .026-inch brass ligature wire through the embrasure between the permanent and primary molars. The brass ligature wire is formed in a semiarc, threaded through the embrasure, and looped around the contact area of the molars with a No. 110 pliers. The twisted terminal ends of the brass ligature wire are cut to 3 mm. lengths and folded into the gingival crevice to eliminate irritating projections into the buccal tissue. The brass ligature wire should be tightened approximately every 3 days to encourage the distal tipping of the first permanent molar. Subtle changes in the repositioning of the teeth should be noted since in cases of marked root destruction of the second primary molar or major unlocking of the first permanent molar tightening of the brass ligature wire results in mesiocclusal tipping of the second primary molar or mesial tipping of both primary molars instead of the desired distal tipping of the first permanent molar. During the period of adjustment the brass ligature wire may become markedly loosened and may need retightening, insertion of a .028-inch brass ligature wire, or possibly doubling of the .026-inch brass ligature wire before reinserting it between the primary molar and the permanent molar.

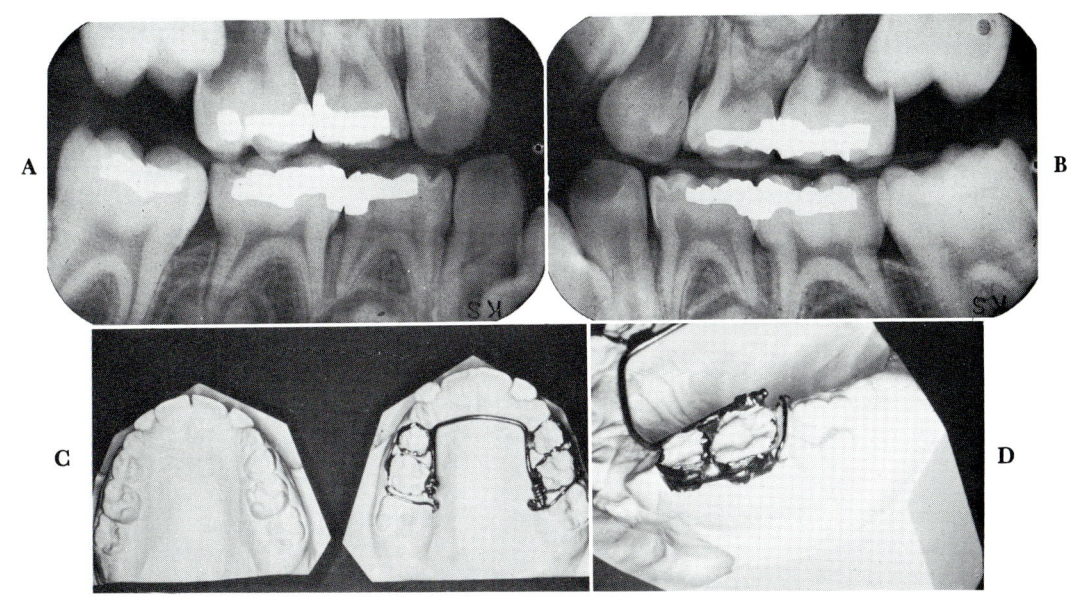

Fig. 8-12. **A** and **B**, Right and left posterior bite-wing radiographs demonstrating ectopic eruption of the maxillary first permanent molars with severe destruction of the distal portion of the second primary molars. **C**, The upper study model on the left shows the pretreatment relationship of the ectopically erupting maxillary first permanent molars. The upper study model on the right is the posttreatment model demonstrating the maxillary lingual arch appliance with activating wires used to deflect the first permanent molars distally from their position of ectopic eruption. **D**, Buccal view of the upper posttreatment model demonstrating the pointed activating wire as it is positioned in the embrasure to deflect the maxillary right first permanent molar from the position of ectopic eruption.

Occasionally the markedly mesially inclined first permanent molar will have destroyed an extensive amount of tooth structure for the second primary molar; the construction of a fixed appliance with an activating wire that transverses the erupting first permanent molar will be indicated (Fig. 8-12).

The ectopically erupting first permanent molar may be successfully tipped distally by placing a soldered lingual arch appliance with an activated spring wire. This appliance may be particularly indicated if the permanent molar is severely locked beneath the primary tooth. The principle of the lingual arch appliance with the activating wire is to secure maximum anchorage of the appliance, so that when the force is applied to the mesial of the first permanent molar, the reciprocal force is dispersed to combinations of other teeth in the arch. The purpose is to minimize mesial tipping of the affected second primary molar and possibly mesial tipping of the first primary molar on the side of the ectopic eruption. In fact, the first permanent molar is tipped distally to secure an adequate path of eruption and is not unlocked at the expense of tipping the second primary molar mesially and occlusally.

Bands are formed around the first and second primary molars with .003 by .015 stainless steel band material. If the affected second primary molar is markedly mobile a band is formed for the primary cuspid on the side of the ectopic eruption. Preformed seamless stainless steel bands may be used, if stock sizes closely approximate the circumference of the primary molars. An upper alginate impression is taken, and the bands are removed from the teeth. The impression is thoroughly dried in the areas of primary molars, the bands are secured in the impression with sticky wax, and a stone working model is poured.

A lingual arch is formed from .036-inch stainless steel wire or .040-inch gold wire and soldered to the four bands. To add rigidity the bands on each side are connected to one another by soldering a .025-inch stainless steel wire to the buccal of each band. A .025-inch stainless steel wire is wound around the lingual arch in the region of the ectopic eruption, and a lingual loop with helix is formed on the activating wire. The terminal portion of the wire is bent toward the buccal to transverse and conform closely to the occlusal surface of the ectopic permanent molar, with engagement of the pointed terminal end in the embrasure of the first permanent molar. The terminal end rests against the mesial-buccal surface of the first permanent molar. The activating wire is soldered to the lingual arch in the region of the wrapping.

Bilateral ectopic eruption of the first permanent molars may occur, and the fixed appliance with activating arms can provide effective mechanics for tipping the permanent molars distally.

Because of the severe amount of tooth loss for the second primary molar during ectopic eruption, the tooth may be lost prematurely. After successfully tipping the first permanent molar distally, the resorption pattern for the second primary molar must be kept under frequent surveillance to permit interception with a space management appliance if the second primary molar begins to loosen during the exfoliation process. If the second primary molar is inadvertently lost between recall examination visits, the arch circumference will be diminished; efforts to prevent an arch length inadequacy because of ectopic eruption will be unsuccessful.

An alternative method for guiding the ectopic first permanent molar to proper position is the placement of a fixed guide plane (Fig. 8-18). In cases where the second primary molar will require extraction or immediate exfoliation is expected, a chrome steel crown is placed on the first primary molar and a gold band with loop and intragingival extension is constructed to provide a mesial guide plane for the first permanent molar. The intragingival extension will be formed to the distal loop with an acute angle to provide the proper guide plane for distally deflecting the mesially tipped ectopic molar. As with any space management appliance, the intragingival extension will require periodic surveillance to evaluate the proper guidance of the first permanent molar during its path of eruption. Consideration for both removing the intragingival extension and adding additional dimension onto the superior aspect of the intragingival extension will be required in subsequent evaluations.

**Local factors affecting delayed eruption**

Occasionally the primary dentition will demonstrate a marked deviation from the usual sequence and age range of eruption. A review of the medical history and intraoral radiographs is appropriate to establish a correlation with the varied eruption pattern. Obscure reasons frequently mask the peculiar sequence of erupting primary teeth.

Supernumerary teeth may prevent the eruption of teeth or influence ectopic eruption of adjacent permanent teeth. A follicular cyst may occasionally develop in association with an unerupted supernumerary tooth. Supernumerary primary teeth occur less frequently than supernumerary permanent teeth. Studies[37-39] have indicated that supernumerary permanent teeth occur in approximately 2 to 3 percent of school-age children. The most common location for supernumerary permanent teeth is the maxillary incisor region (Fig. 8-13). Diagnosing the presence of the extra teeth and outlining a treatment plan may prevent the malalignment of the maxillary anterior teeth.

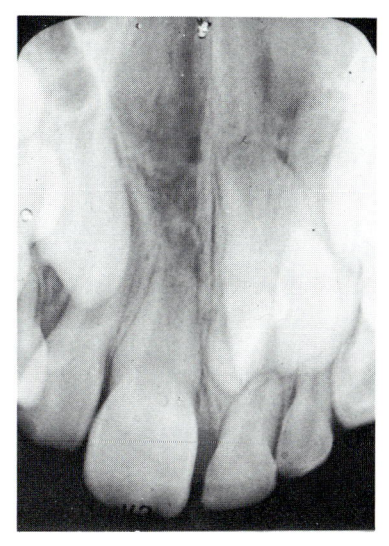

Fig. 8-13. Radiograph of the maxillary permanent incisor region showing the prolonged retention of the maxillary left primary central and lateral incisors and the delayed eruption of their successors by the interference of a supernumerary tooth located to the left of the midline.

**196** *Improving dental practice through preventive measures*

Removal of the unerupted supernumerary tooth is the ultimate treatment. Immediate surgical intervention may be indicated if the oral surgeon believes that the supernumerary tooth can be removed without damage to the adjacent normal teeth. The surgeon may elect to postpone removal of the extra tooth until the adjacent teeth have additional root development and their possible injury during surgery is lessened. During the surgical procedure the soft tissue and bone should be removed from the incisal third of the teeth that are delayed in their eruption. Even after the permanent teeth that have been delayed by a supernumerary tooth have been uncovered and adequate space has been secured in the arch, many months may elapse before the permanent teeth erupt into proper position.

Additional local factors may delay the eruption of permanent teeth. Developmental anomalies such as an odontoma overlying an erupting permanent tooth should be diagnosed and removed early to prevent continued retarded eruption of the permanent tooth (Fig. 8-14). All odontomas should be submitted to an oral pathologist for microscopic examination to confirm the diagnosis. As indicated previously, ankylosis of the primary molar may cause delayed eruption of the succeeding permanent tooth.

Prolonged retention of primary teeth may result in the deflection of the erupting permanent teeth (Fig. 8-15).

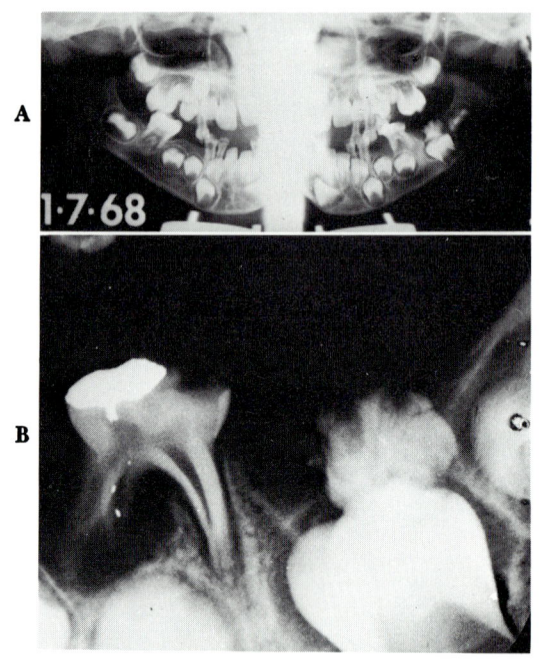

Fig. 8-14. **A,** A panoramic radiograph provides a survey of the unerupted tooth mass and convenient comparison of the right and left dental structures. The mandibular left first permanent molar is delayed in eruption by an overlying odontoma. **B,** A periapical intraoral radiograph provides an additional diagnostic view in cases of suspected pathology or anomalies observed in the panoramic radiograph. Earlier diagnosis and treatment of the odontoma overlying the unerupted mandibular first permanent molar may have prevented the delayed eruption of this tooth.

Trauma to an anterior primary tooth may produce pulpal necrosis and delayed resorption of the primary root. The permanent successor can be deflected to the lingual in a position of crossbite; appliance therapy is indicated to reposition the tooth (Fig. 8-16). Preventive care includes close surveillance of the traumatized primary tooth to ensure normal root resorption.

Posterior bite-wing radiographs taken periodically to diagnose interproximal decay also may give clues as to the possible deflection of permanent teeth. If the bite-wing radiograph indicates a malposed inclination of the unerupted permanent tooth crown a periapical radiograph can confirm the diagnosis of delayed resorption for the primary tooth and deflection of the permanent successor. If resorption is

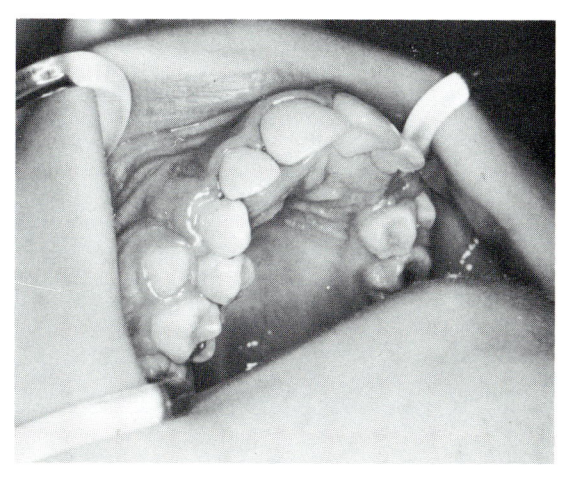

Fig. 8-15. The maxillary right and left first primary molars are over-retained, resulting in the buccal deflection of the maxillary first bicuspids.

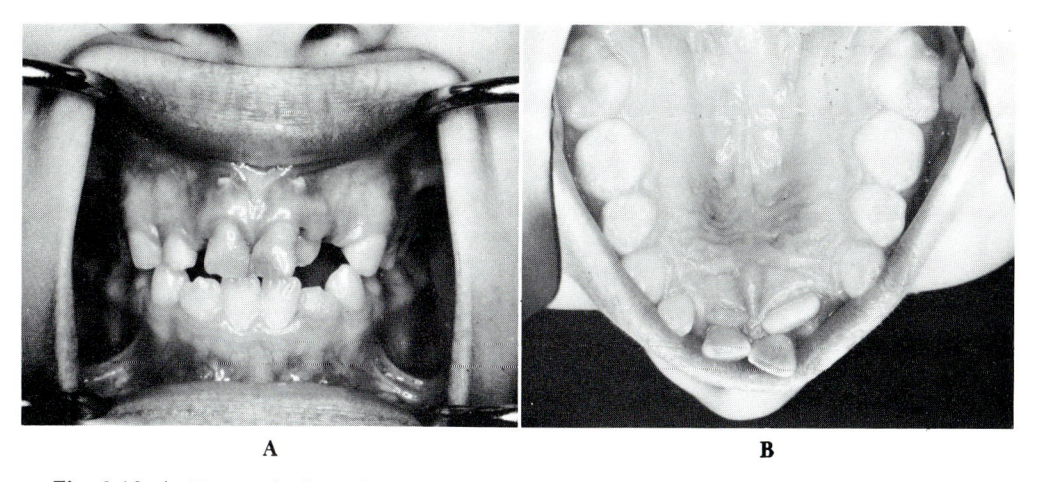

A  B

Fig. 8-16. A, Traumatized maxillary primary central incisors usually show some degree of discoloration; frequently the roots of these nonvital teeth do not resorb normally. B, The prolonged retained primary incisors may cause the erupting permanent incisors to be deflected lingually into an abnormal alignment.

tardy with a normal primary tooth, extraction may be indicated and an immediate space maintainer placed in primary molar or cuspid regions for the unerupted permanent tooth.

**Premature loss of primary molars and cuspids**

Proper management of the developing occlusion after the premature loss of the primary molars and cuspids during the period of either the primary or mixed dentition is an important aspect of preventive care.[40] Partial loss of the primary molars and cuspids during the period of the primary or mixed dentition provides an environment for a decrease in the length of the arch (Fig. 8-17). In a study of school children Jarvis[41] compared mixed dentitions that demonstrated proximal contacts in primary molars destroyed by dental caries with dentitions that maintained their proximal contacts. Statistically the mixed dentitions with deficient interproximal contacts as a result of caries had a significant potential for a decrease in arch length.

Rosenzweig[42] studied the effect of premature loss of primary molars on the resulting space. Spaces between the embrasures of the adjacent teeth were measured in sixty-one instances. Using analogous points of reference, a lineal measurement was completed on the opposite side of the arch for the remaining paired tooth. A comparison of the lineal space between the side of the extraction and the non-

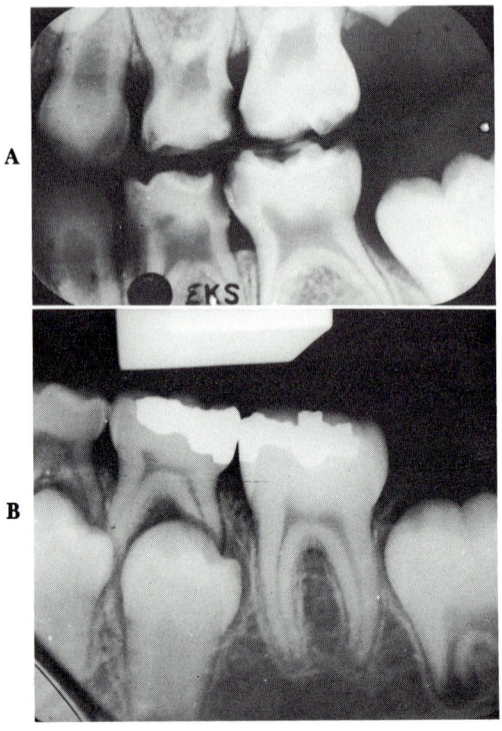

Fig. 8-17. **A,** Posterior bite-wing radiograph demonstrating the encroachment of maxillary and mandibular primary molars into areas of tooth loss resulting from unrestored proximal carious lesions. **B,** Radiograph demonstrating restored areas of interproximal decay in primary molars. Diagnosing proximal carious lesions early and placing properly contoured restorations will prevent the loss of arch length.

extracted side revealed that fifty-three of the sixty-one instances resulted in loss of space ranging between 0.5 mm. and 8.0 mm.

The ignored premature loss of the second primary molar may result in the mesial tipping of the permanent molar with a decrease in arch circumference, which is not altered by the erupting bicuspid. Whenever permanent teeth begin to enter the oral cavity they can be influenced by the tongue and facial muscles to migrate into spaces resulting from caries or extraction. Eruption of the first permanent molar during the absence of the second primary molar provides a vulnerable environment for mesial tipping of the permanent molar. Clinical observations indicate that the mesial inclination of the first permanent molar may occur before and during its emergence whenever the primary molars are lost prematurely. During this period consideration should be given to immediate replacement of mesial support for the erupting molar. A solid V shaped intragingival extension supported by the first primary molar has been advocated by Roche[40] (Fig. 8-18). If the first primary molar is to be lost in addition to the second primary molar, Starkey[43] has recommended a removable acrylic appliance with an intragingival acrylic guide plane for the unerupted or partially emerged first permanent molar (Fig. 8-19). These fixed and removable appliances are methods to direct the first permanent molar into a plane of eruption similar to the guidance provided by the distal surface of the second primary molar.

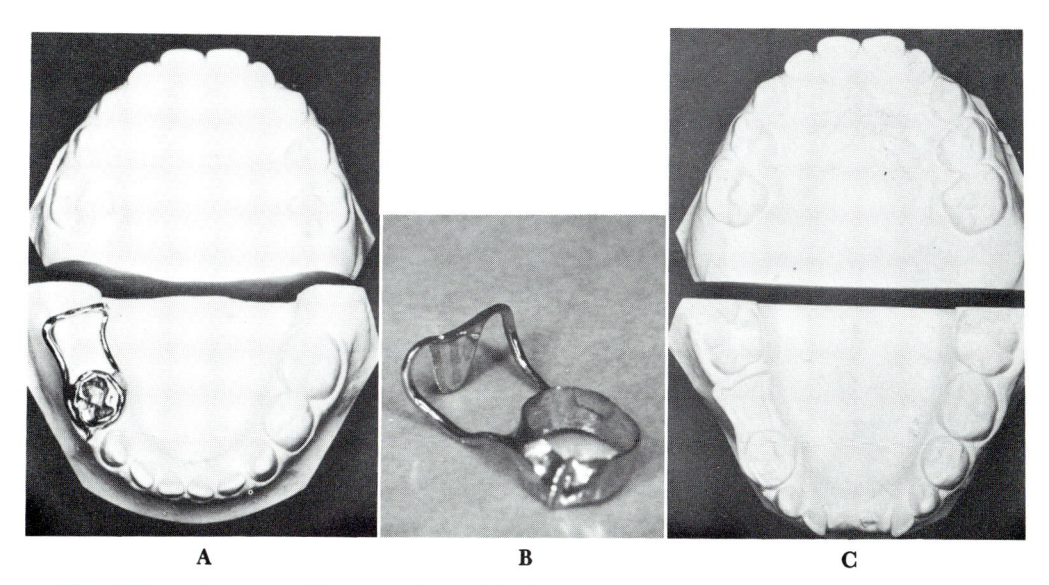

Fig. 8-18. A, Upper and lower study models demonstrating the type of fixed space management appliance used to guide the unerupted mandibular right first permanent molar into occlusion following the premature loss of the mandibular right second primary molar. B, Gold band and distal loop with intragingival extension, which is cemented onto the chrome steel crown of the mandibular right first primary molar. Prior to cementation the soft tissues are anesthetized and the sterilized appliance is poised on the chrome steel crown and crest of the alveolar ridge. The child forces the band and knife-edged solid V shaped intragingival extension into the gingival tissue overlying the alveolar ridge by firmly biting on two tongue blades. A bite-wing radiograph is taken to evaluate the correct position of the intragingival extension in its relation as a mesial guide plane for the unerupted first permanent molar. C, Post-treatment study models demonstrating the successful guidance of the unerupted mandibular right first permanent molar with the use of a fixed intragingival extension.

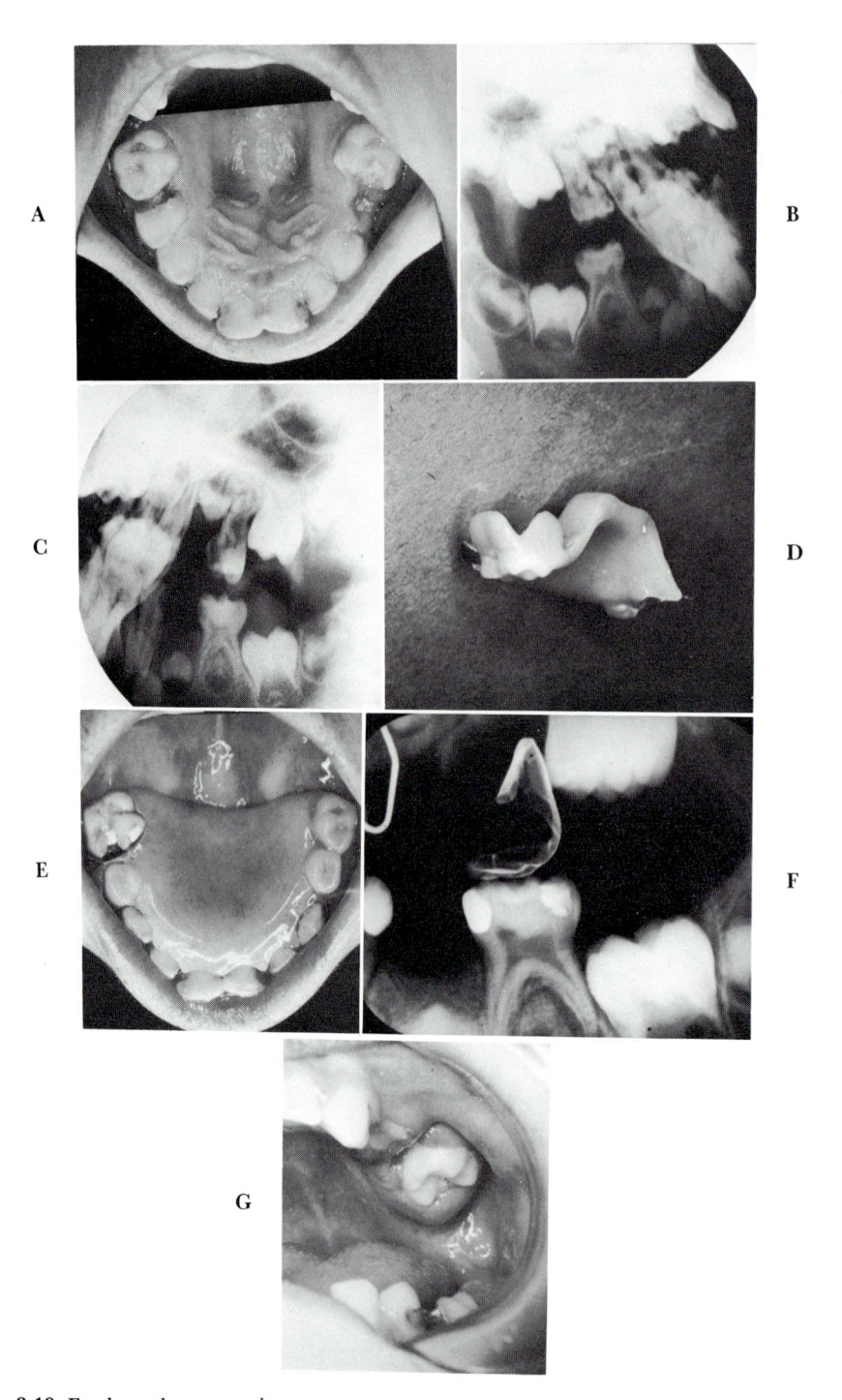

200  *Improving dental practice through preventive measures*

**Fig. 8-19.** For legend see opposite page.

If the first primary molar is lost while the first permanent molar is in the process of emergence the second primary molar tends to tip mesially. Subsequently during the eruption of the first permanent molar into occlusion the axial inclination, accompanied by forces of the buccinator and closing musculature of the mandible, results in mesial tipping. This condition can be prevented by placing a chrome steel crown on the second primary molar with a soldered mesial loop contacting the distal convexity of the primary cuspid. The chrome crown provides a durable, retentive, and anticariogenic abutment for the wire loop arch maintainer.

Preventive care in arch length management can be enhanced by comparing the eruptive positions of the second bicuspid and second permanent molar. Speidel[44] presented sample instances and proposed that, if the second permanent molar is erupting while the first permanent molar does not have mesial contact support, the first molar will tend to tip mesially. If the second permanent molar is markedly advanced to the eruptive level of the second bicuspid, a holding appliance such as a lingual arch may be indicated to preserve the arch length (Fig. 8-20).

After the early loss during the mixed dentition of either the first or second primary molar or both, surveillance of the length of the arch should usually be combined with the placement of preventive appliances. If radiographs indicate that the succeeding permanent tooth has not gained access through osseous tissue, a lingual arch or a removable acrylic appliance may be placed to maintain the length of the arch. The recommendation for these appliances is based on an attempt to maintain the same lineal dimension that would have been provided by the primary molar had it remained in the mouth in good condition. Obviously the proper management of the space and the importance of the appliances cannot be determined adequately without periodic evaluation.

The effects of the early loss of the maxillary primary cuspids have not been clearly substantiated. However, permanent incisors, especially in a crowded arch, may tip toward the area of the premature cuspid loss and may influence the permanent cuspid to erupt in a labially deflected alignment.

Early loss of the primary mandibular cuspid frequently occurs from atypical resorption of its root, which has been precipitated by the force of the adjacent erupting permanent lateral incisor. When the primary cuspid is lost for this reason,

---

Fig. 8-19. **A,** Occlusal view of the maxillary primary dentition demonstrating several extensive carious lesions. Right (**B**) and left (**C**) lateral jaw radiographs included in the preschool survey. Extraction was planned for the maxillary left second primary molar since pulpal necrosis was present as a result of the carious process. **D,** Since the maxillary left first primary molar was prematurely missing, an upper removable acrylic space management appliance was constructed with an acrylic intragingival guide plane to support the unerupted maxillary first permanent molar during eruption. **E,** The upper acrylic appliance in place immediately following the necessary extractions. Note the sedative dressing previously placed in the maxillary right second primary molar as an indirect pulp treatment. Usually, as in this situation, the extensive lesions require redressing during the convalescent period. **F,** Left posterior bitewing radiograph showing the image of the lead foil taken from a radiographic film packet temporarily placed around the acrylic intragingival extension at the time of delivery to evaluate the correct positioning of the guide plane. **G,** Intermediate result of the acrylic guide plane providing proper mesial support to the erupting first permanent molar and preventing mesial tipping as a result of the premature loss of the primary molars. (Courtesy Dr. Paul E. Starkey.)

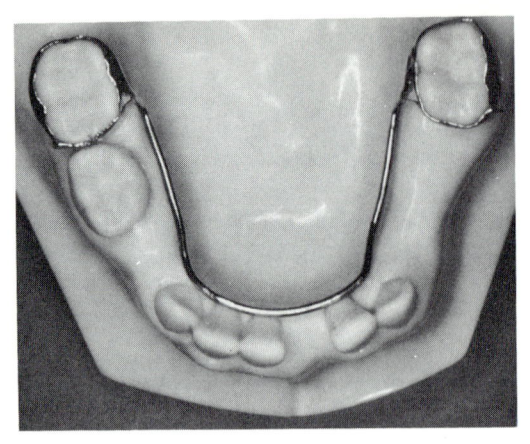

**Fig. 8-20.** For premature loss a holding appliance placed to preserve the arch length is represented by the lower lingual arch on a technic model showing the contact of the anterior portion of the arch wire resting on the cingulum area of the lower permanent incisors. The heavy arch wire is contoured approximately 2 mm. inferior to the crest of the adjacent alveolar ridge to diminish distortion of the wire during mastication. The arch wire is contoured approximately 1 mm. lingually to the adjacent ridge in the regions of premature loss to prevent the unerupted bicuspids from being deflected buccally during eruption.

the loss has often been interpreted as a signal of a forthcoming deficiency in the length of the arch. A basic inadequacy in the length of the arch can be described as a congenital discrepancy between the size of the group of permanent teeth and the size of the jaw and its enveloping structures. This probable deficiency in the circumference of the arch can receive further deficit from a break in the continuity of the arch. Therefore absence of the primary cuspid can easily contribute to an additional decrease in circumference of the arch by permitting lingual tipping of the permanent incisors from the force of the orbicularis oris and its associated muscles. Accordingly, efforts should be made to prevent the mandibular permanent incisors from tipping lingually by cementing a lower lingual arch appliance.

When the early loss of a primary cuspid has occurred as a result of insufficient length of the arch, removal of the opposite primary cuspid may be considered to permit the permanent incisors to tip toward a symmetrical alignment. The stability of the resultant symmetry of the incisors may be changed if one of the erupting permanent cuspids exerts lateral pressure many months before the opposite cuspid has begun to erupt. Wire stops placed on the lingual arch or removable acrylic appliance may aid in preventing this asymmetrical shifting of the permanent incisors.

The presence of supernumerary permanent incisiors can initiate the early loss of the primary cuspid and can result in a problem of arch length. Preventive management calls for removing the supernumerary incisor and regaining and maintaining symmetry of the permanent incisors.

When the primary cuspid in an uncrowded arch is prematurely lost because of trauma or caries, mesial tipping of the primary and permanent molars is unlikely. An awareness of the possibility of distal and lingual tipping of the permanent incisors may be valuable in planning management of the space. Loss of the primary cuspid before the adjacent permanent lateral incisor has erupted presents a particular concern, since it may encourage distal deflection of the lateral during eruption.

The immediate placement of a removable acrylic appliance or a lower lingual arch using wire stops can prevent the undesirable tipping of the incisors.

A bizarre early loss of the mandibular primary cuspid and first primary molar may occur from the erratic eruption of the mandibular permanent lateral incisor. The severe distal and lingual axial inclination of the erupting incisor may force premature loss of the primary cuspid and first primary molar. The crown of the permanent lateral may approach the area of contact with the primary second molar. Malposition of the lateral's crypt may be the cause of the eccentric eruptive pattern. The distolingual position of the crown of the permanent mandibular lateral incisor, as related to the unerupted permanent mandibular cuspid, is extremely hazardous to the alignment of the developing permanent dentition; a diagnosis of this condition warrants immediate orthodontic consultation.

Early loss of the primary molars because of caries may indicate a different management from that for loss by trauma. Loss induced by decay may have been preceded by encroachment of the adjacent teeth into the areas of contact and a resultant decrease in length of the arch. If the mesiodistal widths of the unerupted teeth are predicted to be greater than the lineal space available between the first permanent molar and permanent lateral, an appliance for regaining space should be considered.

The problem of early loss of primary molars or cuspids can be complicated further when teeth appear to be absent in a mouth that already exhibits a trend to malocclusion. When there is a deficiency in length of arch or mesiodistal disharmony of the arches during the early period of the mixed dentition premature losses are an indication for earlier than usual orthodontic consultation. Placing static appliances for guidance of teeth in malaligned arches may be difficult to justify if the child is to receive comprehensive orthodontic treatment in the periods of late mixed or early permanent dentition. Determining whether the child will ultimately receive corrective therapy insofar as parental attitudes are concerned may be as unreliable as predicting whether the arch will be inadequate. Efforts to prevent mesial tipping of the first permanent molar or lingual shifting of the permanent incisors in the arches that demonstrate dental-skeletal disharmonies may result in a less seriously crowded dentition than otherwise would develop. If orthodontic treatment is subsequently performed, these static appliances may serve to maintain the axial inclinations that the lost primary tooth would have provided.

**Anterior crossbite**

Anterior crossbite may indicate a developing skeletal Class III malocclusion or frequently may be the result of local factors such as the presence of a supernumerary tooth, over-retained primary incisors, or arch length deficiency. The deflection of one or more permanent maxillary incisors can be prevented by early diagnosis, if the skeletal growth pattern is not the cause of the crossbite. Unfortunately the child may not be examined by the dentist until after the maxillary permanent incisors have been tipped lingually and are occluding in a crossbite relationship with the mandibular incisors (Fig. 8-21). Several serious disturbances such as marked abrasion of the labial-incisal surface of the inlocked incisor, loss of arch length as the adjacent permanent teeth tip into the area, and marked gingival inflammation and recession on the labial area of the opposing mandibular incisor can be prevented by promptly correcting the crossbite.

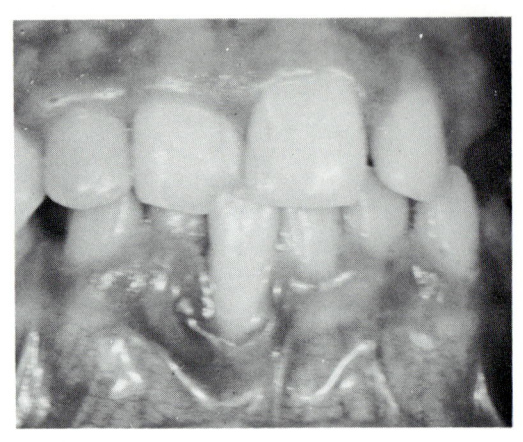

**Fig. 8-21.** Anterior crossbite of a maxillary permanent incisor can contribute to severe recession and inflammation of gingival tissue on the labial area of the mandibular incisors.

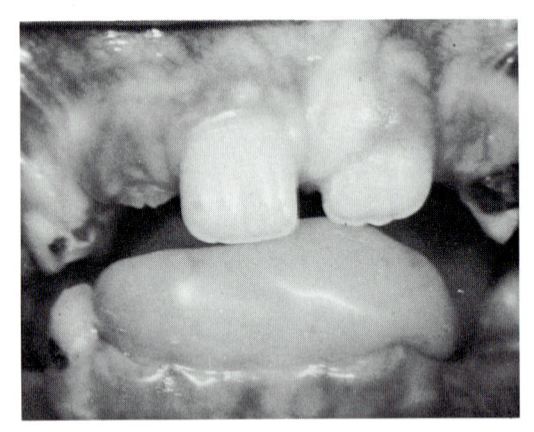

**Fig. 8-22.** An acrylic bite plane is cemented onto the lower anterior teeth to provide an inclined plane for the correction of an upper permanent incisor positioned in crossbite.

Properly ground study models, complete mouth radiographs, and possibly lateral cephalometric films should be used in the differential diagnosis. If the analysis indicates that the crossbite is the result of local factors, sufficient mesiodistal space should be present so that the inlocked tooth can be moved labially.

An acrylic bite plane cemented onto the lower anterior teeth is an effective appliance to position the inlocked central incisors labially (Fig. 8-22). A lower alginate impression is taken, a stone model is formed, and self-curing resin is applied to the model. The lower incisors and possibly the cuspids are covered with resin. An inclined plane is constructed at a 45-degree angle to the axial inclination of the lower incisors. The inclined plane contacts only the inlocked incisor, and the acrylic is adjusted in the mouth to permit the posterior teeth to have an open occlusion of approximately 3 mm. After the bite plane has been cemented the child should return within 1 or 2 days so that the inclination of the plane can be adjusted to continue the single contact with the inlocked tooth. In 7 to 14 days the inlocked

Preventive pedodontics 205

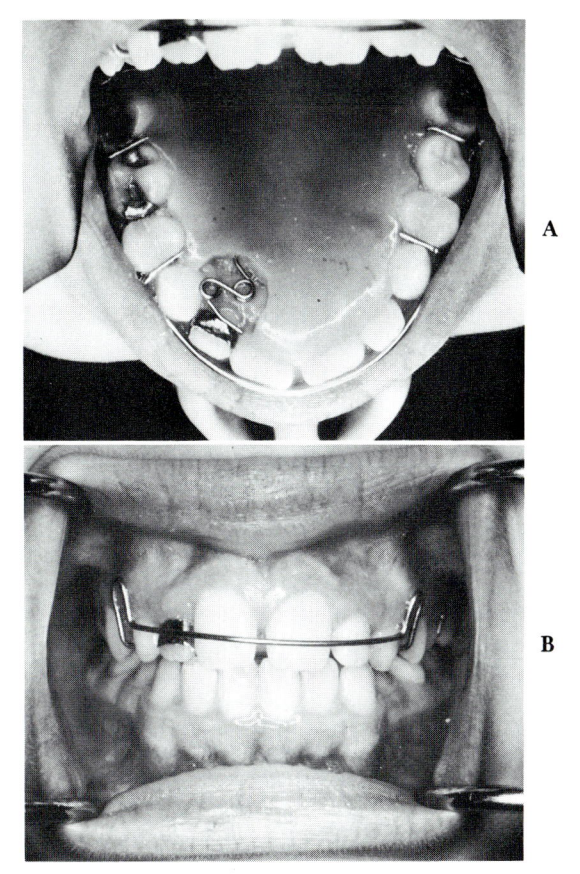

Fig. 8-23. **A**, An upper removable appliance can be placed to correct a maxillary permanent incisor positioned in crossbite. The occlusal view demonstrates the appliance in place after the maxillary right permanent lateral incisor had been tipped labially from a crossbite position. An activating .022-inch wire was held in position by a wire lug attached to the band. **B**, Labial view of the corrected maxillary right permanent lateral incisor showing the position of the labial arch wire used for retention of the appliance.

tooth should be in proper labial version and the bite plane should be removed, since the posterior teeth will have shown continued eruption with a tendency toward an anterior open bite. If there is insufficient overbite to retain the corrected incisor an immediate fixed or removable retainer will need to be placed for a posttreatment period.

A removable acrylic palatal appliance with a retentive anterior labial arch wire, posterior clasps, and S shaped .022-inch stainless steel activating wire may be used to correct an inlocked maxillary permanent incisor, particularly a lateral or a central when there is insufficient overbite for retention (Fig. 8-23).

The maxillary soldered lingual arch is an alternative appliance for correcting the maxillary inlocked incisor. Johnson loop gold bands or stainless steel seamless bands are fitted onto the maxillary permanent molars. An alginate impression is taken, a stone model is constructed, and a passive lingual arch wire is formed from .036-inch stainless steel wire or .040-inch gold wire. The arch wire is soldered to the molar bands and a .022-inch stainless steel activating wire is soldered to the anterior portion of the lingual arch. The activating wire is adjusted by applying a lingual force against the inlocked incisor. The cemented lingual arch appliance should be removed every two or three weeks and the activating wire adjusted.

**RECALL EVALUATION**

Recall of the child patient can be the key to preventive dental care. If the receptionist schedules the appropriate recall visit at the time when the child's current treatment plan is completed, the dentist can adequately fulfill his obligation to the parent and further ensure the appropriate supervision of the child's oral health. Children whose oral tissues have been free of disease for repeated recall periods may be placed in recall categories of longer than 6 months, but the dentist should bear in mind the various conditions mentioned in this chapter which could adversely affect the developing occlusion and could possibly be prevented by diagnosis at the proper time.

**REFERENCES**

1. The American Academy of Pedodontics: Guidelines for advanced education in pedodontics: definition of pedodontics, Chicago, 1969, The Academy.
2. Schaefer, A. E.: The National Nutrition Survey, Presentation at the 51st Annual Meeting of The American Dietetic Association, San Francisco, October 17, 1968.
3. Rayner, J.: Dental hygiene and socioeconomic status, I.A.D.R. Abstract 576, 1969.
4. Moore, R. M.: A study of the effect of water fluoride content and socioeconomic status on the occurrence of gingivitis in school children, Indiana University School of Dentistry, 1963 (master's thesis).
5. Hennon, D. K., Stookey, G. K., and Muhler, J. C.: Prevalence and distribution of dental caries in pre-school children, J.A.D.A. **79:**1405-1414, 1969.
6. Murray, J.: Caries experience of five-year-old children from fluoride and non-fluoride communities, Brit. D. J. **126:**352-354, 1969.
7. Herman, S. C.: Surveys from the American Academy of Pedodontics for their members and the Association of Pedodontic Diplomates, Survey of Pedodontic Practices, 1968 (mimeographed).
8. Shafer, W. G., Hine, M. K., and Levy, B. M.: Tumors and cysts of odontogenic origin. In Shafer, W. G., editor: A textbook of oral pathology, ed. 2, Philadelphia, 1963, W. B. Saunders Co.
9. Tasanen, A.: General and local effects of the eruption of deciduous teeth, Helsinki, 1969, Annales Paediatriae Fenniae.
10. Ravn, J. J.: Sequelae of acute mechanical traumata in the primary dentition, J. Dent. Child. **35:**281-289, 1968.
11. Fass, E. N.: Is bottle feeding of milk a factor in dental caries? J. Dent. Child. **29:**245-251, 1962.
12. Robinson, S., and Naylor, S. R.: The effects of late weaning on the deciduous incisor teeth, Brit. D. J. **115:**250-252, 1963.
13. Kroll, R. G., and Stone, J. H.: Nocturnal bottle-feeding as a contributory cause of rampant dental caries in the infant and young child, J. Dent. Child. **34:**454-459, 1967.
14. Finn, S. B.: Dental caries in infants, Current Dent. **1:**35-38, 1969.
15. Michal, B. C.: "Bottle-mouth" caries, J. La. Dent. Assn. **27:**10-13, 1969.
16. Kelley, G. E., Stookey, G. K., and Muhler, J. C.: Laboratory study concerning the development of a stannous fluoride-phosphate prophylactic paste, J. Dent. Child. **36:**31-38, 1969.
17. Arnim, S. S.: How the dentist can help people learn to prevent and control dental disease, North-West Den. **45:**3-15, 1966.
18. Kimmelman, B., and Tassman, G. C.: Research in designs of children's toothbrushes, J. Dent. Child. **27:**60-64, 1960.

19. Starkey, P. E.: Toothbrushing and oral hygiene instruction. In McDonald, R. E., editor: Dentistry for the child and adolescent, St. Louis, 1969, The C. V. Mosby Co.
20. McClure, D. B.: A comparison of toothbrushing techniques for the preschool child, J. Dent. Child. 33:205-210, 1966.
21. Conroy, C. W., and Melfi, R. C.: Comparison of automatic and hand toothbrushes: cleaning effectiveness for children, J. Dent. Child. 33:219-225, 1966.
22. Huff, G. C., and Taylor, P. P.: Clinical evaluation of toothbrushes used in pedodontics, Texas Dent. J. 83:6-11, 1965.
23. Hall, A. W.: Toothbrushing for pre-school children: comparison of automatic and hand toothbrushing by the child and when parent assisted, Ohio State University College of Dentistry, 1966 (master's thesis).
24. Ritsert, E. F., and Binns, W. H., Jr.: Adolescents brush better with an electric toothbrush, J. Dent. Child. 34:354-358, 1967.
25. Womack, W. R., and Guay, A. H.: Comparative cleansing efficiency of an electric and a manual toothbrush in orthodontic patients, Angle Orthodont. 38:256-267, 1968.
26. Holloway, P. J., Booth, E. M., and Wragg, K. A.: Dietary counselling in the control of dental caries, Brit. D. J. 126:161-165, 1969.
27. Richmond, N. L.: Patient education through the use of caries activity tests and diet analysis, J. Ind. Dent. Assn. 48:314-316, 1969.
28. Rust, B. K.: Special problems of nutrition for children, J. Ind. Dent. Assn. 42:7-11, 1963.
29. Matlock, J. F.: Radiographic techniques for children. In McDonald, R. E., editor: Dentistry for the child and adolescent, St. Louis, 1969, The C. V. Mosby Co.
30. Brown, W. E.: The utilization of radiology in a children's practice, New Jersey Dent. Soc. J. 23:17-27, 1962.
31. MacRae, P. D., and others: Detection of congenital dental anomalies—how many films? J. Dent. Child. 35:107-114, 1968.
32. Lamb, K. A., and Reed, M. W.: Measurement of space loss resulting from tooth ankylosis, J. Dent. Child. 35:483-486, 1968.
33. Pulver, F.: The etiology and prevalence of ectopic eruption of the maxillary first permanent molar, J. Dent. Child. 35:138-146, 1968.
34. Cheyne, V. D., and Wessels, K. E.: Impaction of permanent first molar with resorption and space loss in region of deciduous second molar, J.A.D.A. 35:774-787, 1947.
35. Young, D. H.: Ectopic eruption of the first permanent molar, J. Dent. Child. 24: 153-162, 1957.
36. Carr, G. E.: Ectopic eruption of the first permanent maxillary molar in cleft lip and cleft palate children, J. Dent. Child. 32:179-188, 1965.
37. Luten, J. R., Jr.: The prevalence of supernumerary teeth in primary and mixed dentitions, J. Dent. Child. 34:346-353, 1967.
38. Castaldi, C. R., and others: Incidence of congenital dental anomalies in permanent teeth of a group of Canadian children aged 6-9, Canad. D. A. 32:154-159, 1966.
39. Osorio-Sanchez, O.: Supernumerary teeth in 900 German children, Dent. Abstr. 9:371, 1964.
40. Roche, J. R.: The management of the early loss of primary molars and cuspids during the period of the mixed dentition, J. Dent. Child. 30:170-179, 1963.
41. Jarvis, A.: The role of dental caries in space closure in the mixed dentition, Toronto, 1952, University of Toronto.
42. Rosenzweig, K. A., and Klein, H.: Loss of space of extraction of primary molars, J. Dent. Child. 27:275-276, 1960.
43. Starkey, P. E.: The management of space maintenance problems. In McDonald, R. E., editor: Dentistry for the child and adolescent, St. Louis, 1969, The C. V. Mosby Co.
44. Speidel, T. D.: Diagnostic implications of the sequence of eruption, Amer. Dent. A. J. 38:5-15, 1949.

# Chapter 9 Preventive periodontics
## Irving Glickman

Etiology of gingivitis and periodontal disease
    Dental plaque
    Acquired pellicle
    Calculus
    Materia alba
How to prevent gingival and periodontal disease
Plaque control—a definitive program for periodontal health
    Patient education and motivation
    Plaque control with the toothbrush
    The kind of toothbrush and bristles
    Toothbrushing methods
    Manual or electrically powered toothbrushes?
    Interdental cleansing
        Dental floss
        Rubber and wooden interdental cleansers
        Water irrigation under pressure
    Chemical plaque and calculus inhibitors
    Plaque control by hard fibrous foods
    Plaque control by limiting sucrose-containing foods
Other preventive measures against gingival and periodontal disease
        prevention by systemic measures
    Systemic measures to counteract plaque and bacteria
Dental restorations in preventive periodontics
Orthodontics in preventive periodontics
Trauma from occlusion
Preservation of periodontal health
Conclusion

Preventive periodontics is a multifaceted cooperative program performed by the dentist and patient for the preservation of the natural dentition; it involves prevention of the onset, progression, and recurrence of gingivitis and periodontal disease.

## ETIOLOGY OF GINGIVITIS AND PERIODONTAL DISEASE

Gingivitis, periodontal disease, and tooth loss caused by them can usually be prevented because they are caused by local irritants that are accessible, correctable, and controllable. The local factors cause inflammation, which is the predominant if not the sole pathologic process in most gingival disease. Periodontal disease is an extension of gingivitis and is caused by the same local factors plus trauma from occlusion. Trauma from occlusion is a codestructive factor that shares the responsibility for periodontal breakdown in some cases.

Identifying local factors as the principal causes of periodontal disorders is not an oversimplification. Systemic influences affect the response of the periodontal tissues to local irritants, but in the cases in which systemic factors are suspected, it is difficult to establish what they are. There are no forms of gingivitis or periodontal disease, regardless of how severe or how remote their total etiology, in which the removal of local irritants and prevention of their recurrence do not (1) reduce the severity of the disease, (2) lessen the rapidity of the destructive process, and (3) prolong the usefulness of the natural dentition.

Neglect is to blame for most if not all gingival and periodontal disease—neglect of the healthy mouth that permits disease to occur, neglect of early disease that permits it to destroy the tooth-supporting tissues, and neglect of the treated mouth that permits disease to recur. Poor oral hygiene which permits plaque,[1, 2] calculus, and materia alba[3, 4] to accumulate overshadows all other local factors responsible for gingival disease. The status of the individual oral hygiene determines the prevalence and severity of gingivitis.[5-8]

### Dental plaque

Dental plaque is the most important cause of oral disease. It is the principal etiologic factor in gingivitis and dental caries. The products of the bacteria in the plaque penetrate the gingiva and start gingivitis, which if untreated leads to periodontitis and tooth loss. Acid build-up in dental plaque initiates caries.

Dental plaque is a soft accumulation of multiplying bacteria in a sticky intercellular matrix that adheres to the tooth surface, from which it can be detached only by mechanical cleansing. Plaque is transparent and colorless and ordinarily escapes detection unless it absorbs pigment from within the oral cavity or is stained by disclosing solutions or wafers. It occurs supragingivally, mostly on the gingival third of the teeth and subgingivally,[9] with a predilection for surface cracks, defects, and roughness. It accumulates in greater amounts on the facial and proximal surfaces than on the lingual.[10] The location and rate of formation vary in different individuals and in different teeth in the same mouth.

Dental plaque is not a food residue. Food debris left on the teeth after meals is liquified by enzymes and cleaned from the oral cavity in a relatively short time. The formation of plaque is not related to the consumption of food. Most plaque forms between meals and during the night. If anything, the mechanical action of chewing and the increased salivary flow during mastication are deterrents to plaque formation.

### Acquired pellicle

Dental plaque is different from the acquired pellicle (acquired cuticle),[11, 12] which is a thin, smooth, bacteria-free film that accumulates on the tooth surface. Plaque usually forms over pellicle, although it may also form directly on the tooth surface. Pellicle is adherent to the tooth, transparent, and colorless. When stained with disclosing agents it appears as a thin sheen over the entire tooth surface, in contrast with plaque, which is thicker and granular and concentrated in the gingival third of the crown (Figs. 9-1 and 9-2). Pellicle forms on a previously cleaned tooth surface within minutes,[13] whereas plaque usually develops in approximately 24 hours.[14]

### Calculus

Dental plaque is also important because it is the initial stage in the formation of calculus. Plaque begins to calcify from the second to the fourteenth day after it is

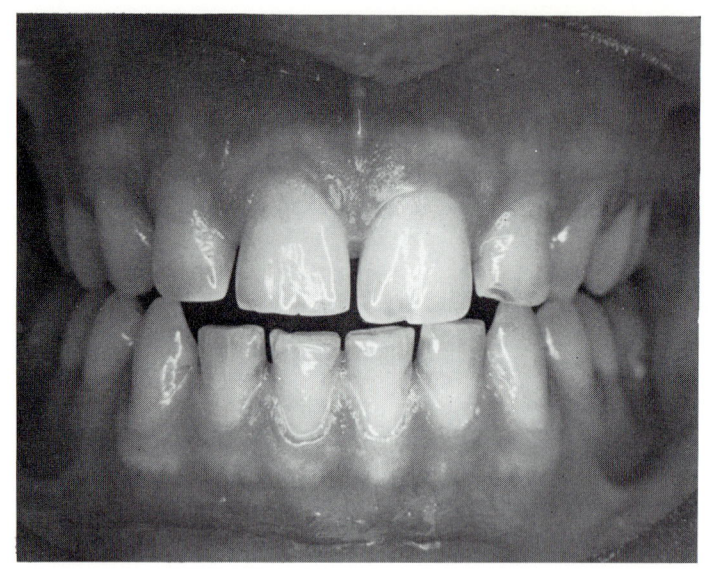

**Fig. 9-1.** Unstained teeth.

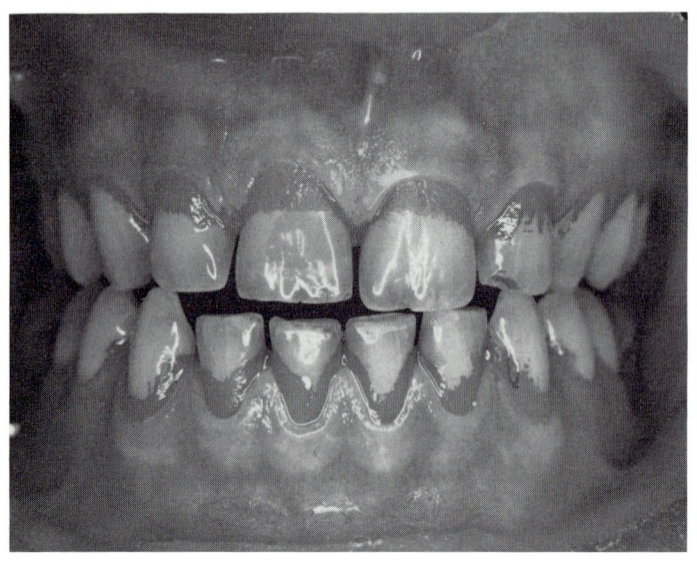

**Fig. 9-2.** Rinsing with 6 percent basic fuchsin reveals plaque and diffuse film not visible on unstained teeth.

formed.[15-17] All plaque does not develop into calculus, but calculus cannot form unless plaque is present, except under experimental conditions in germ-free animals. Calculus perpetuates gingival inflammation and leads to the deepening of periodontal pockets. However, it is the newly added surface layer of plaque, more than the inner calcified portion of the calculus, which is the responsible irritant.

The undesirability of calculus lies in the fact that it is hard, firmly adherent to the tooth, and difficult to remove. It provides a fixed nidus for the accumulation and retention of plaque close to the gingiva and subgingivally.

### Materia alba

Another common accumulant on the tooth surface, particularly near the gingival margin and interproximally, is materia alba. Materia alba is a yellowish or grayish white pablum-like mass that is somewhat less adherent than plaque. Long considered to be a conglomerant of stagnant food debris, it is now recognized to be a concentration of bacteria and cellular debris with little or no food particles.[122] Materia alba is irritating to the gingiva but less insidious than plaque in that it is visible and is more easily removed.

## HOW TO PREVENT GINGIVAL AND PERIODONTAL DISEASE

The best way to prevent gingival and periodontal disease is to prevent plaque formation. Despite intensive research on the subject, methods of completely preventing the formation of plaque have not as yet been discovered, but considerable progress has been made in the control of plaque. Plaque control means retarding or preventing the accumulation of dental plaque and other deposits on the tooth surface. Plaque control prevents gingivitis and the development of plaque into calculus. Plaque control and calculus control are interrelated. The most effective way of controlling dental plaque is by mechanical cleansing.

## PLAQUE CONTROL—A DEFINITIVE PROGRAM FOR PERIODONTAL HEALTH

Preventive periodontics consists of many interrelated procedures, but plaque control is the keystone of the prevention of gingival and periodontal disease. Every patient in every dental practice should be on a plaque control program. For the patient with a healthy periodontium plaque control means the preservation of health, for the patient with periodontal disease it means optimal posttreatment healing, and for the patient with treated periodontal disease plaque control means the prevention of recurrence of disease.

### Patient education and motivation

Plaque control is basic to the practice of dentistry; without it oral health can be neither attained nor preserved. It is a cooperative effort between the dentist and the patient. Instructing the patient in proper oral hygiene procedures is not enough. The patient must understand why he is being taught to clean his teeth properly. The dentist must make it clear that the goal is oral health and not simply the development of manipulative skills.

Most patients think that the toothbrush is only for cleansing the teeth[19]; its importance in the prevention of disease of the periodontium must be explained. Toothbrushing is a most important patient-administered preventive and adjunctive therapeutic procedure. In no other field of medicine can the patient so effectively assist in preventing and reducing the severity of a disease as can be done in relation to gingivitis by toothbrushing, supplemented according to individual needs by interdental cleansing with dental floss, rubber and wooden interdental cleansers, and water irrigation under pressure. If a person maintained good oral hygiene from 5 to 50 years of age, he very likely could avoid the destructive effects of periodontal disease during this major period of his life.[3]

Patients must be made to understand that periodic scaling and cleansing of the teeth in the dental office are helpful preventive measures but that they do not give the continuous protection against disease they themselves can provide by daily oral hygiene procedures at home. Explain that dental visits come two or three times a year, but continuous preventive dental care is available at home on a daily basis. Time spent in the dental office teaching the patient how to cleanse his teeth is a more valuable health service than cleansing his teeth for him. Ideally both services should be provided.

Chairside instruction is more than a cursory demonstration in the use of a toothbrush and oral hygiene aids. It is a painstaking, repetitive procedure that must be checked and rechecked until the dentist is sure the patient can provide the care they require. Underlying every instruction sssion must be the constant theme of oral health, the incentive that makes all the effort worthwhile.

The first step in removing dental plaque is locating it. Materia alba is clearly visible so that its removal should present no problem. Disclosing solutions or chewable wafers[20] are necessary to locate the plaque. The disclosing solution (6 percent tincture of basic fuchsin) is applied to the teeth with a pledget of cotton or diluted in water as a mouthwash. The wafers (erythrosin or other dyes) are chewed and swished around the mouth for about 1 minute. Disclosing solutions stain plaque and pellicle which previously could not be seen (Figs. 9-1 and 9-2). Dental restorations do not take up the stain, but the oral mucous membrane does.

Show the patient the stained plaque and calculus in a hand mirror. Let him try to remove it with his usual toothbrushing. Then demonstrate more effective toothbrushing; after this there will still be some stain interproximally. To remove this, show the patient how to use dental floss and interdental cleansers, followed by water irrigation. To check on the effectiveness of the total process, restain the teeth with disclosing solution (Fig. 9-3).

**Plaque control with the toothbrush**

The most effective way of controlling dental plaque is by mechanical cleansing with a toothbrush and adjunctive cleansing aids. A toothbrush does not cleanse effectively without the cleansing action of a dentifrice. Toothbrushing reduces plaque and materia alba[21-25] and calculus formation[26] and in so doing it reduces the onset and incidence of gingivitis.[27-30] Removal of plaque leads to resolution of gingival inflammation,[31] and cessation of toothbrushing leads to recurrence of gingivitis.[14, 32]

**The kind of toothbrush and bristles**

Toothbrushes vary in size, design, and bristle hardness, length, and arrangement. A toothbrush should clean efficiently and provide maximum accessibility to all areas of the mouth. The choice is a matter of individual preference rather than a demonstrated superiority of any one type. Ease of manipulation by the patient is an important factor in brush selection.

Natural (hog bristle) and nylon bristles are equally satisfactory. The question of the most desirable bristle hardness has not been settled. Bristle hardness is proportional to the square of the diameter and inversely proportional to the square of bristle length.[33] Bristle diameters in common use range from .007 inch (soft), to .012 inch (medium), to .014 inch (hard). Findings regarding the relative cleansing effect of hard and soft bristles are not conclusive. Medium bristles are preferred by many who suspect that hard bristles may traumatize the gingiva and abrade tooth substance and restorations, and soft bristles may not clean effectively. Some prefer

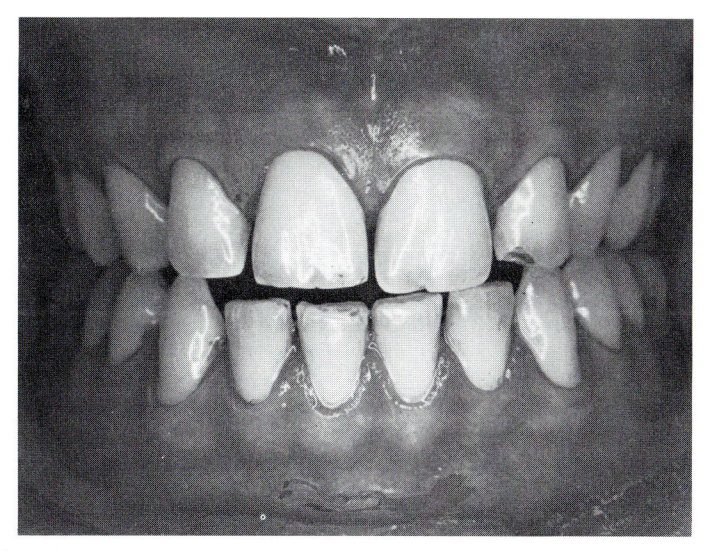

**Fig. 9-3.** After cleansing teeth, mouth rinsed again with 6 percent basic fuchsin indicates that plaque has been completely removed.

soft bristles because they can reach more of the tooth surface with greater ease and provide sulcular cleaning beneath the gingival margin.[34] A matting effect produced particularly by soft bristles embedded in dentifrice increases tooth surface–dentifrice contact and adds to the cleansing action but could also be a factor in toothbrush abrasion.[33]

The manner in which the brush is used and the abrasiveness of the dentifrice affect the cleansing action and abrasion produced by a toothbrush to an equal if not greater degree than the bristle hardness.

Pending definitive research the matter of relative effectiveness and potential harm of different types of toothbrushes and bristles is largely a matter of opinion.

## Toothbrushing methods

There are many methods of toothbrushing. With the exception of overtly traumatic techniques, thoroughness rather than technique is the important factor in determining the effectiveness of toothbrushing. Carefully performed, most toothbrushing methods in common use can accomplish the desired results. Instruction in proper use is necessary to obtain maximum effectiveness of manual or powered toothbrushes.[35] Regardless of the technique you teach, patients usually develop individualized modifications of it.

Patients should be reminded that toothbrushes are expendable and should be replaced periodically. Otherwise, they tend to use a brush as long as it lasts. This often means the bristles are disorganized and frayed, the brush does not cleanse effectively, and the bristles may be injuring the gingiva.

## Manual or electrically powered toothbrushes?

Some have found electrically powered toothbrushes superior to the manual brushes in terms of removing plaque, reducing plaque and calculus accumulation, and improving gingival health.* Others claim that manual and electric brushes

---
*See references 23, 24, 26, and 28.

are equally effective.[1, 36, 37] Electric brushes produce less abrasion of tooth substance and restorative materials than manual brushes[38, 39] but the situation is reversed if the manual brush is used in a vertical rather than a horizontal direction.[33]

There are many types of electric toothbrushes—those with arcuate motion, those with modified elliptical motion, and those with back and forth reciprocal action are examples. Regardless of the type of electric brush, the patient should be instructed in its use. As a rule, patients who can develop the ability to use a toothbrush properly do equally well with a manual or electric brush. Less diligent brushers do better with an electric brush, which compensates somewhat for their inadequacy. Electric brushes are more effective for handicapped individuals and for cleaning around orthodontic appliances.

**Interdental cleansing**

Dental plaque cannot be completely removed by toothbrushing and dentifrice alone because bristles do not reach the entire proximal surface. Thorough removal of plaque interproximally is essential because most gingival disease starts in the interdental papillae and the prevalence of gingivitis is highest there.[40-45] For maximum plaque control it is necessary to supplement toothbrushing with one or more of the other cleaning aids such as dental floss, rubber tips, wooden points, and water irrigation. The supplemental aids required depend on the individual rate of plaque formation, smoking habits, tooth alignment, and the special attention required for cleansing fixed prosthesis.

**Dental floss.** The most effective way of cleansing the proximal tooth surface is with unwaxed nylon dental floss. The floss is passed gently past the contact area to the base of the sulcus then back along the tooth surface to the contact area, after which it is pulled sideways from the interproximal space. The floss is then placed at the base of the adjacent gingival sulcus, and the process is repeated on the other proximal tooth surface. The dental floss must not be snapped past the contact point into the gingiva with such force as to produce injury.

The principal purpose of dental floss is to remove plaque from the proximal tooth surfaces, not to dislodge fibrous shreds of food wedged in the contact area and impacted into the gingiva. Food impaction should be treated by correcting proximal contacts and "plunger" cusps and should not be perpetuated by habitual flossing.

**Rubber and wooden interdental cleansers.** Rubber tips are also effective for interdental cleansing. Interdental gingival inflammation can be reduced by as much as 26.3 percent by interdental cleansing plus toothbrushing, as compared with 6.6 percent reduction obtainable by toothbrushing alone.[46] Keratinization of the interdental gingiva is also increased by combining the rubber tip with toothbrushing.[47, 48] Wood points are useful for cleansing interdental spaces too small to permit the use of a rubber tip.

**Water irrigation under pressure.** Water irrigation devices, of which there are many types, generally consist of a pump that forces a steady or pulsating stream of water under pressure through a nozzle. Water irrigation when used in addition to toothbrushing provides benefits beyond those attainable by toothbrushing alone. It can be used without damage to soft or hard oral tissues or restorations,[49] and without inducing bacteremia in patients with healthy mouths or periodontitis.[50] It does not detach plaque from the teeth but reduces plaque[51] and materia alba formation and gingival inflammation,[52] increases gingival keratinization,[53] and also cleans bacteria from the oral cavity more effectively than toothbrushing and rinsing.[54]

Opinions differ as to whether the improvement in gingival health provided by improved oral hygiene is derived from cleansing action alone or whether a massaging effect also plays a role. Increased keratinization of gingival epithelium produced by toothbrushing[55-59] and interdental cleansers[47, 48] is interpreted as providing greater protection against local irritation, but this has not been established.

Even with diligent brushing and supplemental oral hygiene aids, the control of plaque to a level that will not cause gingival disease is a tedious and demanding task. It is a constant battle, and if the thoroughness of cleansing is relaxed, plaque accumulation and gingival disease follow.

### Chemical plaque and calculus inhibitors

Chemicals that would prevent or significantly reduce the rate of plaque and calculus formation and lessen dependence upon mechanical cleansing would significantly advance the prevention of gingival and periodontal disease. Many substances have been incorporated in toothpastes, mouthwashes, chewing gum, and lozenges for this purpose. Different degrees of effectiveness have been reported, but only few consumer products have been developed. Some of the agents demonstrated capable of inhibiting plaque and/or calculus are: pyridinium chloride,[60] sodium ricinoleate,[61] antibiotics such as vancomycin,[62] erythromycin,[63] and "cc 10232[64]; enzymes[65] such as mucinase,[66] hyaluronidase[67]; other chemicals such as beryllium nitrate and acetates of zinc, manganese, and copper,[68] urea,[69] and Victamine C, a cationic surface-active agent.[70, 71]

### Plaque control by hard fibrous foods

As part of the plaque control program patients should be advised to include hard fibrous foods in their diet, particularly at the end of meals. Although some investigators disagree, it is the general opinion that hard fibrous foods reduce plaque accumulation and gingivitis on tooth surfaces exposed to their mechanical cleansing action during mastication.[20, 73-77] Coarse fibrous foods also provide functional stimulation required for maintenance of the periodontal ligament and alveolar bone.

### Plaque control by limiting sucrose-containing foods

Of all the information thus far developed regarding plaque, the fact that the ingestion of sucrose increases plaque formation is of the greatest clinical importance.[78] A major component of the intercellular matrix of plaque is the polysaccharide dextran. It is produced by streptococci as a sticky substance that envelops the plaque bacteria and attaches them to the tooth surface. The bacteria require sucrose to form dextran; reducing the sugar intake reduces plaque formation.

## OTHER PREVENTIVE MEASURES AGAINST GINGIVAL AND PERIODONTAL DISEASE

Critical though it is, plaque control is only one phase of total service required to prevent periodontal disorders. The following meaningful procedures must also be included on a regular periodic basis.

Thorough supragingival and subgingival cleansing and scaling in the dental office should include the removal of plaque, stain, and calculus and the smoothing and polishing of the surfaces of all teeth, restorations, and prostheses with rubber cups, dental floss, a polishing brush, and polishing paste. Improved polishing agents such as zirconium silicate[79] create smoother surfaces upon which plaque is less likely to be deposited. The incidence of gingivitis has been reduced by 50 to 90 percent by subgingival scaling followed by controlled patient-administered oral hygiene measures.[80]

The earliest signs of gingival and periodontal disease should be noted and treated. It is paradoxical that oral examinations careful enough to employ bite-wing radiograms to detect pinpoint caries sometimes overlook gross gingival disease. By arresting destruction of the periodontal tissues early treatment prevents unnecessary tooth loss. Gingival and periodontal diseases must be recognized early and treated as soon as they are discovered. It is simpler to treat slight gingivitis than severe gingivitis, to eliminate shallow pockets than deep pockets, and to prevent bone destruction and osseous defects than correct them. Tooth loss at 50 years of age can often be prevented by appropriate measures at 30 years of age. Periodontal bone destruction can be arrested by local periodontal treatment.[81]

Mucous membrane disease should be diagnosed and treated. Oral exfoliative cytology should be used as a diagnostic aid.

Sources of local irritation such as overhanging, improperly contoured restorations, and areas of food impaction should be corrected.

Removable prostheses should be cleansed and checked for proper fit, settling, and gingival irritation in relation to clasps and tissue-borne sections.

The most carefully adjusted dentitions undergo changes, and cuspal relationships of dental restorations are modified by wear. Teeth and restorations should be inspected for wear of cusps and marginal ridges that lead to food impaction and altered occlusal forces. Radiograms should be taken periodically.

## PREVENTION BY SYSTEMIC MEASURES

Another approach to the prevention of gingival and periodontal disease is by systemic measures to (1) control or counteract local injurious agents and (2) improve the capacity of the periodontal tissues to resist local injurious agents. Little has been accomplished in these phases of prevention because systemic effects on the periodontium are not as clearly defined as are the changes produced by local factors.

No one questions the fact that the systemic condition of the patient affects the metabolic processes responsible for the preservation of periodontal health. Animal experiments indicate that the injurious effects of local irritants and abnormal occlusal forces are aggravated by nutritional deficiency[82] or other systemic disorders.[83] It may even be hypothesized that local irritants not severe enough to cause clinically detectable disease could produce gingivitis if their effect were enhanced by systemically induced debility of the tissues. But there are no systemic conditions that of themselves cause gingivitis or periodontal pockets. What must be determined are the limits beyond which the systemic condition of the patient must change in order to significantly alter the periodontium or increase its susceptibility to disease.

The information thus far available regarding prevention of periodontal disorders by systemic means has been provided by clinical studies. The evidence that nutritional supplements (protein,[84, 85] multivitamin, trace minerals,[86] and water-soluble bioflavinoids[87]) effectively prevent or treat gingival or periodontal disease or improve the response to local treatment procedures is provocative but not conclusive, and in some phases researched by different groups the findings disagree.[88] Some clinical studies[89] indicate that scaling and polishing reduce the severity of gingivitis by 30 percent, while a significantly greater reduction (45 percent) is obtained by the systemic administration of synthetic vitamin C alone, and more improvement (67 percent) follows the combination of scaling and polishing with systemic synthetic vitamin C. Others[90] find no significant relationship between either whole blood or urine ascorbic acid levels and the periodontal status. Some[91] note that increasing the plasma ascorbic acid levels by dietary supplements in patients with gingival disease and below-average plasma ascorbic acid levels does not improve the condition of the gingiva. Others[92] report that dietary supplementation that elevates the ascorbic acid level of the blood does not affect the ascorbic acid level of locally treated or untreated inflamed gingival tissue, nor does it influence the outcome of the treatment.

## Systemic measures to counteract plaque and bacteria

This aspect of prevention is in the formulative stage but it provides stimulating necessary guidelines for relevant research. For example, saliva could be converted into a potent preventive agent by secreting systemically introduced selective antimicrobial substances such as antibiotics, immunoglobulins, and antienzyme agents. Plaque accumulation and gingival infection have been controlled by antibiotics in the diet,[93] and healing following local periodontal treatment has been improved by systemic antibiotics.[94] In experimental animals the rate of calculus formation has been altered by systemic means.[95-97] Systemically administered drugs that modify the saliva so as to inhibit plaque and calculus formation could be a logical outgrowth of current research on antiplaque and anticalculus agents.

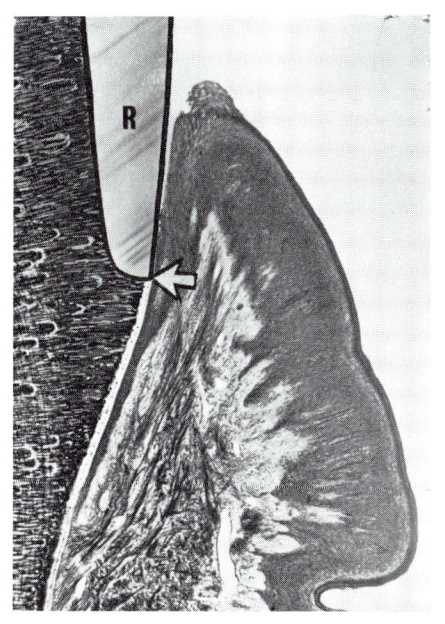

Fig. 9-4. Proper location of crown, **R**, margin at base of gingival sulcus indicated by white arrow. (From Glickman, I.: Clinical periodontology, ed. 3, Philadelphia, 1964, W. B. Saunders Co.)

The crevicular fluid[98-100] could be an excellent vehicle to convey systemically administered substances to counteract the noxious effects of plaque and reinforce the periodontal tissues to better resist them.

Vaccines to provide immunity against periodontal infection and catabolic hormones to reverse the aging of periodontal tissues and resist the cumulative effects of local irritants and alterations in occlusion are not unreasonable prospects.

## DENTAL RESTORATIONS IN PREVENTIVE PERIODONTICS

Dental restorations contribute significantly to gingival and periodontal health.[101] Attention to the following details of construction will add to the longevity of the natural dentition by reducing the likelihood of periodontal irritation and injury.

The margins of crowns should be located at the base of the gingival sulcus at the coronal level of the epithelial attachment (Fig. 9-4). The restoration should not be forced into the attached tissues nor should it terminate at the crest of the marginal gingiva.

Full crowns are important in restorative dentistry, but even when perfectly constructed their surface tends to attract plaque that is irritating to the gingiva.[102] Inlays that do not encroach upon the gingival third of the tooth[103, 104] reduce the risk of gingival irritation (Fig. 9-5).

Proximal surfaces of crowns should be contoured to preserve the gingival embrasures and properly locate the contact zones so as to avoid encroaching upon the interdental papilla. Overcontoured and undercontoured buccal and lingual surfaces should be avoided. The former create ledges that protect irritating debris from the cleaning action of the cheek.[105] The latter may deflect food *into* rather than *over* the gingival sulcus.

The occlusal surfaces of restorations and pontics should restore occlusal dimensions and cuspal contours in harmony with the remainder of the natural dentition. The occlusion should be adjusted before the teeth are prepared for dental restorations.

Self-curing acrylic resin should not be used in restorations close to the gingiva. Irritating plaque tends to accumulate on their surface.[106]

In addition to being functionally and aesthetically acceptable, pontics should

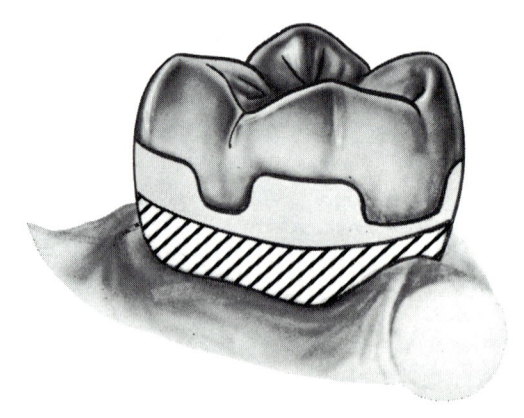

**Fig. 9-5.** Restoration constructed without intruding upon gingival third of tooth. (From Glickman, I.: Clinical periodontology, ed. 3, Philadelphia, 1964, W. B. Saunders Co.)

Preventive periodontics 219

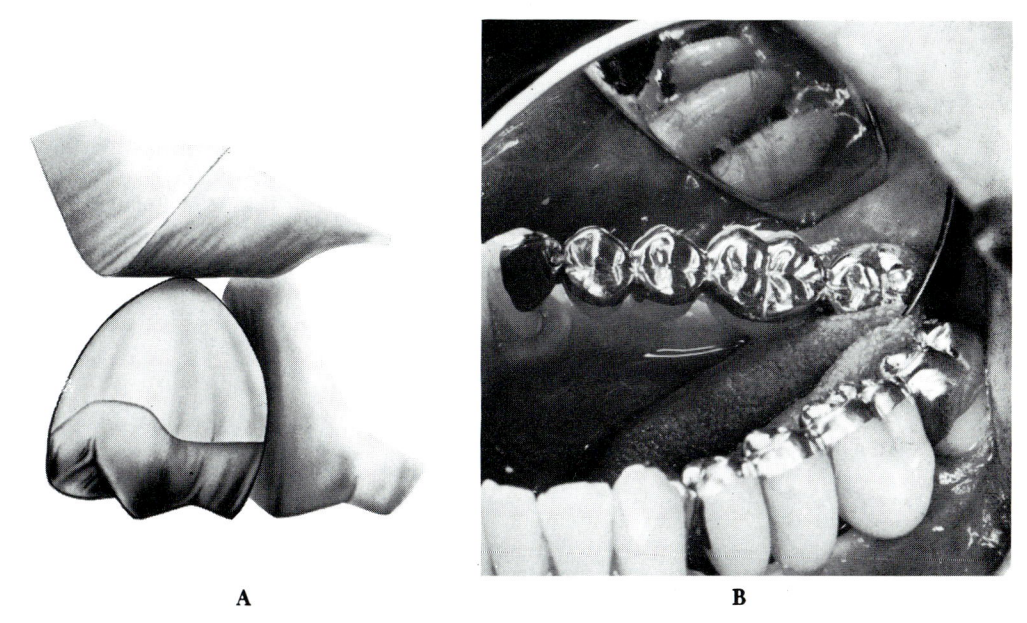

Fig. 9-6. **A,** Spheroidal pontic provides embrasures for food clearance. **B,** Lingual view of spheroidal pontics and healthy surrounding mucosa. (From Glickman, I.: Clinical periodontology, ed. 3, Philadelphia, 1964, W. B. Saunders Co.)

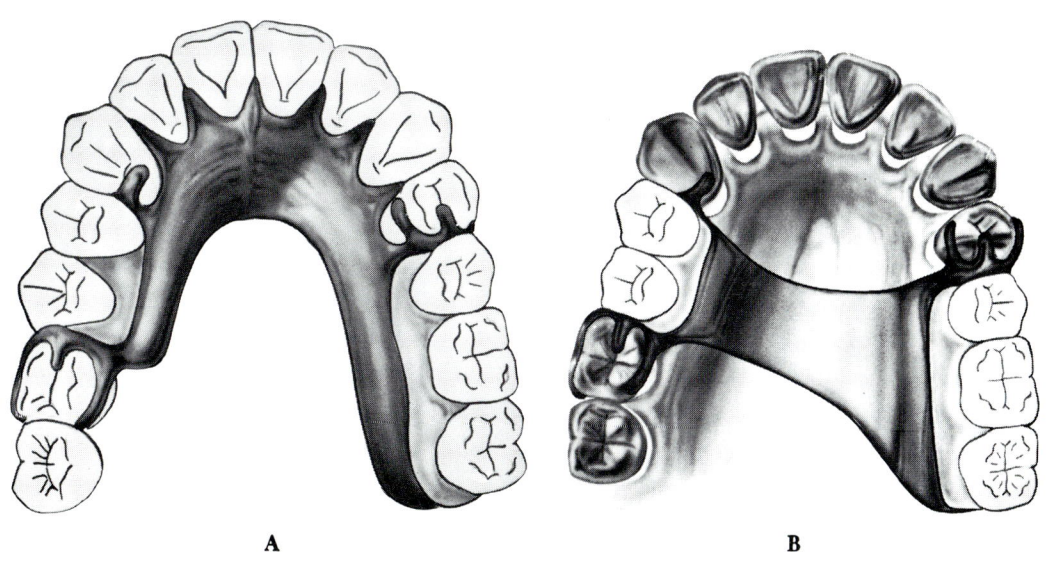

Fig. 9-7. **A,** Interdental projections on improperly designed maxillary partial denture causes gingival irritation. **B,** Properly designed partial denture does not impinge upon gingival margin. (From Glickman, I.: Clinical periodontology, ed. 3, Philadelphia, 1964, W. B. Saunders Co.)

create a hygienic environment for the mucosa and gingiva of the adjacent teeth. The egg-shaped, spheroidal pontic that provides embrasures for food passage and cleansing is most acceptable to the periodontium (Fig. 9-6). The sanitary-type bridges with an occlusal connection without a pontic create even less risk of the accumulation of irritating plaque. However, the health of the soft tissues depends more on thorough mechanical cleansing than on the pontic design. No pontic shape can overcome the effects of poor oral hygiene.

In a removable partial prosthesis there should be no fingerlike projections between the teeth (Fig. 9-7). Wide major connectors on the palate that do not encroach on and irritate the gingiva are preferred.

Clasps should rest passively on abutment teeth without injurious pressures or tensions.[107] Torque can be minimized by using thin wrought wire facial arms.

All clasps should have occlusal rests that extend sufficiently onto the occlusal surface to prevent tipping action.[108, 109] Clasps on anterior teeth should have incisal rests or should be fitted into prepared ledges on the lingual surface to prevent settling.

## ORTHODONTICS IN PREVENTIVE PERIODONTICS

Correction of malocclusion can be an important preventive measure against periodontal disorders, provided it includes the establishment of a stable functional relationship essential to the preservation of the periodontal tissues. Removable Hawley appliances create periodontal risks when used as permanent retainers for teeth that tend to migrate. Usually worn at night, they cause injury to the periodontium and loosen the teeth by the interplay between day and night pressures in opposite directions. The best interest of the periodontium is served when the occlusion is adjusted and the migrating teeth are stabilized in proper alignment by a permanent fixed splint.

## TRAUMA FROM OCCLUSION

Trauma from occlusion, injury to the periodontium produced by occlusal forces, is an important contributing etiologic factor in periodontal disease. The dentist must differentiate between anatomic aspects and functional aspects of occlusion. The anatomic aspect is the relationship of the teeth and arches to each other when the jaws are closed. Anatomic abnormalities are described as malocclusions, of which there are many types. The functional aspect of occlusion refers to the forces created on the periodontium in chewing and swallowing or by aberrations such as bruxism or clenching. The periodontium is the principal indicator of the functional aspect of occlusion. Occlusal function is satisfactory if it meets the needs of the periodontium. Dentitions that appear satisfactory from an anatomic viewpoint are functionally abnormal if they are injurious to the periodontium. Temporomandibular joint disturbances and impaired function or spasm of the masticatory musculature are additional signs of abnormality in the functional aspect of occlusion.

Periodontal findings that suggest the presence of trauma from occlusion should be noted and their location used as a guide to the responsible functional abnormalities, such as occlusal pathway prematurities, bruxing, and clamping. Periodontal signs of trauma from occlusion include widening of the periodontal space often accompanied by thickening of the lamina dura, tooth mobility in excess of that explainable by inflammation and reduced periodontal support, vertical and angular

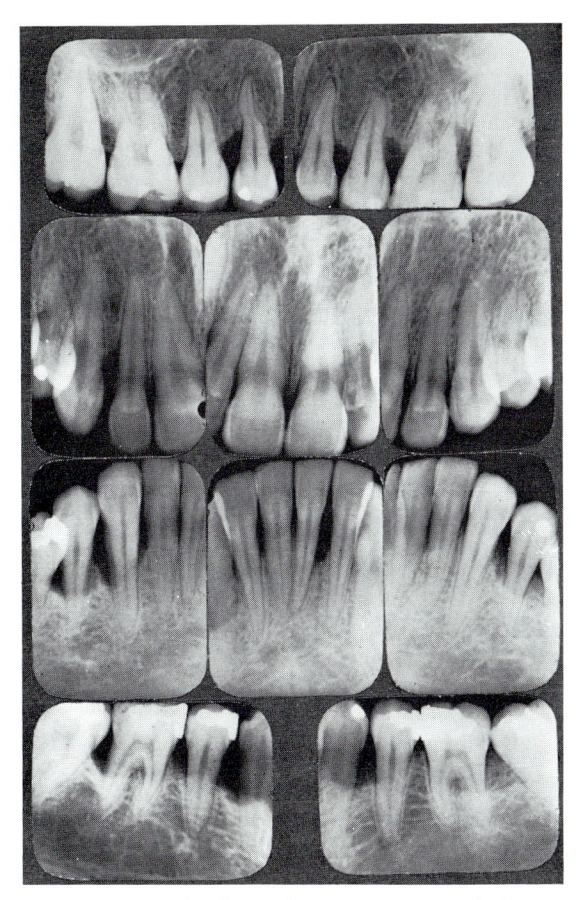

**Fig. 9-8.** Radiograms showing classic signs of trauma from occlusion such as angular bone loss, thickening of the periodontal space, thickening of the lamina dura, and bifurcation and trifurcation involvement. (From Glickman, I.: Clinical periodontology, ed. 3, Philadelphia, 1964, W. B. Saunders Co.)

bone destruction, infrabony pockets, bifurcation and trifurcation involvement, and pathologic migration, particularly of the anterior teeth (Fig. 9-8). Detection and correction of the responsible occlusal abnormalities along with elimination of local irritants are essential for the prevention of progressive bone destruction and tooth loss.

Special mention should be made of pathologic migration of the anterior teeth as a sign of trauma from occlusion. Although a tongue-thrusting habit is often a causative factor, premature tooth contacts in the posterior region that deflect the mandible anteriorly are often responsible for injury to the periodontium and pathologic migration of the maxillary anterior teeth. Therefore the combination of angular bone loss in relation to a molar or premolar combined with bone destruction and pathologic migration of maxillary anterior teeth is a common syndrome caused by trauma from occlusion (Fig. 9-9).

Prophylactic occlusal adjustment in the absence of evidence of trauma from occlusion in anticipation of possible future damage is not recommended. Trauma from occlusion is the tissue injury produced by occlusal forces, not the forces them-

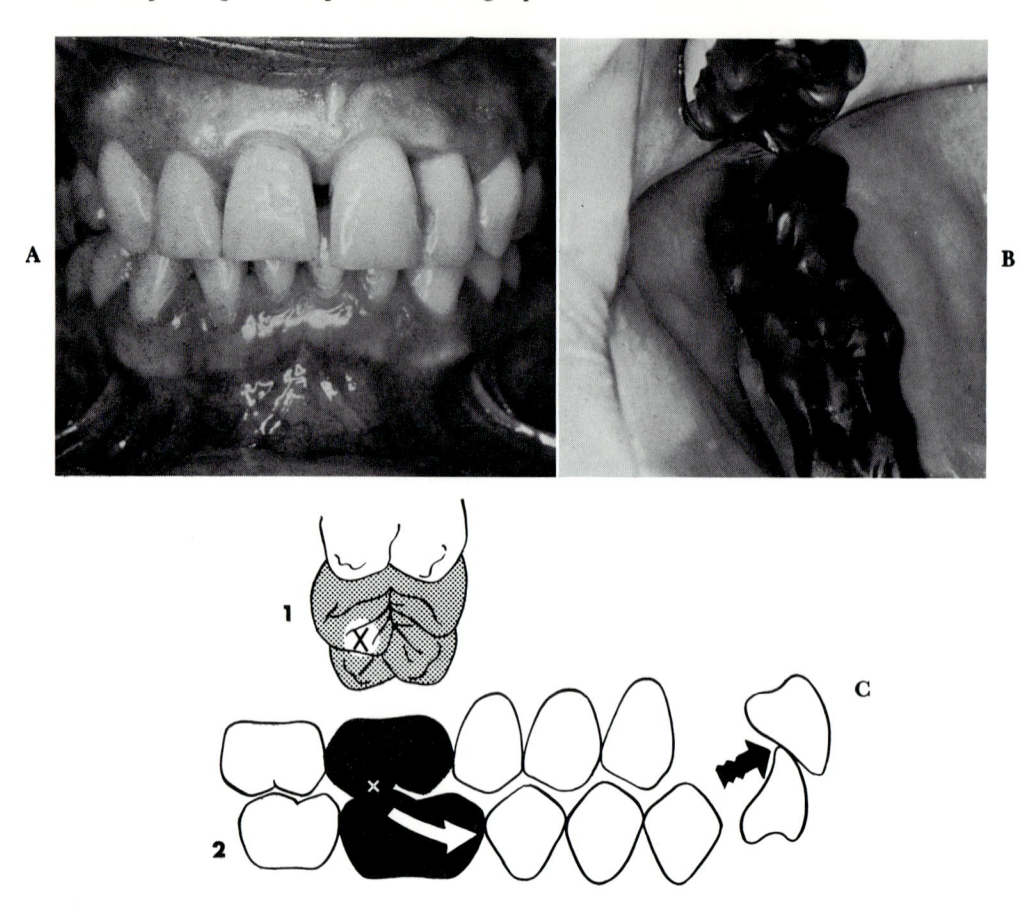

**222** *Improving dental practice through preventive measures*

Fig. 9-9. Pathologic migration associated with trauma from occlusion. **A,** Migration and extrusion of maxillary central incisor. **B,** Occlusal prematurity marked in wax on anterior aspect of the lingual cusp of maxillary molar (mirror view). **C,** Diagrammatic representation of prematurity on maxillary molar, 1, causing anterior glide of mandible and, 2, with impact against maxillary anterior teeth. (From Glickman, I.: Clinical periodontology, ed. 3, Philadelphia, 1964, W. B. Saunders Co.)

selves. Cuspal relationships that are abnormal according to anatomic standards of ideal occlusion are not necessarily injurious to the periodontium. The presence of anatomically abnormal cuspal relationships without evidence of periodontal injury indicates that the periodontium had adapted to the existing occlusal forces. Interfering with a well-adapted functional relationship to create an anatomic ideal may precipitate the type of periodontal injury that the occlusal adjustment aims to prevent.

### PRESERVATION OF PERIODONTAL HEALTH

The maintenance of periodontal health in the treated patient requires as positive a program as the elimination of periodontal disease. Prevention of recurrence is the joint responsibility of the patient and the dentist. The patient must adhere to the prescribed regimen of oral hygiene and periodic recall visits. The dentist must make each recall visit a meaningful preventive service.

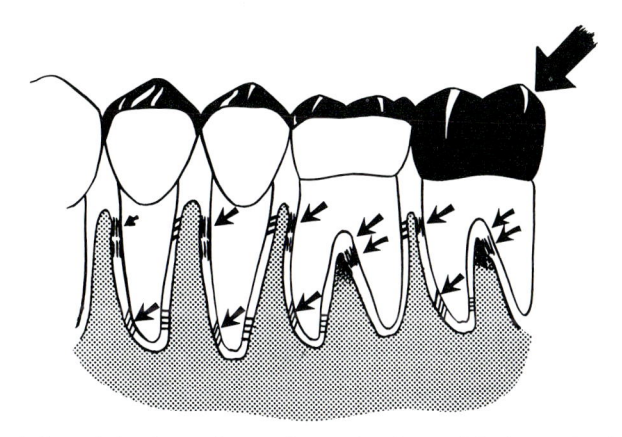

**Fig. 9-10.** Transmission of the forces in a splint makes it possible for occlusal prematurity on one of the teeth (large arrow) to injure the periodontium of all splinted teeth. (From Glickman, I.: Clinical periodontology, ed. 3, Philadelphia, 1964, W. B. Saunders Co.)

In patients with periodontal disease the aim of treatment should extend beyond the arrest of tissue destruction. Provision must be made for preventing further mutilation of the dentition. An environment of periodontal health and optimal occlusal function should be maintained.

Periodontal splints should be used to prevent the loss of teeth weakened by periodontal disease. They are primarily functional catalysts rather than simply devices for holding loose teeth tightly. By stabilizing weakened teeth, they maintain satisfactory relationships between occlusal forces and the periodontium.

Occlusal forces applied to a splint are shared by all the teeth within it, even if the force is applied to only one section of the splint (Fig. 9-10). Teeth weakened by periodontal disease benefit from support provided by adjacent teeth with an intact periodontium. But a weakened tooth in a splint is not completely relieved of the burden of occlusal forces, nor is it immunized against injury from excessive occlusal forces. The functioning surfaces of the firm teeth should be at least one and one-half to two times that of the mobile teeth.

The occlusion of the entire dentition should be adjusted before the splint is prepared, and the splint must be in harmony with the corrected occlusion. A rigid splint in occlusal disharmony accelerates the destruction of the periodontium of all of the splinted teeth, not simply the tooth that is being traumatized.

## CONCLUSION

Most gingival and periodontal disease and tooth loss caused by them can be prevented because they are caused by local factors that are accessible, correctable, and controllable. There are no forms of gingivitis or periodontal disease, regardless of how severe or how remote their total etiology, in which the removal of local irritants and prevention of their recurrence do not (1) reduce the severity of the disease, (2) lessen the rapidity of the destructive process, and (3) prolong the usefulness of the natural dentition.

Dental plaque, a concentration of multiplying bacteria in a matrix that adheres to the tooth surface, is the principal cause of gingivitis and periodontal disease.

Preventive periodontitis is a multifaceted cooperative program of procedures performed by the dentist and the patient to prevent the onset, progression, and recurrence of periodontal disorders. Plaque control, retarding or preventing the accumulation of dental plaque and other deposits on the tooth surface, is the keystone of preventive periodontics. Mechanical cleansing is the most effective method of plaque control. In no other field of medicine can the patient so effectively assist in preventing and reducing the severity of disease as in preventive periodontics; gingivitis can be reduced and/or prevented by toothbrushing, supplemented according to individual needs by interdental cleansing with dental floss, interdental rubber and wooden cleansers, and water irrigation under pressure.

Prevention of gingival and periodontal disease by systemic measures presents many interesting but as yet unexplored possibilities. The evidence that nutritional supplements prevent gingival or periodontal disease or improve the response to local periodontal treatment procedures is provocative but not conclusive.

**REFERENCES**
1. Ash, M. M., Gitlin, B. N., and Smith, W. A.: Correlation between plaque and gingivitis, J. Periodont. **35**:424, 1964.
2. Theilade, E., and others: Experimental gingivitis in man, II, a longitudinal clinical and bacteriological investigation, J. Periodont. Res. **1**:1, 1966.
3. Greene, J. C.: Oral hygiene and periodontal disease, Amer. J. Public Health **53**:913, 1963.
4. Littleton, N. W.: Dental caries and periodontal diseases among Ethiopian civilians, Public Health Rep. **78**:631, 1963.
5. Lovdal, A., and others: Tooth mobility and alveolar bone resorption as a function of occlusal stress and oral hygiene, Acta Odont. Scand. **17**:61, 1959.
6. Heydings, R. T.: A study of the prevalence of gingivitis in undergraduates in Leeds University, D. Pract. **12**:129, 1961.
7. James, P. M. C., and others: Gingival health and dental cleanliness in English school children, Arch. Oral Biol. **3**:57, 1960.
8. Schei, O., and others: Alveolar bone loss as related to oral hygiene and age, J. Periodont. **30**:7, 1959.
9. Fundak, C. P., and Ash, M.: Correlation between supragingival plaque, subgingival plaque and gingival crevice depth, I.A.D.R. Abstract 276, 1969.
10. Jenkins, G. N.: The chemistry of plaque, Ann. N. Y. Acad. Sci. **131**:786, 1965.
11. Bjorn, H., and Carlsson, J.: Observations on dental plaque morphogenesis, Odont. Revy **15**:23, 1964.
12. Leach, S. A., and Saxton, C. A.: An electron microscopic study of the acquired pellicle and plaque, Arch. Oral Biol. **11**:1081, 1966.
13. Lenz, H., and Muhlemann, H.: Repair of etched enamel exposed to the oral environment, Helv. Odont. Acta **7**:47, 1963.
14. Loe, H., Theilade, E., and Jensen, S. B.: Experimental gingivitis in man, J. Periodont. **36**:177, 1965.
15. Turesky, S., Renstrup, G., and Glickman, I.: Histologic and histochemical observations regarding early calculus formation in children and adults, J. Periodont. **32**:7, 1961.
16. Mandel, I. D.: Plaque and calculus, Alabama J. Med. Sci. **5**:313, 1968.
17. Schroeder, H. E.: Formation and inhibition of dental calculus, Berne, 1969, Hans Huber Medical Publisher.
18. Parfitt, G. J.: Summary of the problem of the prevention of periodontal disease, Alabama J. Med. Sci. **5**:395, 1968.
19. Linn, E. L.: Oral hygiene and periodontal disease: implications for dental health programs, J.A.D.A. **71**:38, 1965.
20. Arnim, S. S.: The use of disclosing agents for measuring tooth cleanliness, J. Periodont. **34**:227, 1963.
21. Chilton, N. W., Didio, A., and Rothner, J. T.: Comparison of the clinical effectiveness of an electric and a standard toothbrush in normal individuals, J.A.D.A. **64**:777, 1962.

22. Elliott, J. R.: A comparison of the effectiveness of a standard and an electric toothbrush, J. Periodont. 34:375, 1963.
23. Lefkowitz, W., and Robinson, H. B. G.: Effectiveness of automatic and hand brushes in removing dental plaque and debris, J.A.D.A. 65:351, 1962.
24. Quigley, G. A., and Hein, J. W.: Comparative cleansing efficiency of manual and power brushing, J.A.D.A. 65:26, 1962.
25. Toto, P. D., and Farchione, A.: Clinical evaluation of an electrically powered toothbrush in home periodontal therapy, J. Periodont. 32:249, 1961.
26. Sanders, W. E., and Robinson, H. B. G.: Effects of toothbrushing on deposition of calculus, J. Periodont. 33:386, 1962.
27. Hoover, D. R., and Lefkowitz, W.: Reduction of gingivitis by toothbrushing, J. Periodont. 36:193, 1965.
28. Lobene, R. R.: The effect of an automatic toothbrush on gingival health, J. Periodont. 35:137, 1964.
29. Berman, C. L., and others: Observations of the effects of an electric toothbrush: preliminary report, J. Periodont. 33:195, 1962.
30. Smith, W. A., and Ash, M. M.: Effectiveness of an electric toothbrush, I.A.D.R. 41:86, 1963.
31. Brandtzaeg, P., and Jamison, H. C.: The effect of controlled cleansing of the teeth on periodontal health and oral hygiene in Norwegian army recruits, J. Periodont. 35:28, 1964.
32. Larato, D., and others: The effect of a prescribed method of toothbrushing on the fluctuation of marginal gingivitis, J. Periodont. 40:22, 1969.
33. Harrington, J. H., and Terry, I. A.: Automatic and hand toothbrushing abrasion studies, J.A.D.A. 68:343, 1964.
34. Bass, C. C.: An effective method of personal oral hygiene, J. Louisiana Med. Soc. 106:100, 1954.
35. Ash, M. J.: A review of the problems and results of studies on manual and power toothbrushes, J. Periodont. 35:202, 1964.
36. Toto, P. D., and others: A study on the uninstructed use of the electric brush, J.A.D.A. 72:904, 1966.
37. McKendrick, A. S. W., Barbenel, L. M. H., and McHugh, W. D.: A two year comparison of hand and electric toothbrushes, J. Periodont. Res. 3:224, 1968.
38. McConnell, D., and Conroy, C. W.: Comparisons of abrasion produced by a simulated manual versus a mechanical toothbrush, J. Dent. Res. 46:1022, 1967.
39. Manly, R. S., and others: A method for measurement of abrasion of dentition by toothbrush and dentifrice, J. Dent. Res. 44:533, 1965.
40. Schour, I., and Massler, M.: Prevalence of gingivitis in young adults, J. Dent. Res. 27:733, 1948.
41. Black, A. D.: Something of the etiology and early pathology of the diseases of the periodontal membrane with suggestions as to tooth treatment, Cosmos 55:1219, 1913.
42. King, J. D.: Gingival disease in Dundee, D. Record 65:9, 32, 55, 1945.
43. Schour, I., and Massler, M.: Gingival disease in postwar Italy (1945), I, prevalence of gingivitis in various age groups, J.A.D.A. 35:475, 1947.
44. Massler, M., Ludwick, W., and Schour, I.: Dental caries and gingivitis in males 17-20 years old (at the Great Lakes Naval Training Center), J. Dent. Res. 31:195, 1952.
45. Stahl, S. S., and Goldman, H. M.: The incidence of gingivitis among a sample of Massachusetts school children, Oral Surg. 6:707, 1953.
46. Glickman, I., Petralis, R., and Marks, R.: The effect of powered toothbrushing plus interdental stimulation upon the severity of gingivitis, J. Periodont. 35:519, 1964.
47. Glickman, I., Petralis, R., and Marks, R.: The effect of powered toothbrushing and interdental stimulation upon microscopic inflammation and surface keratinization of the interdental gingiva, J. Periodont. 36:108, 1965.
48. Cantor, M. T., and Stahl, S. S.: The effects of various interdental stimulators upon the keratinization of the interdental col, Periodontics 3:243, 1965.
49. Lobene, R. R., and Soparkar, P. M.: Effect of a pulsed water pressure cleansing device on oral health, I.A.D.R. Abstract 344, 1969.

50. Tamimi, H. A., Thomassen, P. R., and Moser, E. H., Jr.: Bacteremia study using a water irrigation device, J. Periodont. 40:424, 1969.
51. Hoover, D. R., Robinson, H. B. G., and Billingsley, A.: The comparative effectiveness of water-pic in a non-instructed population, J. Periodont. 39:43, 1968.
52. Cantor, M. T., and Stahl, S. S.: Interdental col tissue responses to the use of a water pressure cleansing device, J. Periodont. 40:292, 1969.
53. Krajewski, J., Giblen, J., and Gargiulo, A. W. J.: Evaluation of a water pressure cleansing device as an adjunct to periodontal treatment, Periodontics 2:76, 1964.
54. Phillips, J. E.: Effect of water irrigation on oral flora and gingival health, Marquette University, Milwaukee, Wisconsin, 1967 (master's thesis).
55. Castenfelt, T.: Toothbrushing and massage in periodontal disease, Stockholm, 1952, Nordisk Rotogravyr.
56. Robinson, H. B. G., and Kitchin, P. C.: The effect of massage with the toothbrush on keratinization of the gingiva, Oral Surg. 1:1042, 1948.
57. Stahl, S. S., and others: The effect of toothbrushing on the keratinization of the gingiva, J. Periodont. 24:20, 1953.
58. Stanmeyer, W. R.: A measure of tissue response to frequency of toothbrushing, J. Periodont. 28:17, 1957.
59. Carter, S. B.: The masticatory mucosa and its response to brushing: findings in the Merion rat, Meriones libycus, at different ages, Brit. D. J. 101:76, 1956.
60. Sturzenberger, O. P., and Leonard, B. J.: The effect of a mouthwash as an adjunct in tooth cleansing, J. Periodont. 40:292, 1969.
61. Schroeder, H. E., Marthaler, T. M., and Muhlemann, H. R.: Effects of some potential inhibitors on early calculus formation, Helv. Odont. Acta 6:6, 1962.
62. Mitchell, D. F., and Holmes, L. A.: Topical antibiotic control of dentogingival plaque, J. Periodont. 35:202, 1964.
63. Lobene, R. R., Brion, M., and Socransky, S. S.: Effect of erythromycin on dental plaque and plaque forming microorganisms of man, J. Periodont. 40:287, 1969.
64. Volpe, A. R., and others: Antimicrobial control of bacterial plaque and calculus and the effects of these agents on oral flora, J. Dent. Res. 48:832, 1969.
65. Packman, E. W., and others: Effect of enzyme-chewing gums upon oral hygiene, J. Periodont. 34:255, 1963.
66. Aleece, A. A., and Forscher, B. K.: Calculus reduction with a mucinase dentifrice, J. Periodont. 25:122, 1954.
67. Wasserman, B. H., Mandel, I. D., and Levy, B. M.: In vitro calcification of dental calculus, J. Periodont. 29:144, 1958.
68. Amdur, B., Brudevold, F., and Messer, A. C.: Observations on the calcification of salivary sediment, I.A.D.R. 40:18, 1962.
69. Belting, C. M., and Gordon, D. L.: In vitro effect of a urea containing dentifrice on dental calculus formation, J. Periodont. 37:26, 1966.
70. Turesky, S., Gilmore, N. D., and Glickman, I.: Reduced plaque formation by the chloromethyl analogue of victamine C, J. Periodont. (In press.)
71. Turesky, S., Gilmore, N. D., and Glickman, I.: Calculus inhibition by topical application of the chloromethyl analogue of victamine C, J. Periodont. 38:142, 1967.
72. Lindhe, J., and Wicen, P. O.: The effects on the gingivae of chewing fibrous foods, J. Periodont. Res. 4:193, 1969.
73. Baer, P. N., Stephan, R. M., and White, C. L.: Studies on experimental calculus formation in the rat, I, effect of age, sex, strain, high carbohydrate, high protein diets, J. Periodont. 32:190, 1961.
74. Stewart, W. H., and Burnett, G. W.: The relationship of certain dietary factors to calculus-like formation in albino rats, J. Periodont. 31:7, 1960.
75. Burwasser, P., and Hill, T. J.: The effect of hard and soft diets on the gingival tissues of dogs, J. Dent. Res. 18:389, 1939.
76. Haydak, M. H., and others: A clinical and biochemical study of cow's milk and honey as an essentially exclusive diet for adult humans, Amer. J. Med. Sci. 207:209, 1944.
77. Egelberg, J.: Local effect of diet on plaque formation and development of gingivitis in dogs, I, effect of hard and soft diets, Odont. Revy 16:31, 1965.

78. Carlsson, J., and Egelberg, J.: Effect of diet on early plaque formation in man, Odont. Revy **16:**112, 1965.
79. Muhler, J. C., Dudding, N. J., and Stookey, G. K.: The clinical effectiveness of a particular particle size distribution of zirconium silicate for use as a cleaning and polishing agent for oral hard tissues, J. Periodont. **35:**481, 1964.
80. Lovdal, A., and others: Combined effect of subgingival scaling and controlled oral hygiene on the incidence of gingivitis, Acta Odont. Scand. **19:**537, 1961.
81. Rateitschak, K. H., Engelberger, A., and Marthaler, T. M.: Therapeutic effect of local treatment on periodontal disease assessed upon evaluation of different diagnostic criteria, III, radiographic changes in appearance of bone, J. Periodont. **35:**263, 1964.
82. Miller, S. C., Stahl, S. S., and Goldsmith, E. D.: The effects of vertical occlusal trauma on the periodontium of protein deprived young adult rats, J. Periodont. **28:**87, 1957.
83. Glickman, I., Smulow, J. B., and Moreau, J.: Effect of alloxan diabetes upon the periodontal response to excessive occlusal forces, I.A.D.R. **43:**53, 1965.
84. Ringsdorf, W. M., Jr., and Cheraskin, E.: Periodontal pathosis in man, IV, effect of protein versus placebo supplementation upon gingivtis, J. Dent. Med. **18:**2, 1963.
85. Cheraskin, E., and Ringsdorf, W. M., Jr.: Periodontal pathosis in man, X, effect of combined versus animal protein supplementation upon sulcus depth, J. Oral Ther. **1:** 497, 1965.
86. Ringsdorf, W. M., Jr., and Cheraskin, E.: Periodontal pathosis in man, VI, effect of multivitamin-trace minerals vs. placebo supplementation on gingivitis, J. West. Soc. Periodont. **11:**85, 1963.
87. Carvel, R. I., and Halperin, V.: Therapeutic effect of water-soluble bioflavinoids in gingival inflammatory conditions, Oral Surg. **14:**847, 1961.
88. Glickman, I.: Nutrition in the prevention and treatment of gingival and periodontal disease, J. Dent. Med. **19:**179, 1964.
89. El-Ashiry, G. M., Ringsdorf, W. M., Jr., and Cheraskin, E.: Local and systemic influences in periodontal disease, II, effect of prophylaxis and natural versus synthetic vitamin C upon gingivitis, J. Periodont. **35:**250, 1964.
90. Shannon, I. L., and Gibson, W. A.: Intravenous ascorbic acid leading in subjects classified as to periodontal status, J. Dent. Res. **44:**355, 1965.
91. Parfitt, G. J., and Hand, C. D.: Reduced ascorbic acid levels and gingival health, J. Periodont. **34:**347, 1963.
92. Glickman, I., and Dines, M. M.: Effect of increased ascorbic acid blood levels on the ascorbic acid level in treated and non-treated gingiva, J. Dent. Res. **42:**1152, 1963.
93. Keyes, P. H., and Jordan, H. V.: The effect of two diets and an antibiotic on periodontal disease in hamsters, I.A.D.R. **43:**53, 1965.
94. Winer, R. A., Chauncey, H. H., and Cohen, M. M.: Antibiotic therapy in periodontal disease, I.A.D.R. **43:**72, 1965.
95. King, J. D., and Gimson, A. P.: Experimental investigations of paradontal disease in the ferret and related lesions in man, Brit. D. J. **83:**126, 1947.
96. Becks, H., Wainwright, W. W., and Morgan, A. F.: Comparative study of oral changes in dogs due to deficiencies of pantothenic acid, nicotinic acid and unknowns of the vitamin B complex, Amer. J. Orthodont. **29:**183, 1943.
97. Kakehashi, S., Baer, P. N., and White, C.: Studies on experimental calculus formation in the rat, II, effect of calcium, phosphate, bicarbonate, J. Periodont. **33:**186, 1962.
98. Brill, N., and Bjorn, H.: Passage of tissue fluid into human gingival pockets, Acta Odont. Scand. **17:**11, 1959.
99. Bissada, N. F., Schaffer, E. M., and Haus, E.: Human crevicular fluid flow: a 24 hour quantitative study, I.A.D.R. **43:**72, 1965.
100. Weinstein, E., Green, G., and Villus, O. R.: Studies of gingival fluid, I.A.D.R. **43:**72, 1965.
101. Glickman, I.: Clinical periodontology, ed. 3, Philadelphia, 1964, W. B. Saunders Co.
102. Waerhaug, J.: Effect of rough surfaces upon gingival tissues, J. Dent. Res. **35:**323, 1956.
103. Stein, R. S., and Glickman, I.: Prosthetic considerations essential for gingival health, Dent. Clin. N. Amer., March, 1960, p. 177.

104. Shooshan, E. D.: A pin-ledge casting technique—its application in periodontal splinting, Dent. Clin. N. Amer., March, 1960, p. 189.
105. Morris, M. L.: Artificial crown contours and gingival health, J. Prosth. Dent. **12**:1146, 1962.
106. Waerhaug, J., and Zander, H. A.: Reaction of gingival tissues on self-curing acrylic restorations, J.A.D.A. **54**:760, 1957.
107. Steffel, V. L.: Clasp partial dentures, J.A.D.A. **66**:803, 1963.
108. Ito, H., Inoue, Y., and Yamada, M.: Three dimensional photoclastic studies on the clasp-rest and tooth extraction, J. Dent. Res. **38**:203, 1959.
109. Plitzner, J.: Role of occlusal rest lug as transmitter of masticating stress, Dentist. Reform. **42**:77, 1938.
110. Draus, F. J., Leung, S. W., and Miklos, F.: Toward a chemical inhibitor of calculus, D. Progress **3**:79, 1963.
111. King, J. D., and Glover, N. E.: The relative effects of dietary constituents and other factors upon calculus formation and gingival disease in the ferret, J. Path. Bact. **57**:353, 1945.
112. Ivy, A. C., Morgan, J. E., and Farrel, J. I.: Effects of total gastrectomy, Surg. Gynec. Obstet. **53**:602, 1931.
113. Pelzer, R.: A study of the local oral effect of diet on the periodontal tissues and gingival capillary structure, J.A.D.A. **27**:13, 1940.
114. Glickman, I.: Preventive periodontics—a blueprint for the periodontal health of the American public, J. Periodont. **38**:361, 1967.
115. Villa, P.: Degree of calculus inhibition by habitual toothbrushing, Helv. Odont. Acta **12**:31, 1968.
116. Brandtzaeg, P.: The significance of oral hygiene in prevention of dental disease, Odont. T. **72**:460, 1964.
117. Bjorn, H., and Lindhe, J.: On the mechanics of toothbrushing, Odont. Revy **17**:9, 1966.

# Chapter 10 Preventive orthodontics

## Charles J. Burstone

Prevalence of malocclusions
Genetic factors
Environmental factors
    Trauma to jaws
    Deleterious habits
    Premature loss and missing teeth
    Retained primary teeth
    Malocclusion produced by the dentist
Interceptive orthodontics
    Advantages
    Disadvantages
Conclusion

## PREVALENCE OF MALOCCLUSIONS

In most animals the prevalence of malocclusion and dentofacial deformity is relatively low, yet in man, along with dental caries and periodontal disease, malocclusion presents the dentist with one of his major treatment problems. Since it is difficult to define normal occlusion, estimates as to the prevalence of malocclusion in the United States vary. Some studies show that as high as 90 percent of all children have some type of malocclusion. However, a more conservative estimate of malocclusions requiring treatment will range from 20 to 30 percent of the population.

If orthodontic needs are to be adequately met, there is no argument that preventive measures must be employed whenever feasible. The question is therefore inescapable: Which malocclusions can and cannot be prevented?

From an etiologic point of view, malocclusions can be divided into two categories—genetic and environmental. Genetically produced malocclusions, almost by definition, are not subject to preventive measures unless we are able to alter the gene structure of the individual or to control mating by a eugenic program. On the other hand, environmentally produced malocclusions might possibly be altered by preventive measures.

## GENETIC FACTORS

Many dentofacial deformities are genetic in origin. Recognition of this fact can help the dentist differentiate between many conditions that require preventive measures as opposed to those in which corrective procedures are required.

To a large extent the size and form of the teeth are genetically determined. Patients who exhibit arch length inadequacies or crowded and rotated teeth many times have teeth with larger than average mesiodistal diameters. Crowded teeth in such patients are nothing more than a symptom of a basic problem involving large tooth size, which is under genetic control. Attempts to treat the crowding sympto-

230 *Improving dental practice through preventive measures*

matically rather than the basic tooth size–arch length problem will result in failure. As a result, malocclusions produced by tooth size discrepancies cannot be prevented.

Skeletal patterns are also primarily genetically determined. For example, many patients with Class II and Class III malocclusions have a malrelationship of the maxilla to the mandible.

Three different skeletal patterns are seen on the lateral headplates shown in Fig. 10-1. An arbitrary facial plane has been drawn from the nasofrontal suture (nasion) to the anterior portion of the mandible (pogonion). In a typical profile this line will touch the anterior aspect of the maxilla at the subspinale (Fig. 10-1, *A*). A Class II, Division 1, and a Class III malocclusion in which the facial plane does not run

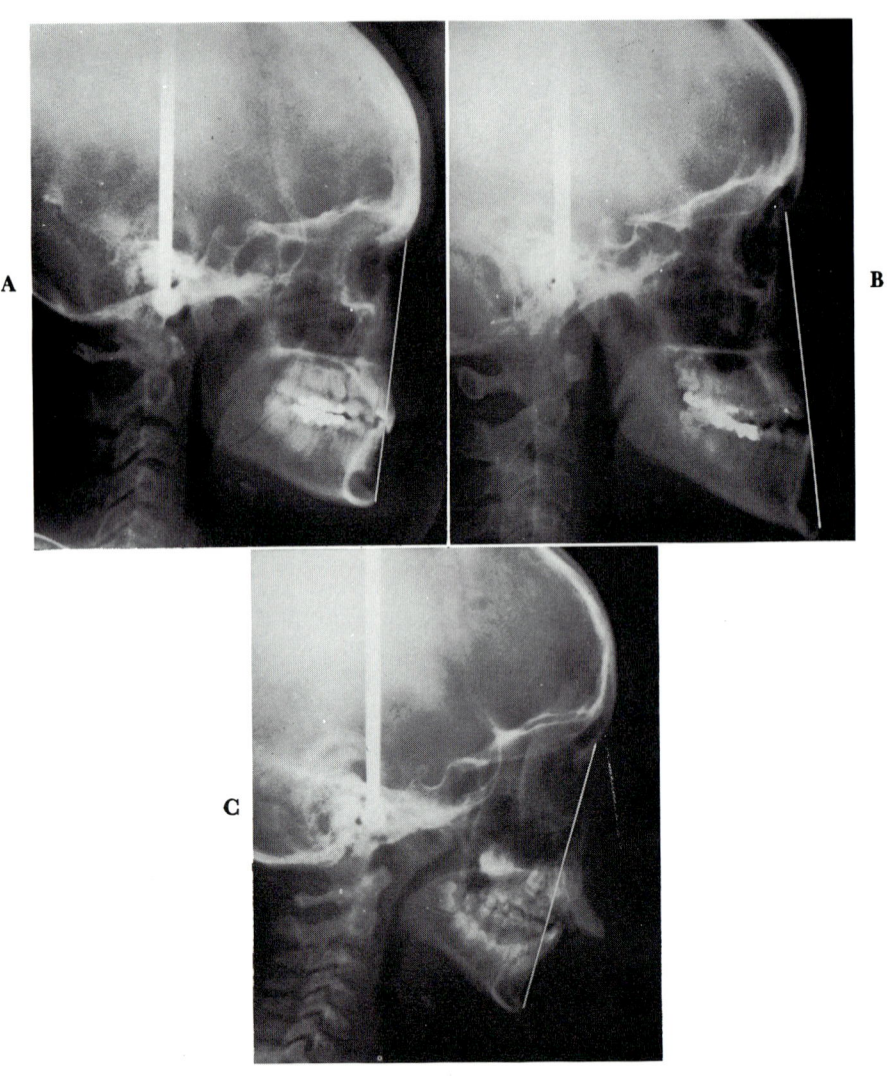

Fig. 10-1. **A,** Normal skeletal pattern. **B,** Prognathic skeletal pattern. **C,** Retrognathic skeletal pattern. A line connecting the nasofrontal suture and the most prominent part of the chin will normally touch the anterior part of the maxilla.

through subspinale are shown in Fig. 10-1, *B* and *C*. The anterior portion of the maxilla is relatively forward in the Class II malocclusion and relatively posterior in the Class III (Fig. 10-1, *B* and *C*). The reason that these patients possess a malocclusion is not that teeth have erupted abnormally but rather that a skeletal discrepancy exists. Preventive measures aimed at the teeth alone cannot succeed since the problem lies with the jawbone. The development of the jaws to a large extent is genetically determined, and no accepted method is available for preventing the development of skeletal discrepancies.

The skeletal pattern can be somewhat modified by orthodontic appliances. Although this is not prevention, since the condition exists at the time of treatment, therapy may minimize the difficulty or may prevent it from becoming worse. Treatment aimed at correction or prevention of skeletal problems is best termed dentofacial orthopedics—for example, sutural expansion of the maxilla, increasing or decreasing the vertical dimension, and redirecting maxillary and mandibular growth. In respect to redirecting jaw growth, the efficiency of currently used treatment is not known. Headgears have been shown to produce maxillary changes at the sutures in experimental animals, but it is not certain how important these changes are in the human or how permanent they are after a headgear is removed. An orthopedic device for the correction of scoliosis (the Milwaukee Brace) can inhibit mandible growth, yet the typically designed chin cap may not deliver the magnitude or constancy of force to produce the same result.

Just as we inherit our tooth size and facial skeleton, we also inherit our basic muscular pattern. This does not mean that function or exercise cannot alter this pattern somewhat. Some examples of neuromuscular problems include discrepancies in lip length and tonus, abnormal tongue size, and atypical swallowing and mastication.

Muscles can exert a broad influence on the development of a malocclusion. Muscle forces can directly influence the position of the teeth, or they may work indirectly by altering the form or the structure of the supporting jawbones. Although it is possible to alter certain neuromuscular patterns and hence prevent or influence the development of the malocclusion, it should be recognized that some muscular problems are inherent in nature and are not easily changed by environmental means. For example, some types of abnormal swallowing with anterior open bites are associated with general lack of muscular coordination and hence originate in the central nervous system. A more stable orthodontic result is usually produced if the malocclusion is treated in harmony with the existing musculature rather than altering the neuromuscular pattern to accommodate the teeth.

The genetic basis of a malocclusion is easily demonstrated by twin studies. Although monozygotic twins are not identical dentofacially in every respect, the observance of marked similarity is striking. Twin boys with almost identical dentoskeletal and facial patterns are shown in Fig. 10-2. Note the remarkable similarity in overjet, overbite, and Class II occlusion. Even the crossbite on the right side and the rotations are identical.

Many of the most commonly found malocclusions that require orthodontic treatment, such as Class II cases, Class III cases, and Class I arch length problems, apparently are determined to a large extent by genetic factors. This does not mean that these cases are untreatable, but they are not suitable for preventive procedures.

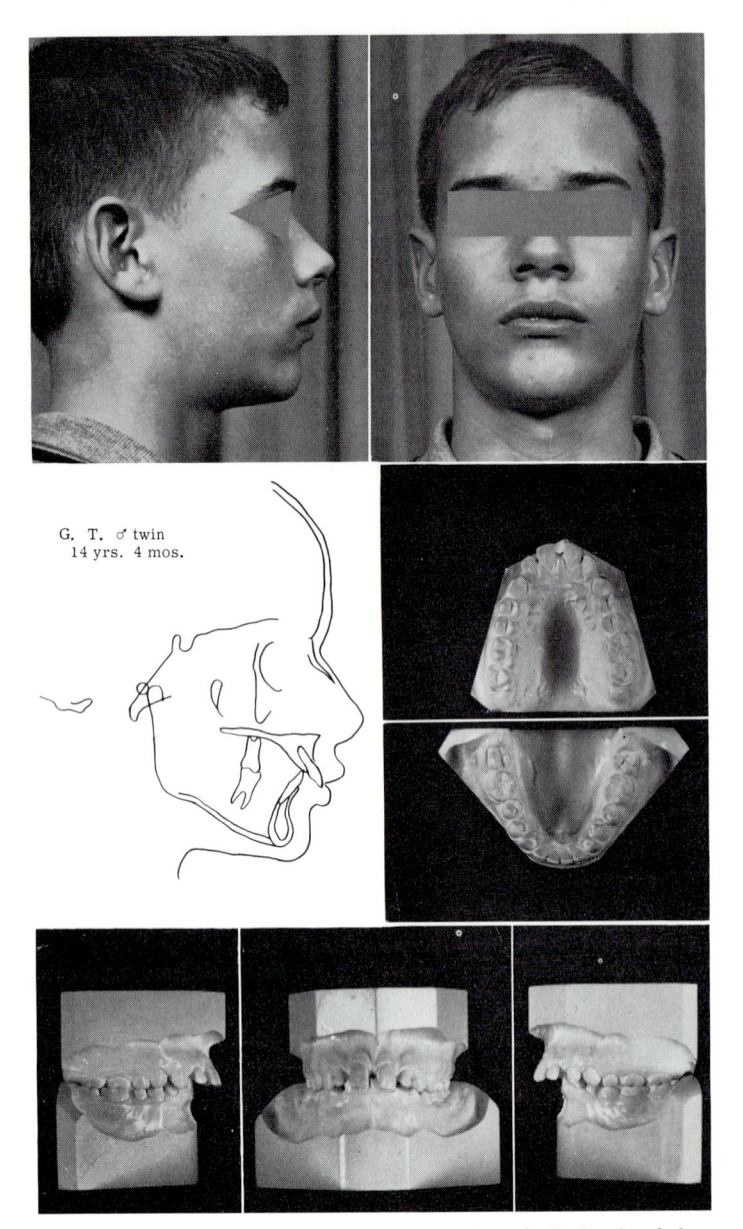

**232** *Improving dental practice through preventive measures*

**Fig. 10-2.** Class II, division 1, malocclusion in twins. Note similarity in skeleton, face, and arrangement of teeth.

## ENVIRONMENTAL FACTORS

Let us consider some environmental factors that may influence the development of the malocclusion. It is in this realm that the hope for preventing dentofacial malformations may be found.

### Trauma to jaws

A prime growth center of the face is at the condyle of the mandible. A traumatic injury to the condyle may result in a marked facial asymmetry, mandibular

*Preventive orthodontics* 233

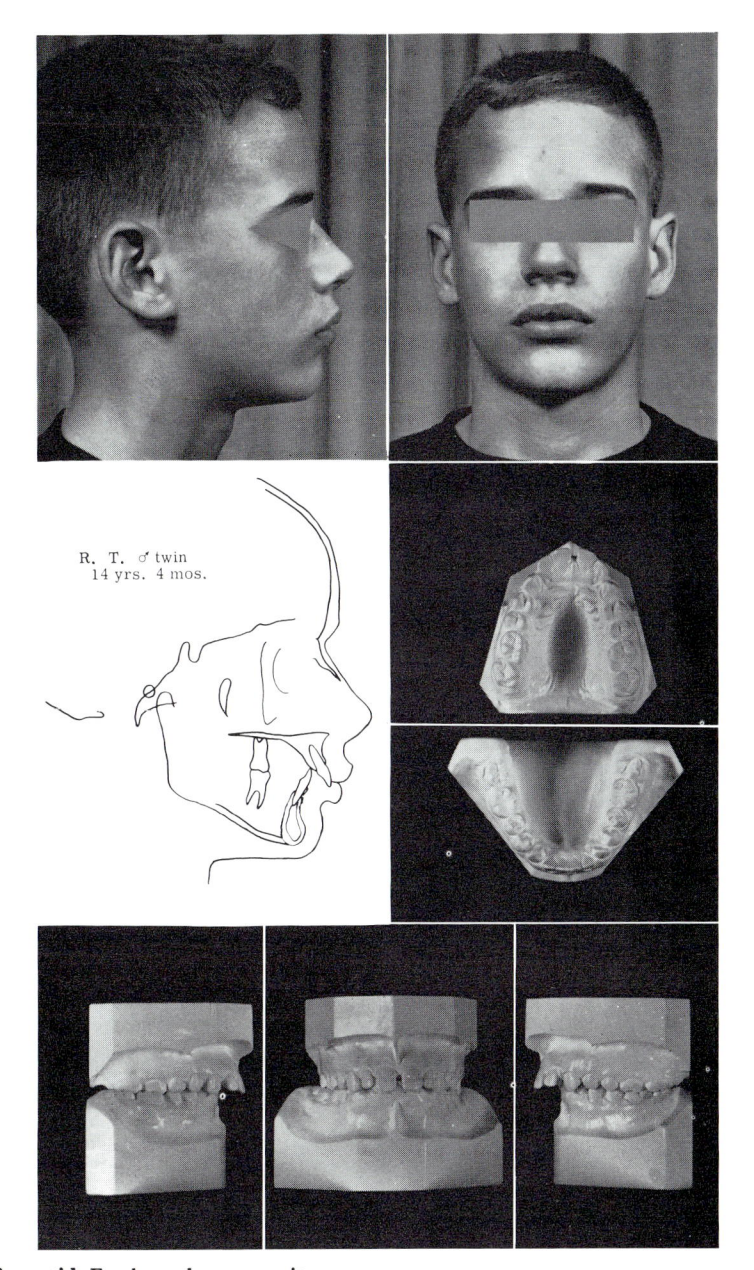

**Fig. 10-2, cont'd.** For legend see opposite page.

retrognathism, and a concomitant malocclusion. Trauma of this type can be produced by a blow to the mandible or occasionally by toxins associated with osteomyelitis. Characteristically, trauma to the condyle with inhibition of condylar growth will lead to the development of a Class II malocclusion with severe retrognathism of the face. A unilateral injury adds to the complication of both mandibular and dental asymmetries (Fig. 10-3).

Since the increments of mandibular growth during childhood are greater than those in other areas of the face, injury to the condyle most likely will lead to a mal-

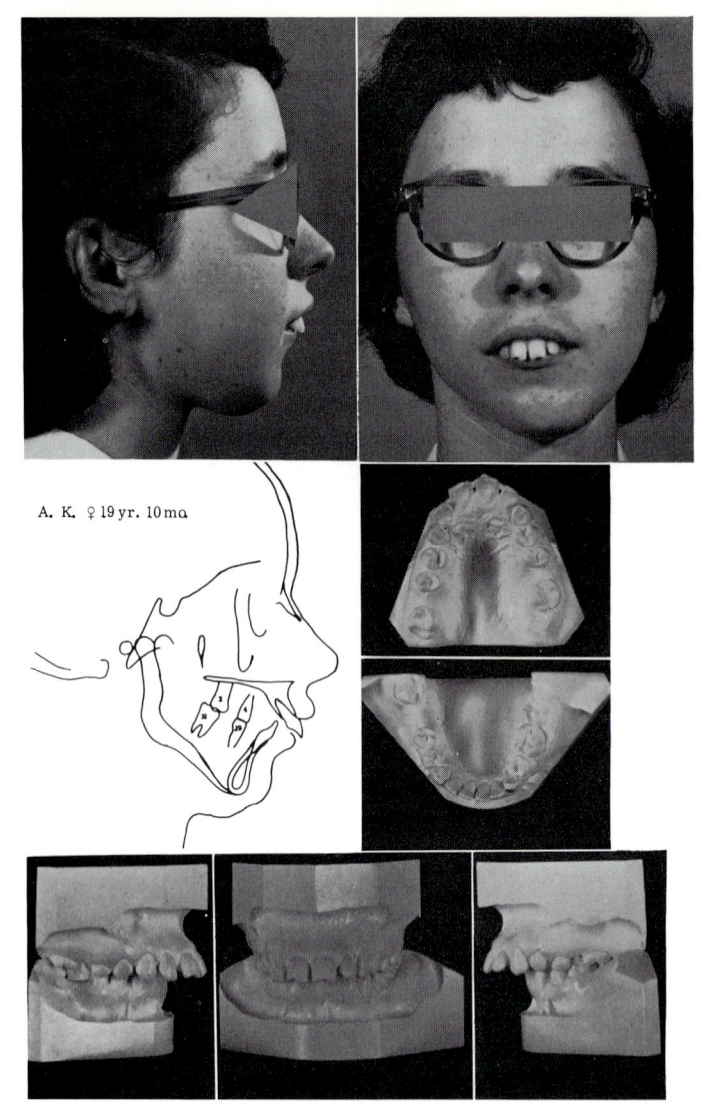

**234** *Improving dental practice through preventive measures*

**Fig. 10-3.** Unilateral condylar inhibition (left) associated with an osteomyelitis. The chin and the lower midline are displaced to the left. Marked retrognathism, overbite, and overjet.

occlusion; a facial deformity becomes progressively worse. Although malocclusions produced by trauma to the mandibular condyles are not frequently observed, the deforming nature is so extreme that care should be taken to minimize the chance of condylar trauma in the early formative years of the child. Immediate attention should be given to any mandibular injury if it does occur.

Sometimes malocclusion is associated with an improperly reduced fracture of the mandible and maxilla. It is important for the surgeon to be particularly "occlusion conscious" in reducing fractures so that a skeletally based malocclusion is not present later in life. Malocclusion that is produced by bone fragments that are allowed to heal in improper positions is difficult to correct since the discrepancy is not in the

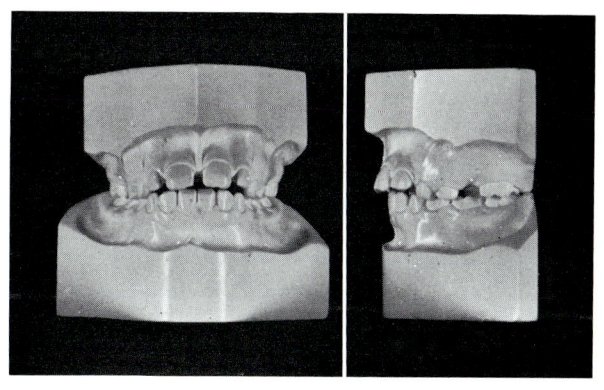

Fig. 10-4. Patient B. S., female, 8 years, 10 months of age. Anterior overjet and open bite produced by a thumb-sucking habit. The cuspids are in a normal position (Class I).

teeth but in the jaw itself. The use of improperly directed intermaxillary elastics to help stabilize a fractured jaw can be an etiologic factor in production of a malocclusion.

**Deleterious habits**

Thumb-sucking and finger-sucking can influence both the teeth and supporting alveolar process. In our society thumb-sucking is common among children, yet not all children who suck their thumbs exhibit a malocclusion. Patients who exhibit a Class II, Division 1 malocclusion seem to be more susceptible to the deleterious effects of thumb pressures.

Characteristically a thumb-sucking habit will produce flaring of the maxillary anterior teeth and many times retrusion of the mandibular anteriors (Fig. 10-4). An open bite will be present in the region where the thumb lies. There is little evidence to suggest that the posterior occlusion is influenced by the thumb-sucking habit, although it is true that a habit of this type can make a potential Class II, Division 1 case become worse by allowing the lower lip to assume a postural position behind the maxillary incisors.

One should not be too concerned about this habit until the eruption of the permanent central incisors at about 6 years of age. Even after this time discontinuance of the habit in a good skeletal pattern with no other malocclusion will usually cause the anterior teeth to return to a normal position.

Several methods are commonly used to correct thumb-sucking. One approach is to forcibly prevent the child from placing the thumb in his mouth either by attaching something to the thumb or by the placement of a suitable crib within the palate. This approach may be questioned since equal success can be obtained by certain psychologic approaches to the child. A consultation with the child and with someone outside of the family, such as the dentist, with whom the problem is sympathetically discussed and the undesirable effects of thumb-sucking shown may be all that is required. It is helpful to have the child keep a daily record of the number of times he has sucked his thumb with the idea of reducing this number daily. In any event, if the patient is not psychologically ready to discontinue the habit, it might be doubted if forcibly eliminating the habit is desirable as far as his psyche is concerned. Other undesirable habits may be substituted or psychologic damage may occur if an an attempt is made to eliminate the habit in a child with a deep-seated emotional problem.

Abnormal swallowing is often listed as a habit when in reality it might better be considered a deep-seated neuromuscular pattern. In order to better understand abnormal swallowing, let us first describe the normal swallow. The mandible is elevated and the teeth are tightly closed; the tongue moves upward and backward in a sphincter-type action toward the throat, carrying saliva or the bolus of food with it; and the lips are lightly closed with very little apparent perioral activity.

By contrast, in abnormal swallowing the action of the mandible, tongue, and lips is altered. The teeth are apart with the mandible depressed, and the tongue will be found between the teeth either anteriorly or posteriorly (Fig. 10-5). If a definite tongue thrust is present, the tongue will move forward as a fang between the anterior teeth. Unlike the normal swallow, the lips may forcibly contract and give rise to a typical facial grimace. Abnormal swallowing is not an entity in itself since all of these characteristics may not be observed in the same child. Considerable variation in abnormal swallowing is the rule rather than the exception.

Abnormal swallowing can be an etiologic factor in the production of malocclusion. The tongue can flare the maxillary anterior teeth and thereby increase the anterior overjet. Simultaneously, mentalis contraction may retrude the lower anteriors, further increasing the overjet. Furthermore, tongue placement between the teeth can produce either an anterior or a lateral open bite. A low-tongue position during rest or function will not give adequate support to the maxillary arch, and hence may contribute to the formation of a posterior crossbite. Although there is no question that tongue and lip action during abnormal swallowing can contribute to a malocclusion, it is an oversimplification to assume that the abnormal function is the only or primary cause of the problem. In many patients the swallowing pattern is secondary to such other problems as a maxillary constriction, an atypical mandible with a steep mandibular plane, or a nasal obstruction. Unless treatment aims at the prime etiologic factor, any attempt to retrain the swallowing pattern will prove most disappointing.

To further complicate the picture, statistical studies have shown that, in the

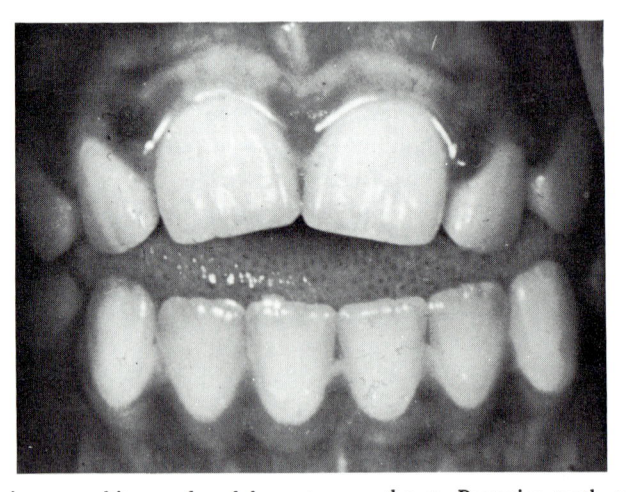

Fig. 10-5. Anterior open bite produced by a tongue thrust. Posterior teeth are in occlusion.

Preventive orthodontics 237

period of the mixed dentition, a high percentage of children have abnormal swallowing with or without malocclusion. Many of these children will begin to swallow normally without any treatment or retraining whatsoever. Other studies also show that Class II, Division 1 malocclusions have a higher incidence of abnormal swallowing. Many of these children will begin to swallow normally after the correction of the malocclusion without any attempt at retraining.

The retraining of the swallowing pattern takes considerable time and effort on the part of the dentist, patient, and speech therapist. Retraining procedures seem to work the best in patients who are well motivated and in those in whom the abnormal swallowing is residual to a thumb-sucking habit. Patients who have atypical skeletal

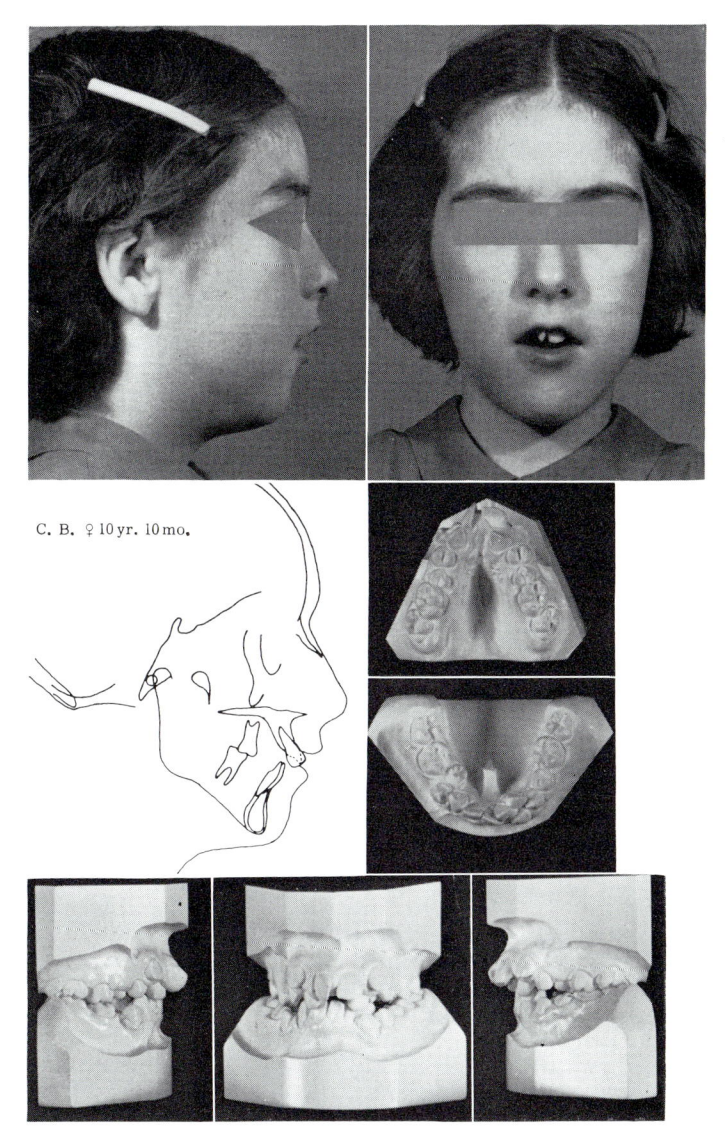

Fig. 10-6. Large interlabial gap (space between relaxed upper and lower lips) associated with a short upper lip and dental protrusion. Severe arch length inadequacies in both arches.

patterns that predispose to abnormal swallowing are the most difficult to retrain. The success of treatment in the atypical swallower is therefore highly dependent on very careful diagnosis.

Another culprit that has been blamed for malocclusion is mouth breathing. Scientific evidence of mouth breathing and its influence on the position of the teeth is sharply lacking. Nevertheless, it seems logical that mouth breathing can produce certain conditions that may well influence the development of occlusion. If the nasal airway is obstructed, a number of neuromuscular changes can be noted. The mandible is depressed and the tongue lowered in order that an airway is created through the oral cavity. It has been suggested that the tighter buccal pressures from the cheek and the greater outward pressures from a low tongue on the mandibular teeth can be responsible for a posterior crossbite. Certainly with the presence of a dental crossbite the possibility of mouth breathing should be considered and corrected whenever possible.

Many children normally carry their lips apart during their daily activities and during sleep. Not all of these children are mouth breathers. If the lips are relatively too short for the vertical dimension of the face, or if the teeth are protruding with or without overjet, the child may make no effort to close his lips. It is futile to berate the child to keep his lips closed for usually the malocclusion is so great that this is not easily accomplished. If protrusion and overjet are present they should be reduced first by orthodontic means so that the child can have a normal dental alveolar environment that will enable him to close his lips normally (Fig. 10-6).

Numerous other habits have been suggested as possible causes of malocclusion: these include sleeping habits, breast feeding, and leaning the head against the fist. No reliable data have shown that these factors are particularly significant in production of malocclusion and hence should not be actively considered in a preventive orthodontic program. They should be reserved for future investigation.

**Premature loss and missing teeth**

Despite the great amount that has been said and written concerning the mutilation of a dentition that can occur by premature loss of primary molars, many primary teeth are still lost because of negligence. With the loss of primary molars, a number of undesirable sequelae can be observed.

1. The posterior segments can move forward.
2. If the loss is unilateral, asymmetries of the posterior and anterior segment may be produced.
3. The anterior teeth may drift around the arch and retract, particularly if the primary first molar is lost.
4. The teeth in the opposing arch can supra-erupt.

Mutilations of this type, particularly when posterior segments have come forward, are very difficult to correct even with the most comprehensive types of orthodontic care since one of the most challenging orthodontic tooth movements is the retraction of posterior teeth (Fig. 10-7). If premature loss and subsequent drift of teeth are superposed upon an already existing malocclusion, the problems of further treatment are even more complicated.

Space maintenance is needed in situations in which the permanent anterior teeth are lost by an accident or extracted for any reason. Unless the space is held, the anterior teeth may erupt into the extraction site and leave inadequate space for an

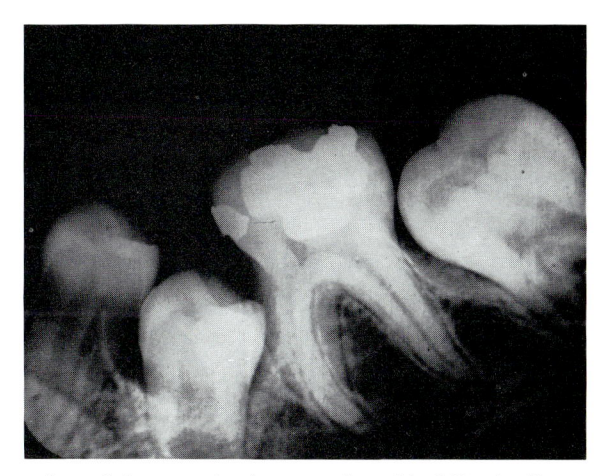

**Fig. 10-7.** Premature loss of the second primary molar with drift of adjacent teeth. Insufficient space is available for the eruption of the second premolar.

anterior bridge. Drift into the extraction site will be particularly noticeable in cases in which crowding already exists in the anterior segment. Even though the importance of space maintenance has been reiterated by the profession time and time again, probably no area of preventive orthodontics is as important as the preservation of the primary teeth and the use of adequate space maintenance. (See pp. 201-202.)

The soldered lingual arch with bands on the permanent first molars is an excellent space maintainer when primary molars are prematurely lost. A unilaterally placed band and loop space maintainer may not be as successful since greater care is needed in contouring the loop, and mesial drift may occur when primary teeth are subsequently shed.

**Retained primary teeth**

Many believe that overretention of primary teeth can lead to misplaced eruption of the permanent teeth. However, it is difficult to establish a definite cause-and-effect relationship between retained primary teeth and the subsequent eruption of the permanent teeth. Ectopically erupting permanent teeth will bypass primary teeth and hence they will fail to resorb. Primary teeth that have been overretained should be removed, but there is a good chance that this will have little effect on the pattern of eruption of the permanent teeth.

There is no question that ankylosed primary teeth may cause deflection of the permanent teeth. Since the normal eruption of teeth is necessary for the development of alveolar process, ankylosis will also inhibit the formation of alveolar process. Generalized ankylosis involving more than one primary molar will create a space between the occlusal surfaces of the teeth since the ankylosed teeth appear to submerge as the jaws develop. The space that is found between the upper and lower teeth is particularly undesirable since it can predispose to a lateral tongue thrust.

The best policy is to extract ankylosed primary molars as soon as possible and make sure the space is adequately held with a space maintainer. Before any primary teeth are removed, a full-mouth roentgenogram should be carefully studied to make sure that the permanent successors are not missing. It is true that many times ankylosed primary teeth will resorb spontaneously; nevertheless, it is wise to extract them as soon as possible so that the deleterious effects on other teeth and the alveolar process can be avoided.

**Malocclusion produced by the dentist**

Nonorthodontic procedures can produce a malocclusion or can make an existing one worse. One group of malocclusions is characterized by arch-length problems in which there is insufficient arch length for all of the permanent teeth. The arch length can be further foreshortened by improper operative procedures if deficient contact areas are placed. If the contact area is insufficiently contoured, space will usually close by posterior segments moving forward.

Conversely, overly tight contact area, as is sometimes observed where inlays are placed, can also aggravate an arch-length inadequacy. The added forces of newly placed tight contact areas may be all that is needed to rotate and displace anterior teeth, which may have had a slight shortage of available space at the onset of the restorative work.

Overly high or improperly carved restorations can also complicate or initiate a malocclusion. In order to accommodate the newly placed occlusal form of a restoration or group of restorations, teeth can drift into new positions or the mandible may assume a new position in maximal occlusion, producing a so-called pseudocentric position.

Improperly constructed partial dentures can serve as orthodontic appliances by delivering lateral stresses to the teeth. The art of properly designing a partial denture, so that the forces delivered during mastication will not displace the teeth, cannot be overemphasized.

Some malocclusions require the extraction of teeth to effect an acceptable end result. However, nothing is more mutilating to the dentition than the extraction of permanent anterior teeth to "make room" in a crowded arch. Particularly undesirable is an asymmetric extraction in which different teeth are extracted on different sides of the arch. If mutilating extraction of this type is resorted to, it may not be possible at a later time to adequately treat the case orthodontically because a bilateral difference in tooth size will not allow either good esthetics or good function.

## INTERCEPTIVE ORTHODONTICS

There are many orthodontic problems that cannot be prevented (in the true sense of the word) but that can perhaps be intercepted. Interceptive or early treatment refers to tooth movement, tooth guidance, and alteration of the neuromuscular environment or the bony skeleton in order to prevent a developing malocclusion from becoming worse. Some malocclusions benefit by early treatment, while others may actually be more difficult to treat if therapy is started too early. Thus a careful case analysis and diagnosis of the existing problems are necessary. Let us consider some of the advantages and disadvantages of interceptive orthodontics.

**Advantages**

A malocclusion may produce particular psychologic problems in a child if there is overjet and protrusion of the maxillary anterior teeth. Reduction of this protrusion can be quite important psychologically to certain children in their formative years.

*Preventive orthodontics* 241

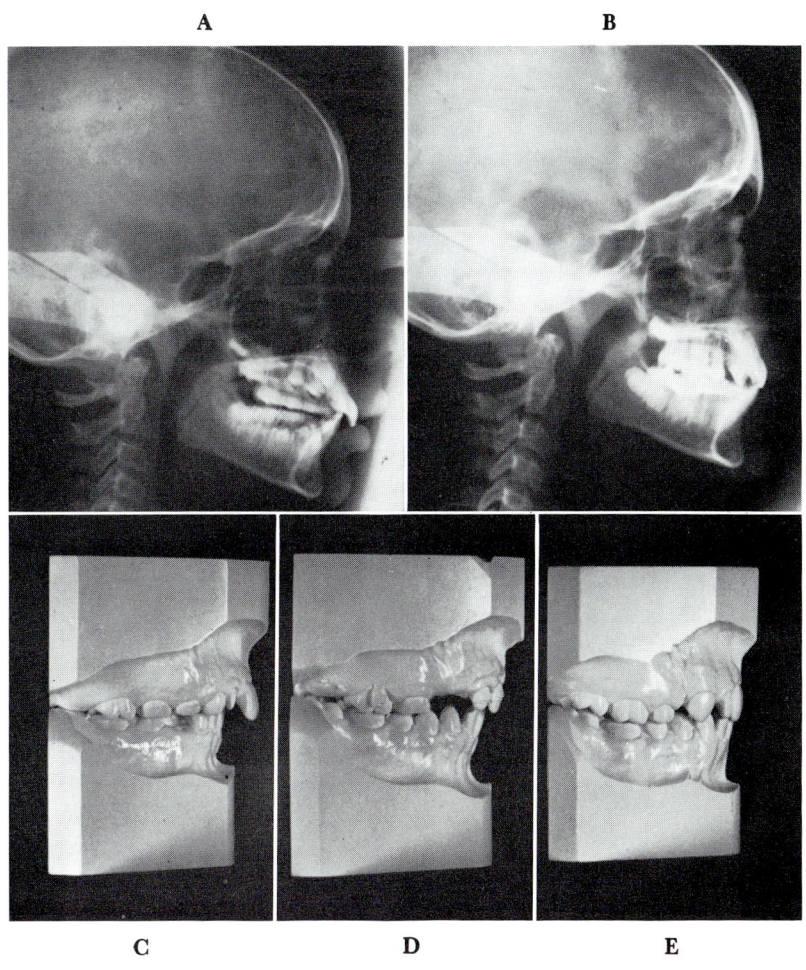

**Fig. 10-8.** Serial extraction of upper first premolars. As the anterior teeth were retracted with an orthodontic appliance, the cuspid was guided posteriorly into position. **A** and **C**, Before treatment. **D**, After anterior retraction, as cuspid has started to emerge. **B** and **E**, After cuspid eruption.

Protruding maxillary anterior teeth are also very commonly fractured as the result of an accident involving the mouth. Hence reduction of overjet, if possible, can minimize the need for extensive restorative or endodontic procedures and prosthetics.

If one waits to treat a malocclusion until it becomes "full blown," it is usually necessary to move teeth over a considerable distance. Early procedures act in many instances to guide teeth to a more favorable position. For example, if serial extraction is successfully accomplished, an erupting cuspid can be guided posteriorly so that there will be sufficient room for the alignment or retraction of the anterior teeth (Fig. 10-8). Another example of tooth guidance is found in ectopic eruption of the maxillary first molar in which gentle posterior pressure can be used to guide the first molar back to its normal position. Early treatment can then minimize the amount of tooth movement that would be needed if treatment were delayed until later in life.

**242** *Improving dental practice through preventive measures*

Some malocclusions in the mixed dentition have only dental problems localized in one area of the mouth. Since no basic skeletal or muscular discrepancies exist, these cases can be treated at an early age. A pseudo-Class III malocclusion of this type is shown in Fig. 10-9. An inclined plane was used to flare the maxillary anterior teeth, which allowed the mandible to retrude to its centric position. Since little tooth movement was needed, the underjet was reduced in 4 weeks. A second phase of treatment was needed in the permanent dentition to establish occlusal detail and to solve the problem of the missing maxillary lateral incisors.

Interceptive methods can be utilized to alter the skeletal as well as the dental pattern. Devices for sutural expansion of the maxilla are used to treat the basal width of the maxilla. This not only allows sufficient width for proper development of the maxillary arch, but also tends to increase the available volume of the nasal fossa, thereby aiding respiration in some children. The use of headgear in early treatment of Class II cases will have an influence on the bone as well as on the teeth. Normally the teeth of the maxillary arch tend to erupt in a downward and forward direction (Fig. 10-10). The restraining posterior force of the headgear inhibits this downward and forward eruption and with it the downward and forward development of the alveolar process (Fig. 10-11). There is debate whether headgear influences structures beyond the alveolar process, but there is some evidence to suggest that inhibition of the maxilla and perhaps parts of the cranial base can occur as a result of this type of therapy.

The forces of abnormal muscular action can either produce a malocclusion or can make a developing malocclusion become worse. In the Class II, Division 1 malocclusion, the lower lip lying behind the maxillary incisor causes the incisor to flare even further anteriorly with maturation. Moreover, protruding teeth preventing a

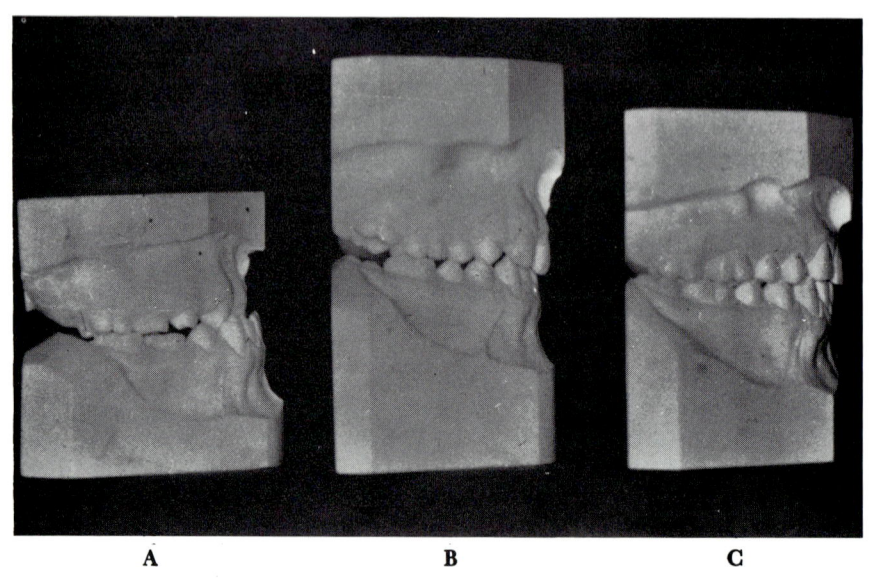

Fig. 10-9. Pseudo-Class III malocclusion. **A**, Before treatment. **B**, After treatment with an acrylic inclined plane. **C**, After comprehensive treatment with a full edgewise hook-up. The bite plane flared the maxillary anterior teeth, allowing the mandible to retrude.

Preventive orthodontics 243

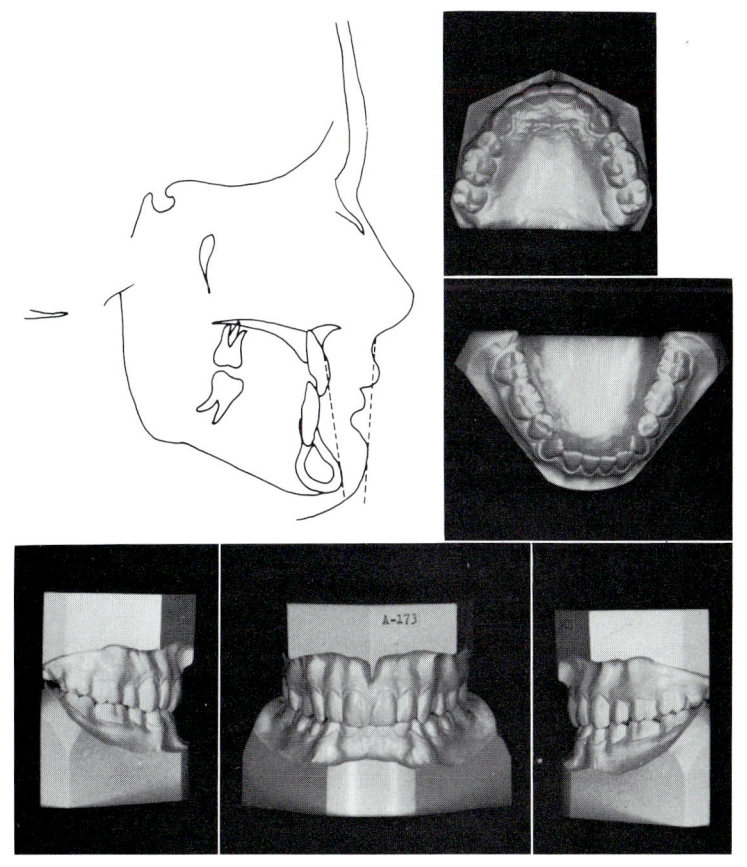

**Fig. 10-10.** Mutilation following serial extraction of four first premolars. Note poor axial inclinations of teeth adjacent to extraction site and linguoversion of the anterior teeth. Normally the lower incisor will lie on the dotted line connecting the maxilla and the mandible, and the lower lip will lie in front of the dotted facial line (tracing).

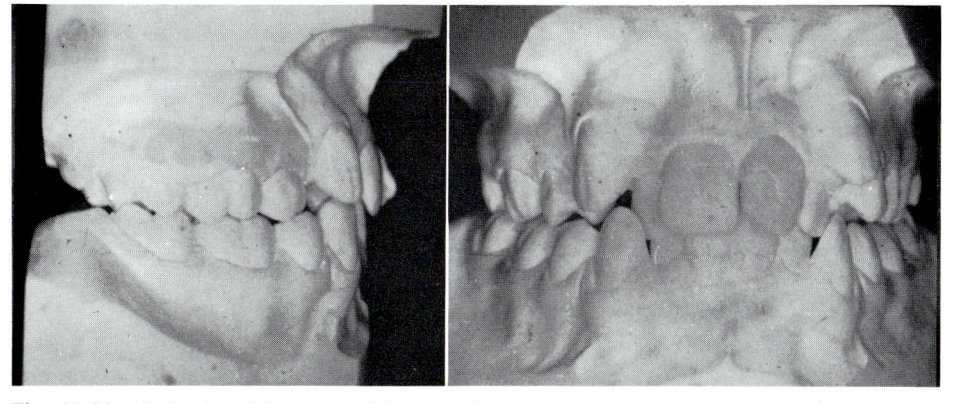

**Fig. 10-11.** Mutilation following serial extraction of three first premolars. Posterior segments have drifted forward. Arch length inadequacy is still present despite extraction of teeth. It will be extremely difficult to regain the space loss through mesial drift.

normal lip seal with loss of restraint of the perioral musculature may flare the maxillary incisors. It is evident that one of the advantages of early interceptive procedures would be to produce a more normal neuromuscular environment for the teeth. This would include the establishment of normal patterns of lip closure, swallowing, mastication, and speech.

**Disadvantages**

It would appear from the preceding discussion that interceptive orthodontics would be highly desirable. Unfortunately, there are many risks to be found in early treatment that contraindicate the widespread application of interceptive procedures to all malocclusions.

One of the major problems of early interceptive orthodontic treatment is the many unknowns that make treatment planning very difficult. For example, consider a 9-year-old child with a Class II, Division 1 malocclusion. Obviously the treatment plan devised at 9 years of age must take into consideration the future growth of the patient to maturity. Even with newer methods of growth prediction, a prediction made at this time cannot be expected to be accurate. It is evident that from 9 years of age to maturity considerable change will take place in the vertical and horizontal relationships of the jaws and in the size and form of the dental arches. If a patient at 9 years of age with a Class II malocclusion has precocious mandibular growth that improves the skeletal pattern, nonextraction treatment methods can easily be employed. On the other hand, if the skeletal pattern becomes worse, it may be necessary to employ an extraction procedure. It cannot be emphasized too strongly that it is difficult at an early age to make definitive decisions about many occlusal problems, particularly the decision to extract permanent teeth. A decision of this kind is made better as the child approaches maturity.

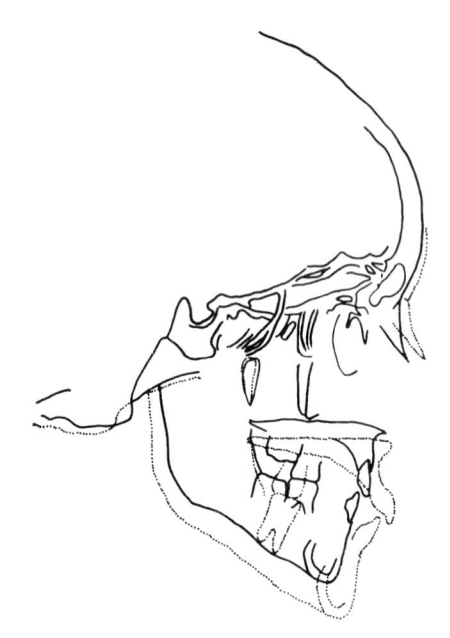

Fig. 10-12. Normal growth pattern; solid line, 5 years of age; broken line, 8 years of age. The maxillary teeth and alveolar process develop in a downward and forward direction.

A facial mutilation produced by early serial extraction is shown in Fig. 10-12. A dentist extracted four bicuspids based only on the measurement of the arch length and the mesiodistal diameters of the teeth. Unfortunately, he did not take into consideration future dental arch changes as well as the facial esthetics of the patient. Following serial extraction the lips are markedly retruded; the patient therefore has an overly flattened, dished-in appearance.

Early procedures may also be problematic from a mechanical point of view. With more and more teeth present in the mouth, it is possible to design appliances that give control over tooth movement and over anchorage. During the primary and mixed dentition it is not so easy to control these teeth. For example, during serial extraction posterior segments can drift forward. If the bicuspids are extracted, the posterior segments are then able to drift forward (Fig. 10-13). The patient may end up with arch length problems and crowding of the anterior teeth with four bicuspids removed. Holding arches with a lingual arch by itself does not ensure that posterior teeth will not drift forward into the extraction site after the loss of the bicuspid.

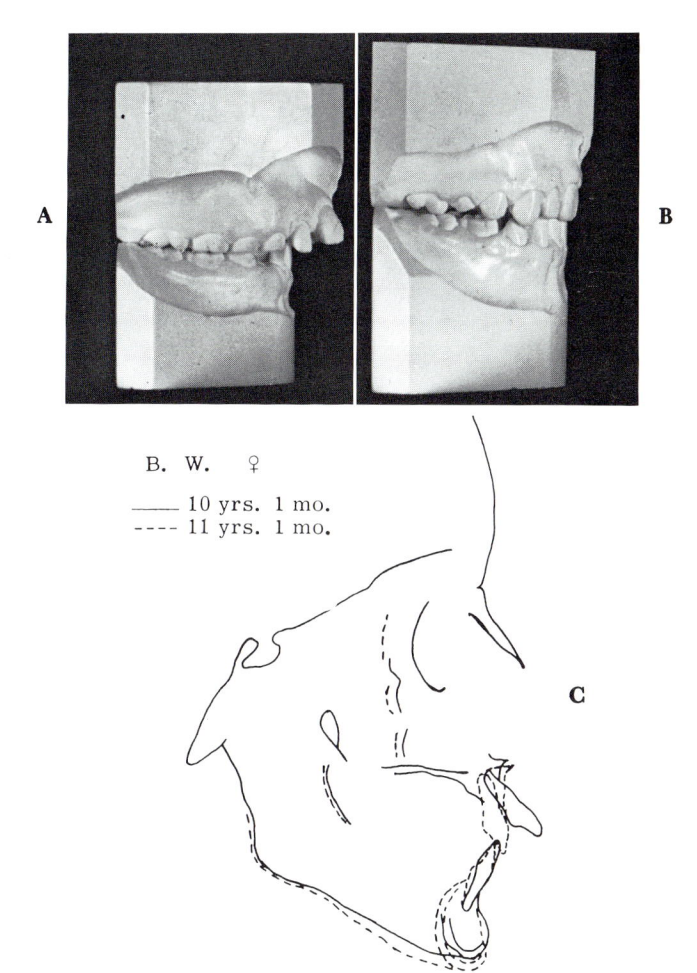

Fig. 10-13. Cervical headgear to the maxillary arch was used to intercept a developing Class II, division 1 malocclusion. A, Before treatment. B, After treatment.

One of the difficulties of early interceptive procedures is that the period of active treatment and observation usually will last a number of years. In other words, a long period of supervision is required. Psychologically this can wear out many patients so that, if comprehensive treatment is needed at a later time, cooperation may not be as good as one would like. In many children there are certain advantages in minimizing the length of the time that they must be under active treatment with an orthodontist. It is discouraging to many children and their parents that retaining devices must be continually made and that retreatment may be required as new teeth erupt and as growth proceeds toward maturity.

One last disadvantage of early treatment should be mentioned. It is desirable in some types of cases, particularly Class II malocclusions, to start treatment at the time of the pubertal growth spurt. Since at this time more improvement in the spatial relationship of the maxilla to the mandible can occur, less tooth movement is needed to correct the Class II occlusion and to reduce the deep overbite. Thus orthodontic treatment is simplified and the amount of tooth movement is reduced if treatment is started at those times when the mandible is growing at a rapid rate, provided, of course, the direction of growth will aid the skeletal pattern. Treatment that is started too early, particularly certain types of headgear treatment, is not as likely to be successful since the amount of mandibular growth is too small and the correction must be accomplished by tooth movement followed by a longer period of retention. On the other hand, corrections that occur mainly because of beneficial growth changes appear to be more stable.

Whenever possible, the family dentist and orthodontist should be interested in intercepting a malocclusion in order to minimize the magnitude of the dentofacial deformity. Although there are many advantages to be found in currently used interceptive procedures, it should be remembered that there are also many disadvantages. Greater knowledge and skill in case analysis and treatment planning are required in interceptive therapy than in treating a patient approaching maturity. In some instances, improper interceptive procedures may make a malocclusion more difficult to treat or almost untreatable at a later time. As the dentist learns more about growth and development and is able to predict with greater accuracy the changes that may be expected, the number of cases that are suitable for interceptive procedures will increase. Until that time care should be exercised before instituting any interceptive procedure, particularly of a radical nature such as the extraction of permanent teeth, at an early age.

## CONCLUSION

To a large extent many malocclusions are genetically determined. These malocclusions cannot be prevented in the usual sense of the word, but at times early interceptive procedures may minimize the degree of dental deformity. On the other hand, malocclusions that are primarily produced by environmental factors, such as trauma to the jaws, deleterious habits, premature loss of primary teeth, and improper operative dental procedures, can be prevented. Early or interceptive orthodontic procedures cannot be recommended for all orthodontic problems since in many instances early treatment may complicate or make more difficult treatment at a later age. As more and more knowledge is made available for the prediction of growth and development of bones, muscles, and dental arches, it will then become possible to treat a greater number of cases during the primary and mixed dentitions.

**REFERENCES**

1. Broadbent, B. H.: Ontogenetic development of occlusion, Angle Orthodont. **11:**223, 1941.
2. Brodie, A. G.: Consideration of musculature in diagnosis and treatment, Amer. J. Orthodont. **38:**823, 1952.
3. Brodie, A. G.: Late growth changes in the human face, Angle Orthodont. **23:**146, 1953.
4. Brodie, A. G.: On the growth of the jaws and the eruption of the teeth, Angle Orthodont. **12:**109, 1942.
5. Cleall, J. F.: Deglutition; a study of form and function, Amer. J. Orthodont. **51:**566-594, 1965.
6. Dewel, B. F.: A critical analysis of serial extraction in orthodontic treatment, Amer. J. Orthodont. **45:**424, 1959.
7. Kaplan, M. J.: Note on psychological implications of thumbsucking, J. Pediat. **37:**555, 1950.
8. Kjellgren, B.: Serial extraction as a corrective procedure in dental orthopedic therapy, Tr. European Orthodont. Soc., pp. 134-160, 1947-1948.
9. Kraus, B. S., Wise, W. J., and Frei, R. H.: Heredity and the craniofacial complex, Amer. J. Orothodont. **45:**172, 1959.
10. Lundstrom, A.: Tooth size and occlusion in twins, Stockholm, 1948, A. B. Fahlcrantz Boktryckeri.
11. Moorrees, C. F. A.: The dentition of the growing child, Cambridge, Massachusetts, 1959, Harvard University Press.
12. Speidel, T. D.: Jaw growth and tooth eruption in their relation to space maintenance, J.A.D.A. **45:**541, 1952.
13. Stockard, C. R., and others: The genetic and endocrine basis for differences in form and behavior, Amer. Anat. Memoirs, Philadelphia, 1941, Wistar Institute.

# Chapter 11 Preventive operative dentistry
## David L. Moore

Introduction
Diagnosing and treating enamel caries
    Diagnosing enamel caries
    Treating enamel caries
Preventing defective restorations
    Isolating the operating field
    Preventing recurrent caries
        Controlling the cariogenic flora
        Extension for prevention
        Preparing the enamel walls
        Fluoride in the preparation
        Cavity varnish
        Adapting the restorative material to the walls of the preparation
        Finishing the restoration
    Preventing physical failure of the restorative material
        Retention form
        Resistance form
    Preventing periodontal involvement
Preventing the loss of pulpal vitality
    Pulp protection
    Pulp capping
        Direct
        Indirect
        Teeth with vital pulps and periapical lesions
    Pulpotomy
Preventing the loss of the tooth
    Conventional endodontics
    Endodontic surgery
Preventing crown and bridge failures
Conclusion

## INTRODUCTION

The role played by restorative dentistry in prevention begins after the caries attack. Before the turn of the century, G. V. Black initiated many principles of prevention. The application of these principles to the daily routine of practice remains an important part of a preventive program.

Preventive dentistry has added a new approach to restorative therapy. The preventive approach requires the use of counseling sessions, visual aids, toothbrushing demonstrations, dental floss, topical fluorides and recall systems, as well as carbide burs, diamond instruments, amalgam, silicate, and gold. The materials, skills, and techniques for primary prevention enable the dentist to achieve a continual reduction of the caries activity in the mouths of his patients. Therefore enamel caries can be treated chemically rather than restoratively, restorations can be placed in less hostile environments, and recurrent caries can be prevented. Thus increasingly complex restorative therapy and tooth loss can be avoided.

## DIAGNOSING AND TREATING ENAMEL CARIES

Preventive restorative dentistry requires the treatment of dental caries at the earliest time the lesions can be detected. With rare exception, the initial attack of dental caries is on enamel; therefore early diagnosis of enamel caries is important in determining the appropriate treatment.

Historically, the accepted "treatment" for caries confined to enamel was either to label it incipient and watch and wait or to restore all incipient lesions before they had a chance to progress into the dentin.

Preventive dentistry now provides a third and better choice of treatment for enamel caries. Enamel caries need no longer progress into dentin. Fluorides applied to the tooth surfaces can inhibit enamel caries and arrest the progress of incipient lesions.[1] A preventive program that includes fluoride therapy provides the initial treatment for dental caries.

### Diagnosing enamel caries

Smooth surface enamel caries begins as a white spot of demineralization. The area may subsequently become stained and present some cavitation in the enamel. Enamel caries of the gingival third of the tooth is diagnosed by clinical examination. A sharp explorer tine pressed into the lesion will not penetrate; the area is hard. The lesion should be diagnosed as enamel caries, notwithstanding the histologic changes in the dentin that accompany the affected enamel.

Pit caries and fissure caries are also diagnosed by clinical examination. Roentgenograms seldom show occlusal caries before the condition is clinically obvious. The following method, described by G. V. Black, remains the procedure of choice.[2]

The discovery of pit and fissure decays is usually a simple procedure. As the examination proceeds, the surfaces of the teeth in each bicuspid-molar region should be dried with blasts of air in order that the best view may be had. An exploring tine, with a small, sharp pointed end, should be used to test the positions of all pits, even though they appear not to be decayed. The point should be applied with some pressure, and if it enters the enamel a little, so that a very slight pull is required to remove it, the pit should be marked for a restoration, even though there is no sign of decay.*

Although the sticky fissure usually indicates dentin caries, the decision of whether or not the probe actually enters the dentin is subjective. Stained, questionable pits and fissures may be considered enamel caries.

Interproximal enamel caries is diagnosed by periapical and bite-wing roentgenographic examination. Some interproximal carious lesions will appear confined to enamel. Others will appear to reach the dentinoenamel junction but will be questionable. Still others will show definite penetration into the dentin. Unless there is evidence of definite penetration into the dentin, the interproximal lesion should be diagnosed and treated as enamel caries.

---

*From Black, G. V.: Operative dentistry, ed. 7, Chicago, 1936, Medico-Dental Publishing Co., p. 31.

250  *Improving dental practice through preventive measures*

**Treating enamel caries**

The preferred treatment for enamel caries is *not* restorative therapy. The treatment consists of: (1) removing bacterial plaque from all enamel surfaces; (2) impregnating the enamel with fluorides; (3) helping the patient to reduce the ingestion of cariogenic foods; (4) teaching the patient a method of effective home care; and (5) continuing the therapy through periodic recall. Each of these treatment measures is dealt with in depth in other chapters of this text.

This preventive treatment of enamel caries requires continued application and evaluation. A progressive radiographic history mount is a helpful tool (Fig. 11-1). It is a visual progress report that aids in evaluating the effectiveness of the conservative therapy and in determining the appropriate time for surgical (operative) intervention.

In a preventive practice many patients will have incipient enamel lesions that progress extremely slowly if at all. Consider the following case history.

The bite-wing roentgenograms of a first-year dental student at the University of Missouri at Kansas City were made in 1952 (Fig. 11-2). The roentgenograms revealed occlusal caries and eight incipient proximal lesions. Indeed some of the

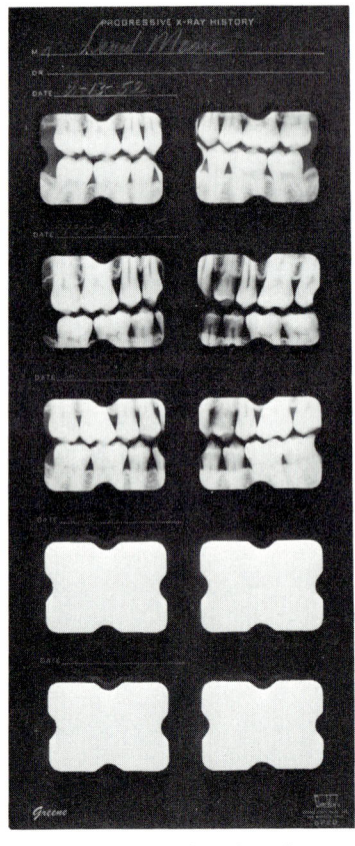

Fig. 11-1. A progressive x-ray history mount for bite-wing roentgenograms (Greene Dental Products, Inc., Los Angeles, California). A record such as this provides a chronologic report on the progress of interproximal enamel caries and helps to determine the appropriate time for restorative therapy.

proximal caries appeared to reach the dentinoenamel junction, prompting the opinion that compound amalgam restorations were indicated. After much discussion among the dental school instructors, it was decided to treat the occlusal carious lesions with Class I amalgam restorations. The proximal enamel lesions were managed with preventive therapy, which included topical fluorides. Seventeen years later the occlusal amalgam restorations remained intact (Fig. 11-3). Two of the proximal lesions had progressed into the dentin and were restored. The other six proximal lesions remained in enamel. Indeed two of the previous

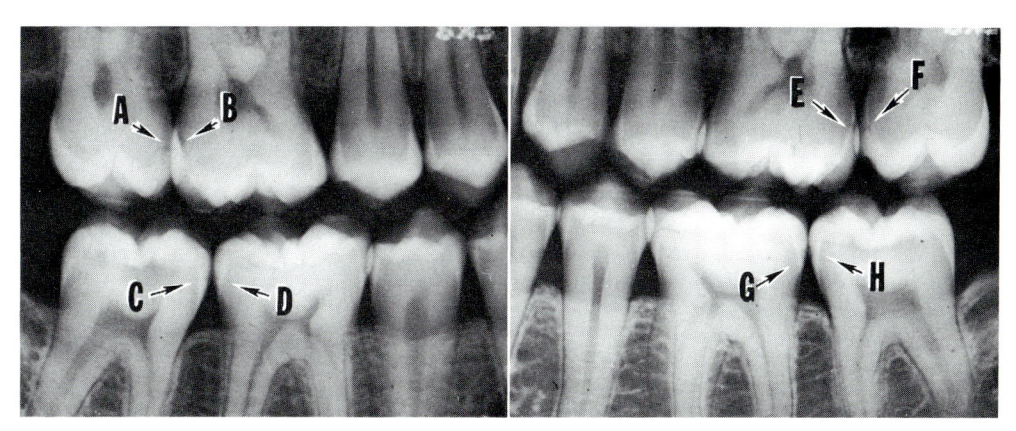

Fig. 11-2. Bite-wing roentgenograms of a 21-year-old patient, taken in 1952. Note the occlusal caries of the mandibular second molars and the interproximal caries at **AB, CD, EF,** and **GH**. The caries at **AB, EF,** and **GH** appears to have reached the dentin. Clinical examination revealed occlusal caries in each of the molars. Occlusal amalgam restorations were placed and the interproximal caries was treated with a preventive program that included topical fluoride therapy.

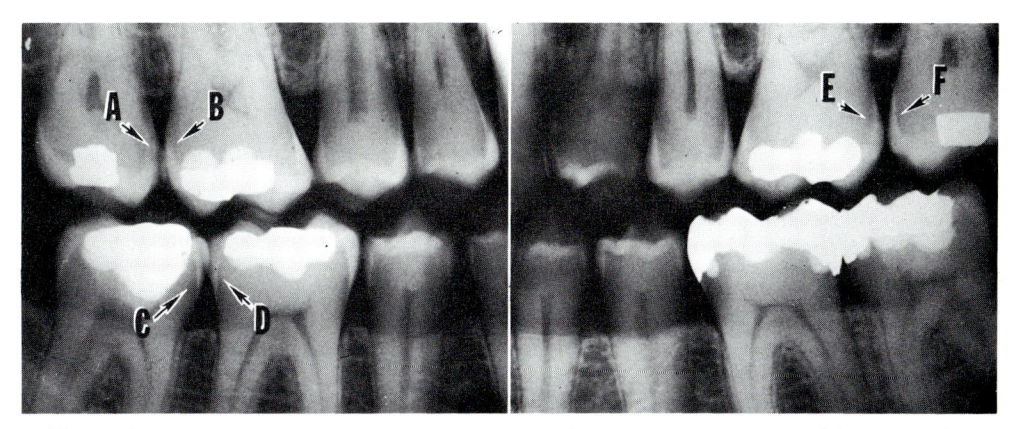

Fig. 11-3. Bite-wing roentgenograms of the same patient as in Fig. 11-2, taken in 1969. After 17 years the interproximal caries on the mandibular right molars had progressed into dentin. Inlay restorations were placed. The remaining interproximal lesions had not progressed. The caries apparent in Fig. 11-1, **EF**, is not apparent in Fig. 11-2, **EF**, and may represent the remineralization of the carious lesion. The patient responded to conservative restorative and positive preventive therapy.

**252** *Improving dental practice through preventive measures*

lesions were not apparent on the later roentgenograms and may represent remineralized enamel caries (Fig. 11-3, *E* and *F*). This patient responded to conservative restorative and positive preventive therapy.

As in other forms of therapy, the success of preventive treatment of enamel caries depends on the response of the patient; when the patient begins to respond to preventive therapy, more and more carious enamel lesions will remain in enamel.

## PREVENTING DEFECTIVE RESTORATIONS

When caries has progressed into the dentin, cavity preparation and restoration become the treatments of choice. The purpose of this treatment is to prevent further extension of the disease and to prevent the ultimate loss of the tooth. Unlike other forms of therapy, the treatment of dental caries does not rely on biologic replacement of the diseased tissue. Restorative dentistry replaces the lost tissue with a foreign body that is retained by mechanical means. The therapy usually is an immediate success. However, the complex oral environment defies permanence in restorative therapy; restorations fail.

The magnitude of the problem of defective restorations is not known. One report indicated that more than a third of the operative effort for 907 patients was consumed replacing defective restorations.[3] Fig. 11-4 shows the percentage of failure of the various restorative materials. If the failure rate of restorative therapy only approaches this magnitude, the problem deserves careful consideration by the dentist committed to the philosophy of prevention.

### Isolating the operating field

The principle of the isolated operating field for restorative procedures needs no defense. Adequate access and vision are prerequisites for proper cavity preparation. The exclusion of saliva is necessary for the proper placement of all restorative materials. An isolated operating field provides the optimum working environment for restorative procedures and is therefore basic to preventing the failure of restorations.

The rubber dam is the best method for maintaining an isolated operating field. Its advantages have been expounded with considerable emotion for many years,[4-6] yet this helpful tool has been largely neglected by the dental profession. Results from a survey indicate that, for operative procedures throughout the United States, the rubber dam was used routinely only 5.3 percent of the time.[7]

| PERCENTAGE OF FAILURE | |
|---|---|
| AMALGAM | 42.4 |
| SILICATE | 67.5 |
| INLAY | 31.4 |
| FOIL | 20.9 |

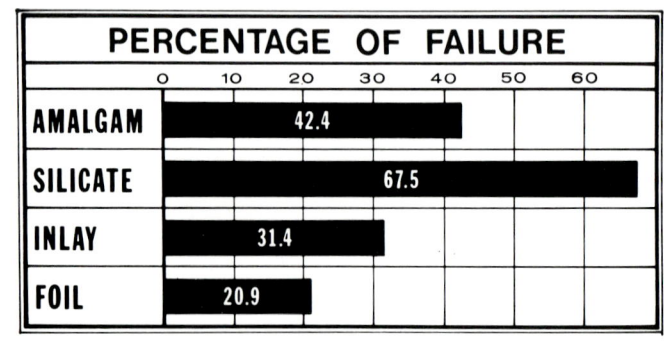

**Fig. 11-4.** Percentage of failure of various restorative materials, from a study of 3,817 restorations that required replacement.

Notwithstanding the general nonacceptance, the dentist interested in improving dental practice through preventive measures should consider a return to the use of the rubber dam. Here are some suggestions that may help to turn this mental hazard into a helpful tool.

1. Decide to relearn the use of the rubber dam. This will be the most difficult part of incorporating the rubber dam into your practice. The inertia of established routines is difficult to overcome.

2. Begin by selecting easy cases. Make the relearning period as atraumatic as possible. Isolate only the maxillary anterior teeth, or one or two posterior teeth, until you have built up speed and confidence.

3. Isolate a minimum number of teeth. The difficulty and time of placement increase in direct proportion to the number of teeth isolated. For a single occlusal restoration one hole for the tooth to be restored is adequate. When the contact is involved, include the proximating teeth. If you find that you need or desire more access, include additional teeth until you learn what is minimum for you.

4. Don't try for a masterpiece. Fully isolated and ligated quadrants or arches displaying beautiful symmetry require an inordinate amount of time to achieve. After all, the restoration and not the rubber dam is the goal.

5. Ligate only when necessary. A heavy-gauge rubber dam material retracts tissue and in many cases requires no ligation. Ligation is usually necessary only when additional retraction is needed. Remember that ligatures take time and are traumatic to gingival tissue.

6. Use a simple rubber dam holder such as the Young's rubber dam frame or the Nuggaard-Ostby (N-O) rubber dam holder. These holders can be placed quickly and are adequate for the purpose. They are readily accepted by patients.

7. Don't let the psychic trauma of unassisted fumbling while learning to use the rubber dam in dental school deprive you of the advantages of the rubber dam. Work out the routine with your assistant. As with other procedures, the assistant helps to make the placement of the rubber dam quicker and easier.

The rubber dam functions well for ultraspeed, washed field operations. Evacuation of water and debris is facilitated and the hazard of aspirating instruments and debris is decreased. When the air turbine drill is used, large numbers of organisms are liberated into the surrounding air.[8] The rubber dam reduces the bacteria in the aerosols and thus becomes a factor in protecting the dentist.[9]

An isolated operating field can be obtained and good restorative dentistry can be accomplished without the use of the rubber dam; however, the dentist who is serious about implementing a preventive philosophy of dentistry should give the rubber dam an honest try. It provides the most efficient means for maintaining an isolated operating field, which is basic to sound restorative procedures.

**Preventing recurrent caries**

Recurrent caries is a major cause for the failure of restorations. A report of amalgam failures assigned 53.5 percent of the total failures to recurrent caries.[10] Once dental caries has attacked the tooth at the margins of restorations, there is no good alternative to increasingly complex restorative therapy. Recurrent caries is demoralizing to the patient, dangerous to the pulp, potentially injurious to patient relations, and time-consuming for the dentist.

Recurrent caries can be prevented by providing a less hostile environment in the

254  *Improving dental practice through preventive measures*

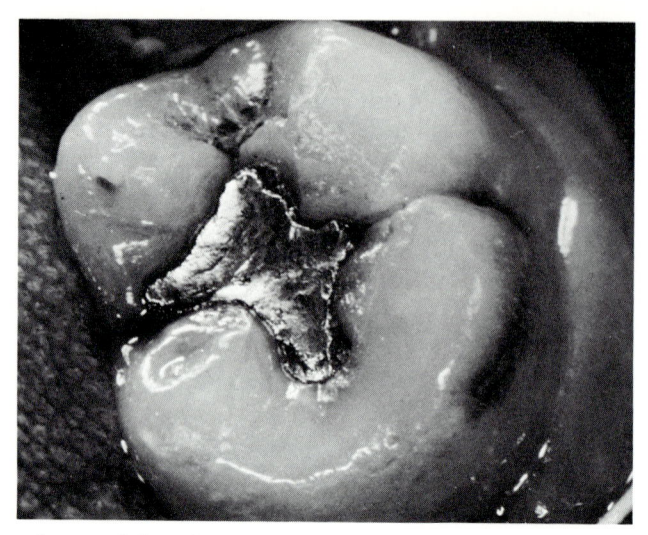

**Fig. 11-5.** An underextended occlusal amalgam restoration. Recurrent caries occurred where the restoration terminated in the fissures. The distal pit was also carious. Note the marginal ditching caused by fracture of the amalgam at the margins.

patient's mouth prior to restorative therapy; such an environment must be provided by the dentist. Restorations placed in an uncontrolled cariogenic environment are doomed to failure from marginal caries. "The half-life of even a good restoration, in a highly cariogenic oral environment is very short—perhaps only 1½ to 2 years."[11]

The dentist's role in preventing recurrent caries continues in the restorative phase. He must place restorations that will not invite recurrent caries. Sound restorative principles coupled with current primary preventive measures can virtually eliminate recurrent caries.

**Controlling the cariogenic flora.** The dentist controls the cariogenic flora in the patient's mouth by (1) removing bacterial plaque from all enamel surfaces, (2) impregnating the enamel with fluorides, (3) helping the patient to reduce the ingestion of cariogenic foods, (4) teaching the patient a method of effective home care, and (5) continuing the therapy through periodic recall. (These same measures comprise the treatment for enamel caries.) Success in preventing recurrent caries hinges on the ability of the dentist to develop his skill in the use of these treatment procedures.

**Extension for prevention.** Placing the margins of a restoration in relatively caries-immune areas is axiomatic. "Extension for prevention" remains a valid principle for the dentist involved in prevention.

Inadequately extended occlusal fissures provide a common site for the attack of dental caries. Fissures are normally considered to be caries-prone. In addition, the margin of a restoration in a fissure increases the hazard of recurrent caries.[12] Therefore a cavity preparation should be extended to include all fissures so that the margins of the preparation do not terminate in fissures. Fig. 11-5 illustrates recurrent caries in fissures that should have been included in the original amalgam restoration.

Underextended proximal margins invite recurrent caries. The buccal and lingual proximal walls must clear the contact area. Margins of a restoration left in a contact area cannot be properly finished by the dentist, nor can they be kept clean by the

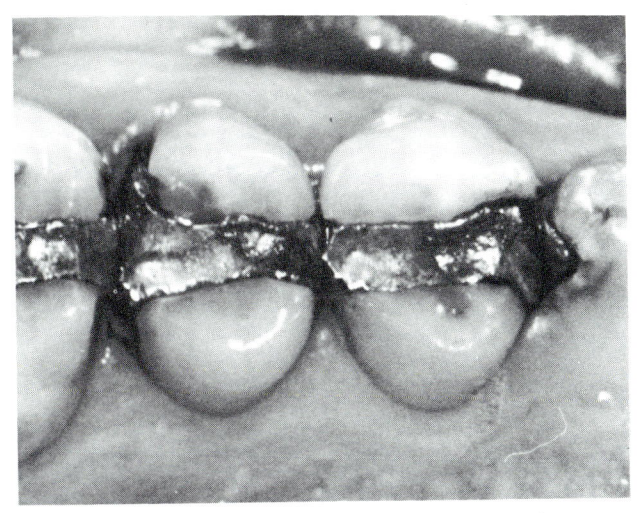

Fig. 11-6. Amalgam failures. Note the underextended buccal proximal margins of the premolars, the marginal breakdown, the displaced Class III restoration, and the poor contour, contact, and finish of the restorations.

patient. Recurrent caries at underextended buccal proximal margins is illustrated in Fig. 11-6. The lingual proximal margins were properly extended, and even though the margins were poorly carved and finished, recurrent caries did not develop. The buccal and lingual proximal margins should be extended at least 0.5 mm. beyond the contact area in order to provide "extension for prevention." A No. 23 explorer provides a handy gauge. The tine is approximately 0.5 mm. in diameter at about 3 mm. from the point.

Underextended gingival margins invite recurrent caries. Margins of restorations, which do not go beyond the contact area gingivally, can neither be properly finished by the dentist nor kept clean by the patient. The gingival extension of the preparation is influenced by the extent of the carious lesion and by the extent of the contact area. The gingival wall should extend at least 0.5 mm. below the contact area.

The practice of routinely placing gingival margins in the sulcus may be more iatrogenic than preventive. The margins of restorations placed in the gingival sulcus irritate the sulcus epithelium and in time become supragingival as a result of gingival recession. Sound tooth structure is the kindest of all materials to the tissues of the gingival sulcus. Leave it there whenever possible.

**Preparing the enamel walls.** Cavity preparations can now be made using a single rotary instrument. One carbide bur or diamond instrument operating at ultraspeeds can rough out the form of almost any preparation in a very short time. These roughed out preparations, however, should not be considered finished preparations.

Special attention must be paid to the enamel walls of the preparation. Properly prepared enamel walls provide a firm foundation for the adaptation of the restorative material. On the other hand, rough enamel margins present unsupported enamel rods that may subsequently break away. The resulting loss of marginal integrity renders the tooth vulnerable to recurrent decay. After the preparation has been roughed out at high speed the enamel walls should then be finished with slow speed rotary instruments and/or hand instruments. The enamel walls should first be smoothed in the direction of the enamel rods. Then, for those restorative materials which permit, the cavosurface angle should be beveled.

Because amalgam and silicate cement are friable materials, amalgam and silicate cement preparations should not be beveled. For these preparations a nonserrated fissure bur running at slow speed is effective for finishing the enamel walls. The bur should be held perpendicular to the enamel surface. Hand instruments should be used in the areas of limited access. For example, a bur should not be used for finishing the proximal box portion of a Class II preparation; the limited access endangers the proximating tooth. Sharp side-cutting hatchets provide a quick and efficient means for finishing the buccal, lingual, and gingival walls of the proximal box.

Direct filling resins are not as friable as amalgam and silicate cement; however, distortion or fracture may occur if the material is thin at the margin, and therefore a bevel is contraindicated. The enamel walls should be finished in the same manner as for amalgam or silicate cement.

Because gold is a burnishable material, beveled preparations are desirable. Bevels for cast gold inlays should be definite enough to be visible to the unaided eye. Small, indefinite bevels fail to provide sufficient gold at the margins for burnishing and finishing. The occlusal bevels may be made with a nonserrated fissure bur or diamond point. Small abrasive discs provide an excellent means for smoothing and flaring the buccal and lingual proximal walls. The gingival bevel is made with a flame-shaped diamond point.

Pure gold is softer and more burnishable than cast gold alloy. Therefore gold foil and powdered gold require smaller bevels than cast gold. A few light strokes with a sharp chisel or hatchet provide a sufficient bevel. The slight bevels thus achieved are generally not visible to the unaided eye.

A return to the routine use of hand instruments in practice may initiate better preparation of enamel walls. The fact that hand instruments are a mental hazard in our age of ultraspeed may be due to the influence of the numerous and dull instruments of student days. In the modern dental practice only a few hand instruments need be used routinely. Side-cutting hatchets, Wedelstaedt chisels, and spoon excavators provide the core. The dental assistant, using an electric instrument sharpener, can quickly provide hand instruments that are both efficient and pleasant to use.

**Fluoride in the preparation.** The protective effect of topical fluorides on enamel is well documented. There is now evidence that topical fluorides have a similar protective effect on freshly cut dentin. Topical fluoride is reported to have increased the acid resistance of dentin and retarded the acid penetration into deeper layers of the tissue.[13] Desensitization of dentin also resulted after fluoride application.[14] In addition, 10 percent stannous fluoride remineralized carious dentin left in the depths of a cavity.[15]

As early as 1949, fluoride applied to freshly cut dentin was shown to be a pulpal irritant.[16] In fact, sodium fluoride crystals, sealed in cavities, produced pulpal abscesses.[17] More recent evidence, however, exonerates fluoride. A solution of 10 percent stannous fluoride applied to freshly cut dentin did not produce untoward pulp reaction.[18] Therefore the routine use of fluoride solutions in cavity preparations should be considered as an additional means of preventing recurrent caries. Bases and liners should be used in the deep areas of freshly cut dentin prior to applying this potential pulpal irritant. Future research will undoubtedly provide more information in this area.

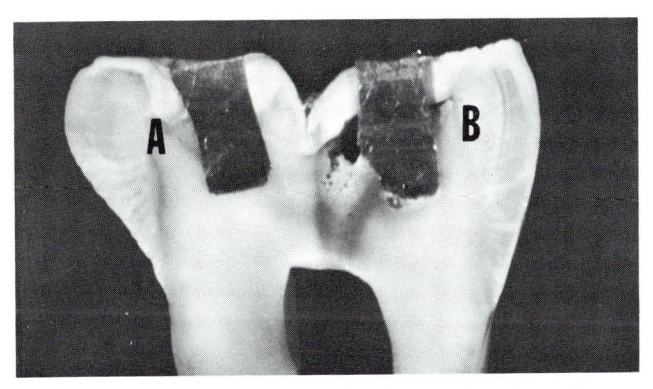

Fig. 11-7. Amalgam restorations exposed to an in vitro cariogenic environment. **A**, Both the dentin and enamel walls of this restoration were lined with cavity varnish. **B**, Caries attacked this unlined restoration. (Courtesy Drs. J. Ellis and L. Brown.)

**Cavity varnish.** Cavity varnish helps to seal the margins of restorations against the marginal penetration of fluids (see p. 256). In addition to preventing marginal penetration of fluids, cavity varnish applied to the enamel walls of preparations may reduce the incidence of recurrent decay.[19] In vitro caries was produced at the margins of unlined amalgam restorations. Lined restorations showed significantly less marginal caries. The amalgam restorations in Fig. 11-7 were a part of the study. They were placed in the same tooth, at the same time, and in a similar manner. One restoration had the enamel margins sealed with cavity varnish prior to insertion of the amalgam. The other restoration was not lined. After 16 weeks of exposure to the in vitro cariogenic environment, the lined restoration showed no recurrent caries but caries attacked the tooth at the margin of the unlined restoration.

Both the dentin and the enamel walls of amalgam preparations should be lined with cavity varnish as a preventive measure for recurrent caries. However, only the dentin wall should be lined for silicate cement restorations; the enamel walls should be in direct contact with the silicate cement. The fluoride flux in the silicate cement can then exert its anticariogenic effect on the enamel. Future research may determine the advisability of using cavity varnish at the margin of direct resins, gold foils, inlays, and crowns.

**Adapting the restorative material to the walls of the preparation.** Incomplete adaptation of the restorative material to the walls of the preparation invites recurrent caries. Discrepancies between the tooth and restoration provide a site for the accumulation of plaque and an avenue for the penetration of fluids.

The dry field is a prerequisite for the proper adaptation of restorative materials to the walls of the preparation. Saliva and blood contamination adversely affect the physical properties of amalgam, silicate cement, plastics, and direct golds. Even the composite resins, advertised as not being affected by moisture, cannot be adequately adapted to the walls of a preparation across a barrier of saliva.

Amalgam is adapted directly to the cavity walls during the condensation procedure. The condensing force should be directed toward all walls and line angles of the preparation. Undercondensation occurs at the walls and margins when amalgam is simply plugged into the preparation. Spherical alloys require less condensing force than that required by conventional alloys. Larger condensers should be used for condensing the spherical alloys and the condensation procedure may be described as pushing, smearing, or buttering the material against the cavity walls.

Direct golds are also adapted to the cavity walls by the condensing force. The force should be directed toward the walls and line angles. Each increment must be completely condensed with overlapping steps of the condenser before the next increment is added. Powdered golds may be adapted by hand condensation, as long as the rules of magnitude and direction of forces are observed.

Silicate cement and restorative resins are best adapted to cavity walls in relatively small increments. Poor adaptation may occur when large bulks of material are forced into the preparation by the matrix strip.

Cast gold inlays and crowns must be adapted to the walls of a preparation by cement. The cement usually used for this purpose, zinc phosphate cement, is soluble in mouth fluids. The solubility is increased when thin, soupy mixes are used. In addition, even slight moisture contamination during the mixing and setting of the cement increases the solubility.[20] Moisture contamination caused the crystal growth in the specimen of zinc phosphate cement shown in Fig. 11-8, *A*. This cement was four times as soluble as the specimen with no moisture contamination seen in Fig. 11-8, *B*. Therefore thick creamy mixes of cement should be used for cementing cast gold restorations. Moisture should be excluded during the mixing of the cement and the dry field maintained as long as possible during the initial set of the cement. Burnishing and finishing the gold margins on the tooth complete the proper adaptation of cast gold to the enamel margins.

**Finishing the restoration.** The goal in finishing a restoration is to provide smooth

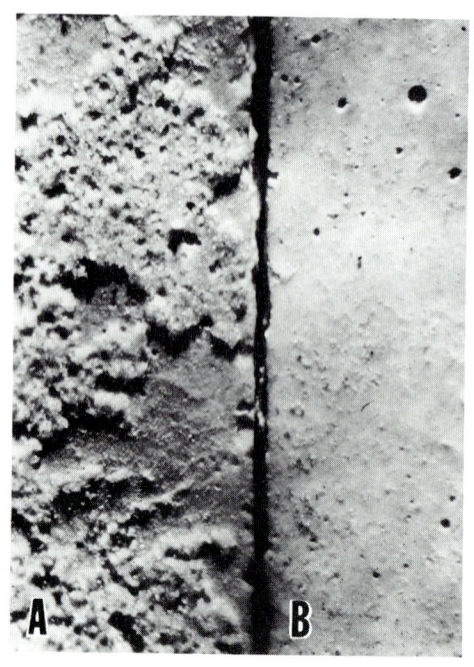

Fig. 11-8. *A*, Moisture contamination during the initial set of zinc phosphate cement caused surface crystal growth and an increase in solubility. This specimen was four times as soluble as specimen **B**. **B**, Surface of zinc phosphate cement with no moisture contamination.

and polished surfaces and margins that may be kept clean with ease. Poorly finished surfaces and interproximal overhangs make flossing and cleaning difficult if not impossible. Unpolished occlusal margins trap debris.

Unfinished amalgam restorations display small spicules of amalgam at the margins that will ultimately fracture away and leave a rough, ditched margin. A round bur will remove the overextensions, and subsequent smoothing and polishing will produce restorations that help the patient in his program of home care. A philosophy of prevention produces finished and polished restorations.

## Preventing physical failure of the restorative material

Restorations fail when the restorative material fails. Attention should be given to the proper manipulation of the materials (see Chapter 17). In addition, cavity preparations should be designed to meet the requirements of the restorative material.

**Retention form.** All restorations are retained by frictional resistance between the restorative material and the walls of the preparation (cast gold restorations are adapted to the walls via the cement). Therefore both proper preparation of the cavity walls and good adaptation of the material to the walls are important factors in retention. A box form of the preparation, finished cavity walls, undercuts, and grooves provide adequate retention for most restorations.

Pins provide additional retention and are indicated when large amounts of tooth structure have been destroyed. The additional retention is gained with minimum destruction of the remaining tooth structure. Pins can be used with all restorative materials.

Pin retention broadens the scope of amalgam therapy. Grossly carious teeth can now be saved for patients who cannot or will not accept cast gold restorations for economic reasons. There is little or no evidence to suggest that properly placed pin amalgams are any more a liability to the patient than large cast gold restorations.

Pins do not reinforce amalgam.[21, 22] Sufficient bulk of amalgam needs no reinforcement. Pins do provide additional retention and reduce the likelihood of the displacement of large restorations.

Cemented pins, friction pins, and self-threading pins offer versatility in pin retention. Each has its advantages and disadvantages.[23-25] The following principles apply to all pin-retained amalgam restorations.

Use the minimum number of pins that will provide adequate retention. Although the retention increases with the number of pins, each pin is potentially hazardous to the pulp. Use the box form of the preparation and accessory grooves for the major retention; pins provide retention when retentive tooth structure is not available.

Use the minimum depth pinhole. The depth of pinhole should usually be 2.0 to 2.5 mm. Deeper pinholes are unnecessary for adequate retention and may encroach upon the pulp.

Use a minimum length of pin extending into the amalgam. The length should usually be 2.0 to 2.5 mm. Bend the pin into the preparation so that maximum bulk of amalgam covers the pin. Pins that approach the surface of the restoration increase the hazard of fracture.

**Resistance form.** Resistance form refers to the form of a preparation that enables the tooth and the restoration to resist the forces of mastication. Fracture of the restoration and/or tooth structure results when sufficient resistance form is not provided.

Cast gold restorations do not fracture. Therefore resistance form for inlays is concerned with protecting weakened tooth structure. For amalgam, silicate, and resin restorations, however, the restoration as well as the tooth structure must be protected from fracture.

The fracture of most restorations can be prevented by sufficient bulk of the restorative material, which is achieved by the proper depth of cavity preparation. The optimal depth in sound tooth structure is 0.5 to 1.0 mm. pulpal to the dentino-enamel junction.

Preparations at the optimal depth need no intermediate base. For preparations deeper than optimal, a base should be used to protect the pulp. The base should be kept at a minimal thickness, however, in order to maintain an adequate bulk of the restorative material. Zinc oxide–eugenol cement bases of 0.5 mm. thickness insulate the pulp and are capable of supporting the condensation of amalgam.[26] Therefore the use of a base to build up an amalgam preparation to ideal box form is unnecessary; this practice may actually weaken the restoration.

Sufficient bulk of the restorative material is achieved at the margins of restorations by providing a cavosurface with no bevel or flare. Marginal fracture is further prevented by removing the small spurs of the restorative material that may extend over the margin.

Fracture of tooth structure at the margins of restorations can be prevented by proper preparation of the enamel walls. Gross fracture of tooth structure is prevented by preserving as much of the sound tooth structure as possible and by covering weakened tooth structure. Large restorations make the remaining tooth structure more vulnerable to destructive forces. Conservatism is a cardinal principle of cavity preparation.

Large cutting instruments invite the excessive removal of tooth structure. For conservative preparations, a No. 34 inverted cone bur or a No. 56 nonserrated bur is indicated for roughing out the cavity. Large burs produce large preparations.

Eccentric cutting instruments also invite the excessive removal of tooth structure. The destructive action of eccentric instruments on tooth structure has been studied.[27] High-speed photography showed tooth structure being "blasted" away by the whipping action of the bur. Diamond instruments were more efficient than burs for the controlled removal of tooth structure.

When preventive restorative dentistry is practiced, sound tooth structure that is destroyed will be destroyed by caries and not by the dental bur. As the caries activity in patients becomes controlled, more and more sound tooth structure can be maintained to support restorations.

**Preventing periodontal involvement**

Restorations fail when they initiate or contribute to periodontal disease. The dentist can prevent this kind of failure by providing good margins, contour, contact, and occlusion for all restorations.

The conservative extension of preparations helps to prevent gingival irritation. Sound tooth structure is the kindest of all materials to the tissues of the gingival sulcus. Leave it there whenever possible. The margins of all restorations irritate the sulcus epithelium.[28] Therefore place the margin of a restoration in the sulcus only when the carious lesion has extended subgingivally or when esthetics is a major factor. Accompany this conservative extension with radical patient education and primary preventive measures.

Smooth margins, good contour, and good contact help the patient to maintain a healthy periodontium; these are achieved by attention to the details of wedging, carving, and finishing. At the completion of restorative treatment, bite-wing roentgenograms are helpful; by means of them gingival overhangs can be detected and corrected before they do damage to the periodontium.

The occlusion should also be checked at the completion of restorative therapy. Shiny wear facets can be detected on restorations in areas of premature occlusal contact. The prematurities can be relieved before they cause trouble. Premature occlusal contact on a single restoration invites fracture and can initiate a cycle of new occlusal interferences.

## PREVENTING THE LOSS OF PULPAL VITALITY

Preserving the vitality of the dental pulp is a part of the preventive philosophy. The vital cells can then continue their reparative function and can continue to maintain the viability of the hard tissues of the tooth.

The pulp has a remarkable capacity for repair. Unfortunately, the repair capacity for a given tooth at a given time cannot be predetermined. Injury that can be tolerated by most pulps may be sufficient to cause the death of others. Therefore the dentist should not unnecessarily injure vital pulp tissue.

### Pulp protection

Sound enamel and dentin are the best protectors of pulpal vitality. The dentist's initial responsibility for pulp protection is the conservation of sound tooth structure. Conservative cavity preparation is the goal. The depth of the preparation is the most critical factor in producing inflammation of the pulp; the inflammation increases with the depth of the cavity (Fig. 11-9).

Much has been written about thermal injury to the pulp. The heat produced

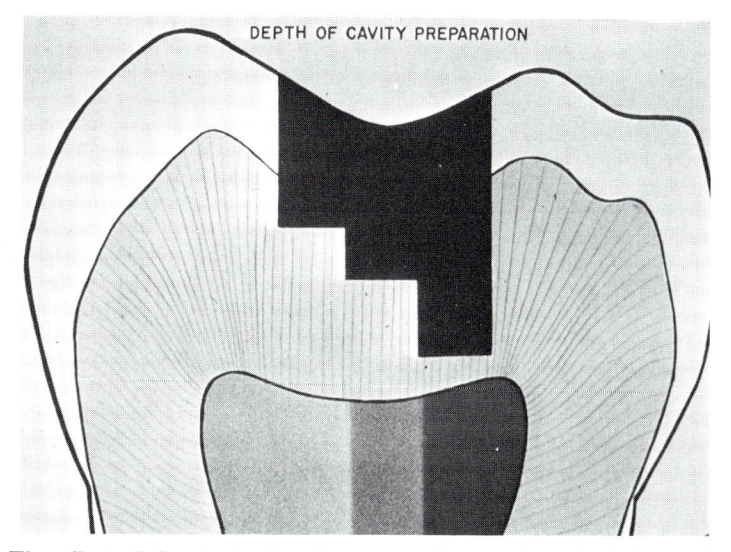

Fig. 11-9. The effect of the depth of cavity preparation on the pulp. Inflammation increases with the depth. Protection is afforded by remaining dentin. (Courtesy Drs. H. B. G. Robinson and W. Lefkowitz.)

262 *Improving dental practice through preventive measures*

while removing sound tooth structure at high speeds can literally burn the pulp to death. Thermal injury can be reduced by using water as a coolant.[29] Air alone also has been shown to reduce the effect of heat on the pulp.[30] More recent evidence indicates that an air-water mist is the most effective coolant for the gross removal of tooth structure.[31] However, the remaining thickness of dentin remains the most critical factor in pulp protection. Intermittent cutting and a few extra minutes of cutting time provide additional protection.

The pulp should also be protected from chemical injury. Harsh medicaments such as phenol, silver nitrate, and the like are contraindicated; these do little more than irritate the pulp. Final debridement is best accomplished by scrubbing the preparation with a pledget of cotton and water.

When the preparation is deeper than optimal, an intermediate base helps to insulate the pulp from further chemical and thermal injury. A cavity liner should precede the use of a zinc phosphate cement base. Both cavity varnishes and calcium hydroxide liners reduce pulpal injury from the acid in the zinc phosphate cement.

In a preventive practice, the pulpal tissue may be debilitated by dental caries, but not by mechanical, thermal, or chemical injury.

## Pulp capping

Pulp capping provides the means for preserving vital pulp tissue and restoring a diseased tooth to a healthy and useful state. Many materials may be used for pulp capping: calcium hydroxide stimulates the formation of reparative dentin; corticosteroids suppress inflammation; antibiotics reduce the number of pathogenic organisms in an infected pulp; certain base materials sedate the pulp. The fact is that many, perhaps most, diseased pulps will recover in the presence of any of these materials used singly or in combination with one another.

More important than pulp capping materials are the following principles of pulp capping therapy.

1. Pulpal vitality is the determining factor in prescribing pulp capping. Every known means including the vitalometer and excavation without anesthesia should be used to establish vitality. When there is pulpal vitality there is *hope* of recovery. The cells of the pulp are the final authority in determining when their repair capacity has been exceeded by injury.

2. The isolated operating field is basic to pulp capping procedures. Adequate vision, access, and exclusion of saliva contribute to success in pulp capping.

3. The sick pulp should not be injured unnecessarily during the excavation procedure. Establish an outline form that provides good vision and access for removing the carious dentin. Then remove the carious dentin cautiously but completely, proceeding from the dentinoenamel junction toward the pulp. Any direct exposure should occur only after the complete removal of the more superficial carious dentin. It is best to expose the pulp in a clean field if it is to be exposed at all.

4. The cavity should be sealed as completely as possible and as soon as possible. Failure of pulp capping results when a restoration leaks or fractures; therefore careful preparation of the enamel walls and an immediate permanent restoration are indicated.

5. The pulp must be given the opportunity to convalesce in an environment as free from trauma as practicable. Occlusal prematurities must be relieved from both the tooth and the restoration. Proximal contact must be achieved to support the

tooth. In addition, the restoration must be contoured, finished, and polished in order to restore the tooth to its normal function.

**Direct.** Historically, the basis for all pulpal therapy was complete removal of the carious dentin. In 1903, G. V. Black stated that "in no case should any decayed and softened material be left. It is better to expose the pulp than to leave it covered only with softened dentin."[32]

This concept produced many exposures and led to the development of direct pulp capping therapy. Early pulp capping technics were recommended for small exposures on young asymptomatic teeth.[33, 34] Subsequent investigation showed the pulp capable of repair in the presence of large exposures and adverse clinical symptoms.[35, 36] Direct pulp capping remains a preventive measure—it prevents the loss of teeth when the pulp is exposed.

**Indirect.** Indirect pulp capping has emerged as a preventative for direct pulpal exposure. As early as 1890, Miller reported "spontaneous healing" of softened dentin left under temporary restorations.[37] The healed dentin was described as being hard and smooth. Subsequent investigations favored leaving a thin layer of softened nondecomposed dentin in order to avoid an exposure of the pulp.[38, 39] Recent evidence continues to favor indirect pulp capping therapy.[40, 41]

Indirect pulp capping embodies the preventive principle of nonembarrassment of vital tissue. The major part of the irritating factor is removed with minimal trauma to the cells of the pulp. The microorganisms left behind do not endanger the integrity of the pulp, provided adequate closure of the cavity is achieved.[42]

**Teeth with vital pulps and periapical lesions.** In the past, teeth with periapical lesions have been excluded from pulp capping therapy. Roentgenographic evidence of a periapical lesion portends a nonvital pulp. The recommended treatment has been endodontic therapy or extraction.[43, 44]

However, roentgenographic evidence of periapical lesions does not necessarily

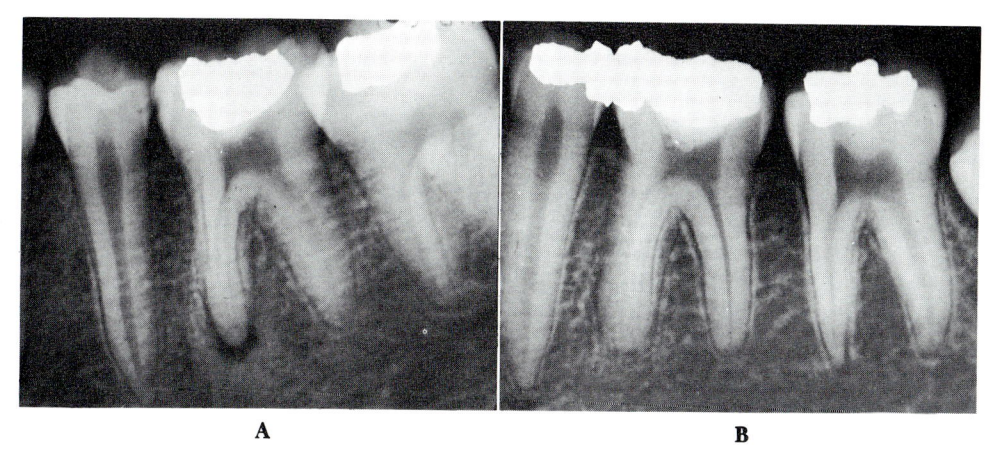

Fig. 11-10. A, A roentgenogram of a lower right first molar of a 15-year-old patient. The tooth responded to a vitalometer. Carious dentin was partially excavated without creating an exposure. The cavity was sealed with zinc oxide–eugenol cement. Note the radiolucency at the apex of the mesial root. B, The same tooth 8 months later. Note the disappearance of the periapical radiolucency and the reappearance of the lamina dura. The asymptomatic tooth responded to a vitalometer.

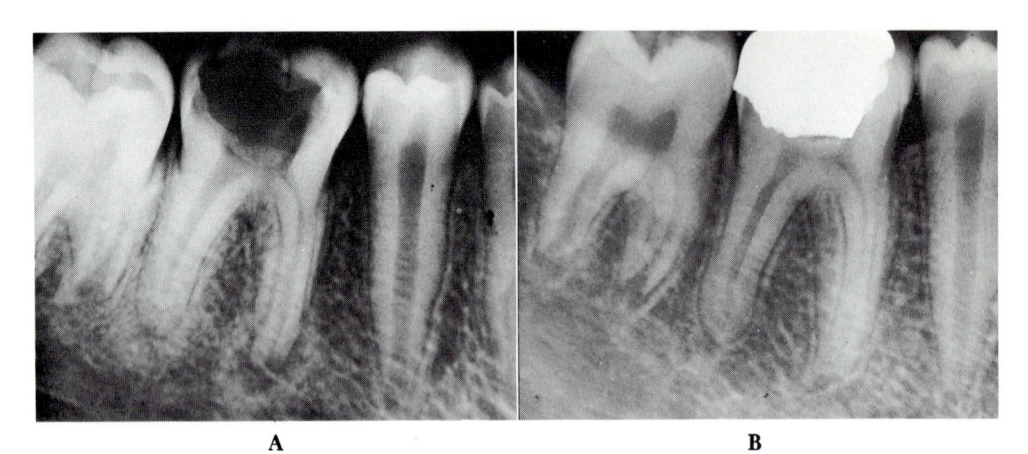

**Fig. 11-11. A,** A roentgenogram of a lower left first molar of a 14-year-old patient. Note the large carious lesion and periapical radiolucencies. The tooth did not respond to a vitalometer. Excavation of caries established pulpal vitality and resulted in a frank pulpal exposure. A base containing calcium hydroxide was placed and the cavity sealed with zinc oxide–eugenol cement. Six weeks later an amalgam restoration was placed. **B,** The same tooth 7 months later. Note the disappearance of the periapical radiolucencies and the reappearance of the lamina dura. The asymptomatic tooth responded to a vitalometer.

indicate a nonvital pulp.[45, 46] Direct and indirect pulp capping were effective in treating teeth with vital pulps and periapical lesions (Figs. 11-10 and 11-11). Roentgenographically the lesions resembled dental granulomas or chronic periapical abscesses, which occur as the sequelae to necrotic pulps. The pulps, however, responded to diagnostic tests, demonstrating vitality. Following the pulp capping procedures the pulps remained vital and asymptomatic and presented roentgenographic evidence of periapical repair.

Therefore the vitality of teeth with periapical lesions should be determined. If pulpal vitality can be demonstrated, pulp capping therapy may preserve the vital pulp tissue. Remember that the cells of the pulp are the final authority in determining when their repair capacity has been exceeded by injury. However, conservative treatment demands careful follow-up. If the pulp succumbs subsequent to pulp capping therapy, endodontic therapy or extraction is indicated.

**Pulpotomy**

Pulpotomy provides an additional means of preserving vital pulp tissue. Coronal pulp amputation has been advocated for treating cariously exposed pulps of both primary and young permanent teeth.[47] Both calcium hydroxide and formocresol are effective agents in maintaining radicular pulp vitality.[48, 49]

Most of the reported successes, however, have been with primary teeth. Long-term studies with a large number of permanent teeth have not been reported. Pulpotomies for permanent teeth demand careful roentgenographic follow-up. Two insidious complications may arise—internal resorption and the development of periapical lesions. Internal resorption has been reported, especially following calcium hydroxide therapy.[50] Fig. 11-12 illustrates extensive internal resorption 4 years after a pulpotomy was performed. The patient reported no symptoms. The tooth was ex-

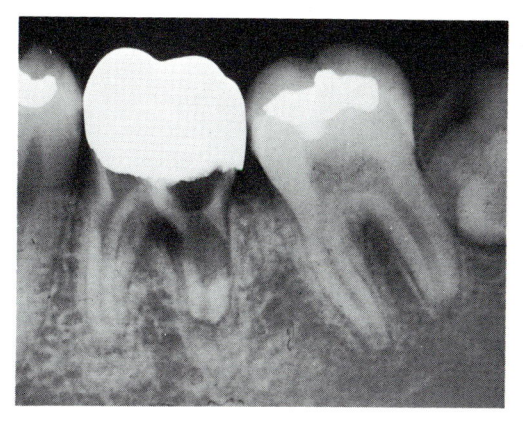

Fig. 11-12. Internal resorption following a vital pulpotomy. This roentgenogram was taken 4 years after the treatment. The tooth was extracted.

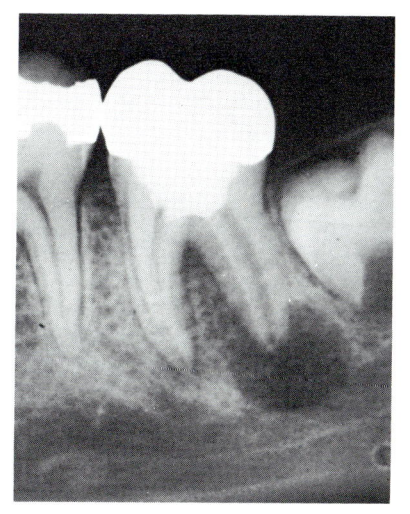

Fig. 11-13. A periapical lesion that occurred 6 months following a vital pulpotomy. Conventional endodontic therapy saved the tooth.

tracted because of the resorption. Fig. 11-13 illustrates the development of a periapical lesion, which was also symptomless, 6 months following a pulpotomy. Conventional endodontic therapy saved the tooth.

## PREVENTING THE LOSS OF THE TOOTH

The preservation of teeth is a concept of preventive dentistry that needs no defense. Each tooth is a keystone to the dental arches. In 1937, the report of Huschfield listed the sequelae of the individual missing tooth.[51] His report might be paraphrased in this way: the loss of one tooth produces 101 complications.

Endodontic therapy provides the means for saving teeth that were once destined for extraction. Research and years of experience have exploded the myth that endodontic therapy produced a "dead tooth" that was a liability to the patient. Improvements in materials and methods have made endodontic procedures easier to perform.

Short courses have become available to the general practitioner which are designed for learning or relearning endodontic techniques. In addition, dentists limiting their practice to endodontics have increased in number and are becoming more readily available for referral services. The dentist concerned with implementing a program of preventive dentistry can now provide endodontic service for his patients.

## Conventional endodontics

Endodontic therapy is indicated only after vital pulp therapy has failed or when the patient presents an already nonvital pulp. When there is vital pulp tissue there is hope of recovery. The first attempt should be to maintain the vitality of the pulp.

When the pulp has succumbed, conventional endodontics is the treatment of choice, even for teeth with periapical lesions. Periapical bone repairs when the irritating factor is removed and the apex of the tooth is effectively sealed. Periapical surgery, sometimes complicated for the general practitioner, is thus avoided. Note the periapical lesions of the first molar in Fig. 11-14, *A*. Periapical surgery was not acceptable to the parents of this teenage patient. The tooth was saved by conventional endodontic therapy. Six months after therapy periapical bone repair was evident. Fig. 11-14, *B,* shows the 3-year postoperative picture.

Endodontic surgery was considered for the lower incisors shown in Fig. 11-15, *A*. The periapical lesion was large. However, the more conservative approach of conventional endodontics was chosen. Periapical repair was complete 7 months after therapy (Fig. 11-15, *B*).

The differential diagnosis of periapical lesions is beyond the scope of this chapter. However, the lesion should be diagnosed as one resulting from pulpal involvement before conventional endodontic therapy is performed. Cementomas, bone tumors, and cysts not associated with pulpal involvement must be ruled out. Careful roentgenographic follow-up should be maintained. If bone repair is not evident, or if

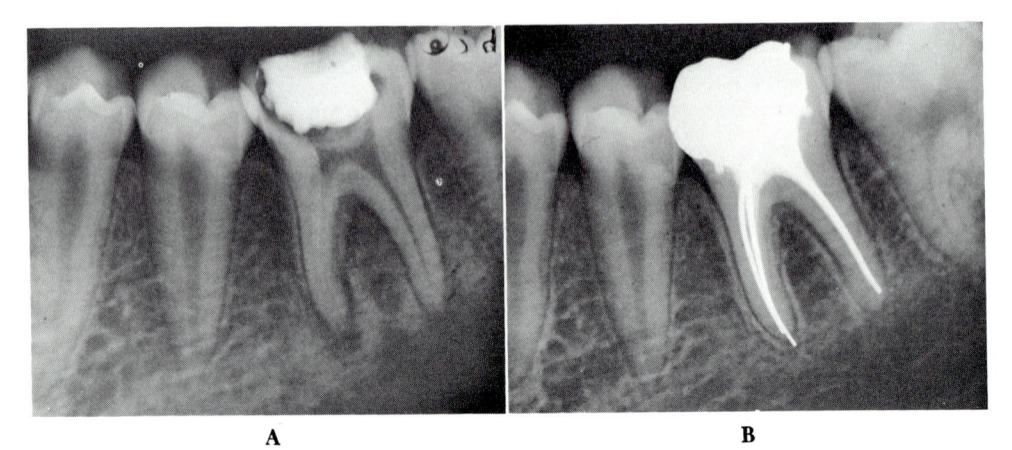

A     B

Fig. 11-14. **A,** A roentgenogram of a lower right first molar of a 15-year-old patient. Note the large carious lesion and periapical radiolucencies. The pulp was necrotic. Conventional endodontics was performed and a pin-retained amalgam restoration was placed. **B,** The same tooth 3 years later. Note the disappearance of the periapical radiolucency and the reappearance of the lamina dura. The tooth was asymptomatic.

symptoms persist following therapy, the more radical procedures of apical surgery or extraction are indicated.

### Endodontic surgery

Conventional or nonsurgical endodontic therapy is the treatment of choice for almost all teeth requiring endodontics.[52] Endodontic surgery, however, as an adjunct to conventional therapy is an important preventative for the loss of teeth.

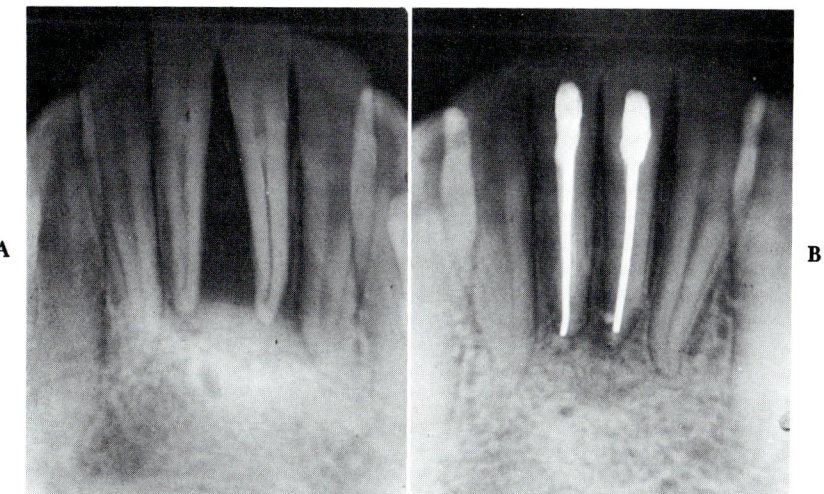

Fig. 11-15. **A**, A roentgenogram of the lower incisors of a 15-year-old patient. The large periapical radiolucency appeared following a fall from a bicycle. The pulps of the central incisors were nonvital. Conventional endodontics was performed. **B**, The same teeth 7 months later. Note the disappearance of the periapical radiolucency and the reappearance of the lamina dura. The teeth were asymptomatic.

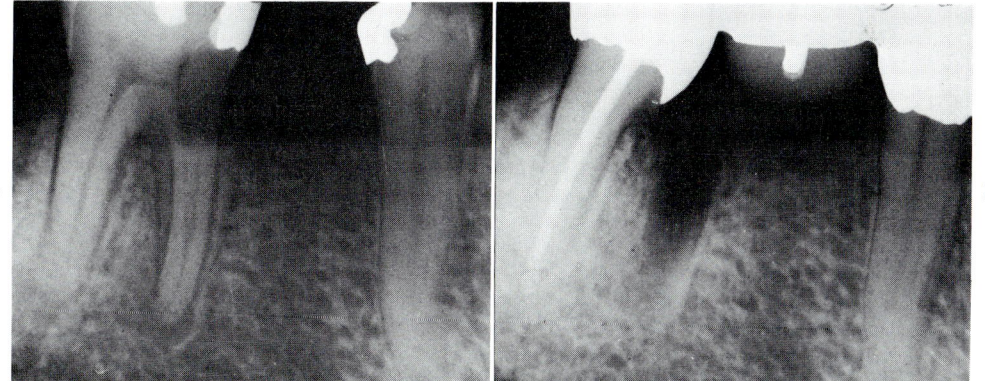

Fig. 11-16. **A**, A roentgenogram of the lower left first molar of a 43-year-old patient. Note the large carious lesion and the periapical radiolucency. The pulp was necrotic. The extensive carious involvement eliminated the coronal approach to the mesial root. Endodontic therapy included mesial root amputation. The remaining half of the tooth provided an abutment for a bridge. **B**, The same tooth immediately following the cementation of the bridge.

268 *Improving dental practice through preventive measures*

Corrective surgery may be necessary subsequent to the failure of conventional therapy or when the conventional approach is impractical—for example, porcelain jacket crowns with retentive dowels interfere with the coronal approach to the root canal.

Extensive caries eliminated the coronal approach to the mesial root of the molar tooth in Fig. 11-16, *A*. Extraction of the tooth would have necessitated a partial denture. The patient expressed a strong aversion to a removable appliance, so endodontic therapy was chosen. The surgery included mesial root amputation. The remaining half of the tooth provided an abutment for a bridge. Fig. 11-16, *B,* shows the tooth immediately after the cementation of the bridge.

The preventive dentist should become familiar with the indications and contraindications for endodontic surgery. These are available, along with the surgical techniques, in recent textbooks.[52, 53] This preventive service can then be made available to the patient either directly or through referral.

## PREVENTING CROWN AND BRIDGE FAILURES

In spite of our best preventive efforts, some teeth will be lost. Treatment planning for patients with missing teeth should provide high priority for early replacement. Missing teeth that have not been replaced initiate a host of undesirable changes. These changes include occlusal prematurities, extrusion of previously opposing teeth, inclination with pocket formation, lack of function, and poor esthetics.

Fixed prosthodontic therapy is excellent for replacing missing teeth. But here, as with other restorative therapy, the principles of prevention must be followed or unexcused failures will surely occur.

Dental caries and mechanical problems caused more than 85 percent of the failures in a study of 791 crown and bridge failures.[54] Dental caries caused 36.8 percent of the failures, and mechanical problems made 49.1 percent of the restorations unserviceable (Fig. 11-17).

Marginal caries results when restorations are placed in a highly cariogenic environment. Even the full coverage afforded by crowns does not eliminate recurrent caries. Reducing the cariogenic flora of the patient's mouth prior to restorative therapy remains tantamount to preventing recurrent caries. This can be accomplished by the dentist who develops skill in primary prevention.

Properly prepared margins of crown preparations provide a firm foundation for adapting cast gold to tooth structure. The margins, whether they be slice, bevel, or chamfer, must be definite and smooth. Indefinite margins of the preparation invite poor marginal adaptation of the restoration and recurrent caries.

The cement, which adapts cast gold restorations to tooth structure, is soluble in mouth fluids. Proper mixing of the cement and the exclusion of moisture help to reduce the solubility. At best, however, cement margins are undesirable. The gold should be adapted to the margins of the preparation as closely as possible.

Full crowns need an avenue of escape for excess cement so that the restoration can be seated completely. A small hole drilled through the crown can be filled with powdered gold following cementation. Holes made with a precision drill can subsequently be filled with self-threading precision pins. More complete seating of the restoration and better margins result when provision is made for the escape of cement. Burnishing the margins further adapts the gold to the tooth structure.

Fluoride solutions applied to crown preparations may help to prevent recurrent

## CAUSES FOR CROWN AND BRIDGE FAILURES

### ORAL DISEASE

| | PERCENTAGE OF FAILURES | LIFESPAN |
|---|---|---|
| CARIES | 36.8 | 11.1 YRS. |
| PERIODONTAL DISEASE | 6.8 | 15.5 YRS. |
| MOBILITY OF ABUTMENT | 4.4 | 10.9 YRS. |
| PERIAPICAL INVOLVEMENT | 2.9 | 5.3 YRS. |
| TOTAL | 50.9 | |

### MECHANICAL PROBLEMS

| | PERCENTAGE OF FAILURES | LIFESPAN |
|---|---|---|
| UNCEMENTED CROWNS | 12.1 | 6.8 YRS |
| DEFECTIVE MARGIN | 11.3 | 9.7 YRS. |
| WEAR OF GOLD OR ACRYLIC | 7.4 | 13.1 YRS. |
| LOST VENEER | 3.7 | 5.1 YRS. |
| POOR ESTHETICS | 3.3 | 9.3 YRS. |
| BROKEN SOLDER JOINTS | 2.9 | 6.5 YRS. |
| BROKEN PONTICS | 2.9 | 9.6 YRS. |
| MISCELLANEOUS | 5.5 | |
| TOTAL | 49.1 | |

Fig. 11-17. Causes for crown and bridge failures. This tabulation is from a study of 791 unserviceable restorations. (Courtesy Dr. N. Schwartz.)

caries. Cavity varnish may also help to prevent the marginal penetration of fluids. In the final analysis, however, recurrent caries can best be prevented by placing restorations that are well adapted at the margins in the mouths of patients who are well indoctrinated in the methods of primary prevention.

Many of the mechanical failures in fixed prosthodontics can be prevented when the dentist assumes a dynamic role in dentist–dental laboratory relationships. The dentist must provide parallel abutments, sufficient interocclusal space, sufficient interproximal reduction to allow for strong solder joints, and sufficient labial or buccal reduction for veneers. He must provide accurate dies with definite margins if he expects accurate castings. An extra amount of time spent in making a margin more definite or retaking an impression may be required. He must then write laboratory prescriptions that are clear, detailed, and explicit. Such prescriptions help the technicians to comply with specifications and leave little room for misunderstandings.

The principles for preventing pulpal and periodontal involvement are valid for all restorative therapy. Atraumatic tooth reduction, pulp production, harmonious contour, contact, and occlusion are among the preventive measures that must be a part of the total preventive program.

## CONCLUSION

Detection of dental caries while the lesion is in enamel is advantageous. The treatment for the less extensive lesion is technically simpler and is associated with less morbidity. The treatment consists of topical fluoride therapy and a continued reduction of the cariogenic flora in the patient's mouth. Confidence in the effectiveness of the treatment develops with the development of the dentist's skill in administering the treatment.

Prevention of defective restorations is an important part of a preventive program. Some of the methods for achieving this goal were presented.

The loss of pulpal vitality can be prevented through conservative tooth reduction and conservative management of teeth with diseased pulps.

Evidence of a periapical lesion does not necessarily indicate a nonvital pulp. After pulp capping therapy, teeth with vital pulps and periapical lesions remained vital and presented roentgenographic evidence of periapical repair.

Conventional endodontics is the treatment of choice for teeth with nonvital pulps—even for teeth with large periapical lesions. Endodontic surgery as an adjunct to conventional therapy is an important preventative for the loss of teeth.

Most failures in fixed prosthodontic therapy result from recurrent caries and mechanical problems. The dentist can control many of the causes for these failures.

The word prevention has a Latin origin meaning "to anticipate." Restorative dentistry can most certainly be improved by anticipating the problems that may reduce the effectiveness of restorative therapy. Problems arise from poor restorative techniques. Therefore technical excellence will prevent many of the problems from developing. Problems also arise when restorations must function in hostile environments. Therefore teaching the patient to exercise control over his oral environment is also a major factor in prevention.

Dentists must continue to develop skills in restorative techniques. They must also develop skills in teaching and motivating patients.

## REFERENCES

1. Scola, F. P., and Ostrom, C. A.: Clinical evaluation of stannous fluoride in naval personnel, I.A.D.R. Abstract 49, 1965.
2. Black, G. V.: Operative dentistry, ed. 7, Chicago, 1936, Medico-Dental Publishing Co.
3. Moore, D. L., and Stewart, J. L.: Prevalence of defective dental restorations, J. Prosth. Dent. 17:372, 1967.
4. Prime, J. M.: Inconsistencies in operative dentistry, J.A.D.A. 24:82, 1937.
5. Murray, M. J.: Value of the rubber dam in operative dentistry, J. Amer. Acad. Gold Foil Oper. 3:25, 1960.
6. Ireland, L.: Rubber dam, its advantages and application, Texas D. J. 80:6, 1962.
7. Going, R. E., and Sawinski, V. J.: Frequency of use of the rubber dam: a survey, J.A.D.A. 75:158, 1967.
8. Larato, D. C., and others: Effect of a dental air turbine drill on the bacterial counts in air, J. Prosth. Dent. 16:758, 1966.
9. Brown, R. V.: Bacterial aerosols generated by ultra high-speed cutting instruments, J. Dent. Child. 32:112, 1965.
10. Healy, H., and Phillips, R. W.: A clinical study of amalgam failures, J. Dent. Res. 28:439, 1949.
11. Massler, M.: Changing concepts in prevention and treatment of dental caries: outline of clinical procedures, New York Dent. J. 39:80, 1969.
12. Gilmore, H. W.: Textbook of operative dentistry, St. Louis, 1967, The C. V. Mosby Co.
13. Selvig, K. A.: The effect of fluoride on the acid solubility of dentin studied by microradiography and electron microscopy, I.A.D.R. 47:160, 1968.

14. Terry, J., and Shannon, I.: Topical application of low concentrate stannous fluoride solutions on the dentin, I.A.D.R. **47:**160, 1968.
15. Wei, S. H., Kaqueler, J. C., and Massler, M.: Remineralization of carious dentin, J. Dent. Res. **47:**381, 1968.
16. Rovelstad, G. H., and St. John, W. E.: The condition of the young dental pulp after the application of sodium fluoride to freshly cut dentin, J.A.D.A. **39:**670, 1949.
17. Lefkowitz, W., and Bodecker, C. F.: Sodium fluoride; its effect on the dental pulp, Ann. Dent. **3:**141, 1945.
18. Evans, J. A., and Massler, M.: Non-reaction of pulp to fluoride application, J. Dent. Child. **35:**91, 1968.
19. Ellis, J. M., and Brown, L. R.: Application of an in-vitro cariogenic technic to study the development of carious lesions around dental restorations, J. Dent. Res. **46:**403, 1967.
20. Moore, D. L.: Unpublished material, University of Missouri at Kansas City School of Dentistry.
21. Going, R. E.: Pin retained amalgam, J.A.D.A. **73:**619, 1966.
22. Welk, D. A., and Dilts, W. E.: Influence of pins on the compressive and transverse strength of dental amalgam and retention of pins in amalgam, J.A.D.A. **78:**101, 1969.
23. Markley, M. R.: Pin-retained and pin-reinforced amalgam, J.A.D.A. **73:**1295, 1966.
24. Dilts, W. E., Welk, D. A., and Stovall, J.: Retentive properties of pin materials in pin-retained silver amalgam restorations, J.A.D.A. **77:**1085, 1968.
25. Moffa, J. P., Razzano, M. R., and Doyle, M. G.: Pins—a comparison of their retentive properties, J.A.D.A. **78:**529, 1969.
26. Chong, W. F., Swartz, M. L., and Phillips, R. W.: Displacement of cement bases by amalgam condensation, J.A.D.A. **74:**97, 1967.
27. Ingram, R., and Harley, J.: High speed techniques evaluated, Dental Times **2**(9):1968.
28. Stein, R. S., and Glickman, I.: Prosthetic considerations essential for gingival health, Dent. Clin. N. Amer., March, 1960, p. 177.
29. Lefkowitz, W., Robinson, H. B. G., and Postle, H. H.: Pulp response to cavity preparation, J. Prosth. Dent. **8:**315, 1958.
30. Schuchard, A., and Watkins, C. E.: Thermal and histologic response to high-speed and ultra high-speed cutting in tooth structure, J.A.D.A. **71:**1451, 1965.
31. Woods, R. M., and Dilts, W. E.: Temperature changes associated with various dental cutting procedures, J. Canad. D. A. **35:**311, 1969.
32. Black, G. V.: Operative dentistry, ed. 2, Vol. 2, Chicago, 1914, Medico-Dental Publishing Co.
33. Rosenstein, S. N.: Pulp capping in children's teeth, J.A.D.A. **39:**658, 1949.
34. Hess, W.: The treatment of teeth with exposed healthy pulps, Int. Dent. J. **1:**10, 1950.
35. Berk, H.: Pulp capping: re-evaluation of criteria based on clinical and histological findings, Int. Dent. J. **13:**577, 1963.
36. Lawson, B. F., and Mitchell, D. F.: Pharmacologic treatment of painful pulpitis, Oral Surg. **17:**47, 1964.
37. Miller, W. D.: Microorganisms of the human mouth, Philadelphia, 1890, The S. S. White Dental Mfg. Co.
38. Besic, F. C.: The fate of bacteria sealed in dental cavities, J. Dent. Res. **22:**349, 1943.
39. Sarnat, H., and Massler, M.: Microstructure of active and arrested dentinal caries, J. Dent. Res. **44:**1389, 1965.
40. Aponte, A., Harsook, J., and Crowley, M.: Indirect pulp capping success varified, J. Dent. Child. **33:**164, 1966.
41. Langeland, K., and Langeland, L.: Indirect capping and treatment of deep carious lesions, Int. Dent. J. **18:**326, 1968.
42. Crone, L.: Deep dentinal caries from a microbiological point of view, Int. Dent. J. **18:**481, 1968.
43. Thoma, K. H., and Goldman, H. M.: Oral pathology, ed. 5, St. Louis, 1960, The C. V. Mosby Co.
44. Miller, S. C.: Oral diagnosis and treatment, ed. 3, New York, 1957, McGraw-Hill Book Co.
45. Sapone, J.: Pulp-capping of vital teeth, D. Progress **3:**51, 1962.

46. Moore, D. L.: Conservative treatment of teeth with vital pulps and periapical lesions: a preliminary report, J. Prosth. Dent. **18:**476, 1967.
47. McDonald, R. E.: Dentistry for the child and adolescent, St. Louis, 1969, The C. V. Mosby Co.
48. Phaneuf, R. A., Frankl, S. N., and Ruben, M. P.: A comparative histological evaluation of three calcium hydroxide preparations on the human primary dental pulp, J. Dent. Child. **35:**61, 1968.
49. Spedding, R. H., Mitchell, D. F., and McDonald, R. E.: Formocresol and calcium hydroxide therapy, J. Dent. Res. **44:**1023, 1965.
50. Doyle, W. A., McDonald, R. E., and Mitchell, D. F.: Formocresol versus calcium hydroxide in pulpotomy, J. Dent. Child. **29:**86, 1962.
51. Hirschfeld, I.: The individual missing tooth: a factor in dental and periodontal disease, J.A.D.A. **24:**67, 1937.
52. Ingle, J. I.: Endodontics, Philadelphia, 1965, Lea & Febiger.
53. Grossman, L. I.: Endodontic practice, ed. 6, Philadelphia, 1965, Lea & Febiger.
54. Schwartz, N. L., and others: Unserviceable crowns and fixed partial dentures: life span and causes for loss and serviceability. (In press.)

# Chapter 12 Preventive prosthodontics (complete dentures)

Frank C. Jerbi

Introduction
Evaluation of the patient
    Choice of prosthesis
        Fixed or removable partial denture
        Removable partial or complete denture
        Contraindications for a prosthesis
    Factors to consider in the decision to retain or extract certain teeth
    The tooth
    The periodontium
    The supporting bone
Complete dentures
    Preparing denture-supporting tissues
        Physical conditioning
        Systemic measures
        Surgical correction
    The impression
        Tissue control
        Maximum extension
        Intimate contact
        Border edges
    Recording interjaw relations
        Occluding vertical dimension
        Centric jaw relation
    Posterior tooth selection and arrangement
        Selection
        Arrangement
    Resilient liners
Immediate dentures
Patient education
    Philosophy of patient education
    Knowledge of the denture and its use
        Denture insertion and removal procedures
        The tongue's acceptance of the denture
        Eating habits
        Diet
        Salivation
        Speech
    Care of the mouth
        The denture should not be worn continually
    Care of the denture
        General
        Armamentarium
    The immediate denture patient
    Recognizing the need for postinsertion therapy
Insertion and postinsertion therapy
    Insertion therapy
    Postinsertion therapy
Conclusion

## INTRODUCTION

The purpose of prosthodontics is to replace missing teeth and their supporting and surrounding structures in appearance, form, and function. Artistic and mechanical considerations are among the factors involved, and they are important, but no phase of prosthodontic therapy is of much importance if the biologic structures and responses are neglected or ignored. A dental prosthesis must be compatible with the remaining dental structures and must not insult their integrity, impair their functions, or foreshorten their life. The practice of prosthodontics must emphasize prevention during the evaluation and education of the patient, during the construction of the prosthesis, and during planned, periodic postinsertion therapy.

## EVALUATION OF THE PATIENT
### Choice of prosthesis

The success of a dental prosthesis in preventing damage to oral tissues and dental function begins with determining which type of prosthesis is best for a given patient.

**Fixed or removable partial denture.** A fixed partial denture is preferred over a removable partial denture replacement except when the former is contraindicated. In respect to the remaining dental tissues and structures, a properly designed and constructed fixed partial denture is the most compatible and least destructive of any dental prosthesis because it performs the following functions.

1. Favors the periodontium by directing the functional forces through the long axis of the supporting teeth
2. Minimizes the destructive forces of torquing and lateral movements
3. Splints the supporting teeth together, causing them to assist each other during function
4. Presents a lower predisposition to caries and periodontal disturbance than does a removable partial denture
5. Does not depend on soft tissue and the bone of the residual ridge for support, bracing, or retention

**Removable partial or complete denture.** The choice of a removable partial denture over a complete denture depends on many factors, some of which are the following.

1. Whether or not a sufficient number of favorable teeth, properly located, can be retained
2. The adequacy of the bone to support the remaining teeth and the periodontium's proved ability to accept the added stresses of a removable partial denture
3. Whether or not caries susceptibility can be controlled
4. The existence of a gross difference in size between the opposing arches (The problems of occlusion and stability associated with complete dentures in these instances give reason to consider a partial denture for at least the smaller arch.)
5. The problems presented by a mouth that has been deformed or mutilated by congenital disturbances, surgery, trauma, or pathosis (Heroic measures of saving teeth, even a single tooth, in order to permit the construction of a partial denture in such circumstances will often assure the success of a prosthesis.)
6. Whether or not the patient's physical and psychologic capabilities better enable him to initially adapt to a removable partial denture rather than a complete denture
7. The patient's ability to practice effective oral hygiene

The choice of recommending a removable partial denture over a complete denture should not be entirely influenced by the possible length of service that the remaining teeth will give with the use of a partial denture. The benefit is measured on the basis of the value such an appliance has as a transitional prosthesis that will "lead" the patient into being a more successful complete denture patient. The most successful complete denture patients are usually those who have become progressively edentulous with the successive wearing of increasingly extensive removable partial dentures.

**Contraindications for a prosthesis.** In some instances the patient and the preservation of the dental mechanism and oral health may best be served by not replacing certain missing teeth. Dentures should not be initiated for the aged and/or debilitated patient who has denture-bearing tissues that lack resiliency, the comfort of thickness, or the proper fluid content, until these tissues have been therapeutically restored to a state of health that will accept the stresses of a prosthesis without injury. Age and certain systemic diseases lower the tolerance that oral mucous membranes have toward the stresses of artificial dentures. Concurrent with the elimination of systemic disease these tissues may be strengthened by correcting all nutritional deficiencies, particularly that of protein.

The loss of a third molar, or a second and a third molar, from one or both sides of either dental arch will not greatly affect the masticatory functions. Therefore these particular teeth need not be replaced for the purposes of improved mastication alone. Their replacement may be indicated to prevent the extrusion of opposing teeth, to prevent disturbances in occlusion or intrajaw relations, or to prevent the periodontium from being adversely affected.

When denture-bearing structures have been subjected to therapeutic doses of radiation, the soft tissues and the bone lose much of their ability to resist stress and trauma and to regenerate when abused. The possibility of osteoradionecrosis suggests a reasonable lengthy delay in the construction of a removable prosthesis after the the conclusion of the radiation therapy. The period of delay will depend on the extent of radiation, the radiation dosage, and the response of the individual patient's oral tissues. There are instances in which the tissues never respond sufficiently to permit the construction of a prosthesis.

### Factors to consider in the decision to retain or extract certain teeth

The decision to retain or extract some or all of the remaining teeth is influenced by whether or not their retention or extraction would be either harmful to the patient or prejudicial to a removable partial denture, or favorable or unfavorable for the preservation of oral and dental tissues and structures. The fate of an individual tooth is determined by the character of the tooth itself, its periodontium, and its supporting bone. The decision can be made only after certain factors have been taken into consideration—the tooth, the periodontium, and the supporting bone.

**The tooth.** The remaining teeth should exhibit an acceptable degree of caries immunity and, if carious, they must be restorable to health, form, function, and relative immunity to decay. The roots of teeth to be utilized as abutments must have the necessary length, form, and bone support to resist tilting and torquing forces. The long axes of abutment teeth should be approximately at right angles to the occlusal plane so that the removable prosthesis can be designed to favorably transmit the forces of occlusion through these long axes. Opposing teeth must be in harmonious occlusion or capable of being adjusted or repositioned to be so.

Nonvital teeth that are required for the success of a removable partial denture may be retained if endodontic therapy and restorations are feasible. The value of unerupted teeth is based on their potential to erupt to a favorable position and to serve a useful purpose.

**The periodontium.** If, in the absence of local etiologic factors, the patient's history indicates an innate susceptibility to alveolar atrophy, it might be assumed that the added stresses placed on the remaining teeth by a removable partial denture may cause their early loss. In conjunction with other extenuating circumstances this condition might contraindicate any prosthesis as a current therapy or dictate the recommendation of a complete denture.

The existing loss of bone supporting the teeth may decide their retention, depending on whether the loss is local or general throughout the dentition; whether the loss is slight, moderate, or severe; or whether the rate of bone loss has been slowly extended over a long period of time or is rapid. If pathologic or mechanical factors exist that are potentially destructive to the periodontium, the possibility of their control or elimination becomes a decisive factor.

The teeth must be sufficiently stable to support a prosthesis without degeneration of the periodontium. If there is minor mobility of a tooth following periodontal therapy, this movement may be able to be controlled by splinting. The tooth must first be capable of normal function as an individual tooth without progressive periodontal involvement. This then makes the primary purpose of splinting that of supporting the tooth against the stresses of the prosthesis and not compensating for its own weakness. The tooth to which the mobile tooth is splinted must be capable of accepting the additional stresses.

For some patients who present periodontal involvement of both the maxillary and mandibular teeth it may be advisable to delay the extraction of the mandibular teeth. The life of periodontally weakened mandibular teeth many be extended in some instances if they are opposed by a complete maxillary denture, instead of being subjected to the greater stresses that would be exerted on them by natural maxillary teeth. If practical, this practice will require the patient to adapt to only a single complete denture rather than to simultaneouly adapt to two dentures. Furthermore, most patients can more readily adapt to a maxillary complete denture than they can to a mandibular complete denture.

**The supporting bone.** A uniform and adequate level of alveolar bone is desirable to support the teeth and the prosthesis against the forces of function. The bone-supported length of the teeth, particularly the abutment teeth, should be in favorable proportion to their nonbone-supported length, that is, the clinical root must be longer than the clinical crown to provide a longer lever arm of resistance to deflecting forces applied to the crown.

The favorable response of alveolar bone to the added stresses of a prosthesis is a key to the success of the prosthesis. The degree of density that bone may portray in a roentgenogram is not a reliable guide to the bone's ability to accept additional stress. Clinical experience records instances of added stresses on bone in which dense appearing bone rapidly failed and bone that appeared less dense was stimulated to a favorable response (Fig. 12-1). A more reliable index for each individual patient is the resistance that his alveolar bone has made to increased loads in specific locations. These index areas include those where teeth have been or are being subjected to deflective or traumatic occlusal contacts, isolated teeth in occlusion, tipped

*Preventive prosthodontics (complete dentures)* 277

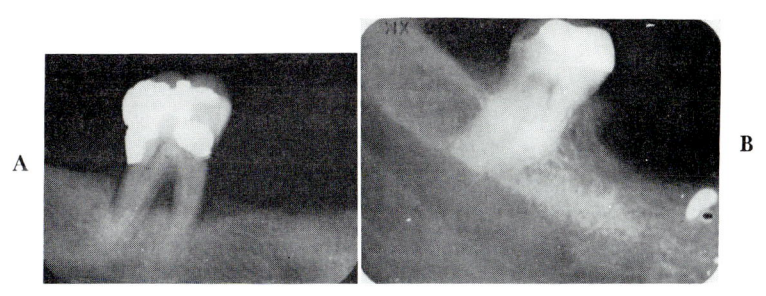

Fig. 12-1. **A,** Gross loss of alveolar bone from around an isolated lower molar, which was caused partly by added stresses. **B,** Favorable response of alveolar bone surrounding an isolated lower molar in the face of added stresses. Radiographically the bone appears less dense than that exhibited in **A**.

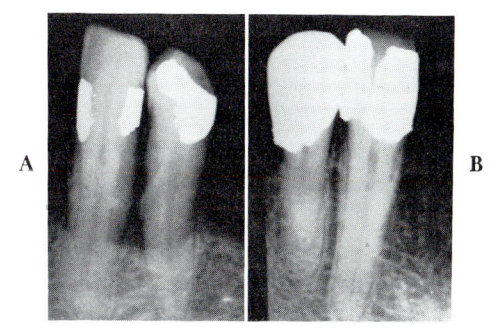

Fig. 12-2. **A,** Loss of alveolar bone surrounding a lower cuspid and first bicuspid serving to support a removable partial denture. **B,** Favorable response of alveolar bone surrounding a lower cuspid and first bicuspid serving to support a removable partial denture. Radiographically the bones appear to be of comparable densities.

or malposed teeth supporting increased loads, teeth serving as abutments for fixed or removable partial dentures, and so on (Fig. 12-2). If there is an area in which overloading is active, how long has this been in effect and what has been the reaction of the bone? Or, what is the residual reaction of supporting structures to a previous period of increased stress? Prognostic proof lies in the roentgenographic evidence of the degree of maintenance of alveolar bone level in these index areas and, of equal importance, in the resistance these teeth exhibit to deflective finger pressure.

## COMPLETE DENTURES

Practicing the principles of preventive dentistry is as important in complete denture therapy as it is in any other aspect of dentistry. The edentulous tissues, soft and bony, that support the denture must be preserved in shape, bulk, and functional ability to permit the patient to continue to wear dentures, which are necessary for his health, appearance, and morale. What is accomplished and how it is accomplished in the construction of the denture and in periodic, postinsertion servicing will largely determine the length of the denture-wearing life of the patient. If attention to these factors increases the denture-wearing life of the patient by way of preventing abuse and loss of denture-bearing tissues and structures, then vital preventive dentistry is being practiced.

**Preparing denture-supporting tissues**

To construct a denture on adverse tissue structures predisposes a prosthesis that will perpetuate and advance pathosis. Healthy tissues resist stress, are less subject to change, assure comfort, and are necessary for the stability and retention of the denture. Pathologic tissue, which includes unacceptable physical features, must be restored to health by local or physical means, systemic measures, and/or surgical correction.

**Physical conditioning.** The methods of physical conditioning chosen to restore tissues to health will depend on the procedures that will best accomplish the purpose in each instance. Choice, following thorough evaluation, is made from a selection of one, several, or all of the following factors.

1. Adjustment and correction of faulty dentures
2. Minimal use of faulty dentures by the patient
3. Stimulation of tissues by the patient with finger pressure, soft toothbrushes, and massaging with the tongue
4. Warm, isotonic saline solution mouth rinses
5. Thermal expansion and contraction of the tissues by alternate hot and cold mouth rinses
6. Repeated use of the temporary, soft reline materials

**Systemic measures.** Systemic measures include the following factors.

1. Establishing adequate medical control of pathologic processes
2. Ensuring proper nutrition and metabolic balance

In appreciating the need for medical control it must be recognized that complete denture patients are usually at that period of life when degenerative tissue changes, particularly bone loss, take place. This bone loss is accelerated in certain systemic disturbances, such as the osteoporosis accompanying menopause and postmenopausal periods, tuberculosis, and others. Soft tissue disturbances, for example, are evident in diabetic and anemic patients.

Proper nutrition is important for tissue repair and resiliency, and a low carbohydrate, high protein diet benefits these requirements. An adequate diet will provide all the required nutrients and water. In some instances dietary supplements might be indicated, such as crude liver extract with vitamin B, vitamin C to complement tissue repair, and vitamin D to help establish calcium-phosphorus balance. (See Chapter 3.)

**Surgical correction.** Surgical procedures may be required to provide a healthy denture-bearing foundation that satisfies physical requirements. The ideal foundation should present an edentulous ridge that, from a cross-sectional view, is U shaped with nearly parallel sides, has adequate bulk and height, and possesses a well-rounded, broad-surfaced crest. The surface of the ridge should be smooth and free of bony projections, pendulous tissue, depressions, and rough areas. The mucous membrane covering the ridges should be firm and firmly attached to the bony substance, uniformly comfortable in thickness, and offer a cushioning yield to pressures. Frena and other tissue attachments should not approximate the crest of the ridge nor should these attachments be excessively broad or heavy. The bony part of the ridge should be stress resistant and free of residual pathosis and foreign bodies. The length of the anterior segment of the ridge should not limit the choice or arrangement of artificial teeth. The distal aspect of the maxillary tuberosity should have a positive projection upward into the hamular notch, and its downward projection should be on a level with or only slightly inferior to the ridge. The alveolar ridges on the opposite sides of each arch should not diverge from one another, and the crests of the right and left side segments of each ridge should approximate a common horizontal plane. The opposing ridges should be symmetrical in size, shape, and arch form. The crests of the maxillary and mandibular ridges should be parallel to each other when the mandible is in the position of vertical dimension of occlusion. When at this position, the ridges should be separated by sufficient, but not excessive, space to permit the positioning of artificial teeth and denture base material.

Corrective procedures for excessive hyperplastic soft tissue should begin with conservative measures, as previously described in the discussion of physical conditioning of soft tissues. Quite often these measures are sufficient in themselves, but if not, then the excess tissue is surgically removed. The amount of soft tissue excised is only that required to provide a surgically sculptured reproduction of a normal ridge in both bulk and shape. Soft tissue should not necessarily be completely excised to the level of its bony base because in the grossly resorbed bony ridge a ridge of dense, fibrous connective tissue is better than none at all. A stable, well-extended denture, balanced in occlusion, and with functional stresses centralized and properly directed, will place the remaining soft tissues in physiologic and physical equilibrium. The loose connective and sometimes hyperemic soft tissue will then be replaced with dense fibrous connective tissue to present the best ridge possible under the circumstances.

Every torus need not be removed, but to prevent tissue abuse from the denture they should be removed if they present the following conditions.
 1. Continual irritation
 2. Interference with insertion and removal of prosthesis
 3. Difficult to maintain good oral hygiene when they are pedicle in shape

Palatal tori should also be removed if they extend into the posterior palatal seal area of the denture. The lack of displaccability of thin tissue overlying the tori will not permit a peripheral denture seal.

## THE IMPRESSION

**Tissue control.** Making the impression, the initial technical procedure in the construction of a complete denture, influences the preventive characteristics of the prosthesis. The relation of the impression to the denture-bearing area should be one of controlled pressure in consideration of the variety of soft tissue consistencies that an individual patient may present. The design of the impression tray for the final impression and the choice of materials should provide an equitable distribution of pressure over tissue areas that are respectively hard and soft, thick and thin, and rigid and displaceable. In this manner the forces directed to each area will be commensurate with each individual tissue area's ability to accept stress and not be abused. For example, the impression should not exert any pressure on either displaceable or thin tissues. In the first instance displaced tissue becomes abused tissue and brings about an unstable denture foundation. In the latter instance thin tissue cannot cushion the periosteum against the stresses that will produce pain as well as bone atrophy.

**Maximum extension.** The impression must cover the maximum area permitted by tissue attachments and tissue functions in order to permit the construction of a fully extended denture base. The stress per unit area upon the denture-bearing

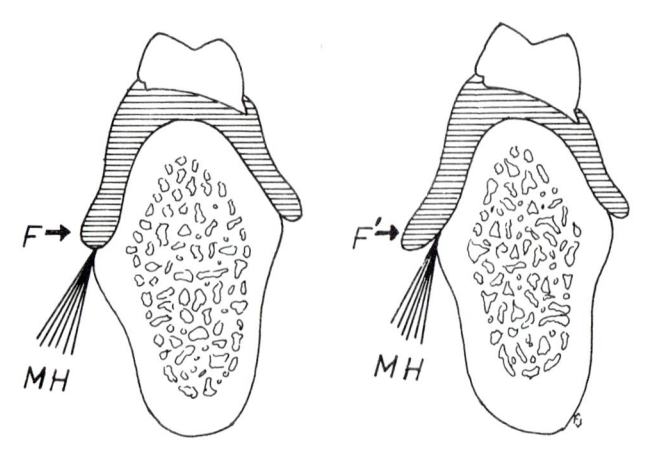

**Fig. 12-3. Left,** lingual flange, **F,** terminates at the insertion of the mylohyoid muscle and will cause discomfort. **Right,** lingual flange, **F',** extends slightly inferior to the mylohyoid ridge to eliminate the event of discomfort.

tissues is indirectly proportional to the denture base extension. The larger the denture base the less stress per unit area will be exerted against the tissues, which will mean less soft tissue abuse and bone atrophy. Also, the amount of biting force it is possible to place on the tissues through the denture is directly proportional to the size of the area covered. In every instance the distal extension of the maxillary or mandibular denture must include, respectively, the maxillary tuberosity and the retromolar pad. By virtue of their composition and architecture both of these anatomic structures offer an advantageous support to vertical movements of the dentures that is superior to the other residual alveolar ridge areas. Furthermore, if completely enveloped by the denture base, each of these structures will help resist anteroposterior movements of the dentures. The border of the lingual flange of the mandibular denture should extend slightly below the mylohyoid ridge to prevent impinging the attachment of the mylohyoid muscle (Fig. 12-3).

**Intimate contact.** The impression must be in intimate contact with the tissues throughout the entire denture-bearing area. If not, the spaces or voids between the denture base and the tissues will invite instability, food- and debris-trapping spaces, and areas of negative pressure that may cause a proliferation of soft tissues in the form of papillary hyperplasia.

**Border edges.** The periphery, or border edges, of the impression must be rounded and smooth and must fill the functional space of the vestibule. These physical characteristics will offer the opportunity to provide a denture base that will be comfortable and compatible with the soft tissues and their attachments. Thin, sharp, rough peripheries will quickly irritate contacting tissues and may even produce traumatic ulcers or lacerations. To avoid irritation, the borders of the denture must be designed to provide space for free movement and not displace frena or other tissue attachments. Filling the functional spaces of the vestibule is necessary to effect the retention seal of the denture, to minimize ingress of food beneath the denture base, to prevent food impaction in areas difficult for the tongue to retrieve, to replace lost dental structures in bulk in order to support muscular and facial tissues for proper function and facial appearance, and to provide the bulk of denture base material required for proper contouring of the polished surfaces of the denture. The buccal surfaces of the denture bases should be contoured to a slight concavity to encourage the natural positioning and actions of the buccinator muscle that complements denture retention and mastication. Essentially, the lingual flange of the mandibular denture should slope medially to approximate a hint of a shelf upon which the tongue may rest and help stabilize and retain the denture. The exception to this is in the retromolar or lateral throat form area, where the denture should slope laterally to allow the tongue to comfortably protrude onto the lingual flange without displacing the denture.

### Recording interjaw relations

**Occluding vertical dimension.** It is necessary to construct complete dentures at an acceptable occluding vertical dimension if the health of the supporting tissues, musculature, and temporomandibular joint is to be preserved. To accurately reestablish the occluding dimension by a complete denture is extremely difficult with current clinical practices and will vary with the many factors that influence it, such as time of day, posture, current health and emotional status, and method of recording the relation. To increase this dimension to the point of depriving the patient of the amount of interocclusal distance he needs will produce a pressure atrophy of the supporting bone, disturb the functional habits and tonicity of the musculature, place the components of the temporomandibular joint in strained relations, promote general soreness beneath the denture and a tired feeling of face and jaws, and cause the denture to be unstable. Nature must either compensate for or be injured by any disturbance to physiology or interference with function. If any latitude is permitted in establishing the occluding vertical dimension, it can only be in the direction of a decreased dimension. This latitude might be indicated for elderly, debilitated patients with little remaining ridge structure and with poor bone and soft tissue surfaces. To judiciously decrease the occluding vertical dimension in these instances will shorten the distance between the origin and the insertion of the muscles and decrease the amount of biting force the muscles will be able to exert upon the denture-supporting tissues. But a gross overclosure will cause lowered masticatory efficiency and the esthetic result may not be pleasing.

The difficulty experienced in attempting to restore the correct occluding vertical dimension emphasizes the importance of preextraction records. Preextraction records should be made whenever possible. Occluding casts of the patient's dentition are a reference for tooth selection and arrangement, and written records or diagrammetric charts indicate the shades of the different teeth and their individual characterizations and provide a record of the vertical dimension of centric occlusion. The occluding vertical dimension record can be made in one of several ways, for example, a soft tissue exposure, lateral head radiogram in a 1 to 1 size reproduction, a cardboard template of the patient's profile made from a bent wire adaption or silhouette projection, an index of plaster of Paris flowed along the vertical length of the midline of the face, a transparent, acrylic resin template of the dental area, or facial measurements made between fixed anatomic landmarks.

**Central jaw relation.** The importance of correctly recording the mandibular position of centric relation in the construction of complete dentures is well known. The need to position opposing artificial teeth in harmonious, maximum intercuspation at this relation is, among other reasons, a requirement for preservation. At this position of centric occlusion are the initial and terminal contact points of the masticatory cycle, the bracing point of the mandible for swallowing, and the location at which the patient subconsciously positions the mandible to "seat" the dentures when they become displaced. If the teeth have been set in maximum occlusal contact at a position other than centric relation, it is obvious that deflective occlusal contacts will become evident and active when the mandible assumes its position of centric relation, for the purposes just mentioned. The resultant effects of the constant displacement of the dentures will be discomfort, irritation to the soft tissues, improper function, and a traumatic atrophy of the supporting bone.

**Posterior tooth selection and arrangement**

There is much controversy about which occlusal surface design of artificial posterior teeth is best for the purpose of all or certain patients. The intent of this discussion is not to perpetuate that controversy. But in the interest of prevention, posterior artificial teeth should be designed or be capable of being modified to favor the stability of the denture and minimize the stresses of mastication that are directed to the supporting tissues.

**Selection.** Considering those authorities who have expressed opinions on the design, specifications, and selection of artificial posterior teeth to favor denture stability and stress reduction the following factors seem to be the consensus.

1. The configuration of the occlusal surfaces should not permit or introduce a locking of the denture into any position. If interference-free, gliding movements are not allowed, then destructive horizontal forces will abuse the soft supporting tissues, precipitate discomfort, and bring about the loss of bone. The design of the tooth should favor the direction of occlusal forces through the long axes of the teeth so that the forces are applied at right angles to the crest of the ridge rather than at a displacing tangent.

2. The effective occluding surface area should be less than that of the individual patient's corresponding natural teeth. The reduction in occlusal surface area minimizes the forces required for mastication and reduces frictional contact. The narrower occlusal area increases chewing efficiency by establishing more of a cutting or shearing action than the crushing action of broad surfaces. The design of chewing elements should provide the cutting efficiency required for shearing fibrous foods and diminishing trauma to the edentulous ridge. The selection of a design of chewing elements for masticatory efficiency will vary from sharp-cusped, anatomic-type posterior teeth for patients with a generally vertical masticatory cycle to monoplane, nonanatomic posterior teeth with efficient subocclusal features for patients with a wide range of lateral excursions. Cusped posterior teeth can be considered appropriate for patients whose natural dentition presented anterior teeth with a deep vertical overlap, those in whom the relationship of the dental arches is of the prognathic type, and those whose posterior inter-ridge relationships present a crossbite situation. The nonanatomic tooth could be considered for patients with the opposite conditions, that is, no anterior vertical overlap and an orthognathic relation (Class II malocclusion).

Chewing efficiency is a must! With natural teeth the forces of mastication are resolved by a tensing of the periodontal ligaments. With complete dentures the patient experiences a compressing of the soft tissues of the ridge and periosteum between an unyielding denture base and the bone of the jaws. This is the reason why the biting force possible with artificial dentures is only about 10 to 12 percent of that possible with natural teeth. This then necessitates efficiency in tooth design to provide kindness to the supporting tissues and to permit the successful acceptance of an adequate diet. Diet and denture success go hand in hand. Proper diet is not possible without a good masticatory mechanism, and healthy, stress-resistant, denture-bearing tissues are not possible without a proper diet.

3. The subocclusal design must permit food to escape from the occlusal surfaces following the penetration of the bolus of food during the chewing cycle. If resistant food is trapped in occlusal surface depressions, a completely flat surface will result and will require greater chewing forces. Therefore channels or grooves, referred to as escapeways or spillways, must lead from occlusal depressions onto the buccal and lingual surfaces of the teeth to keep the function of occlusal depressions active. These escapeways should be in excess of those found in corresponding human dental anatomy, and, if reduced or obliterated during the correction of occlusion by grinding, the escapeways must be recut into the teeth.

**Arrangement.** The positions in which teeth are placed in a denture bear a direct relation to the prevention of abuse to denture-supporting tissues, primarily because these positions have a direct effect on the stability of the denture during function. There is no need to elaborate on the importance of balanced occlusion (maximum or widely separated, harmonious contacts) between teeth during all movements of the mandible and in every position to assure denture stability. This fact is well known and understood, but what about other factors of tooth positioning?

Stability can be complemented by centralizing the forces of occlusion as close to the geometric center of the denture base as possible. In compromise, this means placing the predominate forces of occlusion in approximately the second bicuspid–first molar area. Permitting only slight to no contact between the anterior teeth enhances centralization and minimizes the tilts and torquings that result from hypercontact between the anterior teeth.

The level of the occlusal surfaces to establish the orientation of the plane of occlusion must be given some thought too. This plane should be parallel to the crest of the edentulous ridge in order that forces of occlusion may be directed at right angles to the ridge. The mandibular plane of occlusion should be slightly below the level of the tongue to minimize the opportunity for the tongue to lift the denture and to favor the tongue's action of keeping food on the occlusal table. With

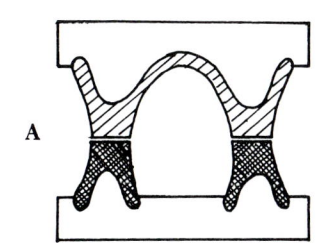

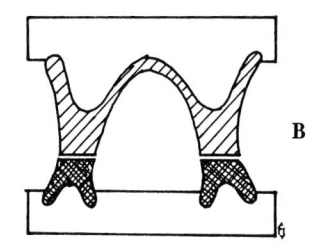

Fig. 12-4. **A**, When the maxillary and mandibular edentulous ridges are approximately equal in size, shape, and strength, the occlusal plane may be positioned equidistant between the crests of the opposing ridges. **B**, When one of the edentulous ridges is appreciably weaker than the other, the weaker ridge will be favored if the occlusal plane is positioned closer to it because the torquing lever-arm distance between the occlusal plane and the crest of the ridge is thereby reduced.

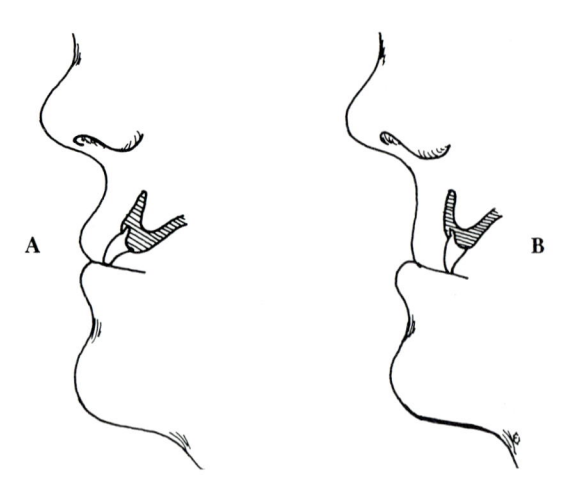

**Fig. 12-5. A,** Placing artificial teeth in the position of their natural predecessors reproduces the natural appearance of both the teeth and the lips. **B,** One common error is to place artificial teeth too far to the lingual in order to approximate the ridge. An unnatural and displeasing appearance of the teeth and lips will result.

patients having one ridge appreciably weaker than the other, the plane of occlusion should be established closer to the weaker ridge in order to shorten the distance between the occlusal plane and the ridge. A shorter, torquing lever arm is the result of favoring the weaker ridge in this manner (Fig. 12-4).

The wider of the two arches of teeth must be set sufficiently "outside" of the narrower arch to provide a horizontal buccal overlap that will push the cheek aside as the teeth are brought into contact. If the posterior teeth are set edge to edge, the possibilities of cheek biting must be expected.

To construct an esthetic denture for an edentulous patient without pre-extraction records requires esthetic judgment, imagination, and experience to select and combine the shape, size, color, arrangement, and characterizations of artificial teeth and the color and contours of the denture base into a natural, personalized denture. But the primary mechanical aspect of providing an esthetic result is to place the artificial teeth in relatively the same position as their natural predecessors. When this is accomplished, not only will the dental appearance be natural, but so will the appearance of the lips and cheeks, whose pleasing contours depend upon being supported in natural positions by the teeth. One word of caution! If, individually, the natural positioning of the maxillary and mandibular artificial teeth is esthetic, but in function these positions are traumatic, then the esthetic result must be compromised to prevent abuse to the supporting tissues (Fig. 12-5).

A natural positioning of teeth will prevent defective speech by permitting the tongue and lips to function in a natural manner as they produce linguodental and labiodental sounds. Natural positioning of the artificial teeth is a vital factor in both esthetics and phonetics.

### Resilient liners

Although resilient denture-lining materials still present some unfavorable technical problems, they have demonstrated that they have a positive application in the preventive aspects of prosthodontics. Further improvement is required in their ability to remain resilient for an acceptable period of time, be color stable, present a minimum of porosity, not support organic growth, permit adjustment, finishing, and polishing with conventional equipment, and lend themselves to a more simple method of processing. Dentures with resilient linings may be indicated for patients with ridges that have thin, soft tissue covering, tissues that have shown low tolerance to the stresses of dentures, poor, denture-bearing tissues resulting from age or debilitation, anatomic defects or deficiencies resulting from congenital disturbances, surgery, or trauma, and with radiated tissues.

## IMMEDIATE DENTURES

The immediate denture is one of the most effective preventive dental prostheses because it permits the accurate duplication of desirable natural factors as they exist in the patient. On the other hand, in the construction of a conventional denture (which is initiated after the extraction of the remaining teeth and the consolidation of the edentulous ridge), jaw positions, occlusion, and esthetics must to some degree be restored via estimations during clinical procedures and to some degree depend on clinical judgment. This fact points out the importance and value of making as many accurate, preextraction records as possible and retaining these records as part of the patient's permanent clinical file.

There are other important preventive features about immediate dentures that can be enumerated.
1. Patients are justifiably reluctant to permit the extraction of all their remaining teeth and to subject themselves to an embarrassing period of edentulousness. When this procrastination amounts to a detrimental retention of diseased teeth and untreated periodontal pathosis, the patient's oral health and structures may be adversely affected and his general health jeopardized. When immediate dentures are offered as the treatment plan, the reasons for procrastination are eliminated.
2. The tonicity of the muscles of mastication, expression, and facial appearance is not lost.
3. The articulatory processes of speech are not disturbed.
4. Because the ridge in the area from which the remaining teeth have been extracted is immediately put into functional stimulation, the ridge is of better shape, size, and tone than if it were subjected to a period of edentulousness.[1]
5. The patient is not obliged to unlearn his lifelong habits of dental functions in order to learn those new habits necessary to accommodate to a period of edentulousness, and then have to unlearn his edentulous habits while going through the difficulties of learning how to function with dentures. This can be confusing to young patients and an insurmountable problem to some of the aged and debilitated patients.
6. An immediate denture maintains the postural position or vertical dimension, whereas a period of edentulousness might disturb the mechanism that regulates the position of the mandible.[2]

## PATIENT EDUCATION
### Philosophy of patient education

The introduction and the explanation of prosthodontics to the patient is an important phase in the preventive aspects of prosthodontic therapy. Complete knowledge about his dentures and what they will do for him will result in patient appreciation for the prosthesis that will encourage proper care, usage, and satisfaction. The approach to this education must be through the presentation of the preventive aspects as well as the other benefits of the dentures and not by emphasizing the source, cost, or advantages of certain materials. Prevention is a health service, not a commodity.

Every prosthesis has its own peculiar advantages and disadvantages that the patient must be made to understand. The pessimistic patient should be made to appreciate the advantages, and the optimistic patient should not be allowed to forget the disadvantages. Patient education must begin with the first appointment and be continual throughout both the preconstruction and construction phases of the dentures. The patient's interest in the dentures being constructed for him should and can easily be developed by enthusiastically satisfying his natural curiosity of the "whys" and "hows" of the technical procedures as they are being accomplished during each appointment. If patient education is postponed until the patient presents postinsertion complaints about his denture, then he might well accept the explanations as excuses rather than education. Possible eventualities must be anticipated and explained before they occur. This does not mean that all the requirements of instruction are met by the time of insertion because it is equally important to reiterate and to continue patient education during postinsertion therapy.

Patients will vary in their ability to learn to use removable prostheses. These differences must be recognized, and the dentist must be prepared to employ several methods of explanation and demonstration. Patience and repetition are usually the keys to successful patient education.

### Knowledge of the denture and its use

Both removable partial and complete dentures can do much for the patient, including the restoration of an esthetic appearance, the return of a masticatory mechanism, the preservation of proper speech functions, and the maintenance of healthy tissues and mandibular-maxillary relations; also they can be a decided factor in the patient's morale. In addition the removable partial denture will benefit the remaining teeth and the periodontium, as previously discussed. But if the patient does not have a respectful knowledge of the dentures and their use, the dentures might have an adverse effect upon the remaining dental structures, speech, comfort, and chewing functions.

A dental prosthesis is an artificial substitute. It can be referred to as an oral crutch that provides the means to simulate, to a lesser degree, the functions of lost dental structures. It can be compared to any external body prosthesis to which the patient must devote hours of practice and experience before reaching an acceptable degree of mastery. If the patient is not educated in the things he should know about the dental prosthesis, and if his learning period is not properly guided, he may well abuse dental tissues and structures while attempting to learn, and he could develop harmful habits. It is easier to learn a good habit than it is to unlearn a bad one.

An explanation of some of the problems a patient can expect with removable dentures is in order.

**Denture insertion and removal procedures.** The insertion and removal of complete dentures are neither as precise or complicated nor as difficult to learn as with removable partial dentures, but there are some things that the patient should be taught. Immediately prior to insertion the tissue contact surfaces of the complete denture must be clean and moist to assist in establishing a surface tension adhesion between the denture and the tissues. In general, the maxillary denture is inserted with a gentle movement that is simultaneously upward and backward to comfortably follow a path that is dictated by the contours of the residual ridge. The final phase of insertion is to ensure that the denture is in uniform contact with the tissues. To do this the denture is firmly seated by pressing upward with the ball of the thumb at the center of the palate or with a similar movement by the thumbs simultaneously applied to the occlusal surfaces of the second bicuspids and first molars. The mandibular denture is positioned while the tongue is slightly elevated and then uniformly seated in a downward and backward movement by pressing the balls of the index fingers against the occlusal surfaces of the second bicuspids and first molars. For this procedure to be comfortable the path of insertion must follow the dictates of the contours of the residual ridge.

The maxillary denture is removed by sliding the tip of the index finger distally along the buccal aspect of the denture until it engages the periphery of the denture base above the tuberosity. Then to release the tension of the musculature, the mouth is closed to a position just prior to where the teeth would contact. Finally, the index finger is pulled downward and forward to "break" the atmospheric seal along the posterior palatal border, and the denture is dislodged. The mandibular denture is removed in a similar manner with a lifting, rotating movement of the tip of the index finger applied to the buccal periphery of the denture in the molar area. Although some people quickly develop the ability to dislodge the maxillary denture by forcing air between the denture and the palate and to dislodge the mandibular denture with the tongue, neither practice should be advised for the particularly nervous type of patient. It is quite possible that this patient will use these procedures as a nervous habit to "play" with the dentures while they are in the mouth, which might result in degenerative changes in the denture-supporting tissues.

**The tongue's acceptance of the denture.** The tongue is an extremely sensitive organ. It reacts rapidly to any stimulus, and it tends to relay an exaggerated impression of size and shape of objects and of motion. The tongue will immediately object to the denture occupying the space into which the tongue has expanded coincident with the loss of teeth. Fortunately, the tongue is also a highly adaptive organ and in a short time it will retrain and reposition itself to accommodate the denture.

If the patient's natural tongue position is one of retraction or if the tongue's reaction to the denture is to assume such a position, then the stability and retention of the lower denture will be adversely affected. In either event the patient must be taught a series of tongue exercises in order to regain or establish the normal tongue position. Normal tongue position, observed while the mouth is slightly open, reveals the tongue as fully occupying the floor of the mouth, with its tip covering the lingual surfaces of the mandibular anterior teeth and with the dorsum of the tongue above the occlusal plane. The following tongue exercises[3] are of value in establishing the normal tongue position, helping the patient adjust to dentures, and promoting stability of the mandibular denture.
   1. Thrusting the tongue in and out of the mouth as rapidly as possible
   2. Rapidly swinging the tongue from side to side, during which the tongue is extended about one-half inch beyond the lower lip

3. Thrusting the tongue out as far as possible and then quickly pulling it back into the mouth
4. Articulating the sound of "eeyuh" with the tongue raised to its highest position well forward in the mouth (the "ee" should be spoken at a high pitch before saying the "yuh")

**Eating habits.** The denture is an important part of the chewing mechanism, but it will be of little value and it will harm the mouth if it is not used properly. A reasonable degree of skill is required for the act of chewing with dentures. These skills are sometimes slow to develop and may cause disappointments, if not frustrations, during the learning stages. The patient must employ planned, concentrated effort in learning to use the other elements of the chewing mechanism, namely, his lips, cheeks, and tongue in unison with the functional movements of the dentures. With the knowledge that the best artificial dentures are only 20 percent as efficient as natural teeth, the need for good eating habits becomes apparent.

The denture-bearing tissues should be gradually conditioned to the stresses of mastication. To avoid overuse and abuse to the oral tissues it is good practice for the patient to initially eat only small amounts of food frequently during the day rather than to attempt full meals at regular mealtime intervals. Also, only small portions, one-fourth to one-half of the habitual normal, should be placed into the mouth for each cycle of chewing and swallowing.

Chewing food with artificial teeth should be accomplished slowly and deliberately, in order to maintain the proper denture-to-tissue relationship. Hurried and exaggerated movements may displace the denture, and if a chewing force is applied to a displaced denture, the resulting trauma can be painful and tissue abusing. With a similar occurrence the patient would be embarrassed to have a displaced denture mixed in with incompletely chewed food. It is a good habit for the patient to occasionally employ some "extra" swallowing actions to ensure the proper seat of the dentures prior to inserting food into the mouth.

Although incision is possible with artificial dentures, denture stability and the supporting tissues in the anterior part of the mouth will benefit if this action is kept to a minimum. In general, incision should be accomplished on the dinner plate with a fork and knife and the food placed into the mouth and onto the chewing surfaces of the posterior teeth.

**Diet.** The substitution of lost teeth with artificial dentures does not change dietary requirements, but it does require a change in the consistency and the preparation of foods used during the initial experiences with dentures. Except in the use of immediate dentures the patient should take a day or so to simply become accustomed to having the dentures in his mouth before attempting to use them in eating. Then his dietary progression should be from liquid foods (eggnogs, milk shakes) to soft foods (custards, pureed foods, baby foods, gelatin preparations) and finally into ground or finely chopped foods before attempting his normal diet. During the learning period it is advisable to avoid foods that are hard to chew, that fill and occlude the teeth's spillways, and that are difficult to swallow or tend to dislodge the dentures. Such foods are fruit with small seeds, sticky or doughy foods, fibrous, stringy meats, and "dry" foods such as peanut butter. Chewing gum should always be avoided because it is a source of constant trauma.

**Salivation.** A denture is a foreign body and, as with any foreign object when placed into the mouth, it will trigger an increase in salivary flow. This is only a temporary reaction and will continue until compensatory mechanisms and habits develop to accommodate this phenomenon. The patient should be advised that when he becomes aware of an accumulation of saliva in his mouth he should bring the dentures together into a light centric occlusion contact and gently swallow. He should be cautioned against developing the habit of expelling saliva and wiping it away from the corners of the mouth with a handkerchief or facial tissue. This habit prevents the patient from developing confidence in the prosthesis and delays the formation of good denture control and habits.

**Speech.** Any dental prosthesis will temporarily interfere with the articulatory mechanism of speech, particularly with the labiodental and linguodental sounds. The difficulties in speech that may be encountered with dentures can be eliminated with perseverent practice. One of the best means of quickly developing good speech habits with dentures is to read aloud as much as possible or to silently form words with the lips and tongue, performing all of the actions that would be necessary for audible speech. Corrective and optimum tongue and lip positions and movements should be sought and practiced. Initially the pronunciations should be with simple words, and the motions should be slow, deliberate, and somewhat exaggerated until the patient achieves the confident "feel" of speech. Words that are difficult to pronounce should be avoided when talking in social or public circumstances during the period when accommodating to dentures.

### Care of the mouth

The patient's effectiveness in the care of his mouth and dentures is directly related to the thoroughness with which the dentist demonstrates and explains the procedures involved.

Oral hygiene is important for the edentulous mouth even though there are no teeth present. Several times during the day, particularly following eating and while the dentures are out for cleaning, the edentulous ridge and the surface of the tongue should be cleaned and stimulated with a soft toothbrush. There is a stimulating, massaging benefit in the periodic use of mouth rinses, such as warm isotonic saline solution or alternate hot and cold rinses.

**The denture should not be worn continually.** The denture is a foreign and unnatural mechanical device that continually exerts unnatural forces and influences the tissues and structures it contacts. In many instances these forces will eventually exceed the physiologic tolerance of the dental tissues, and whenever such a situation exists upon any tissue or part of the body, an adverse reaction is inevitable. Then, there is a need to rest these tissues periodically to permit them to "rebound" to healthy, normal shape and tone.

Usually the most advantageous period of the day during which the dentures can be kept out of the mouth is at night while sleeping, because during this time the dentures serve no useful function. In addition to some instances of vanity, there are other exceptions to this suggestion.

1. A removable partial denture patient with some residual mobility of the remaining teeth following periodontal therapy. (If the partial dentures are designed to provide the additional service of a periodontal splint, the periodontium might be abused during sleep if the patient has the habit of bruxing.)
2. An edentulous arch opposed by either an arch of natural teeth or a partially

edentulous arch. (If the patient bruxes, it is possible that the tissues covering the edentulous ridge will be traumatized by the opposing teeth.)
3. If a protracted period (6 to 8 hours) of being without the dentures fatigues the muscles of mastication and facial expression

There is no need to insist that the period to be without the dentures is either at night while sleeping or for a continual period of 6 to 8 hours. The important thing is that the denture-bearing tissues should be rested for a daily cumulative period of approximately that amount of time. This resting can be accomplished during multiple, short periods of time during the day. Certainly the patient can take advantage of the relaxing periods in the evenings and the free time he has on weekends and holidays.

The only real objection that some patients have to the practice of resting denture-bearing tissues is that, after the denture is inserted, it takes a few minutes for the denture to feel as if it is properly seated. But this is proof of the need for resting the tissues involved because it indicates that rested tissues will "rebound" by regaining cellular volume and intercellular spaces and in the process promote tissue stimulation and tone.

To strengthen this premise, clinical experience has shown that the majority of denture patients who present papillary hyperplastic palatal tissues admit to the habit of not removing their dentures at any time except for cleansing. Uninterrupted use of the maxillary denture causes a regression of the palatal glandular tissues. Frequent removal of the prosthesis, resting the tissues, and rinsing with an astringent initiates glandular activity and promotes a better physiologic state. Markov, showing that keratinization of the oral mucosa supporting a denture increased if the dentures were regularly removed from the mouth at night, concluded that rest makes it possible for the oral mucosa to recover from the effects of wearing dentures.[5]

## Care of the denture

**General.** By keeping the dentures as clean as possible at all times, the accumulation of stains and deposits will be kept to a minimum; tissue irritation will not be invited; the original appearance of the denture will be preserved; denture odors and denture breath will be reduced; and objectional tastes can be prevented from occurring. Complete dentures should be cleansed following any incident of eating, at the end of the day, and immediately prior to inserting them in the morning. If the cleansing armamentarium is not available following eating, the patient should at least remove the dentures, rinse them thoroughly with running water, and vigorously rinse out his mouth.

The procedure of cleansing dentures begins with covering the bottom of the lavatory basin with a small towel or wash cloth, filling the basin half-full with water, and holding the denture close to the surface of the water while brushing and rinsing. This precaution is taken to prevent fracturing or distorting the denture in the event it is accidentally dropped. The denture should be held firmly but not in an ever-tightening grip. Some mandibular complete dentures have been fractured by an overzealous grip.

**Armamentarium.** The patient should have a special, different type of brush for cleaning his dentures in addition to the toothbrush he uses for the care of his mouth. The complete denture brush is purchased as such, and it should have sections of bristles of different lengths to permit cleansing all of the various depths of the inner

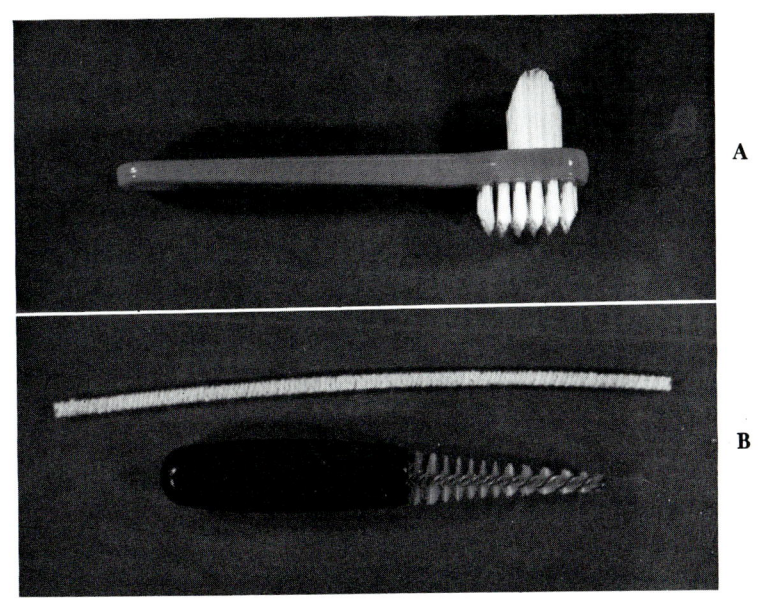

**Fig. 12-6. A,** Type of denture-cleansing brush that is particularly suitable for complete dentures and removable partial denture bases. **B,** Pipe cleaner and removable denture brush for cleansing confined areas and the inner and outer surfaces of removable partial denture clasps.

surface of the denture, the confined spaces between the teeth, and the pits and grooves of the artificial teeth. Whatever the type of brush used, its effectiveness will depend upon how thoroughly it is used, that is, if its bristles are made to enter all the depths and crevices of the denture (Fig. 12-6). Patients who have their vision corrected by eyeglasses should be advised of the necessity of using their glasses whenever they clean their dentures. This point is mentioned because many patients have the habit of cleaning their dentures after they have removed their glasses for the day, just prior to bedtime. Many times the same patient will cleanse his dentures as a part of his morning toilet before putting on his glasses.

The mechanical action of the brush is the most important aspect of cleaning dentures. This cleansing is made more effective when used along with a low-abrasive cleansing medium, such as a good dentifrice, liquid or castile soap, or sodium bicarbonate and water, but not abrasive scouring powders. Immediately after brushing, the denture should be rinsed thoroughly under a stream of warm (not hot) water.

In addition to the mechanical cleansing of dentures, as just described, the patient should occasionally use some type of immersion cleaner. The commercially available types of immersion cleaners are effective, or the patient may wish to prepare his own cleaner, such as one of the following.

1. A solution of one teaspoonful of 28 percent ammonia in a glass of water
2. A solution of one tablespoonful of white vinegar in a glass of water (effective in removing films of hard deposits)
3. A mixture, commonly referred to as the University of Michigan denture cleaner, made up of one tablespoonful of a liquid household laundry bleach and two tablespoonfuls of Calgon detergent in a glass of water

The frequency and the length of time that dentures are allowed to remain in an immersion type of cleaner will depend upon the strength of the cleaner and the rate at which stains and foreign material tend to accumulate on the dentures of each individual patient.

**The immediate denture patient**

In addition to the instructions that are given to those patients who are to use conventional dentures, there are several, specific instructions that should be given to a patient for whom an immediate denture is being constructed.
1. The patient should not remove the immediate denture between the insertion appointment and the follow-up appointment, which should be approximately 24 hours later, except in an emergency circumstance. This precaution is taken to preclude any difficulty that the patient may have in comfortably reinserting the denture during the edematous phase.
2. The use of cold packs to the outside of the face is advised to minimize edema and to promote comfort. For the same reasons some patients benefit from the use of cold foods and drinks during the healing stages.
3. The patient is advised to use a high-caloric, high-vitamin liquid or soft diet.
4. Analgesics are prescribed to alleviate postoperative pain.
5. The patient should rest at home during the first 24 hours. Rest benefits the initial healing processes, and it offers the patient an opportunity to develop confidence in the prosthesis prior to entering social or vocational activities.
6. Gently applied warm normal saline mouth rinses during the healing period are indicated to maintain good oral hygiene and to stimulate the tissues. These rinses should be used with the denture in place during the first 24 hours and thereafter with the dentures removed.

**Recognizing the need for postinsertion therapy**

The denture-bearing tissues are biologic structures that will change in character, size, and shape simply by virtue of the passing of time. Dentures are mechanical devices and are not subject to appreciable changes in either size or shape. These facts, among others, make it important for the patient to know that prosthodontic therapy does not end with the insertion of the denture. Therapeutic, corrective, and/or maintenance procedures are continually necessary to prevent abuse of the dental tissues and to maintain the comfort and function of the dentures. The importance of periodic, postinsertion, recall appointments must be emphasized. Because the mouth or the denture may require evaluation or attention at times other than that scheduled at recall appointments, the patient should be taught to recognize such needs when he becomes aware of any of the following experiences with his dentures.
1. Difficulty or pain during insertion or removal of the denture
2. Pain during eating or from any movements or pressures of occlusion
3. Any persistent soft tissue lesion, such as ulcerations associated with the borders of the denture
4. An increase in the contact and pressures between the anterior teeth in conjunction with a diminishing contact and pressures between the posterior teeth
5. An unusual increase in the accumulation of food and debris beneath the dentures
6. An obvious decrease in the denture's stability or retention
7. Evidence of distortion or fracture of any element of the denture

Educating the patient to recognize the need for denture adjustments does not give him the prerogative to make these adjustments. The patient should be forcefully advised that any personal attempt to correct his denture may result in harm to his mouth, impair the comfort and function of the denture, or require an additional expense to correct any error he might make.

## INSERTION AND POSTINSERTION THERAPY
### Insertion therapy

Following the careful attention given to the professional and technical procedures to construct the best possible denture, it is equally important that the same attention be given the denture during the insertion appointment. During this appointment it is necessary to thoroughly and completely examine the denture to determine the presence of any discrepancies. The errors that are found must be corrected immediately and should not be allowed to remain until a future appointment. It is not justified to permit the "settling" of the dentures to "erase" certain denture discrepancies. The disappearance of any discrepancies by "settling" usually means that the supporting structures have been abused in some manner in order to accommodate the discrepancy.

During the insertion appointment the following procedures must be accomplished and preferably in the sequence listed:

1. Minutely examine the tissue-contacting surfaces of the denture for the presence of sharp protuberances, blebs of denture base material, and porous areas that must be corrected prior to the initial insertion.

2. Examine the relation of the frena and other tissue attachments to the denture. If necessary, the periphery of the denture is contoured to permit these attachments to assume their natural position and freedom of movement.

3. Evaluate the shape, size, and projection of the border extensions of the denture. This is accomplished with the tip of the index finger while the denture is in place and while viewing muscular movements and the tissues and the tongue in function. Necessary adjustments are made immediately.

4. Areas of the denture base that may exert unacceptable pressures on the tissues are detected with the use of a pressure-indicating medium applied to the inner surface of the denture. Properly applied finger-seating pressure will reveal the offending areas that are relieved by the removal of an appropriate thickness of the denture base material. Testing and relieving are continued until uniform contact is evident.

5. Accurate, appropriate, interjaw relation, check records are made, and the dentures are remounted in an articulator. Any tooth-contacting discrepancies in centric occlusion, occluding vertical dimension, or the eccentric positions are corrected.

6. The dentures are returned to the mouth, and the evaluation and the correction of tooth contacts, as accomplished with the articulator, is made. Some dentists prefer to attach a central-bearing device to the dentures during this procedure.

7. The correction of occlusal contacts may eliminate or minimize the number of spillways or sluiceways that the food must have to escape from the occlusal surfaces. The spillways must be restored by sculpturing the teeth with sharp stones or discs.

8. After a uniform, simultaneous contact has been established between the teeth in the various positions of the mandible, the use of a pressure-indicating medium is repeated. At this time the pressure of various occlusal contacts is employed to produce any evidence of excessive pressure.

9. Any adjustments to improve the esthetic result are performed at this time.

This may include shortening teeth, modifying their facial contours, producing interdental embrasures, and characterizing incisal edges or cusp tips.

The completion of the procedures described and any other adjustments that may be peculiar to the individual prosthesis should make the dentures comfortable and functional. The patient is dismissed after a definite follow-up appointment is made for a date within 2 to 5 days following the insertion appointment. The purpose of the follow-up appointment is to correct any faults that use may reveal. In addition, any objections or complaints that the patient may have as a result of having used the dentures for a few days are evaluated and corrected if necessary. It is usually found necessary to repeat some of the adjustment procedures that were accomplished during the insertion appointment, with particular attention to refining the occlusion. If an unusual number of adjustments is required at a follow-up appointment it is advisable to have another postinsertion appointment within a week.

When both the dentist and patient are satisfied with the dentures, a definite recall appointment is made to follow within 6 months. In the event of an immediate denture, or if the patient has had his remaining teeth extracted shortly before the dentures were constructed, it is advisable to make the first recall appointment within 3 months following the insertion of the denture. Some patients, particularly some immediate denture patients, have the unfortunate faculty of overadapting to their dentures and not returning for recall appointments. Patients must be made to realize the value of timely corrections or adjustments on a periodic basis in preventing abuse and maintaining the health of the denture-bearing tissues.

**Postinsertion therapy**

A removable dental prosthesis is correct, proper, and therapeutic only at the time of the initial insertion. From that moment on, physiologic, pathologic, and/or physical changes act to progressively bring about disturbances in supporting or related dental tissues and structures. The rapidity and the degree of disturbance will vary with the type of appliance and the individual patient. Whether or not these changes are clinically significant depends upon what the changes are and to what magnitude they occur. Therefore a removable denture patient and his prosthesis must be periodically examined to determine which if any preventive or maintenance procedures are necessary for dental health and denture serviceability.

The use of so-called home relining kits that are available for direct purchase by patients is condemned. Without a knowledge of the biomechanical principles involved the patient will invariably produce a malrelation between the denture and the supporting tissues. The results will include unhygienic surfaces, malocclusions, and ultimately an unacceptable increase in the vertical dimension of occlusion. Unfortunately, the size and shape of the edentulous ridges are rapidly reduced and the tissues abused, bringing about a condition that makes successful prosthodontic therapy difficult to achieve.

A loss of posterior occlusion between opposing dentures (be it either between complete dentures or between a complete maxillary denture and natural mandibular teeth or a mandibular removable partial denture) causes the mandible to arc into protrusion and closure. This brings a hyperocclusal force to bear against the anterior maxillary ridge, causing a loss of bone and hyperplastic mucosal tissue. The denture becomes unstable and loses retention, and the process compounds itself. The denture then must be relined, occlusion must be corrected, and, if necessary, the denture must be remade.

The initial procedure in postinsertion therapy should be that of listening to any constructive information that the patient has to offer about his dentures. Valid complaints must be sympathetically received and corrections made in order to maintain an atmosphere of mutual responsibility and cooperative effort. When this responsibility has been met, the denture and the denture-bearing tissues must be minutely examined.

Corrections should not be impulsively made. The conditions that indicate the need for correction must be carefully studied, and the cause or causes positively determined before any change in the denture is made. The cause for a particular area of tissue abuse may not be due to that part of the denture approximating the site of the abuse. The cause can actually be far removed from the abused area. For example, a premature occlusal contact in the mandibular posterior area may produce a soft tissue lesion on the lingual aspect of the anterior mandibular ridge because this prematurity can force the denture into a traumatizing, anterior shift.

It would be repetitive at this time to describe the procedures of making denture adjustments and the sequence in which they should be practiced, and it is suggested that, in general, the procedure of denture evaluation and adjustment during postinsertion therapy be as described in the previous section concerning insertion therapy. Emphasis must be given to the all-important investigative procedure of critically studying the nature of any changes that may have occurred in the occlusion. Many tissue reactions, patient discomforts, the loss of denture stability and retention, and the impairment of function are often directly attributed to an unacceptable change in the occlusion.

It is of *vital* importance to be suspicious of any long-standing tissue lesions, small or large, that refuse to respond to resting the tissues by not wearing the dentures and/or to repeated denture adjustments or corrections. Procrastination or reluctance to perform a biopsy on such lesions cannot be condoned. Any such lesions that persist, particularly in the floor of the mouth, must be regarded as extremely dangerous because of their highly malignant potentialities.

## CONCLUSION

In the modern practice of prosthodontics there is a tremendous opportunity to contribute as never before to positive, long-range, continuing dental health. This can be accomplished by careful evaluation of the patient, an intelligent treatment plan, an ever-present attention to the preventive aspects of technical procedures, a thorough patient education, and scheduled, periodic postinsertion evaluation and therapy.

The following statement by G. B. Shillington places preventive prosthodontics in its deserving and proper perspective: "The success of prosthetic treatment must be examined from four aspects, namely comfort, esthetics, efficiency and tissue preservation. The first three concern the observations of the patient; the fourth is largely determined by the dentist and should constitute his main interest. The preservation of the supporting tissues, furthermore, presents the greatest challenge to his professional ability."[6]

## REFERENCES

1. Kelly, E. K., and Sievers, R. F.: The influence of immediate dentures on tissue healing and alveolar ridge form, J. Prosth. Dent. 9:738, 1959.

2. Carlsson, G. E., and Persunn, G.: Morphological changes of the mandible after extraction and wearing dentures, Odont. Revy 18(1):27-54, 1967.
3. Wright, C. R., and others: Facts you should know about your dentures, Toledo, Ohio, 1963, Healthcare, Inc.
4. Butcher, E. O., and Mitchell, O. G.: Effect of dentures and astringents on palatal mucosa, J. Prosth. Dent. 20(1):3-7, 1968.
5. Markov, N. J.: Cytologic study of keratinization under complete dentures, J. Prosth. Dent. 20(1):8-13, 1968.
6. Shillington, G. B.: Handbook of the fundamentals of partial denture planning, Ottawa, Ontario, Canada, 1957, The Queen's Printer.

# Chapter 13 Preventive adult space maintainers (partial dentures)

Wayne L. Harvey

Introduction
Partial dentures and caries and periodontal disease
The adult space maintainer
    Patient education program
    Preventive diagnosis and preventive prescription program
        Crowns of the teeth
        Investing tissue
        Soft tissues
        Classification
        Continuum between easy and difficult cases
        Treatment program
    Preventive mouth preparation and construction program
        Rest preparations
        Contour of natural tooth surfaces
        Units of the adult space maintainer
        Units of tooth-supported and tissue-supported prostheses
        Functional impression procedure
    Instructions for home care program
    Dependable recall system
Conclusion

## INTRODUCTION

Some dental educators have divided preventive dentistry into two categories: primary prevention and secondary prevention. "Primary prevention" implies the use of agents or technics that will prevent a disease process before therapy is needed. "Secondary prevention" implies the use of therapy to arrest further progress and recurrence of disease. Removable partial dentures fall into the category of secondary prevention.

The concept of the partial denture as a secondary preventive appliance is relatively new. The more recent concepts of removable partial dentures are based upon preventive dentistry,[1, 2] and since prevention is a dynamic process, the comments expressed in this chapter should add fuel to the burning desire to prevent disease.

In order to adequately discuss the role of partial dentures in preventive dentistry, there is need to add a new phrase to existing partial denture terminology. This is needed because some patients and some dentists consider partial dentures disreputable prostheses.

The public has learned, rightly or wrongly, that the partial denture invites the loss of teeth.[3] Patients believe that a partial denture is the makeshift between not enough natural teeth for satisfactory chewing and acceptable esthetics and complete dentures. But a partial denture need not be a stepping-stone to a complete denture, provided it is properly diagnosed and made. Above all, patients must learn their role in prevention. Much more clinical research is needed in prosthetic dentistry; much of what has been written in dental literature is based on common sense.[4]

There are two kinds of removable partial dentures—one preventive, the other destructive. We have new preventive concepts in partial dentures, but we need a new term so that the preventive partial denture regains the confidence of the patient. It is proposed that the preventive partial denture be known as an *adult space maintainer.*

Space maintenance is the most important function of a removable partial denture. Restoration of esthetics and masticatory function are important but too often are sought at the expense of space maintenance.

If the spatial relationship of each remaining tooth to its antagonist, to its supporting tissue, and to other remaining teeth is desirable, then these relationships should be preserved as they are. If there is no disease present, then the spatial relationships are desirable and should preserve the remaining structures for the longest possible time.

## PARTIAL DENTURES AND CARIES AND PERIODONTAL DISEASE

The relationship of the destructive partial denture to caries and periodontal disease must be understood. Let us consider each briefly.

Caries control per se is discussed elsewhere. The remarks here concern the hygienic problem created for the patient who is wearing a removable partial denture. Caries that destroys the invaluable tooth contacts and contours allows the tooth too frequently to migrate, thus upsetting space maintenance. Tooth movement can result from a destructive triad of a loss of support from proximal tooth contact, food trapping, and unfavorable occlusal relationships. Therefore caries, by supplying some of the necessary conditions, can indirectly cause periodontal disease.

Partial dentures retain food debris around abutment teeth and marginal gingiva. The amount of trapped food is related to the construction of the partial denture. Food traps may be present almost anyplace about a removable partial denture. However, the most important areas to prevent food impaction are between minor connectors and abutment teeth, saddle borders and abutment teeth, and lingual (palatal) bar major connectors and underlying tissues.

A food trap can be created by the dental laboratory. Excess space between a cast framework and abutment teeth can be made by excess relief of the master cast prior to duplication and casting (Fig. 13-1). In the same place a food trap can result if the dentist fails to remove overhanging enamel from a tipped tooth (this situation will be discussed on p. 316). Dental caries can be initiated or can recur in areas where food collects.

A food trap can supply some of the necessary conditions that may precipitate periodontal disease or aggravate a recovered periodontal lesion. However, a necessary condition associated with the most destructive periodontal disease, is often supplied by a free-end saddle partial denture. If the denture is not equally supported by the base and natural teeth, then the free-end partial denture contributes excess stresses to the abutment teeth. Stresses are usually excessive when a partial denture rotates around a fulcrum line[5] (Fig. 13-2). As the saddle of the partial denture settles under an occlusal load the cast retentive arm more tightly engages the infrabulge of the abutment tooth, rotating it in the alveolus at a pivot point located about mid-

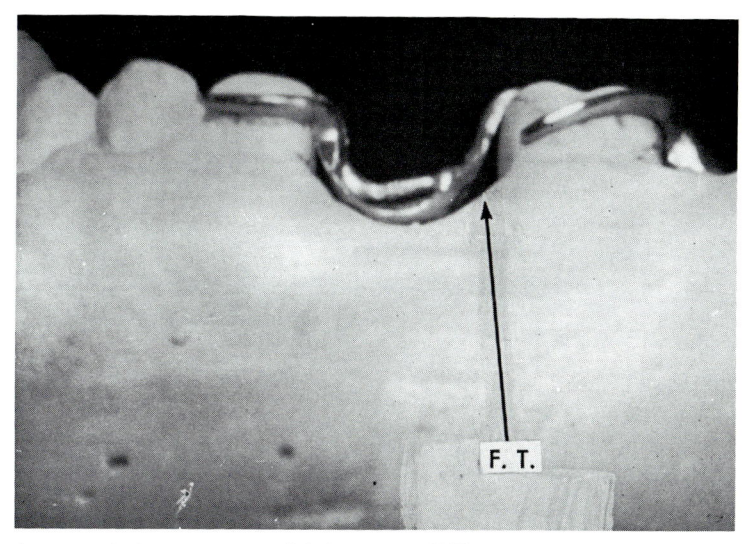

Fig. 13-1. Arrow pointing to a potential food trap, **F.T.**, created by excess relief of a master cast before duplication.

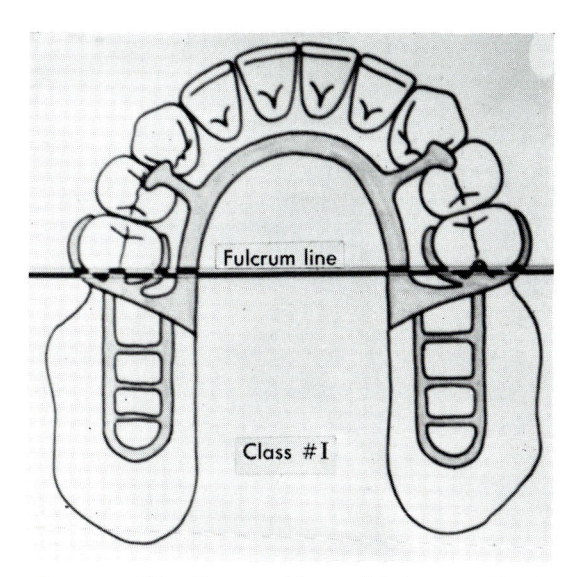

Fig. 13-2. A fulcrum line on a Class I removable partial denture. The free-end saddle rotates vertically around this line.

way in the clinical root (Fig. 13-3). Excess rocking of the partial denture, like a child's seesaw, torques, and tilts the abutment teeth. Excessive stress on abutment teeth and the supporting periodontium can be pathogenic, destroying the supporting tissue faster than the patient can recover. The periodontium cannot readily resist this type of constant stress and remain healthy. The result is the loss of one or more teeth. Therefore the preventive partial denture (adult space maintainer) must control the stresses described.

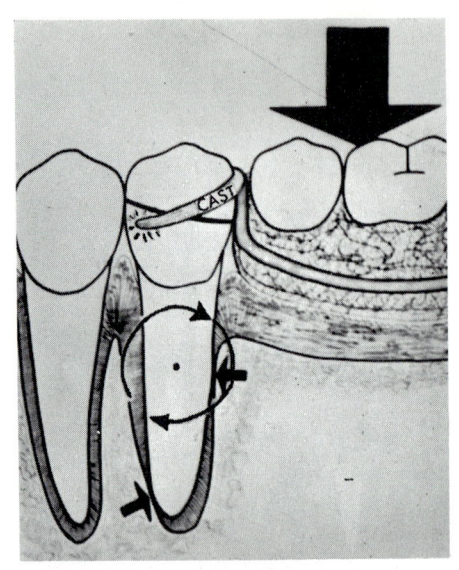

**Fig. 13-3.** The effects of a fulcrum line of a free-end saddle partial denture on an abutment tooth. The larger arrows show the areas of compression created when an abutment is rotated about a pivot point.

## THE ADULT SPACE MAINTAINER

A preventive partial denture must be the result of (1) an enthusiastic and effective patient education program, (2) a preventive diagnosis and preventive prescription program, (3) a correct treatment program, (4) a preventive mouth preparation and construction program, (5) instructions for a home-care program, and (6) a dependable recall system.

### Patient education program

The first preventive step for the dentist is to become friendly with the patient. Friendship develops rapport; strong rapport and a dentist who is enthusiastic about preventive dentistry will help motivate patients to do their part in prevention.

Without complete and enthusiastic cooperation of the patient, preventive dentistry will only be a dream. The patient and dentist must become a team dedicated to the preservation of the patient's oral health. Patient education begins with the first appointment and continues as long as the team effort exists. The varying degrees of success this relationship enjoys in maintaining oral health, once it is established, are directly related to the level of patient education and motivation.

The dentist must "pave his way with words" to succeed. The "chuckholes" in the road to success will be the voids in the patient's knowledge about his role in preventing disease. Often patient education will be the most important part of preventive dentistry. The knowledge that the dentist imparts to a patient about oral health problems is important to the patient; in addition, to teach suggests that learning should be evaluated. In other words, the patient must be tested for the same reasons that students are tested. How else can we find out how much learning has occurred? For example, on the day that the patient is to get his new appliance give him his qualifying exam. Question him about the things you have taught him. One of the many questions I use is, "Why are you getting a new space maintainer?" He should be able to tell you about the value of space maintenance. Your questions should be directed toward the objectives of your patient educational program.

If the patient is not learning, a review is indicated. On the other hand, if the patient cannot learn or refuses to learn, the prognosis for the remaining teeth and tissues is poor. Patients who cannot learn to care for their mouths should be offered an alternate prescription, if one exists, or the dentist may be better off if he refuses to accept his portion of the responsibility for the oral health of those patients. For example, if abutment teeth decay, an uncooperative patient might blame the dentist when in fact the patient may have rarely brushed. However, the patient may not have learned about the value of good oral hygiene because the dentist taught too much too fast.

People learn rapidly at first and then reach a plateau.[6] So, concentrate the important part and a larger amount of patient education during the first two visits.

When teaching patients, it is well to remember that, like students, they are likely to forget 75 percent of what you tell them within 2 to 3 days.[7] Therefore effective patient education demands repeating or reviewing areas covered at earlier appointments. Only a small amount of new information should be added after the first two visits. How much a "small amount" of new knowledge is will have to be defined by the dentist as he talks with his patients and estimates their intelligence and motivation.

## Preventive diagnosis and preventive prescription program

This chapter cannot cover the entire subject of oral examination and diagnosis. Diagnosis is important because it is the foundation of the prescription work order. Every dentist should have a modern textbook on oral diagnosis[8-11]; teeth are saved every day that 20 years ago would have been unfit to be retained.

The first part of all preventive prescriptions and therapy for all patients will be a thorough stannous fluoride prophylaxis[12] and stannous fluoride topical application.[13] A clean mouth is easier to diagnose. Also, the stannous fluoride arrests carious lesions and prevents further lesions from developing.

The preventive diagnosis and prescription includes weighing many factors, which collectively will prevent loss of teeth under the preventive partial denture. To diagnose patients' problems the dentist must make accurate radiograms and diagnostic casts mounted in centric occlusion. Also, the patient should complete a health chart (Fig. 13-4).

The dentist must visualize all of the preliminary treatment and then the classification of removable partial denture that is possible for the patient. The preventive prescription is the prescription of choice. It is made as if the dentist were the patient with the same diagnostic picture. With the roentgenograms, diagnostic casts, and the patient at hand, the dentist should consider each of the following areas: (1) the crowns of the teeth, (2) the investing tissues, (3) the soft tissues, and (4) the classification of the partially edentulous situation.

**Crowns of the teeth.** The examination of the clinical crowns of the teeth is probably the strongest part of any dentist's diagnosis. Dental caries, both frank and

**University of Missouri at Kansas City**
SCHOOL OF DENTISTRY

________________________________
Student Signature

**DEPARTMENT OF ORAL DIAGNOSIS**
(Student Diagnosis)

Patient________________ Address ________________
Date of birth________ Referred by________________ Phone No.________
Reason for present visit ________________________
Abnormalities noted:________________________

**DIAGNOSIS:**

| | 1 | 2 | 3 | 4 | 5 | 6 | 7 | 8 | 9 | 10 | 11 | 12 | 13 | 14 | 15 | 16 | |
|---|---|---|---|---|---|---|---|---|---|---|---|---|---|---|---|---|---|
| **R** | | | | | | | | | | | | | | | | | **L** |
| | 32 | 31 | 30 | 29 | 28 | 27 | 26 | 25 | 24 | 23 | 22 | 21 | 20 | 19 | 18 | 17 | |

| TREATMENT PROGRAM | TREATMENT PROGRAM |
|---|---|
| 1 ________ | 32 ________ |
| 2 ________ | 31 ________ |
| 3 ________ | 30 ________ |
| 4 ________ | 29 ________ |
| 5 ________ | 28 ________ |
| 6 ________ | 27 ________ |
| 7 ________ | 26 ________ |
| 8 ________ | 25 ________ |
| 9 ________ | 24 ________ |
| 10 ________ | 23 ________ |
| 11 ________ | 22 ________ |
| 12 ________ | 21 ________ |
| 13 ________ | 20 ________ |
| 14 ________ | 19 ________ |
| 15 ________ | 18 ________ |
| 16 ________ | 17 ________ |

**Write a short treatment prescription for this case**________________

**Additional diagnostic information:**

**Fig. 13-4.** Examination record and prescription form for use in diagnosis and treatment planning for the adult space maintainer.

## GENERAL HEALTH CHART

### CARDIOVASCULAR SYSTEM
*Circle One*

| | |
|---|---|
| Has a physician ever said you had heart trouble? | Yes No *DK |
| Do you get out of breath easily? | Yes No DK |
| Has a physician ever said your blood pressure was too high or too low? | Yes No DK |
| As a child did you have rheumatic fever, growing pains, or twitching of the limbs? | Yes No DK |
| Have you fainted more than twice in your life? | Yes No DK |
| Do you have spells of dizziness? | Yes No DK |
| Have you ever had rheumatic heart disease or Saint Vitus' dance? | Yes No DK |
| Are your ankles often badly swollen? | Yes No DK |
| Have you at times had bad nose bleeds? | Yes No DK |
| Do you get out of breath readily? | Yes No DK |

### NERVOUS SYSTEM

| | |
|---|---|
| Do you suffer badly from frequent severe headaches? | Yes No DK |
| Has a physician ever told you that you had neuralgia? | Yes No DK |
| Has a physician ever told you that you had neuritis? | Yes No DK |
| Has a physician ever told you that you had neurosis? | Yes No DK |
| Have you ever had a nervous breakdown? | Yes No DK |
| Has a physician ever told you that you had epilepsy? | Yes No DK |

### RESPIRATORY SYSTEM

| | |
|---|---|
| Is your nose continually stuffed up? | Yes No DK |
| Do you have asthma? | Yes No DK |
| Do you have hay fever? | Yes No DK |
| Have you ever had tuberculosis? | Yes No DK |
| Do you have frequent sore throat? | Yes No DK |
| Do you have sinusitis? | Yes No DK |

### GASTROINTESTINAL TRACT

| | |
|---|---|
| Do you suffer from stomach trouble? | Yes No DK |
| Do you have frequent diarrhea? | Yes No DK |

### ENDOCRINE SYSTEM

| | |
|---|---|
| Are you frequently thirsty? | Yes No DK |
| Has a member of your family had diabetes? | Yes No DK |
| Have you ever taken thyroid tablets? | Yes No DK |
| Have you ever had diabetes? | Yes No DK |
| At what age did you reach puberty? ........ Age | |
| Are you menstruating regularly? | Yes No DK |
| At what age did your menstruation cease? ........ Age | |

### GENITOURINARY TRACT
*Circle One*

| | |
|---|---|
| Did a physician ever say that you had kidney or bladder trouble? | Yes No DK |

### SPECIAL ORGANS

| | |
|---|---|
| Have you ever been treated for ear trouble? | Yes No DK |
| Have you ever been treated for eye trouble other than corrective glasses? | Yes No DK |

### OTHER

| | |
|---|---|
| Are you sensitive to any particular medicine (aspirin........, antibiotics ........, sulfa drugs ........, barbiturates ........, others ........)? | Yes No DK |
| Have you gained or lost much weight recently? | Yes No DK |
| Have you ever had syphilis or bad blood? | Yes No DK |
| Have you ever been treated for bad blood? | Yes No DK |
| Have you ever had X-Ray treatments? | Yes No DK |
| Have you ever had an operation? | Yes No DK |
| Have you ever had a series of "needles," "shots," or injections? | Yes No DK |
| Has a physician ever told you that you had a tumor or a cancer? | Yes No DK |
| Have you ever had an anesthesia? Local? Yes No General? | Yes No DK |
| Have you ever had an undesirable reaction to an anesthetic? | Yes No DK |
| Are you receiving any treatment with anticoagulants? | Yes No DK |
| Are you taking any cortisone type of treatment? | Yes No DK |
| Are you receiving any treatment by any physician now? | Yes No DK |
| If so, by whom............................................................... | |

### BLOOD

| | |
|---|---|
| Have you ever had anemia? | Yes No DK |
| Have you ever had abnormal bleeding following extraction of teeth or from a cut? | Yes No DK |

### SKIN

| | |
|---|---|
| Have you ever been treated for a skin disease? | Yes No DK |
| What disease? ............................................................. | |

### BONES AND JOINTS

| | |
|---|---|
| Are your joints often painfully swollen? | Yes No DK |
| Have you ever had more than one fracture? | Yes No DK |
| Have you ever had more than one dislocation? | Yes No DK |
| Do you have arthritis? | Yes No DK |

### SPECIAL DENTAL

| | |
|---|---|
| Have you often had severe toothaches? | Yes No DK |
| Have you ever had severe pains of the face or head? | Yes No DK |
| Do your gums bleed when you brush your teeth? | Yes No DK* |
| Have you ever had gum treatments? | Yes No DK |
| Have you ever had an acute sore mouth? | Yes No DK |
| What was your last dental treatment and when? ........................ | |

PHYSICIAN'S REPORT AND GENERAL STATEMENT ...........................................

..............................................................................................................................

*DK—don't know.

Fig. 13-4, cont'd. For legend see opposite page.

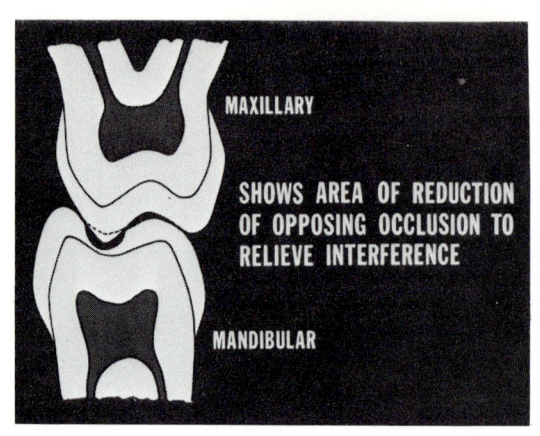

**Fig. 13-5.** We are assuming that an adequate rest area has been prepared in the mandibular abutment. However, a wax bite was taken of the patient in centric occlusion and, when examined against a light, showed insufficient space available for the lug rest. Therefore the opposing cusp tip should be reduced as illustrated.

recurrent, often receives first attention when the patient comes to the dental office. The location of dental caries should be recorded as part of the prescription. Defective restorations will, of course, be recorded and replacement prescribed.

The teeth must be tested for vitality.[14] Endodontic therapy should be prescribed for any nonvital tooth that can be used in restoring oral health.

Examine the chewing surfaces of the abutment teeth. The occlusal surface of each abutment tooth will be prepared to receive an occlusal rest. To accommodate the partial denture occlusal rest a preparation must be made. The mechanics of this will be considered later. There must be adequate room or space for the occlusal rest. If there is inadequate space, it must be indicated on the prescription for correction. Correction means that either the location of the lug rest must be changed, or a gold restoration must be placed, or the opposing tooth must be reduced (Fig. 13-5).

All proximal abutment restorations must be made of gold since this metal has good edge strength. Note that all wax patterns for abutment restorations must be contoured with the aid of a surveyor. Surveying is a nebulous area for dentists. However, every dentist can learn to survey by buying a surveyor, reading how to survey[15] in a textbook, and practicing with the surveyor, with the help of a technician, until he becomes competent and at ease with the instrument.

It is the dentist's responsibility to survey and design each removable partial denture. Only after a comprehensive oral diagnosis and survey can a dentist write a preventive prescription that includes the indicated partial denture design.

With a diagnostic cast on a surveyor table, examine the buccal surface of each abutment tooth. Conceive a path of insertion that is a mean of all of the proximal surfaces. Next, visualize the restoration or contouring needed to make the proximal surface of each abutment that borders an edentulous space parallel to the path of insertion (Fig. 13-6). Minor correction should be included as part of the prescription. It might indicate that grinding and polishing the enamel of a restoration may be necessary. If the contour is excessive on either the buccal or proximal surface the prescription should include grinding the surface and polishing the enamel. Insuffi-

*Preventive adult space maintainers (partial dentures)* 305

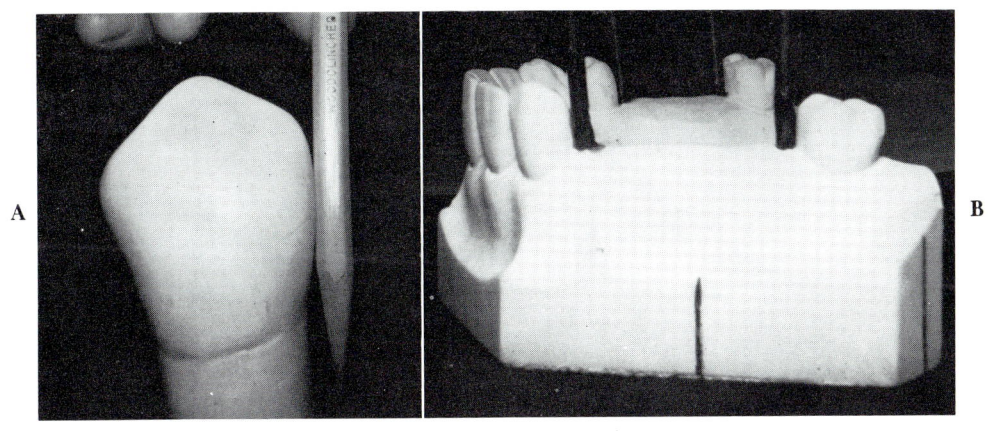

**Fig. 13-6. A,** The proximal surface of each abutment tooth must be ground or restored to be parallel with the path of insertion. **B,** The proximal surfaces of all the abutment teeth have been ground or restored to be parallel with the path of insertion. Note the path of insertion lines on the base of the cast.

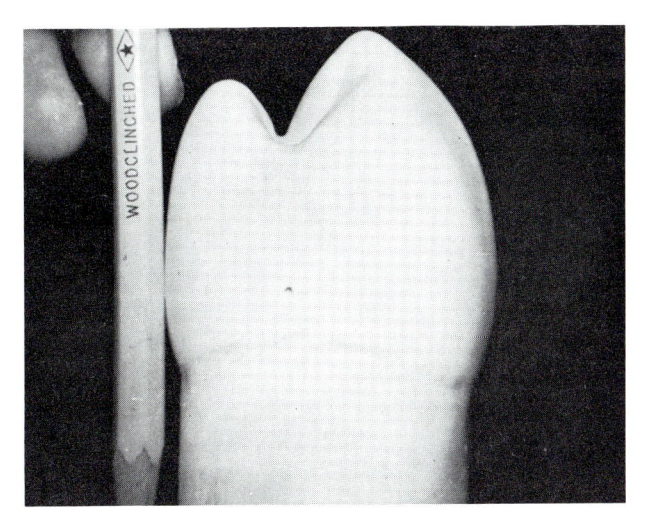

**Fig. 13-7.** The lingual surface of each abutment tooth must have a low survey line to provide adequate room above it for the nonretentive reciprocal arm.

cient retentive contour will require prescribing a three-quarter crown with lingual undercut or a full crown on the abutment.

The lingual surface of each abutment tooth must be examined for contour. The reciprocal arm must lie opposite the retentive arm but above the greatest tooth convexity (Fig. 13-7). A preventive prescription often includes preparing this surface to adjust the contour. Ideally, the lingual surface should be parallel to the proximal surface; this can always be achieved if the abutments are crowned.

To complete the survey, place three widely separated lines that are parallel to the path of insertion on the capitol or base of the cast for future reference (Fig. 13-8).

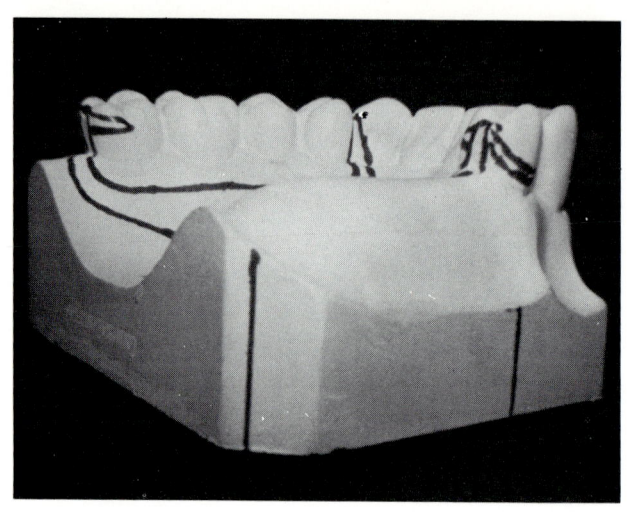

**Fig. 13-8.** The three widely separated vertical lines on the base of each surveyed study cast are parallel to the path of insertion. The lines aid the laboratory technician in duplicating the identical path of insertion that the dentist used to prepare the guiding planes.

Malposed teeth present the greatest complexity in abnormal contour; they must be crowned unless it may enhance the results to extract them.[17] However, before you extract a tooth visualize the difficulty of the situation you would create (Fig. 13-12).

Contact of the teeth should be either tight or far enough apart that the spaces created are self-cleansing. Examine the marginal ridges above each contact point. Marginal ridges help hold the bolus of food on the chewing surfaces of teeth and should be of equal height to produce a satisfactory occlusal table. If the proximal tooth contact and marginal ridges are not satisfactory, include in the preventive prescription simple grinding or placement of corrective restorations.

The clinical crowns of teeth should be examined for premature occlusal contacts. The occlusion should be meticulously examined in patients with temporomandibular joint disorders. A preventive prescription would include equilibration of the occlusion to eliminate various types of occlusal disharmonies.[18] The occlusion should be examined before, during, and after all therapy.

**Investing tissue.** The dentist should complete a periodontal chart[16] (Fig. 13-9), palpate the teeth for mobility, and record the movement of each tooth horizontally and longitudinally. If excess mobility[19] can be demonstrated, examine the health chart for systemic influences. Indicate preventive periodontal therapy as a part of the preventive prescription.

Bone maintenance of each patient is a nebulous area. Glickman[20] says that bone is the least stable component of the periodontium. Bone is in a constant state of flux.[21] A preventive diagnosis would consider the crown-root ratio. If less than half the original bone remains, the prognosis for the tooth as an abutment might be questioned.[22] However, the health of the periodontium is probably more important than generalizations about crown–root–alveolar bone ratio. The responsibility must rest with the dentist whether or not to prescribe multiple tooth splints for partial denture abutments. If a dentist would routinely prescribe multiple tooth splinting for lower bicuspid abutments that are to support a free-end partial denture, the prognosis for the abutments and the partial denture would be much improved. If a patient has vertical bone loss in the absence of gingivitis, he may have periodontosis. If the systemic error in bone metabolism cannot be treated, prescribe a transitional appliance.[23]

**Soft tissues.** Soft tissues should be examined for pathoses.[24] Question the patient about abnormalities about the face, lips, and oral cavity. Palpate the tissues for firm masses. Look for unusual radiolucencies and opacities on the radiographs. Record any suspicious lesion in the preventive prescription for future observation or biopsy. If there is any doubt about the diagnosis of a lesion, biopsy it. (See Chapter 15.)

Surgical therapy must be prescribed to correct the following anomalies: tori, embedded tooth remnants, bony ledges, and hyperplastic tissue. Unerupted third molars should not be routinely extracted for all younger patients. They may need these teeth as a bridge abutment later in life. Enlarged tuberosities should be removed to provide space for one or two removable partial dentures. Excess leverage on abutment teeth and resorption of subbasal tissues will result from the occlusion of a tuberosity with a free-end saddle partial denture.

**Classification.** Classification is the key to preventive partial denture design and construction.[1] Each partially edentulous situation dictates a specific design and the materials best suited to control the stresses on the abutment teeth.

If more than a single edentulous space is present, the basic classification identifies the most difficult situation. For example, classify free ends first, which would be Classes I, II, and V. They would take precedence over Classes III, IV, or VI, which would be called modification spaces. If all of the posterior teeth were missing from a posterior quadrant with only bicuspid missing from the opposite side of the jaw, the classification would be Class II-P.

**Support for the removable partial denture.** The six classes of the Applegate-Kennedy Classification System for partially edentulous situations are divided into two basic categories: tooth-supported removable (bridges) partial dentures (Fig. 13-10) and tooth-supported and tissue-supported prostheses (Fig. 13-11). Tooth-supported prostheses are preferable. They transmit the stresses of mastication through the teeth to the supporting tissues. Within physiologic limits, the tensile stress maintains bone by tension on the periodontal ligaments. Tooth-tissue–supported removable partial dentures also receive part of their support from the subbasal tissue. Here the stress is compressive and transmits pressure through the underlying soft tissues to bone. If beyond physiologic limits, compressive stress causes the edentulous ridge to resorb. It is rare for a patient to not have some tissue change under a tissue-supported prostheses. Our attempts are directed toward minimizing and delaying the change as long as possible.

The ease with which a removable partial denture can be made and worn is important to the dentist and patient. The difference between the two categories of partial dentures is often one key tooth. For this reason I have devised a visual aid for identifying key teeth. The aid shows a continuum between "easy" and "difficult" and places each of the six classes in their respective locations.

**Continuum between easy and difficult cases.** A helpful visual aid for patient education is to place all six classes of the Applegate-Kennedy Classification System on a continuum between easy and difficult cases. "Easy" means that the removable partial denture, usually tooth supported, creates few problems for the dentist and few problems for the patient. Tooth-supported removable partial dentures require

308 *Improving dental practice through preventive measures*

### UNIVERSITY OF MISSOURI AT KANSAS CITY
### SCHOOL OF DENTISTRY
## DEPARTMENT OF PERIODONTICS

Name_____ Birthdate_____ Date_____
Occupation_____ Student_____ Jr.
Race_____ Sr.

| CHIEF COMPLAINT | SIGNIFICANT MEDICAL HISTORY |
|---|---|
| HISTORY OF PRESENT ILLNESS | HABIT HISTORY |
|  |                                     1st Visit Quest      2nd Visit Quest. |
|  | CLENCHING |
|  | GRINDING |
|  | BRUXING |
|  | LIP-CHEEK BITING |
|  | TONGUE THRUSTING |
|  | OTHER_____ |
| PAST DENTAL HISTORY |  |
|  | DIET EVALUATION |
| SOCIAL HISTORY | LABORATORY TESTS |
|  | Date_____ Type_____ |
|  | Date Received_____ |
| PATIENT ATTITUDE | OCCLUSAL OBSERVATIONS |
| Visit No. 1_____ |  |
| Visit No. 4_____ |  |
| Visit No. 10_____ |  |
| Completion_____ |  |
| First Recall_____ |  |

| ORAL HYGIENE | First Examination | Recom. |
|---|---|---|
| Brush type (how many): |  |  |
| Dentifrice: |  |  |
| Technic: |  |  |
| When Brushed: |  |  |
| Interdental Stim: |  |  |

REMARKS

Fig. 13-9. Examination forms for recording, classification, and diagnosis of periodontal disease.

# Preventive adult space maintainers (partial dentures)

## EXAMINATION CHART

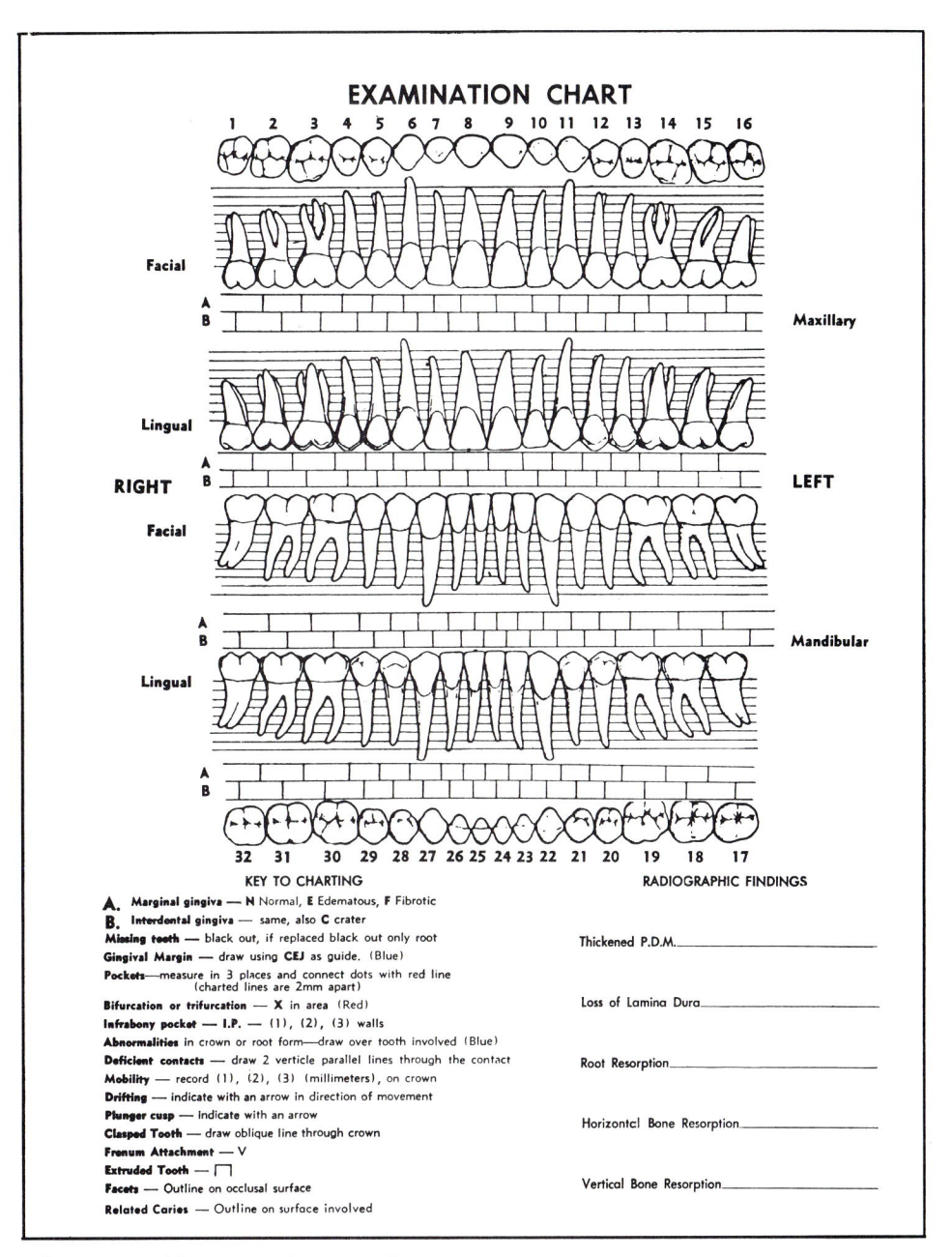

**Facial** — Maxillary
**Lingual**
**RIGHT** — **LEFT**
**Facial** — Mandibular
**Lingual**

### KEY TO CHARTING

**A.** **Marginal gingiva** — **N** Normal, **E** Edematous, **F** Fibrotic
**B.** **Interdental gingiva** — same, also **C** crater
**Missing tooth** — black out, if replaced black out only root
**Gingival Margin** — draw using **CEJ** as guide. (Blue)
**Pockets**—measure in 3 places and connect dots with red line (charted lines are 2mm apart)
**Bifurcation or trifurcation** — **X** in area (Red)
**Infrabony pocket** — **I.P.** — (1), (2), (3) walls
**Abnormalities** in crown or root form—draw over tooth involved (Blue)
**Deficient contacts** — draw 2 verticle parallel lines through the contact
**Mobility** — record (1), (2), (3) (millimeters), on crown
**Drifting** — indicate with an arrow in direction of movement
**Plunger cusp** — indicate with an arrow
**Clasped Tooth** — draw oblique line through crown
**Frenum Attachment** — V
**Extruded Tooth** — ⊓
**Facets** — Outline on occlusal surface
**Related Caries** — Outline on surface involved

### RADIOGRAPHIC FINDINGS

Thickened P.D.M._____

Loss of Lamina Dura_____

Root Resorption_____

Horizontal Bone Resorption_____

Vertical Bone Resorption_____

**Fig. 13-9, cont'd.** For legend see opposite page.

## ETIOLOGY

**Local Environmental Factors**

Calculus_____
Food Retention_____
Food Impaction_____

Overhang_____
High frenum attachment_____
Malposed tooth_____
Improper embrasure_____
Denture irritation_____
Inadequate Oral Hygiene_____

Occlusal trauma_____
Underfunction_____
Other_____

**GENERAL ORAL & SYSTEMIC FACTORS**

**OCCLUSAL FACTORS**

**DIAGNOSIS**

**KEY TO BELOW CHART**

Curettage — C
Gingivectomy — G.V.
Gingivoplasty — G.P.
Vest. Ext. — V.E.
Ging. Ext. — G.E.
Osteoplasty — O.P.
Osteoectomy — O.E.
Reattachment — R.A.
Minor tooth move — M.T.M.
Occlusal Adjust. — O.A.
Extraction — X.
Prognosis Doubtful — ? (Red)

## TREATMENT & PROGNOSIS

R | 1 | 2 | 3 | 4 | 5 | 6 | 7 | 8 | 9 | 10 | 11 | 12 | 13 | 14 | 15 | 16 | L
32 | 31 | 30 | 29 | 28 | 27 | 26 | 25 | 24 | 23 | 22 | 21 | 20 | 19 | 18 | 17

**RESTORATIVE RECOMMENDATIONS ADJUNCTIVE TO PERIODONTAL THERAPY**

**TREATMENT PRESCRIPTION**   Instructor

___ Emergency Treatment_____
___ Preliminary Prophylaxis_____
___ History & Charting (Diagnosis)_____
___ Scaling & Root Planing_____
___ Oral Physiotherapy_____
___ Temp. Stabilization_____
___ Surgery (Type)_____

___ Occ. Adjustment_____
___ Minor Tooth Movement_____
___ Bruxism Splint_____
___ Re-evaluation_____
___ Other_____

**REGISTER EACH COMPLETED PHASE FOR CREDIT**

Fig. 13-9, cont'd. For legend see p. 308.

Fig. 13-9, cont'd. For legend see p. 308.

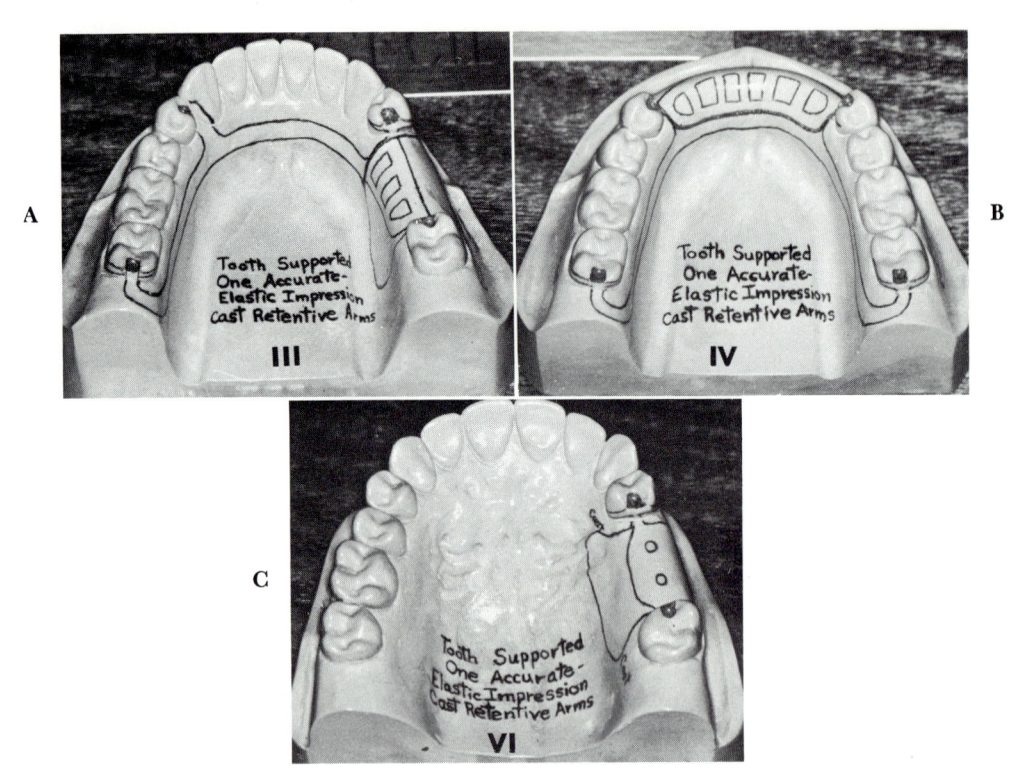

**312**  *Improving dental practice through preventive measures*

Fig. 13-10. **A,** Tooth-supported Class III partially edentulous situation and removable partial denture design. The abutment teeth cannot withstand the entire work load of chewing. Therefore the framework design must use cross-arch splinting. The direct retainers are made up of one cast retentive arm, a cast nonretentive reciprocal arm, and an occlusal rest. Direct retainers are on abutments 18, 28, and 31. **B,** Tooth-supported Class IV partially edentulous situation and removable partial denture design. The anterior space crosses the midline of the mouth. The Class IV partial denture is indicated following extensive bone loss in the anterior part of the mouth. Use cast clasp direct retainers on the most anterior abutments and most posterior molars. **C,** Tooth-supported Class VI edentulous situation and removable partial denture design. The abutment teeth are sound. Prescribe a fixed bridge for the Class VI edentulous space if possible. The direct retainers must have both buccal and lingual cast retentive arms.

few postinsertion adjustments. Comfortable prostheses are usually more preventive than uncomfortable ones. "Difficult" means that the construction of the prosthesis is more complicated and more postinsertion adjustments are needed because of the dual support. A general arrangement along the continuum from easy to difficult is: Classes III and VI are the easiest; Classes I and IV are moderately easy; finally, Classes V and II are difficult (Fig. 13-12). For example, a Class II removable partial denture (free-end base) is difficult because the patient compares the natural teeth on one side with the artificial teeth on the other. This is not a fair comparison, but patients consciously or unconsciously make the comparison each time they swallow, chew, or brux. I suspect that fewer Class II appliances are worn by patients for whom they are made than any other removable partial denture. If possible, difficult

Preventive adult space maintainers (partial dentures) 313

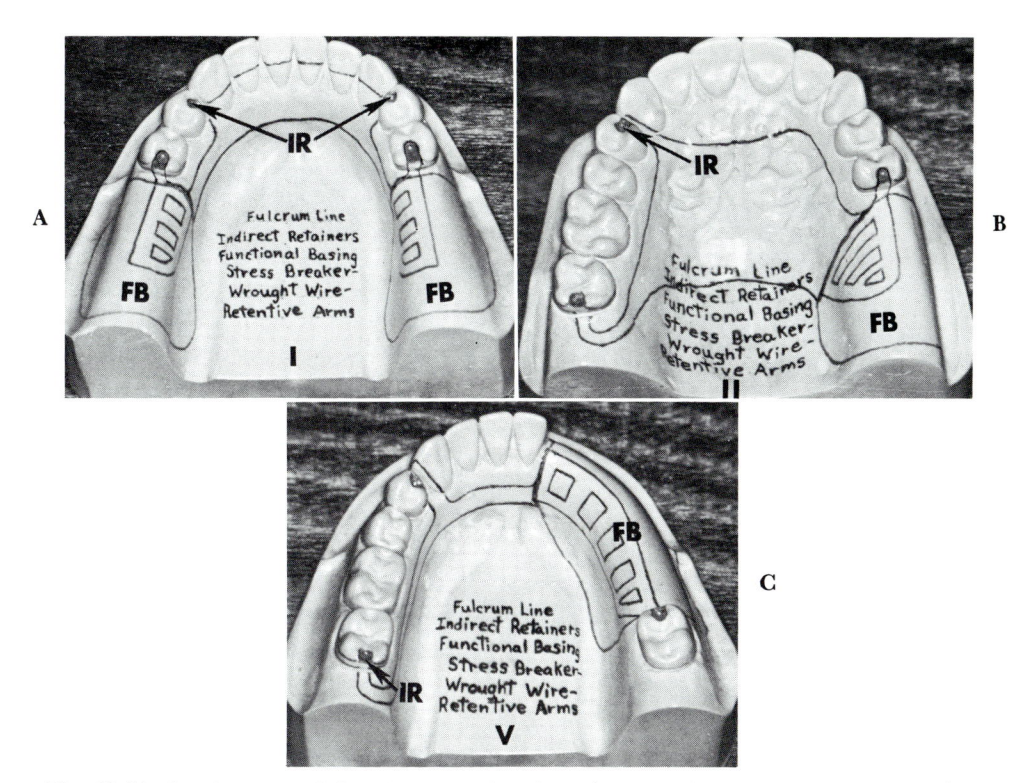

Fig. 13-11. A, Class I partially edentulous situation with its design has two *free-end* saddles. Class I is the most common type of removable partial denture. Free-end removable partial dentures have a fulcrum line. Fulcrum lines dictate the use of an indirect retainer, **I.R.**, a direct retainer composed of a wrought wire retentive arm, reciprocal arm, and an occlusal rest, and functional basing, **F.B. B**, Class II partially edentulous situation with its design has one *free-end* saddle. Free-end removable partial dentures have a fulcrum line. Fulcrum lines dictate the use of an indirect retainer, **I.R.**, a direct retainer composed of a wrought wire retentive arm, a cast reciprocal arm, and an occlusal rest, and functional basing, **F.B. C**, Class V partially edentulous situation with its design. Class V is similar to a Class II in that it has one *free-end* saddle. However, the single free-end saddle is to the anterior portion of the arch. Class V also looks much like Class III except the anterior abutment is not suited for abutment service. Direct retainers are located on abutments 18, 21 or 22, and 31. (Additional edentulous spaces beyond each basic classification may occur. They are anterior and posterior modification spaces. Occlusal rests, mesial and distal, to each space are sufficient.)

classes, such as Class V, should be "pushed" toward the easy area by prescribing multiple tooth splinting. Then a Class III could be made. Both the dentist and patient will be happier. Occasionally a patient will demand that a single molar in a posterior quadrant be extracted. If the patient and dentist are unaware of the continuum the dentist may change a potentially easy Class III into a difficult Class II.

To complete the diagnosis and prescription the dentist should make a final classification of the partially edentulous situation and draw the framework outline onto the diagnostic cast.

**Treatment program.** The correct sequence for oral rehabilitation or maintenance is one in which the maximum results are achieved in the shortest possible time with the minimum effort for both the dentist and the patient. The treatment program

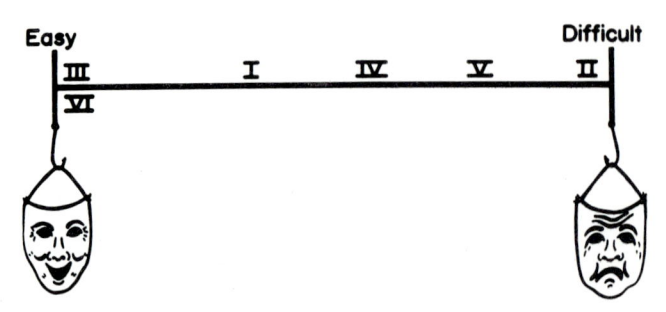

314 *Improving dental practice through preventive measures*

**CONTINUUM OF EASY-DIFFICULT**

**Fig. 13-12.** Dentists create partially edentulous situations with forceps. This learning model should help the dentist and patient visualize the ease or difficulty of the patient's situation before and after extraction. If extraction of one or more teeth creates a situation that is undesirable, measures such as endodontics, hemisection, and periodontal therapy must be followed by the dentist.

should be tailored to each patient. Usually endodontic therapy or oral surgery should be completed first. Periodontal therapy, operative dentistry, crown and bridge prosthodontics, and removable partial dentures are usually completed in this order. The order can and often should vary. For example, improperly contoured proximal restorations can create some of the conditions necessary for periodontal disease. Operative dentistry would then be completed as an adjunct to periodontal therapy.

Usually the adult space maintainer will be made after all other therapy is completed. Often, all therapy may be completed with the exception of rest preparation and adjusting tooth contour. Alterations in contour, even though noted in the original diagnosis, prescription, and treatment program, must again be considered.

### Preventive mouth preparation and construction program

Since all abutment teeth with inlays and crowns are surveyed to ensure contours receptive to the adult space maintainer, the same technics must be applied to the contours of the other abutment teeth.

**Rest preparations.** Occlusal rest must be present on every adult space maintainer. Absence of a rest from neglect, from some misguided partial denture concept, or from a fracture cannot be allowed in preventive dentistry. Unfortunately for the patients concerned, most dentists have seen the destructive aftermath created by a fracture of an occlusal rest from a removable partial denture.

For the particular class of partial denture on the articulated study casts locate the area of each rest preparation. View each area from the buccal surface and lingual surface in order to determine the best area for the preparation. If the abutment is a bicuspid or molar tooth the rest area may easily be prepared by first exaggerating the fossa and then by reducing the marginal ridge. The fossa is reduced by using a 2 to 3 mm. diameter round diamond rotary instrument. Reduce the fossa to half the diameter of the particular instrument. This will remove only enamel in some teeth but in others it may expose dentin. The matter of exposed dentin will be considered later. Return the stone to the prepared fossa and remove a portion of the enamel from the marginal ridge and then pull the instrument over the marginal ridge of the tooth to create a wedge-shaped preparation (Fig. 13-13). The preparation slopes from the marginal ridge into the prepared fossa. The result is a rest area deep enough to accommodate a strong occlusal rest without affecting the opposing teeth. The completed rest can be described as spoon shaped (Fig. 13-14). If the retentive arms are removed or become broken off the lug rests should be able to retain the partial denture in rest seats as the patient bites down. Polish the rest area and apply stannous fluoride. Exposed dentin under an occlusal rest should be considered in terms of the age of the patient, tooth sensitivity, and caries attack rate. A young patient should have a rest area prepared in a gold restoration if he has a high caries attack rate or tooth sensitivity after a rest area is prepared. Older patients have dead tracts of dentin that are caries resistant and insensitive.[25, 26]

Rest areas prepared on large cuspids may be placed on the cingulum. Prepare the cingulum rest with an instrument comparable to a No. 58 smooth fissure bur. The floor of the completed rest must slope apically toward the long axis of the tooth (Fig. 13-15). Round the sharp gingival cavosurface line angle to prevent fracture of the master cast in this area.

An incisal rest should be made on small cuspids. The rest preparation may be made with a diamond wheel. The rest area is made opposite the edentulous space.

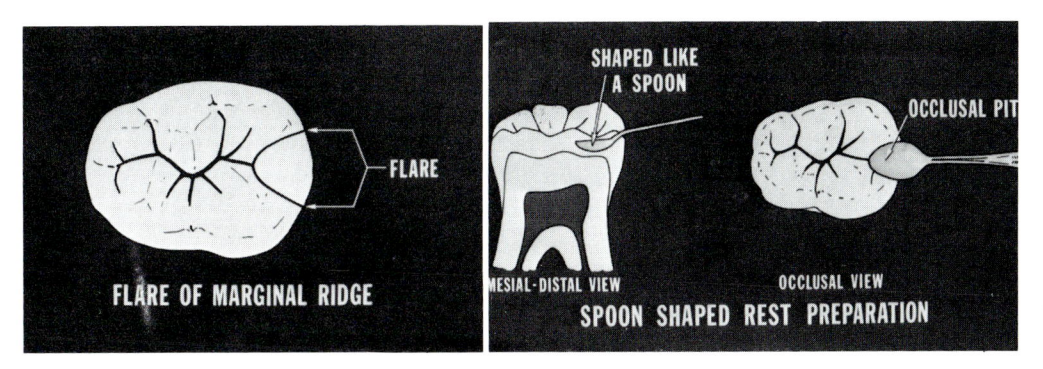

Fig. 13-13

Fig. 13-14

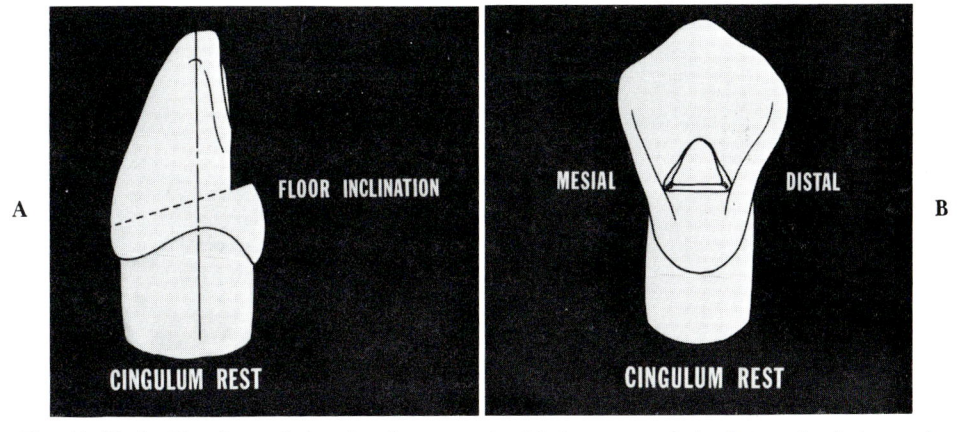

Fig. 13-15. A, The floor of the cingulum rest should slope toward the long axis of the tooth. B, The floor of the cingulum rest should be perpendicular to the long axis of the tooth.

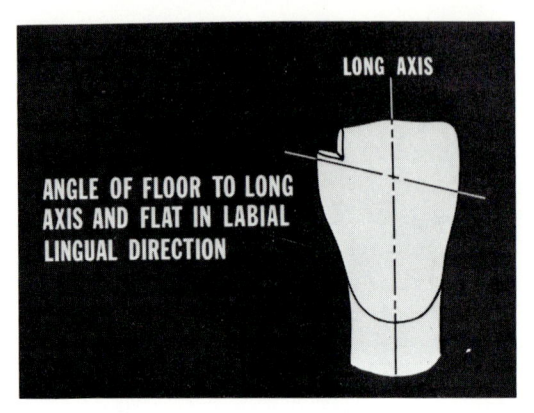

Fig. 13-16. The incisal rest should be opposite the edentulous space. The floor should slope toward the long axis of the tooth. Labiolingually the floor should be flat.

The floor of the incisal rest slopes apically from the incisal corner of the tooth toward the long axis of the abutment tooth (Fig. 13-16).

**Contour of natural tooth surfaces.** Contour of the natural vertical tooth surfaces should be changed at the time rest preparations are made. Reduce those areas of enamel that were noted on the diagnostic cast after it was surveyed and designed. The surfaces are corrected to prevent the partial denture from gaining excessive retention from abnormal tooth contours and from creating food traps. The corrected surfaces are indispensable to the preventive partial denture in space maintenance.

The mouth is now ready for the adult space maintainer. Every possible preventive measure has been taken in the diagnosis, prescription, treatment program, and therapy for the teeth and soft tissue. In order to control the stresses introduced by the prosthesis the dentist must know the function of the units of the preventive prosthesis.

**Units of the adult space maintainer.** Each adult space maintainer is composed of many parts called units.[27] The tooth-supported prostheses are Classes III, IV, and VI. They are composed of a major connector, many minor connectors, two to four direct retainers, one or more bases, and one or more artificial teeth.

A major connector is the largest part of the partial denture cast framework. The major connector may be either a lingual bar connector or a palatal bar connector. This part unites the other units of the partial denture and transmits masticatory stress over as wide an area as possible. A major connector must be rigid to do its job. Minor connectors occur between major connectors and direct retainers, indirect retainers, and saddle connectors. The minor connector must also be rigid to transmit stress from these other components to the major connector.

The extracoronal direct retainers for a tooth-supported space maintainer are composed of one cast retentive arm, a cast reciprocal arm, and an occlusal rest. The final part of the tooth-supported prosthesis is the base. The base may be made from either metal or resin. Extension of the base is determined by the amount of resorbed subbasal tissue in the edentulous area. Contour is restored by the base material. In addition the base attaches one or more restored teeth to the retention webbing. The base of the tooth-supported prosthesis maintains only passive contact with the underlying tissue. The restored teeth will be considered later.

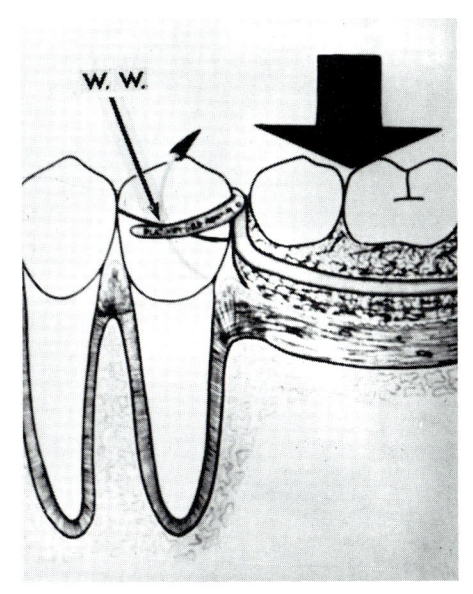

Fig. 13-17. Round wrought wire retentive arm, **W.W.**, dissipating stress by flexing sideways when a saddle settles.

**Units of tooth- and tissue-supported prostheses.** Tooth- and tissue-supported prostheses, Classes I, II, and V, are composed of a major connector, many minor connectors, two to four direct retainers, one or more indirect retainers, one or more bases, and one or more artificial teeth. The major and minor connectors of tooth-supported and tissue-supported prostheses have the same function. On the other hand, the extracoronal direct retainers are different. They are of two types—combination clasps for cuspids and bicuspids and cast clasps for molars. The combination clasp is composed of one alloy wrought wire retentive arm, a cast reciprocal arm, and an occlusal rest. The round wrought wire is 18 gauge. Wrought wire is used as the retentive arm of a direct retainer for its stress-breaking qualities. An added advantage of wrought wire retentive arms is that they do not stay well adapted. If a free-end saddle partial denture settles about its fulcrum into the soft underlying tissue, the retentive arm of the direct retainer must flex vertically to dissipate stress (Fig. 13-17). This is possible for a round wrought wire retentive arm, but impossible for a one-half round cast retentive arm. Another advantage of a round wire is that it has only line contact with the tooth surface. Therefore the chance of caries is lessened. The short reciprocal arm ends 182 degrees from the beginning of the distal third of the retentive arm. The reciprocal arm is cast. The function of the reciprocal arm is to counteract the orthodontic stress created by the retentive arm when the prosthesis is inserted or removed. Also, the reciprocal arm ensures the same function should the retentive arm be accidentally bent. Excessive length of the reciprocal arm adds unnecessary clasp-tooth contact area (Fig. 13-18). Thus there is greater danger of dental caries.

Between the wrought wire retentive arm and the reciprocal tooth is the occlusal rest. The rest is a most important unit of the direct retainer. The adult space maintainer always has the necessary occlusal rests. Fracture of an occlusal rest, even on

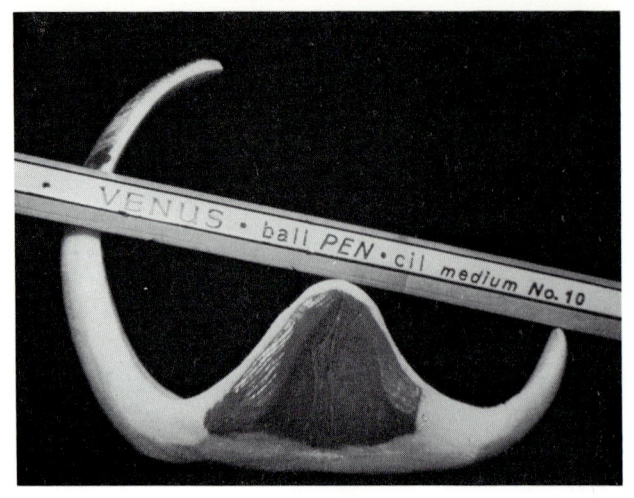

**Fig. 13-18.** A plastic model shows the relationship of a short reciprocal arm to a retentive arm. An excessively long reciprocal arm is unnecessary.

a preventive removable partial denture, allows the prosthesis to become destructive. The occlusal (incisal) rest must prevent the removable partial denture from settling gingivally or laterally a fraction of a millimeter. Settling of the framework can traumatize the underlying tissue, precipitate periodontal disease, and produce ridge resorption.[28-31] Let us briefly consider the intracoronal or precision type of direct retainer.

The support available for the precision attachment partial denture is the same as for the clasp type partial denture. This means that the partial denture must be supported by teeth, tissue, or their combinations. Another similarity is the need for functional basing, which I suspect is rare with precision partial dentures. Functional basing will be mentioned later. In addition to functional basing, a stress breaker should be used for mandibular Classes I and II.

A difference is in classification. For example, Class V partially edentulous situations should always be changed to a Class III, which lies at the easy end of the continuum. A potential Class V is changed to a Class III by the use of multiple fixed crown or horizontal pin splints. Class VI situations should be fixed partial dentures. Therefore precision partially edentulous classification would include only Classes I, II, III, and IV.

The design of the framework would remain the same as for the extracoronal direct retainers. A Class I and II precision prosthesis should have indirect retainers, just like the clasp type partial denture.

An additional unit of both the clasp and precision type extension base adult space maintainer is an indirect retainer. The indirect retainer is located across the fulcrum line from the extension base (Fig. 13-19). The indirect retainer is composed of a minor connector and an occlusal rest. The indirect retainer is a counterlever to the extension base.

Maxillary Class I precision partial dentures should have a base that covers the palate between the ridges, very much like a complete denture, to stabilize the base. Avoid hinge type stress breakers on maxillary precision prostheses; gravity often causes the bases to drop down when the patient opens his mouth.

*Preventive adult space maintainers (partial dentures)* 319

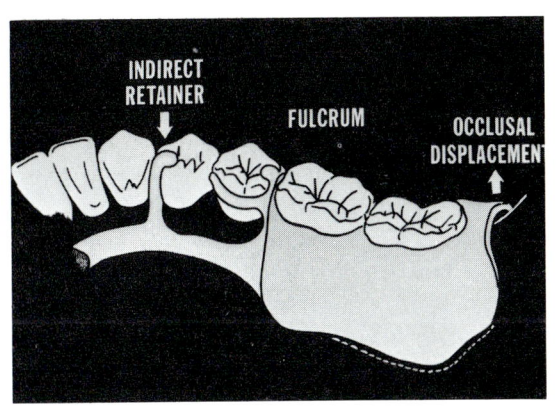

Fig. 13-19. If during mastication the extension base attempts to rise, the indirect retainer prevents the upward movement of the base about the fulcrum.

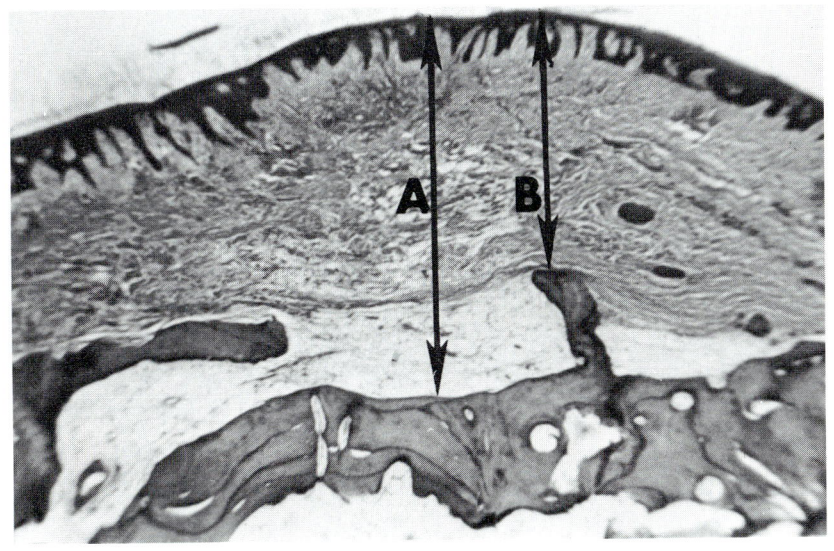

Fig. 13-20. A cross section of a mandibular ridge. Functional basing is needed for the free-end adult space maintainer to equalize the support between the thick (**A**) and thin (**B**) areas of the residual ridge. (Courtesy Dr. D. A. Dean.)

If the type of precision attachment used depends on saddle support, like the Ney attachment, keep the male attachment short of its rest seat to ensure that a fulcrum does not develop during mastication. Thus the chewing forces will be more perpendicular to the ridges.[32] Internal retentive precision devices such as the Sterns attachment should have a hinge stress breaker used with them except when a maxillary Class I is to be made, in which case the full posterior palate should be covered; then the hinge is not needed.

One of the most important parts of the extension base adult space maintainer is the extension base(s). The base carries artificial teeth and transmits masticatory stress into the underlying tissue. All extension bases of the adult space maintainer

**320** *Improving dental practice through preventive measures*

are functionally based. This means that the bases are maximally extended to spread stress over the greatest possible area without restricting the function of the tissue at its borders. The tissues under the bases are adapted to the functional form of the underlying tissue.[32] Functional impressions produce a functional form of the subbasal tissues. Such a form distributes the stress of mastication equally over hard and soft subbasal tissue (Fig. 13-20). Applegate[34] uses the term "placement" to illustrate the nonischemic pressure placed on the softer subbasal tissues during functional basing.

Functional impressions are so important to the adult space maintainer that a method for making one will be described here.

**Functional impression procedure.** Make an accurate elastic impression of the prepared partially edentulous mouth. Pour a master cast. Send it, the surveyed and

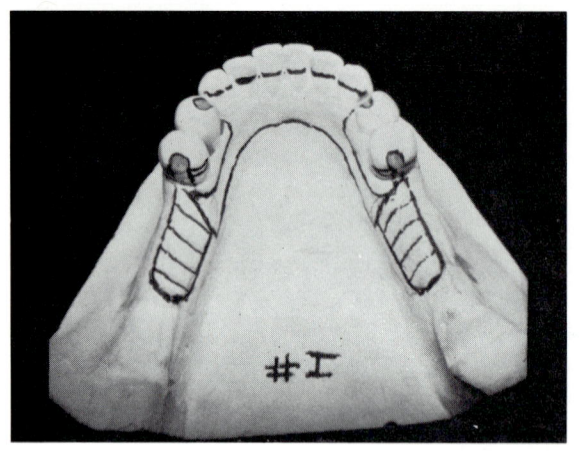

Fig. 13-21. Surveyed and designed Class I study cast, which, with a master cast and written prescription, is ready to be sent to the dental laboratory.

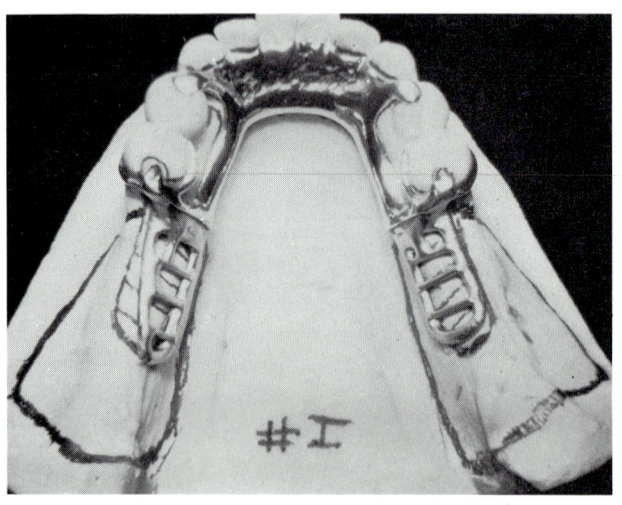

Fig. 13-22. Cast framework returned by the dental laboratory. The limiting and supporting structures have been outlined with a soft lead pencil.

designed study cast (Fig. 13-21), and the written prescription to the dental laboratory. The written instructions state that the framework is to be returned after the appliance is cast and polished. When the cast framework is returned, outline the limiting and supporting structures lying at the denture border with a soft lead pencil (Fig. 13-22). Dip the cast into water, mix a self-curing tray resin, and adapt the dough through the retention webbing. Be sure to hold the casting tightly to the master cast to prevent the indirect retainer from rising (Fig. 13-23). Shorten the cured temporary base to the line which transferred to the tissue side of the base. The completed temporary impression base is shown in Fig. 13-24. Blue or white

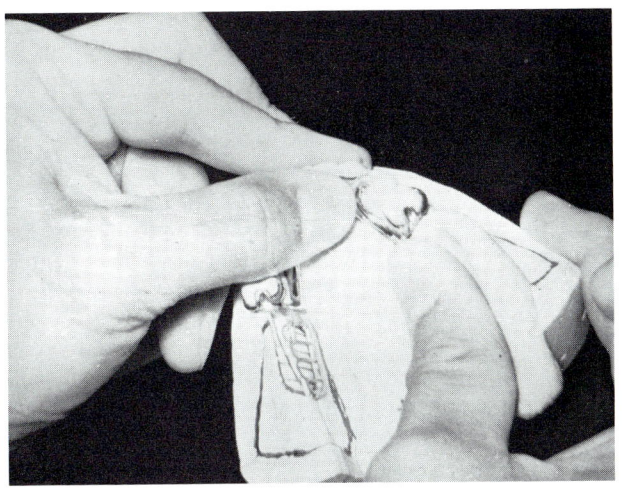

Fig. 13-23. Attaching a temporary self-curing acrylic resin base. Adapt the resin through the framework to lock the material securely to the casting.

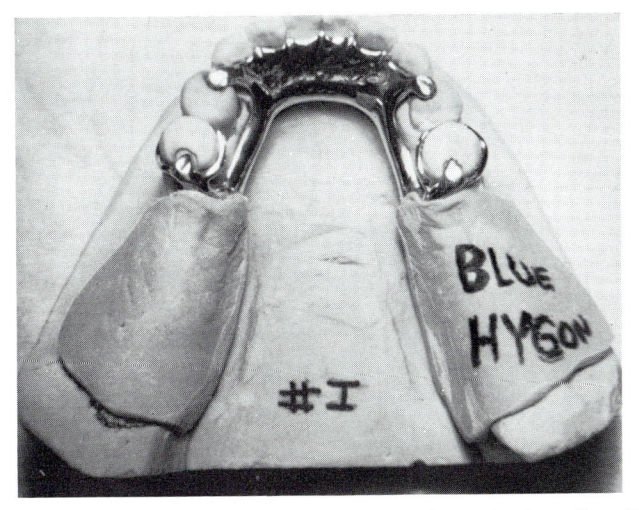

Fig. 13-24. Temporary resin base shortened to the predetermined outline. Blue self-curing acrylic resin is used with a white functional impression material so that pressure spots will show.

**322** *Improving dental practice through preventive measures*

resin may be used. The choice of colored or white resin would depend upon the functional impression material used. Tissue treatment material that is white shows pressure spots best on blue self-curing resin. Mouth temperature wax shows pressure spots better against a white tray material. If there is little residual ridge, wax is the material of choice. Try the casting and temporary bases in the patient's mouth and adjust the retentive units if necessary. Make sure the free-end bases do not come into contact in the tuberosity–retromolar pad area. Now proceed to the impression.

Tissue treatment material is mixed according to the manufacturer's directions unless within 2 to 3 minutes the material seems thin. In this case use two parts of powder to one part of liquid to produce a heavier mix. After the material is mixed,

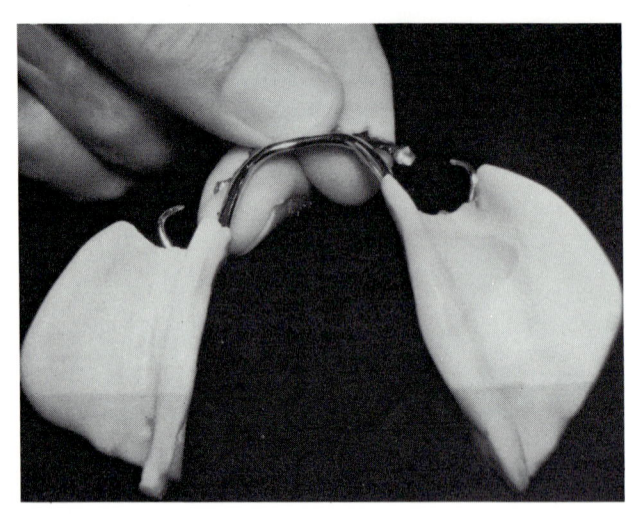

**Fig. 13-25.** Completed functional impression.

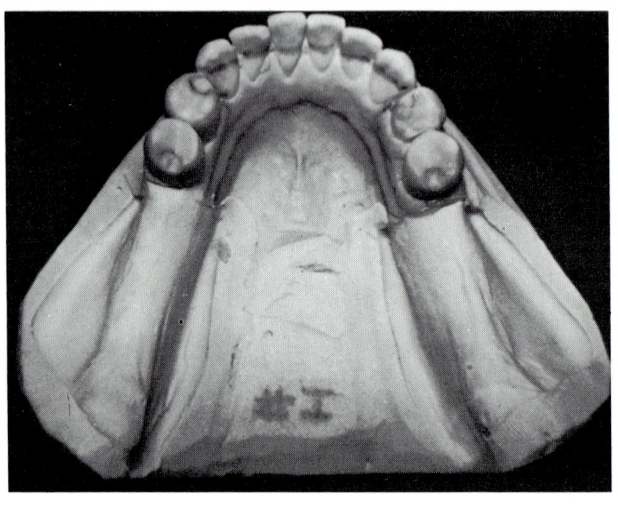

**Fig. 13-26.** A corrected master cast made by removing the edentulous ridge area and then replacing it with one made from the functional impression.

load the tray within 60 seconds, border mold the tray with the same material in another 30 seconds, and then seat it into the mouth. Tripod the casting on the patient's teeth by holding down the direct and indirect retainers. Force the casting completely in place. Remove your fingers from the patient's mouth. Instruct the patient to moisten his lips, open wide, push his tongue into each cheek, and swallow. When necessary, reseat the casting. Remove the impression and casting 5 minutes or more after insertion. Pressure spots show as bare areas and they should be removed by grinding. Repeat the impression. When there are no bare areas in the impression material, trim the retromolar pad area to correct length. Also, be sure to remove any impression material that covers the marginal gingiva. Reinsert the casting and have the patient wear the casting and impression material 30 to 60 minutes. The patient can sit in the reception room while forming the impression. After the prescribed time remove the impression and examine it for desired outline form (Fig. 13-25). If the impression is satisfactory, remove the ridge areas of the cast and correct the master cast (Fig. 13-26) by pouring the new ridge sections.

Let us summarize the preventive prosthodontics that has been practiced through the construction phase of the adult space maintainer. To this point the dentist has removed the immediate possibility of the adult space maintainer developing the excessive stresses associated with a fulcrum line. Again referring to a child's seesaw, the indirect retainer supports one end of the seesaw and the functionally based free-end supports the other end (Fig. 13-27). Also, the dentist has planned for the probability that the free-end prosthesis will develop a fulcrum as the subbasal tissue changes by using stress breaking wrought wire retentive arms. They do not stay well adapted to the abutment teeth. Sometimes they break off after a fulcrum develops. This is good. The retentive arm may or may not need to be replaced.

Posterior artificial teeth should be smaller than the natural teeth they replace. Usually the artificial teeth need to be ground to narrow the occlusal table (Fig. 13-28).

### Instructions for home care program

The partial denture is a debris collector. The patient must prove to the dentist in the office that he can correctly brush his teeth, clean his adult space maintainer, and insert and remove the prosthesis with ease.

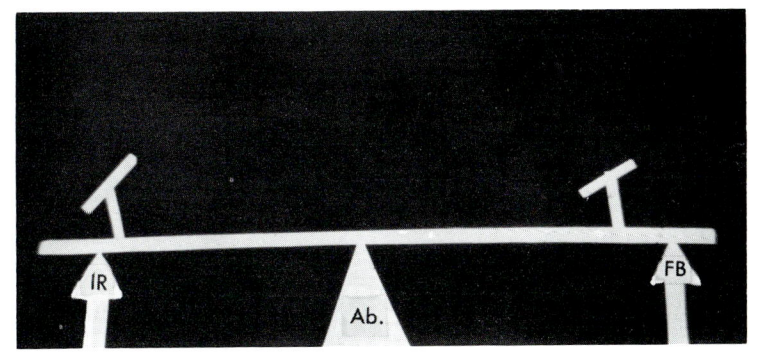

Fig. 13-27. A child's seesaw, which represents a free-end saddle partial denture on abutment tooth, **Ab**, is supported on one end by an indirect retainer, **IR**, and on the other by a functionally based free-end saddle, **FB**.

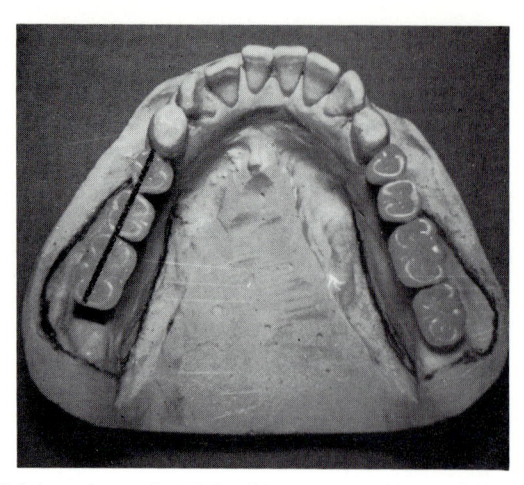

**Fig. 13-28.** The artificial teeth on the right side are too wide mesiodistally. The teeth on the left are correct mesiodistally but should be narrowed from the buccal surface, as shown by the line.

For the adult space maintainer to participate in its important role in preventive dentistry, the patient must become dependent on his prosthesis as soon as possible. The patient will adapt to the new prosthesis more quickly if the dentist instructs him to wear his appliance day and night. Two to four weeks after insertion the dentist must again evaluate the patient and decide if he would benefit from removing the prosthesis at night. If the patient has a high caries index, it would be to his advantage to remove the prosthesis. If the patient removes his partial denture at night, and he is also wearing a complete denture, *both* appliances must be removed (Fig. 13-29). However, in the final analysis only a dentist's clinical judgment can decide when the patient should wear or remove his prosthesis.

Patients should be taught to be watchful for changes in the subbasal tissues. If the base of the prosthesis is a free-end type, the patient should occasionally place his fingers on the saddle connector and press down. If the residual ridge has changed, the saddle connector will settle and the indirect retainer will rise. If the indirect retainer rises 1 to 2 mm., the patient can see this movement. He is educated to call the dental office as soon as possible for the needed functional reline.

After the adult space maintainer is inserted, the patient is responsible for effective caries control and freedom from periodontal disease. This means that he must maintain the routine for good oral hygiene taught him by the dentist.

To facilitate good oral hygiene, most patients would benefit from using an electric toothbrush.[35, 36] Also, an electric toothbrush works well on an adult space maintainer. The patient has less change to drop his prosthesis if the automated brush does the scrubbing. Patients should be instructed to clean the prosthesis over a full basin of water to cushion the fall should the appliance be accidentally dropped.

Calgon in warm water provides a good cleaning solution for the prosthesis. If stains are difficult to remove, the patient is instructed to return to the dental office for correct cleaning of the prosthesis by the dentist. An ultrasonic cleaning machine will aid the dentist in the removal of calculus and stain from adult space maintainers. The patient is also instructed that if he accidentally drops his space

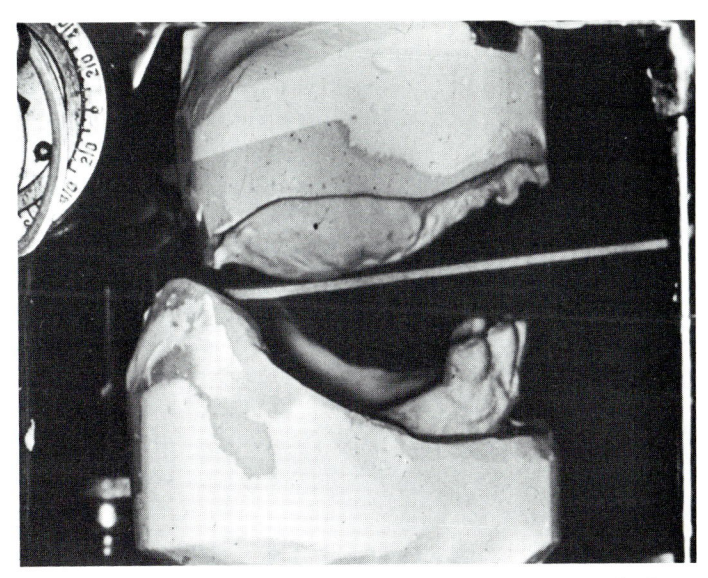

**Fig. 13-29.** If a patient has a maxillary complete denture and a mandibular extension base removable partial denture, then the prostheses should be removed for 8 hours per day. If the patient removes the lower appliance, then he should remove his upper denture to prevent bone from resorbing in the maxillary incisor area.

maintainer he should not wear it, but should return to the dental office. Only the expert judgment of the dentist can decide if the prosthesis has been bent. If the casting is bent, a new one must be constructed. Orthodontic stress produced by a bent casting and periodontal disease are common sequelae. Attempting to straighten a bent casting is a false economy if the act interferes with space maintenance and abutment teeth are lost.

### Dependable recall system

The key to recall is patient education. The patient must be educated to demand preventive dentistry by returning for maintenance services. Recall for maintenance is mandatory to prevent initiation and recurrence of disease.

The dentist and patient must have a dependable recall system. A postcard alerts a patient for recall appointment. The card followed by a phone call will confirm the appointment. (See more concerning this topic on pp. 25-28.) Each patient must have his own recall interval. Some patients will need a prophylaxis every month or two. The space maintainers of some patients will have to be relined a week after insertion. Clinical experience has shown that many adult space maintainers need relining 1 month after insertion.

All preventive dentistry can be ideally conceived and masterfully executed, but unless maintained by both the dentist and patient disease will recur.

### CONCLUSION

The future of dental practice lies in the prevention of disease. Prevention is dynamic since the ideas and methods of preserving health are changed by preventive research.

Prevention can be divided into two categories: primary and secondary prevention. Fabrication of removable partial dentures is a secondary preventive service.

The average patient and some dentists believe that a removable partial denture is not particularly useful or desirable. However, if the patient's needs are correctly diagnosed and he is properly educated and recalled for maintenance, the removable partial denture need not be a stepping-stone to a complete denture.

A new name is needed to help regain the confidence of our patients who need this service; therefore to distinguish between a destructive and preventive removable partial denture I suggest that the preventive prosthesis be called an adult space maintainer.

A detailed account of preventive removable partial denture service from an enthusiastic and effective patient educational program through a dependable recall system was given.

The onus is on the dentist to always provide an adult space maintainer, with all that the phrase implies, whenever a removable partial denture prosthesis is prescribed.

**REFERENCES**

1. Applegate, O. C.: Essentials of removable partial denture prosthesis, ed. 3, Philadelphia, 1965, W. B. Saunders Co.
2. Henderson, D., and Steffel, V. L.: McCracken's partial denture construction, ed. 3, St. Louis, 1969, The C. V. Mosby Co.
3. Eich, F. A.: Role of partial dentures in the destruction of the natural dentition, Dent. Clin. N. Amer., November, 1962, p. 717.
4. Nagel, E.: The structure of science, New York, 1961, Harcourt, Brace and World, Inc.
5. Prothero, J. H.: Prosthetic dentistry, ed. 2, Chicago, 1916, Medico-Dental Publishing Co.
6. Bernard, H. W.: Psychology of learning and teaching, New York, 1954, McGraw-Hill Book Co.
7. Ebbinghaus, H.: Memory; a contribution to experimental psychology, New York, 1913, Teachers College.
8. Thoma, K. H., and Robinson, H. B. G.: Oral and dental diagnosis, ed. 5, Philadelphia, 1960, W. B. Saunders Co.
9. Kerr, D. A., Ash, M. M., and Millard, H. D.: Oral diagnosis, ed. 3, St. Louis, 1970, The C. V. Mosby Co.
10. Burket, L. W.: Oral medicine, ed. 4, Philadelphia, 1961, J. B. Lippincott Co.
11. Mitchell, D., and others: Oral diagnosis and oral medicine, Philadelphia, 1969, Lea & Febiger.
12. Muhler, J. C.: Stannous fluoride as an anticaries agent for topical application in the dental office, J. Indiana Dent. Ass. 39:42, 1960.
13. Muhler, J. C., and Dudding, N. J.: Technique of application of stannous fluoride in a compatible paste as a topical agent, J. Dent. Child. 29:219, 1962.
14. Moore, D. L.: Conservative treatment of teeth with vital pulps and periapical lesions; a preliminary report, J. Prosth. Dent. 18:476-481, 1967.
15. Applegate, O. C.: Use of a paralleling surveyor, J.A.D.A. 27:1397, 1940.
16. McCracken, W. L.: Survey of partial denture designs by commercial dental labs, J. Prosth. Dent. 12:1089-1110, 1962.
17. Murata, S.: Method of measuring mesial tipping of the lower second molar, J. Prosth. Dent. 4:673, 1954.
18. Glickman, I.: Clinical periodontology—the periodontium in health and disease, ed. 2, Philadelphia, 1958, W. B. Saunders Co., p. 712.
19. Muhlmann, H. R.: Tooth mobility, I, the measuring method; initial and secondary tooth mobility, J. Periodont. 25:22, 1954.
20. Glickman, I.: Clinical periodontology—the periodontium in health and disease, ed. 2, Philadelphia, 1958, W. B. Saunders Co., p. 51.

21. Weinmann, J., and Sicher, H.: Bone and bones, ed. 2, St. Louis, 1955, The C. V. Mosby Co.
22. Johnson, J. F., Phillips, R. W., and Dykema, R. W.: Modern practice in crown and bridge prosthodontics, Philadelphia, 1960, W. B. Saunders Co.
23. Harvey, W. L.: A transitional prosthesis, J. Prosth. Dent. **14**:60-70, 1964.
24. Robinson, H. B. G., Kerr, D., and Colby, R.: Color atlas of oral pathology, ed. 2, Philadelphia, 1961, J. B. Lippincott Co.
25. Lefkowitz, W.: The "vitality" of the calcified dental tissues, J. Dent. Res. **21**:423, 1942.
26. Thomas, B. O. A.: Protective metamorphosis of the dentin; its relationship to pain, J.A.D.A. **31**:459, 1944.
27. Applegate, O. C.: Essentials of removable partial denture prosthesis, ed. 2, Philadelphia, 1959, W. B. Saunders Co., Chapter 15.
28. Bauer, W. H.: Effect of a faultily constructed partial denture on a tooth ond its supporting tissue, with special reference to formation of fibro cartilage in the periodontal membrane as result of disturbed healing caused by abnormal stresses, Amer. J. Orthodont. **27**:640-651, 1941.
29. Frechette, A. R.: The influence of partial denture design on distribution of force to abutment teeth, J. Prosth. Dent. **6**:195-212, 1956.
30. Kaires, A. K.: A study of partial denture design and masticatory pressure in a mandibular bilateral distal extension case, J. Prosth. Dent. **8**:340-380, 1958.
31. Holmes, J. B.: The influence of partial design and occlusal loading on partial denture movement, J. Prosth. Dent. **15**:474, 1965.
32. Cohn, I. A.: The physiologic basis for tooth fixation in precision-attached partial dentures, J. Prosth. Dent. **6**:220-244, 1956.
33. McLean, D. W.: The partial denture as a vehicle for function, J.A.D.A. **23**:1272-1273, 1936.
34. Applegate, O. C.: Essentials of removable partial denture prosthesis, ed. 2, Philadelphia, 1959, W. B. Saunders Co., p. 42.
35. Hoover, D., and Robinson, H. B. G.: The effect of automatic and hand toothbrushing on gingivitis, J.A.D.A. **65**:361, 1962.
36. Hoover, D., and Lefkowitz, W.: Reduction of gingivitis by toothbrushing, J. Periodont. **36**:193, 1965.

# Chapter 14 Preventive oral surgery
## Robert B. Shira

Introduction
Prevention of errors in therapy because of improper diagnosis
Prevention of major surgical problems developing from minor surgical problems
    Infections associated with teeth
    Other infections
    Prevention of cysts and ameloblastomas
Prevention of operative and postoperative complications
Prevention of adverse reactions to local anesthetics
Prevention of postoperative hemorrhage
Oral surgery to minimize prosthetic failures
Oral surgery to correct facial deformities
Oral surgery evaluation of orofacial trauma
Early detection of malignant lesions to prevent death
Oral surgery in the diagnosis of leukoplakia and erythroplasia
Conclusion

## INTRODUCTION

The objectives of preventive dentistry are to prevent oral disease and its sequelae.

It may be difficult for some dentists to visualize the role of oral surgery in a preventive dentistry program. Oral surgery is usually considered to be the end of the line as far as dental procedures are concerned; however, it does contribute to the overall objectives of preventive dentistry. It should be the objective of the dental profession to preserve the natural dentition and supporting structures throughout life. It should be axiomatic that no serviceable, useful tooth should be removed—this is preventive dentistry in its truest sense. Removal of teeth should be considered only after all efforts to restore and to maintain the natural dentition in a healthy situation have failed. Should all efforts fail, then oral surgical procedures become necessary. The preventive aspects of oral surgery enter the picture to ensure that timely, appropriate, sound, and conservative procedures are accomplished. This comprehensive approach is the diagnostic and treatment pathway to the prevention of untoward results, unnecessary complications, and needless mutilation.

In discussing the preventive aspects of oral surgery, many problems must be considered. These range from prevention of errors in diagnosis to prevention of death from malignant disease.

## PREVENTION OF ERRORS IN THERAPY BECAUSE OF IMPROPER DIAGNOSIS

Severe mutilation may occasionally occur when oral surgical procedures have been predicted on errors in diagnosis. Mandibles have been resected when dental cysts have been mistaken for more serious pathology.[1] Removal of segments of the maxilla or mandible involved by benign processes such as fibrous dysplasia or reparative giant cell granuloma occurs all too frequently. These mistakes result most frequently from errors in diagnosis or from the failure of the surgeon to be completely familiar with the natural history of the disease process in question.

It is an axiom of good practice that treatment should be predicated upon an accurate diagnosis. If a correct diagnosis is made, the correct treatment will usually follow in logical sequence. However, if an improper diagnosis is made, wrong treatment will usually result. The oral surgeon should obtain all possible information about the patient and the patient's disease before he instigates treatment. He should evaluate the information derived from a comprehensive history, from a thorough examination, from adequate and complete roentgenograms, and from indicated laboratory studies. Consultation with allied specialists in dentistry and medicine may also be indicated. Correlation of this information with the disease processes capable of producing the problems presented by the patient should lead to a correct diagnosis. It is therefore obvious that the dentist must have wide knowledge of the disease processes affecting the oral structures if he is to make an accurate diagnosis. Sir William Osler has said, "You cannot diagnose a condition unless you first know of its existence."[2] Once a correct diagnosis has been established, errors in treatment will usually be avoided.

The first rule of surgery is to "do no harm." If a surgical procedure will not benefit a patient, it should not be performed. It is best that a surgeon not treat a case if he is unable to arrive at a correct diagnosis and cannot determine the correct therapy. It is better that he refer the patient to a consultant with wider experience and depend upon this consultant to solve the problem. In no instance should he proceed merely to be doing something.

## PREVENTION OF MAJOR SURGICAL PROBLEMS DEVELOPING FROM MINOR SURGICAL PROBLEMS

**Infections associated with teeth.** One of the most frequently encountered problems in dental practice is the management of acute infections associated with the teeth. While this infectious process may be minimal and of little consequence, it has the potential of developing into a serious, life-endangering, space infection. However, if the infection is properly treated early in its development, serious complications can usually be avoided.

In the past it was considered hazardous to extract a tooth involved in an acute infection because of the danger of spreading the infection.[3] The condition was usually treated in a conservative manner by waiting for localization of the infectious process in the soft tissue to permit incision and drainage. Only after drainage had been accomplished and the soft tissue swelling had completely resolved was it considered safe to remove the tooth. An adage that is often quoted is "Never extract a tooth until it is getting better." This conservative therapy does little to control the infection but contributes to lowered resistance and debilitation by causing the patient to suffer continual pain, to spend sleepless nights, and to subsist on an altered nutritional intake. Such an infection might spread along facial planes and localize in anatomic spaces, producing serious infections with attendant dangers to life.

Most oral surgeons now believe that the delayed treatment of the acutely infected tooth is no longer tenable and immediate extraction of the tooth, regardless of the length of time the infectious process has been developing or the amount of soft tissue swelling that is present, is the treatment of choice.[4] This has been made possible with the advent of antibiotics, improved anesthetic agents, and refined surgical techniques. Experience has shown that the proper use of appropriate preoperative and postoperative antibiotics and the removal of the offending tooth by a simple, atraumatic procedure will cause resolution of the infectious process without untoward complications. Immediate extraction of the infected tooth usually results in early relief of pain with resolution of the soft tissue swelling within 24 to 48 hours. This procedure fulfills the basic surgical principle of removal of the cause. In this way space infections are often prevented and serious complications are avoided.

When an acutely infected tooth is removed, it should be emphasized that the surgery must be accomplished by a simple, atraumatic procedure. If removal of the offending tooth requires a more complicated procedure, such as the reflection of a soft tissue flap with removal of bone and sectioning of the tooth, removal should be postponed until the infectious process has resolved. However, this condition is seldom encountered. Most acutely infected teeth are easily accessible, and the infectious process has usually loosened the tooth to the degree that removal is not difficult.

**Other infections.** Serious infections arising from sources other than infected teeth are also encountered.[5] Contaminated instruments and supplies, contaminants introduced into open wounds at time of surgery, improper use of antibiotics, and improper postoperative care of the surgical patient occasionally result in serious local or systemic infections. Deep-seated space infections may result, and the systemic infections created by the introduction of contaminants are well known.[6-8] The seriousness of the latter problem is revealed by a recent report of 313 patients who developed infectious hepatitis after receiving treatment at the Municipal Hospital in Palermo, Italy. Of these patients, 91, or 31 percent, developed hepatitis following dental procedures.[9]

Such infections are usually preventable by careful attention to recognized procedures. All instruments, syringes, towels, drapes, and other supplies should be thoroughly sterilized. The use of disposable sterile needles and rubber gloves is encouraged. Every dental office should establish a regimen of clean operating techniques to prevent the introduction of contaminants into surgical wounds. Patients should be observed carefully following surgical procedures to detect any signs of a developing infection. If such signs appear, vigorous treatment with antibiotics and good supportive care will usually abort or minimize the magnitude of the infection. When the use of antibiotics is indicated, they should be prescribed in an intelligent manner, depending, whenever possible, on positive bacteriologic findings to determine the antibiotic of choice. The antibiotic should then be administered in sufficient quantity and for sufficient time to control the infection and to prevent the emergence of resistant strains of the organisms. When intelligently utilized, these procedures will prevent most of the infections associated with dental procedures and will minimize the magnitude of the few that do develop.

**Prevention of cysts and ameloblastomas.** The best way to treat a pathologic condition is to prevent its occurrence. The potential for cyst formation about the crowns of unerupted teeth is well known. It has been demonstrated that the follicles about unerupted teeth often contain epithelial remnants that have the potential to proliferate and to form follicular cysts.[10] These cysts develop slowly, expand along the lines of least resistance, and often become large destructive lesions before they are discovered. In addition there is considerable evidence that a certain number of ameloblastomas originate from the epithelial lining of these cysts and from the epithelial remnants in the follicles about unerupted teeth.[11]

It is well known that some unerupted teeth may be retained for years without

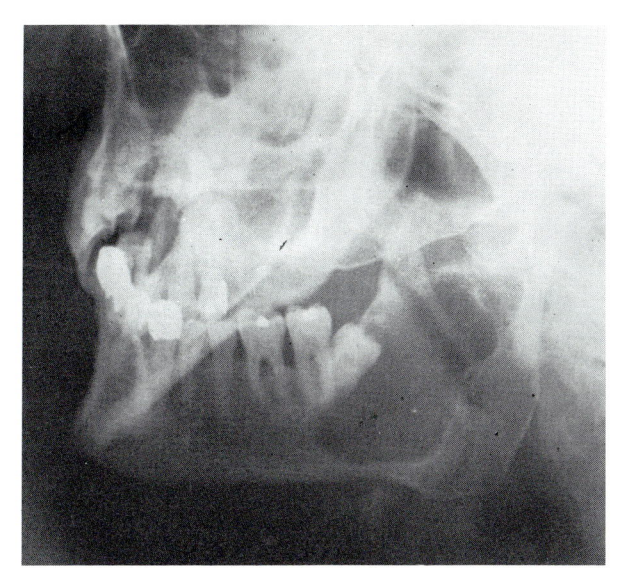

Fig. 14-1. A destructive cyst associated with an unerupted third molar. Early prophylactic removal of the unerupted tooth would probably have prevented the cyst.

creating problems and do not progress to the formation of cysts or ameloblastomas. In these instances the epithelial remnants remain dormant and do not proliferate. However, as mentioned previously, other unerupted teeth do create problems and may lead to the development of cysts and ameloblastomas. In these instances the epithelial remnants do persist and proliferate to produce the pathologic process.

Thus the epithelial remnants in the follicles appear to be the important factor. It is logical to reason that removal of the follicle before proliferation of the epithelium has occurred will prevent the development of a certain number of cysts and ameloblastomas (Fig. 14-1).

This possibility has led many oral surgeons to believe that serious consideration should be given to the prophylactic removal of unerupted teeth that are hopelessly impacted and that cannot possibly erupt and become serviceable.[12] It is recommended that a roentgenographic survey be taken at the time the teeth should erupt (approximately 18 to 21 years of age for third molars); if this survey reveals the teeth to be hopelessly impacted, they should be removed as soon as practicable. Removal of the follicle with its epithelial remnants should be accomplished at the same time. At this age removal of impacted teeth is usually a relatively simple procedure accompanied by minimal postoperative complications. Should the teeth be allowed to remain and, in later years, a cyst, ameloblastoma, or other complications develop, then surgery becomes a major, time-consuming, often traumatic and mutilating experience. The early prophylactic removal of impacted teeth that have no chance of erupting into the dental arch is a forward step in preventive dentistry. These teeth cannot possibly benefit the patient and are capable of producing complications.

## PREVENTION OF OPERATIVE AND POSTOPERATIVE COMPLICATIONS

Operative and postoperative complications are encountered in every dental practice. Most of these complications are minor and of little consequence, while a few may go on to major proportions. It is important that surgical patients be seen post-

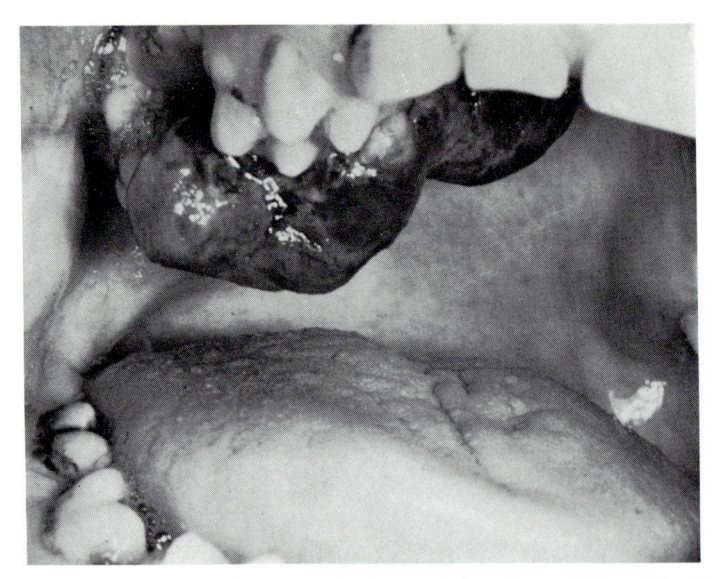

**Fig. 14-2.** Serious bleeding following removal of a tooth in a hemophiliac. The bleeding could have been more readily controlled if the problem had been recognized preoperatively and the patient properly prepared before surgery.

operatively so developing complications can be detected in their incipiency. Vigorous therapy instigated at this time will usually abort or minimize the complications or prevent them from developing into major proportions.

While many postoperative complications are unpredictable and unavoidable, others are undoubtedly self-generated and result from negligence, inadequately planned procedures, or ignorance on the part of the operator. The best way to treat a complication is to prevent its occurrence; the dentist has many methods and procedures at his command to accomplish this.

Before instigating a surgical procedure, a thorough preoperative evaluation of the patient is indicated. Most dental patients are ambulatory and presumably in good health; however, constant vigilance is necessary to discover associated or concomitant conditions that may have an effect upon the problem at hand. A concurrent systemic problem may jeopardize the success of a surgical procedure, or a surgical procedure may be of such magnitude that it would have a deleterious effect upon a systemic problem. An excellent example of the importance of the preoperative evaluation is the serious bleeding problems that arise when surgery is performed on an unprepared hemophiliac. When the bleeding problem is recognized preoperatively, the patient can usually be prepared in such a manner that the subsequent bleeding can be more readily controlled (Fig. 14-2).

The preoperative evaluation should include a careful history, a thorough examination, indicated laboratory procedures, and necessary consultations. Surgery should not be undertaken until it is determined that the patient is capable of withstanding the stress the procedure will produce.

To prevent complications no surgical procedure should be performed on the teeth or their hard and soft supporting structures until adequate roentgenograms are available. The roentgenograms furnish additional information by revealing hidden

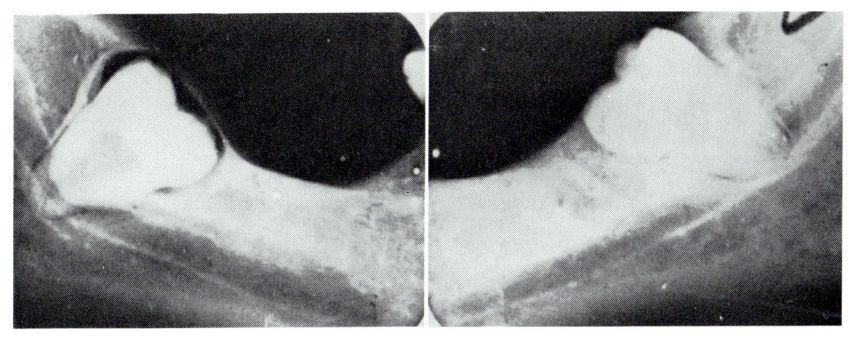

**Fig. 14-3.** Impingement on the mandibular canal by the roots of unerupted third molars. Information derived from the roentgenograms permits a surgical approach that will minimize the danger of injury to the structures in the canal.

pathology, operative complications, and involvement of contingent structures. Roentgenograms also assist the surgeon in determining his surgical approach to the problem. Procedures carried out without roentgenograms may result in fractured roots, fractured bones, involvement of the maxillary sinus, nerve injuries, and other injuries, many of which could be prevented by the intelligent use of good roentgenograms (Fig. 14-3).

As a further step in prevention of complications, the dentist should possess the knowledge to evaluate the magnitude of the problem presented by the patient. If the preoperative evaluation reveals a concomitant systemic condition, he must know the effect of this condition on the problem at hand. He must also be able to evaluate the magnitude and technical difficulty of the surgical procedure. Not all procedures are of the same magnitude; complications frequently arise when a dentist attempts operations that are beyond his capabilities. Serious soft tissue injuries, injuries to other teeth, fractured tuberosities, fractured mandibles, and injury to nerves and vessels are only a few of the complications that may be created. Prevention of these complications calls for an honest appraisal of the problem with referral of those cases that are beyond the comfortable range of operative ability of the dentist. Adherence to the adage "A good doctor knows what he can't do as well as what he can do" will go a long way in preventing complications of operative origin.

Complications will be minimized if a well-regulated surgical plan is formulated before the procedure is started. The adage "Keep your mind ahead of your knife" is always applicable. The surgical plan should provide a step-by-step procedure that will facilitate the operation and yet be flexible enough to allow the management of any unanticipated problem or emergency that may develop. By adherence to a sound surgical plan, the procedure can be so systematized that the operation may be completed with dispatch while ensuring optimal results for the patient (Fig. 14-4).

Once the procedure has been started, adherence to sound surgical principles is essential. These principles include asepsis, complete and profound anesthesia, adequate access to the operative field, hemostasis, use of controlled force, conservative manipulation of tissues, adequate cleansing and closure of the wound, and a well-regulated postoperative regime. These principles have stood the test of time and, if followed meticulously, will minimize postoperative complications. On the other hand, failure to adhere to these principles while resorting to shortcuts often leads to troublesome complications (Fig. 14-5).

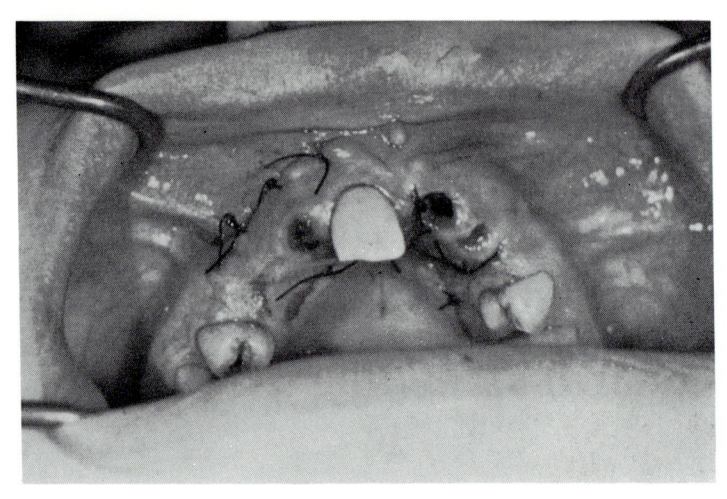

**334** *Improving dental practice through preventive measures*

**Fig. 14-4.** Soft tissue lacerations accidentally produced during removal of residual roots. Failure to adhere to a surgical plan was responsible for this accident.

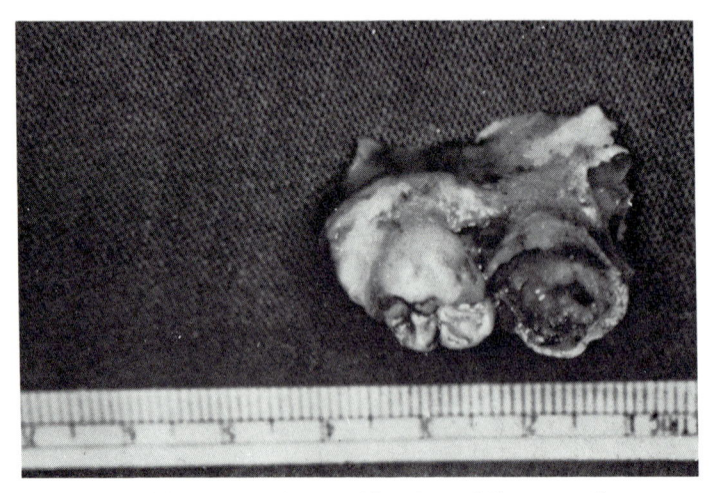

**Fig. 14-5.** Fractured maxillary tuberosity resulting from failure to adhere to sound surgical principles.

## PREVENTION OF ADVERSE REACTIONS TO LOCAL ANESTHETICS

When the frequency with which local anesthetics are administered in dental practice is considered, the incidence of adverse reactions is relatively rare. However, available data indicate that untoward reactions do occur with some regularity.[13, 14] The dentist should utilize every available precautionary method to prevent these reactions and be prepared to administer adequate resuscitative measures should a reaction develop in spite of these precautions.

When the patient's physical limitations are recognized preoperatively, and when the patient is properly prepared before treatment is instigated, an emergency situation can usually be avoided. An adequate history and a physical evaluation will usually disclose these limitations.

A careful history should elicit any allergic reactions to specific anesthetic agents. When a patient has reacted unfavorably to one agent, an alternate anesthetic of a different chemical structure should be used. Since cardiac patients are prone to emergency incidents, they should be carefully evaluated to determine their cardiac status. They should also be premedicated to prevent undue apprehension. Patients with a history of easy and frequent fainting or patients who are abnormally apprehensive or frightened also require careful preoperative management if emergency situations are to be avoided.

A common cause of complications associated with local anesthetics is the psychologic impact of pain or the fear of pain. This problem causes an increased liberation of epinephrine with resultant tachycardia and rise in blood pressure. Fainting occurs frequently, and in patients with an altered cardiovascular capacity the added strain of the increased epinephrine may be sufficient to produce an emergency of major consequence.

Every available precaution should be utilized to allay apprehension. The dentist should maintain a kind, calm, reassuring attitude and at every opportunity assure the patient that all will go well. All office personnel should display a quiet, dignified, professional attitude so the patient will realize he is in competent hands. There should be no display of ominous instruments and equipment. During surgery the patient should receive the undivided attention of the operator and his assistant and be reassured from time to time that he is doing well and that the operation is progressing smoothly. When properly utilized, these steps will do much to allay apprehension.

Perhaps the best means of allaying apprehension and minimizing the adverse effects of local anesthetics is the use of adequate premedication. Barbiturates and narcotics are the agents most frequently prescribed, and the intelligent use of these drugs must be given a paramount place in any regimen to prevent emergencies arising from local anesthetic agents.

Following premedication, additional procedures are available to prevent adverse reactions. *The position of the patient is important.* The semirecumbent or recumbent position is preferable to the upright position for all patients. These positions may be altered by adjustment of the headrest to provide proper lighting and exposure of the oral cavity for the operative procedure. Pain may be reduced at the injection site by the use of topical anesthetics. Extreme care should be exercised when injecting the anesthetic solution. Every injection should be made slowly and with minimal pressure. Too rapid injection of the anesthetic solution produces increased pain in the injection site by rapid distention of confined tissues and increases the untoward response if an inadvertent intravascular injection is made. The smallest quantity of the lowest concentration anesthetic agent compatible with the problem at hand should be used. Minimal amounts of vasoconstrictors should be used. Rarely are concentrations of vasoconstrictors in excess of 1:100,000 required. If multiple injections are required, they should be spaced in time. Following injection, the patient should be observed carefully, and at the first indication of an adverse reaction, oxygen should be administered. If the reaction does not respond to oxygen therapy, other indicated resuscitative measures should be initiated. Every dental office should be equipped with resuscitative equipment and drugs and all personnel trained to act promptly, calmly, and efficiently in emergency situations. No patient should be left unattended following injection of a local anesthetic agent.

As a final step in prevention of reactions to local anesthetics, intravascular injection of the anesthetic agent must be assiduously avoided. Intravascular injection is probably the cause of most local anesthetic reactions in dentistry.[15] Unless they are avoided, concentration of local anesthetics and vasoconstrictors may be inadvertently built up and death or serious cardiovascular complications may result.[16]

Intravascular injections usually may be avoided by using no smaller than a 25-gauge needle, by always aspirating before injecting, and, if the position of the needle is changed during injection, by reaspirating before continuing the injection. It must be remembered, however, that collapse of the wall by back pressure in a small lumen vessel may give a false sense of security. Thus the necessity for repeated aspirations and slow injection of the agent is apparent.

The measures the dentist should utilize to prevent adverse reactions may be summarized as follows:

1. Careful preoperative evaluation of the patient
2. Allay apprehension
3. Adequate premedication
4. Proper positioning of the patient
5. *Aspiration before injection*
6. *Slow injection, with minimum pressure*
7. Smallest amount of anesthetic compatible with problem at hand
8. Spaced multiple injections
9. Low concentration of vasoconstrictor
10. Following injection, close observation of patient
11. Oxygen administration at first sign of emergency
12. Other indicated resuscitative measures if patient does not respond to oxygen therapy

Utilization of these procedures will minimize the problems associated with local anesthetics and to a large extent will prevent the development of serious complications.

**PREVENTION OF POSTOPERATIVE HEMORRHAGE**

One of the annoying and sometimes dangerous complications of surgery is postoperative hemorrhage. Preventive measures with which all members of the dental profession should be familiar are available to minimize this problem.

The majority of postoperative bleeding problems are local in nature and present little difficulty in management. Bleeding problems of a systemic nature, however, are occasionally encountered. Howell and Monto's[17] report that over 25 percent of 250 patients with hemorrhagic disease seen on the hematology service at Henry Ford Hospital at Detroit, Michigan, were referred by the oral surgical group is evidence that patients with bleeding disorders are seen in the dental office. It is important to recognize these patients preoperatively so correct therapy can be instigated to prevent serious bleeding when surgery is necessary.

Every dentist should have a reliable method of screening surgical patients to detect those with hemorrhagic disorders. The history, clinical examinations, and laboratory tests are the most reliable methods of detecting these problems.

A patient with a condition that predisposes bleeding will usually have experienced other episodes of bleeding or extravasations of blood, which will give a clue to the problem. A history of abnormal bleeding following previous surgery or trauma is significant. Abnormal bleeding following previous oral surgical procedures is of particular significance and should arouse the suspicions of the dentist that a bleeding problem may exist. The history should also reveal bleeding tendencies in other members of the family and disclose any systemic disease such as hypertension, liver disease, or intake of anticoagulant drugs that might lead to bleeding if a surgical procedure is performed. The properly controlled anticoagulated patient is amenable to surgery if properly evaluated.

The clinical examination may reveal conditions that suggest hemorrhagic disorders. The pale, weak, lethargic appearance of patients with leukemia, the petechiae and ecchymosis of thrombocytopenic purpura, the enlarged joints of the hemophiliac, the yellow tint of the skin and sclera of the jaundiced patient, and the pale lips, nail beds, and mucosa of anemia are familiar signs that warn of potential hemorrhage in event of surgery (Fig. 14-6).[17]

When the history or clinical findings suggest a bleeding problem, laboratory tests are indicated to establish or rule out a hemorrhagic disorder. These tests are best ordered and interpreted by a hematologist or an internist who is well versed in the hemorrhagic disorders. If a bleeding tendency is confirmed, specialized therapy is indicated to prevent or minimize bleeding when surgery is necessary. Such patients should be referred to a specialized treatment center where adequate facilities and trained personnel are available to manage all aspects of the problem.

Postoperative bleeding in normal patients may also be prevented or minimized. In this regard careful attention to surgical principles is essential. *Soft tissue flaps must be formed in such a manner that incisions do not involve larger vessels.* Sharp bone margins and bone splinters should be removed since they cause irritation and may predispose to secondary hemorrhage. Pathologic soft tissue should be excised at time of surgery, since for the most part this tissue is highly vascular and is conducive to continued hemorrhage if allowed to remain. Bleeding from bone should be controlled before closure of the soft tissue and any intraseptal "spurters" should be controlled by pressure on the bone at the bleeding point with a blunt instrument. Profuse hemorrhage from injury to the inferior alveolar vessels or other large vessels should be controlled by packing with gauze or one of the absorbable hemostatic agents. Soft tissue bleeding encountered at time of surgery should also receive attention. If "spurting" arterial hemorrhage is encountered, the bleeding points should

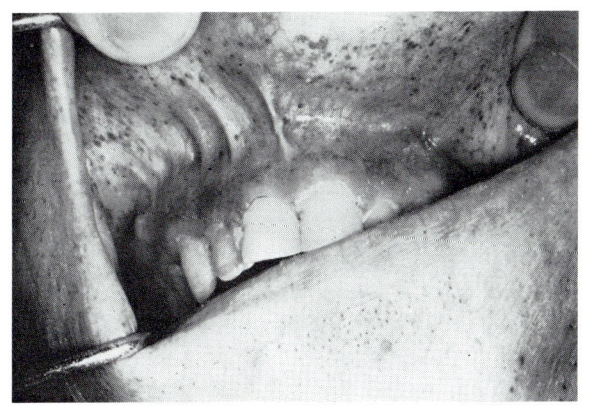

Fig. 14-6. The multiple petechiae of the oral mucosa indicate the possibility of a hemorrhagic disease and warn of potential hemorrhage in event of surgery.

be grasped with a hemostat and tied with a ligature or controlled by the use of the electrocautery. Brisk seepage from granulation tissue should be controlled by excision of this highly vascular tissue. Soft tissue flaps should be returned to their normal position and held firmly in place with sutures. The use of sutures to prevent postoperative hemorrhage cannot be overemphasized. The additional time required to place a few well-situated sutures will often pay large dividends in the prevention of postoperative hemorrhage.

A final measure of prevention is the use of a careful postoperative regime. A large, moistened, gauze pad should be placed over the operative site, and the patient instructed to maintain firm pressure on the gauze for several hours. A properly placed gauze pad will occlude the operative site and still permit the patient to occlude the teeth. The excess gauze should be placed in the buccal vestibule to immobilize the soft tissue flap against the bone. The maintenance of this dressing for several hours will reduce bleeding, reduce postoperative edema, and reduce postoperative discomfort occasioned by a bulky dressing in which the patient cannot close the mouth. The patient should be instructed to go home and rest. Mouth rinsing should not be permitted for at least 24 hours, and measures to protect the blood clot should be taken. These include a soft or liquid diet, no toothbrushing for the first day, and no strenuous exercise. Sedation to control pain and to ensure rest should be prescribed. Instructions to notify the surgeon immediately of any abnormal bleeding that may occur completes the postoperative regime.

## ORAL SURGERY TO MINIMIZE PROSTHETIC FAILURES

When the natural dentition is lost, the replacement prosthesis is seldom as efficient as the natural teeth. However, the prosthesis will have the best chance of success if it is constructed on an adequate base. Surgery is often necessary to provide a firm foundation for the support of the denture.

There are many conditions of developmental, pathologic, and operative origin that interfere with the construction of ideal dentures. Surgical correction of these conditions eliminates some of the associated prosthetic problems and aids in the construction of more satisfactory replacements. Surgical preparation of the ridges to remove undercuts and to provide a broad, flat bearing area at the crest of the alveolar ridge, removal of soft tissue redundancies, hyperplasias, and hypertrophies, removal of bony exostoses, reduction of protruding alveolar processes, reduction of enlarged tuberosities, repositioning of abnormal muscle and soft tissue attachments to provide an adequate sulcus, and the surgical repositioning of the mandible to provide proper ridge relationship are some of the surgical procedures that are useful to prevent or minimize prosthetic failures.

## ORAL SURGERY TO CORRECT FACIAL DEFORMITIES

An aspect of preventive oral surgery that is frequently overlooked is the beneficial result produced by the surgical correction of congenital or acquired facial deformities. These procedures are not only effective in improving function and cosmetic appearance, but also frequently result in a decided improvement in any overriding psychologic problem that may be present. Every human being has an inborn desire to look like other human beings and, when some condition sets an individual apart as being abnormal, it usually produces an adverse psychologic reaction. Patients, particularly children, with defects such as congenital double lip, alveolar protrusion, mandibular prognathism, and cleft lip and palate, are often subjected to ridicule and taunts of their associates to the point where they may become self-conscious and introverted. When the deformity is corrected, the results are not only gratifying, but also often amazing. When these patients look in the mirror and see that they now look like other people, a marked beneficial effect on their outlook on life is produced, and a major contribution is made toward solving their psychologic problems. This is one of the greatest health services that can be provided.

## ORAL SURGERY EVALUATION OF OROFACIAL TRAUMA

Another aspect of preventive oral surgery is the evaluation and treatment of the trauma patient. Facial injuries present functional and psychologic problems that are extremely important since the face is the mirror of the man. Too frequently facial injuries, particularly minimal fractures of the facial skeleton, go undetected for long periods of time. The nature of the bony and muscular architecture predisposes toward occlusal disharmony. This disharmony may be minimal or significant but is always functionally important. Every dentist must be cognizant of this and be prepared to examine the patient to ascertain the extent of the injury and its potential for impairment of function. If the injury is beyond the scope of the practitioner he should refer the patient to the appropriate specialist. Intermaxillary fixation for varying periods of time is desirable in every facial fracture except the true blowout fracture of the orbital floor and the solitary nasal fracture.

## EARLY DETECTION OF MALIGNANT LESIONS TO PREVENT DEATH

Tissue analysis plays an important role in preventive dentistry. Cancer affects the oral cavity and, unless the disease process is controlled, it will kill the patient. The logical approach to control of oral cancer would be to eliminate the disease through discovery of its causes. While progress is being made, the causes of malignant disease are still unknown. At the present time the early detection of the malignant lesion provides the patient with the best chance of survival. It has been estimated that 80 percent of all oral malignancies could be cured if they were detected early. The importance of early diagnosis is emphasized by the work of Dr. Gordon Castigliano of the American Oncological Hospital of Philadelphia. He estimates that 80 percent of the patients with untreated oral malignancies will be dead in a short 18 months as compared to 2 years for carcinoma of the rectum and 5 years for carcinoma of the breast.[18] In dealing with a disease that is so rapidly destructive to life, the importance of early diagnosis is obvious. Biopsy is necessary to establish an accurate, definitive diagnosis of a malignant lesion. Hence oral surgery plays a paramount role in this aspect of prevention.

There can be no question of the importance of the dentist in the control of oral cancer, for he is in an ideal situation to detect the lesions in their early stages. As the dentist examines the oral cavity there are certain clinical signs and symptoms that, if present, should arouse his suspicions that a malignant lesion may be present. These signs and symptoms may be summarized as follows.

1. Local lesions
    a. Insidious onset
    b. Chronic and progressive
    c. Lesions that present induration, ulceration, and fixation of their base
    d. Lesions that do not respond to recognized therapy

**340** *Improving dental practice through preventive measures*

2. Pain
3. Asymmetry of the face
4. Regional adenopathy
5. Loose teeth
6. Roentgenographic evidence of bone changes
7. Paresthesia
8. Trismus, altered mobility of tongue, and difficulty in swallowing
9. Increased salivation, bad breath, and hemorrhage

It must be emphasized that these descriptions of oral malignant lesions are those of advanced, rather than early, cancer. When these findings are present there is a strong possibility that the malignant process has been present for considerable time and has already spread beyond the oral cavity.

To ensure early diagnosis, malignant lesions must be discovered before they produce these signs and symptoms. In other words, they must be discovered before they produce the classic clinical signs and symptoms of cancer—they must be found before they look and feel like cancer. Only when this has been accomplished will any great inroads be made in the control of this disease (Fig. 14-7).

Unfortunately at the present time the only reliable method of discovering oral cancer in its early stages is a thorough clinical examination. To make this examination effective, the examiner must consider three important factors.

*He must be cancer conscious!* The dentist must develop an awareness of cancer and realize that patients can and do develop malignancies of the oral cavity. Whenever he examines a patient he must ask, "Could this patient have cancer?" and rule out this possibility before proceeding with other therapy.

*He must do a thorough oral examination!* The dentist must develop a definite routine for a complete oral examination that includes the visual examination of the lips, cheeks, floor of the mouth, all surfaces of the tongue, the palate, the throat, and the mucosa of the alveolar ridge. This visual examination must be followed

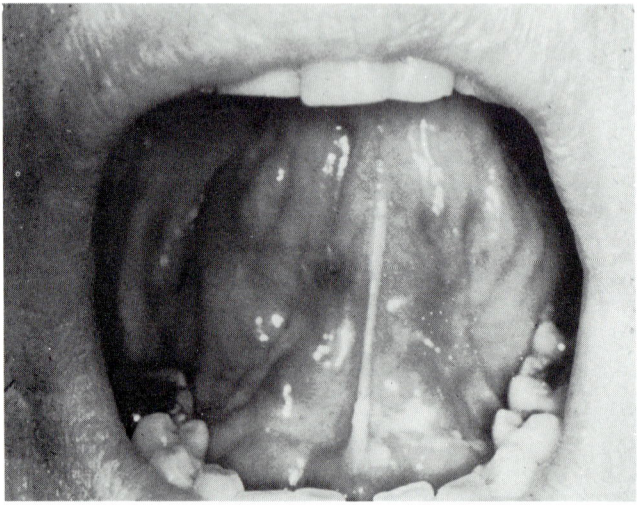

Fig. 14-7. A small innocuous-appearing lesion that proved to be an invasive squamous cell carcinoma on tissue examination.

by a digital examination not only of the mouth but of the cervical areas as well. Only by a thorough and complete examination will it be possible to detect some of the lesions that represent early malignant change.

*He must be suspicious of deviations from the normal!* As the result of being cancer conscious and by completing a thorough oral examination, the dentist must be suspicious of any deviations from the normal. Whenever confronted with a lesion that he cannot readily identify as a benign and innocuous lesion, he must consider it malignant until it is proved otherwise.

When confronted with a suspicious lesion that he cannot recognize, the dentist should do one of two things. He should either do a biopsy immediately to establish a diagnosis or, if he does not include biopsy examinations within the scope of his practice, he should immediately refer the patient to a qualified specialist who will assume the responsibility of establishing the correct diagnosis. *In no instance should he wait to see what happens.*

By assuming this aggressive attitude, early malignant lesions will be discovered and the lives of many patients will be saved. Any dentist who finds a cancer at a time when therapy will result in a cure should be given credit for saving the life of the patient. By early detection of oral cancer the dentist is making a real contribution; this is prevention in its truest sense.

That the efforts of the dental profession are rewarding in this field is revealed by the following studies. In 1956 the Veterans Administration instituted a program whereby all patients admitted to Veterans Administration Hospitals for any reason would, whenever feasible, be given an oral examination by a dentist. Many of these were examined by the ward physician prior to referral to the dental clinic. From 250 to 400 oral malignancies that otherwise might have been overlooked have been detected each year since this program was instigated.[19]

Gilmore[20] made the following statement: "The mortality rate for cancer in Pennsylvania is 173 per 100,000 compared to 147 per 100,000 for the United States: but the mortality rate for cancer of the buccal cavity and pharynx is 2.5 compared to 3.4 for the United States. I am sure this favorable showing is due to the efforts of the dental profession."*

On the other hand, the dentist who overlooks a suspicious lesion and fails to make an early diagnosis of an oral cancer is not fulfilling his professional responsibilities. Failure to locate a small area of dental caries may result in loss of a tooth, but failure to recognize a small cancer may result in death of the patient.[21]

It must be stressed that the primary interest of the dental profession in the field of oral malignancy is detection and diagnosis. While there may be a few dentists who play an active role in the treatment of oral malignancy, it is well recognized that the responsibility for the treatment and management of the cancer patient rests primarily with the medical profession. The dentist has fulfilled his responsibility when he discovers the early malignant lesion. Following discovery the patient should be referred to the proper facilities for definitive treatment.

## ORAL SURGERY IN THE DIAGNOSIS OF LEUKOPLAKIA AND ERYTHROPLASIA

No discussion of preventive oral surgery would be complete without mention of leukoplakia and erythroplasia and the need for an early definitive diagnosis of these

---

*From Gilmore, H.: Personal communication, 1962.

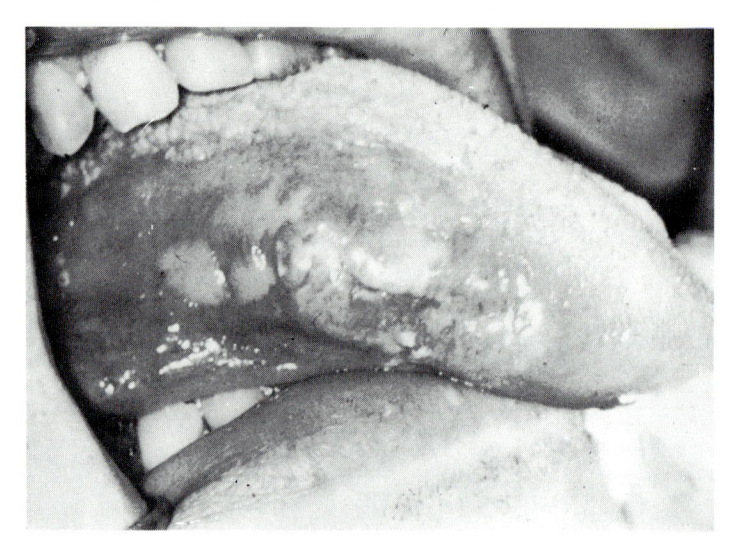

**Fig. 14-8.** A squamous cell carcinoma arising in an area of leukoplakia.

lesions. While there is need to be suspicious of all oral lesions until a definitive diagnosis has been established, leukoplakia and erythroplasia require particular emphasis.

Leukoplakia, a white, keratotic, elevated, roughened lesion that may involve any portion of the oral mucosa, is a common and well-recognized oral lesion. A great deal of attention must be given to the correct diagnosis of this entity. It has been shown by many investigators[22-32] that, while some of these lesions are innocuous, others are dangerous and may go on to malignant transformation (Fig. 14-8). A study by Shafer and Waldron[33] of 332 cases of oral leukoplakia revealed that 17 percent were dangerous, with 7.8 percent demonstrating focal atypia, 1.8 percent demonstrating carcinoma in situ, and 8.1 percent demonstrating invasive squamous cell carcinoma. With this number of dangerous lesions developing in areas of leukoplakia, it becomes evident that early and accurate diagnosis is essential.

Investigators[18, 33-36] have shown that diagnosis of the malignant potentiality of leukoplakia cannot be made on a clinical basis alone and that microscopic examination of the tissue is essential. These investigators have emphasized the importance of biopsy in the diagnosis of this condition. Thus when the clinician is confronted with a white lesion of the oral mucosa which cannot be diagnosed as an innocuous lesion by its clinical characteristics it is essential that a biopsy be performed to disclose its true nature. If the biopsy reveals a dangerous or potentially dangerous lesion, early and energetic therapy is indicated to eradicate the lesion.

Erythroplasia is the second soft tissue lesion that should be given special consideration. Oral erythroplasia has been described by Ackerman and Johnson[37] and by Hertz.[38] It is quite similar to erythroplasia of Queyrat, a malignant or premalignant lesion of the penis. The oral lesions occur anywhere on the oral mucosa and are usually small, rough, innocuous-appearing, slightly raised, granular, red or pinkish red areas. The margins are irregular and small areas of a white, membranous-appearing slough may be present. Induration is usually not a feature. These lesions frequently represent early malignancies, and the clinician must be alert for this condition. When it is encountered, immediate biopsy examination is indicated.

If it proves to be malignant, energetic therapy will usually ensure an excellent chance of survival.

## CONCLUSION

Oral surgery plays an important role in any preventive dentistry program. Timely, sound, conservative oral surgical procedures are indicated to prevent untoward results, unnecessary complications, and needless mutilation in the eradication of oral disease. Oral surgery procedures based on time-tested surgical principles contribute greatly to the comfort, health, and well-being of the patient. The contributions of oral surgery to preventive dentistry may be summarized as follows.

1. Prevention of errors in therapy due to improper diagnosis
2. Prevention of major surgical problems developing from minor surgical problems
3. Prevention of operative and postoperative complications
4. Prevention of adverse reactions to local anesthetics
5. Prevention of postoperative hemorrhage
6. Prevention of minimizing prosthetic failures
7. Prevention of psychological and functional problems associated with facial deformities and injuries
8. Prevention of death by early diagnosis of oral malignancies
9. Prevention of leukoplakia and erythroplasia from progressing into serious lesions

## REFERENCES

1. Waldron, C. A.: Solitary (hemorrhagic) cyst of mandible, Oral Surg. 7:88, 1954.
2. Clark, H. B., Jr.: Practical oral surgery, ed. 3, Philadelphia, 1965, Lea & Febiger.
3. Mead, S. V.: Diseases of the mouth, ed. 5, St. Louis, 1940, The C. V. Mosby Co.
4. Krogh, H. W.: Extraction of teeth in the presence of acute infections, J. Oral Surg. 9:136, 1951.
5. Walker, R. V.: Sterile techniques in everyday practice, Dent. Clin. N. Amer. November, 1959, p. 692.
6. Evans, R. J., and Spooner, E. T. C.: Infections from dental syringes, D. Digest 57:274, 1951.
7. Trumbull, M. and Greiner, D. J.: Homologous serum jaundice, J.A.M.A. 145:965, 1951.
8. Runyan, J., Wright, H. W., and Beebe, R. T.: Homologous serum jaundice; report of 8 fatal cases, J.A.M.A. 144:1065, 1950.
9. d'Angelo, Matteo: Incidenza della virus epatite in rapporto a prestazioni stomatologiche, Ann. Stomat. 13:941, 1964.
10. Conklin, W. W., and Stafne, E. C.: A study of odontogenic epithelium in the dental follicle, J.A.D.A. 39:143, 1949.
11. Small, I. A., and Waldron, C. A.: Ameloblastomas of the jaws, Oral Surg. 8:281, 1955.
12. Henny, F. A.: The impacted third molar, J. Michigan D. A. 40:10, Oct., 1958.
13. Seevers, M. H.: 1949 Symposium: anesthesia in otolaryngolic surgery, J. Amer. Acad. Ophthal. 53:281, 1949.
14. Vital Statistics of the United States, vol. II, p. 30, Washington, D. C., 1956, U. S. Department of Health, Education, and Welfare, U. S. Public Health Service, National Office of Vital Statistics.
15. Management of dental problems in patients with cardiovascular problems; report of working conference, J.A.D.A. 68:333, March, 1964.
16. Chamberlain, F. L.: Management of medical-dental problems in patients with cardiovascular disease, Mod. Concepts Cardiovas. Dis. 13:12, Dec., 1961.
17. Howell, J. T., and Monto, R. W.: Recognition and management of bleeding disorders in oral surgery, J. Oral Surg. 11:129, 1953.
18. Burket, L. W.: Oral medicine, ed. 3, Philadelphia, 1957, J. B. Lippincott Co.
19. Fauber, J.: Personal communication
20. Gilmore, H.: Personal communication.

21. Muhler, J. C., Hine, M. K., and Day, H. G.: Preventive dentistry, St. Louis, 1954, The C. V. Mosby Co.
22. Weisberger, D.: Precancerous lesions, J.A.D.A. **54**:507, 1957.
23. Trieger, N., and others: Cirrhosis and other predisposing factors in carcinoma of the tongue, Cancer **11**:357, 1958.
24. Hobaek, A.: Leukoplakia oris, Acta Odont. Scand. **7**:61, 1946-1947.
25. Eichenlaub, F. J.: Leukoplakia buccalis, Arch. Dermat. Syph. **37**:590, 1938.
26. Martin, E. R., and Sugarbaker, E. D.: Cancer of the floor of the mouth, Surg. Gynec. Obstet. **61**:347, 1940.
27. Sharp, G. S.: Cancer of the oral cavity, Oral Surg. **1**:614, 1948.
28. Ackerman, L. V.: Verrucous carcinoma of the oral cavity, Surgery **23**:670, 1948.
29. Gibbel, M. S., Gross, J. H., and Ariel, I. M.: Cancer of the tongue; a review of 330 cases, Cancer **2**:441, 1949.
30. Wilkins, S. A., Jr., and Vogler, W. R.: Cancer of gingiva, Surg. Gynec. Obstet. **105**:145, 1957.
31. Moertel, C. G., and Foss, E. L.: Multicentric carcinomas of the oral cavity, Surg. Gynec. Obstet. **106**:652, 1958.
32. Smith, J. F.: Carcinoma of the gingivae, J. Tennessee D. A. **39**:236, 1959.
33. Shafer, W. G., and Waldron, C. A.: A clinical and histopathologic study of oral leukoplakia, Surg. Gynec. Obstet. **112**:411, 1961.
34. Bhaskar, S. N.: Synopsis of oral pathology, ed. 3, St. Louis, 1969, The C. V. Mosby Co.
35. Bernier, J. L.: Management of oral disease, ed. 2, St. Louis, 1959, The C. V. Mosby Co.
36. Shira, R. B.: Diagnosis of common lesions of the oral cavity, J. Oral Surg. **15**:95, 1957.
37. Ackerman, L. V., and Johnson, R.: Present day concepts of intra-oral histopathology. In Mast, S. P.: Proceedings of the Second National Cancer Conference, New York, 1954, American Cancer Society, Inc.
38. Hertz, J.: Oral precancerous lesions with special reference to the role played by the dentist in cancer prevention, Oral Surg. **9**:687, 1956.

# Chapter 15 Preventive oral pathology

## Hamilton B. G. Robinson

Introduction
Diagnosis
Lesions of soft tissues
Conclusion

## INTRODUCTION

Oral pathology deals with the essential nature of oral disease.[1] In one sense, oral pathology may be considered as the science of oral diseases—their causes, their courses or natural histories, their effects on local tissues and on the body's economy, their symptoms, and their prognoses. Inevitably complete knowledge of a disease leads to more effective methods for its treatment and prevention. A second consideration of oral pathology is as a part of general practice or as a specialized type of practice that leads to identification of variations from the normal produced by genetic disturbances, by disturbances in development, by disturbances in metabolism, by injuries from physical, chemical, or thermal trauma, by radiant energy, or by living agents. In this practice of oral pathology, which largely is clinical oral pathology, it overlaps with diagnosis, oral medicine, or stomatology. While clinical recognition of a disease obviously comes too late to prevent its occurrence, it may be made early enough to prevent severe local or general effects. Thus early diagnosis is prevention. For example, recognition of cancer at an early stage may prevent mutilation or death, while early recognition of gingivitis and traumatism may prevent periodontitis and loss of teeth.[2]

Preventive oral pathology begins with knowledge and is activated by complete examination. There are no shortcuts in the diagnostic procedure. It begins with taking the history of the patient, continues with general physical evaluation and thorough intraoral examination and x-ray examination, and uses laboratory tests[10] wherever their employment is indicated. These ingredients—history, clinical examination, x-ray examination, and laboratory tests—are then reviewed and evaluated using one's knowledge and experience to arrive at the diagnosis. The diagnostic process leads to recognition of all abnormalities and should thereby permit prevention as well as therapy. The astute diagnostician by his thorough approach and application of knowledge recognizes disease early. The importance of good diagnosis, which recognizes lesions early when they have first become clinically recognizable rather than later when no acumen and little professional ability is required to identify them, is shown in Fig. 15-1. Finding an early decalcification at the margin of an occlusal fissure, an early loss of calcium in interproximal caries, an impinging gingival margin on a restoration, or a potentially irritating clasp may prevent pulpitis, periodontal disease, or carcinoma. This complete dental service is deserved by every patient who has been accepted as a responsibility of any dentist.

The dental profession has motivated its patients to expect preventive treatment —the arrest or repair of carious lesions before pain is a symptom, improvement of

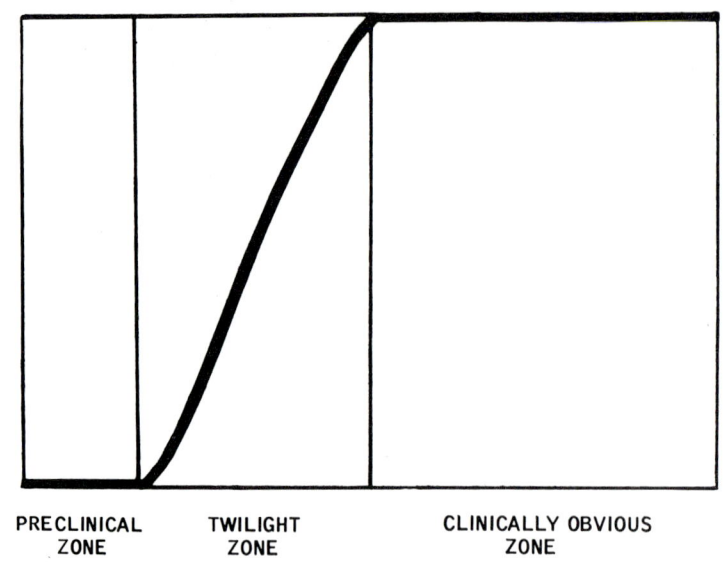

**Fig. 15-1.** Diagrammatic representation of diagnostic zones. As better diagnostic procedures are devised the width of the preclinical zone, where diagnosis is clinically impossible, will be reduced. In the clinically obvious zone the lesions may be apparent even to untrained individuals. The dentist diagnoses in the twilight zone—the more astute and capable he is, the closer he approaches the preclinical zone and preventive diagnosis. (From Thoma, K. H., and Robinson, H. B. G.: Oral and dental diagnosis, ed. 5, Philadelphia, 1960, W. B. Saunders Co.)

occlusion and replacement of lost teeth before the entire dentition is mutilated, and preservation of the periodontium before the teeth are doomed. Dental patients expect the dentist to recall them for periodic examination as a preventive practice. Unfortunately this recognition of the value of preventive dentistry extends to less than 40 percent of the population since only that portion of the American public sees a dentist with any real frequency. Nevertheless, the educational program has motivated a great number of individuals and they have placed the responsibility for diagnosis and prevention of oral diseases and their sequelae on their dentists. The responsibility cannot be assigned to paradental personnel or to other professional people. The dentist is the one trained and educated for this professional responsibility. The diagnostic process must not be limited to exploration for cavities and evaluation of the gingival condition. The dentist practicing prevention must include these examinations, but he must be much more extensive and thorough if he is to fulfill his moral and professional obligations. The procedure of diagnosis must not be viewed as a time-consuming and boring task. It is an opportunity for the dentist to apply his knowledge of oral pathology and his experience from continuing study of patients to allow him to participate as a clinical oral pathologist and to exercise his clinical acumen and brain power for the ultimate benefit of the patient.

Traditionally the dentist has charged for procedures he carries out manually—for placement of restorations, removal of calculus, extraction of teeth, and so on. He has given consultative advice to his patients without charge, and now as patient education, detailed examination, and preventive counseling occupy more of his time he will find it necessary to change his fee structure and charge for this nonmanipulative service just as the physician and psychiatrist have done for many years. The patient expects to pay for such professional service and will appreciate it and respect it more when he is charged for the dentist's time.

## DIAGNOSIS

In preparation for the physical examination of the patient, a history is obtained. A general health chart is a useful approach to evaluation of the general health of the patient (Fig. 15-2; see also Fig. 13-4). It is not a substitute for careful history taking with each individual patient but serves as a portion of the patient's recorded history. The general health chart may yield evidence of systemic disease leading to consultation with the patient's physician on questions such as the status of cardiovascular disease, diabetes mellitus, hypothyroidism, and psychosis. The additional information gained by the dentist through careful and sympathetic questioning should produce relevant facts about the family history, history of general and local disease, nutritional history, occupational history, and attitudes toward prevention and therapy.[4-6]

The usual pattern in medical diagnosis is to learn the chief complaint of the patient, to seek its cause, to diagnose the condition, and to prescribe and render therapy. While there is a certain amount of this diagnosis in dentistry, through expansion of the preventive approach to dental practice, more and more patients seek dental care before a painful symptom or disfiguring sign arises. If a patient does present with a complaint of pain or swelling, thorough examination may lead to prevention of death of the tooth from pulpitis or death of the patient from cancer.

Either after the history is obtained or in coordination with the taking of the history, one should begin the physical examination of the patient. A general assessment of gait, posture, constitution, complexion, and psychic state should have been made as the patient entered the operatory and consulted with the dentist. The facies and lips should have careful examination, not only by visualization but also by palpation. This includes the areas of distribution of the salivary glands and of the orally related lymph nodes. When the intraoral examination is commenced, it should be performed with two tongue blades, one held in each hand, and good lighting. This phase of the examination should not be begun with explorers and mouth mirrors for these inevitably direct the attention of the examiner to the teeth and start a premature search for carious lesions.[9] The oral mucosa of the lips and cheeks, the palate, the tongue, and the floor of the mouth can be visualized when tongue blades are used. The tongue is then extended; now, using the mouth mirror as a pharyngoscope, the posterior portions are visualized. The tongue also should be palpated for any lumps or regions of undue firmness. The gingiva is now examined, retracting the lips and cheeks to permit visualization of the mucolabial and mucobuccal folds. A moderate air blast blown into the gingival sulcus will permit useful visualization of it. Finally, with an explorer, periodontal probe, and mouth mirror, the teeth and gingival sulci are examined. One must remember that final diagnosis of caries will be carried out after prophylaxis, which greatly increases the opportunity to discover early carious lesions without cavitation, and with bite-wing roentgenograms, which are necessary to identify 60 percent or more of the proximal carious lesions. Moreover, the periodontium will be examined by the roentgenogram as well as by the eye, palpation, and probing, so it is good practice to reexamine after the roentgenograms are available. The tooth surfaces should be studied for evidence of abrasion, attri-

### GENERAL HEALTH CHART

**Cardiovascular system** — Circle one

| | |
|---|---|
| Has a physician ever said you have heart trouble? | Yes No DK* |
| Do you get out of breath easily? | Yes No DK |
| Have you had rheumatic fever, growing pains, or twitching of the limbs? | Yes No DK |
| Have you fainted more than twice in your life? | Yes No DK |
| Do you have spells of dizziness? | Yes No DK |
| Have you ever had rheumatic heart disease or Saint Vitus' dance? | Yes No DK |
| Are your ankles often badly swollen? | Yes No DK |
| Have you at times had bad nosebleeds? | Yes No DK |
| Do you get out of breath rapidly? | Yes No DK |

**Nervous system**

| | |
|---|---|
| Do you suffer badly from frequent severe headaches? | Yes No DK |
| Has a physician ever told you that you had neuralgia? | Yes No DK |
| Has a physician ever told you that you had neuritis? | Yes No DK |
| Has a physician ever told you that you had neurosis? | Yes No DK |
| Have you ever had a nervous breakdown? | Yes No DK |
| Has a physician ever told you that you had epilepsy? | Yes No DK |

**Respiratory system**

| | |
|---|---|
| Is your nose continually stuffed up? | Yes No DK |
| Do you have asthma? | Yes No DK |
| Do you have hay fever? | Yes No DK |
| Have you ever had tuberculosis? | Yes No DK |
| Do you have frequent sore throat? | Yes No DK |
| Do you have sinusitis? | Yes No DK |

**Gastrointestinal tract**

| | |
|---|---|
| Do you suffer from stomach trouble? | Yes No DK |
| Do you have frequent diarrhea? | Yes No DK |

**Endocrine system**

| | |
|---|---|
| Are you frequently thirsty? | Yes No DK |
| Has a member of your family had diabetes? | Yes No DK |
| Have you ever taken thyroid tablets? | Yes No DK |
| At what age did you reach puberty? ___ Age | |
| Are you menstruating regularly? | Yes No DK |

**Genitourinary tract**

| | |
|---|---|
| Did a physician ever say that you had kidney or bladder trouble? | Yes No DK |

*DK — don't know

Fig. 15-2. A general health guide.

**Special organs**     **Circle one**

| | |
|---|---|
| Have you ever been treated for ear trouble? | Yes No DK |
| Have you ever been treated for eye trouble other than corrective glasses? | Yes No DK |

**Other**

| | |
|---|---|
| Are you sensitive to any particular medicine (aspirin..., antibiotics..., sulfa drugs..., barbiturates..., others...)? | Yes No DK |
| Have you gained or lost much weight recently? | Yes No DK |
| Have you ever had x-ray treatments? | Yes No DK |
| Have you ever had an operation? | Yes No DK |
| Have you ever had a series of "needles," "shots," or injections? | Yes No DK |
| Has a physician ever told you that you had a tumor or cancer? | Yes No DK |
| Are you receiving any treatment with anticoagulants? | Yes No DK |
| Are you taking any cortisone type of treatment? | Yes No DK |
| Are you receiving any treatment by any physician now? | Yes No DK |
| If so, by whom _____ | |

**Blood**

| | |
|---|---|
| Have you ever had anemia? | Yes No DK |
| Have you ever had abnormal bleeding following extraction of teeth or from a cut? | Yes No DK |

**Skin**

| | |
|---|---|
| Have you ever been treated for a skin disease? | Yes No DK |
| What disease? _____ | |

**Bones and joints**

| | |
|---|---|
| Are your joints ever painfully swollen? | Yes No DK |
| Have you ever had more than one fracture? | Yes No DK |
| Have you ever had more than one dislocation? | Yes No DK |

**Special dental**

| | |
|---|---|
| Have you often had severe toothaches? | Yes No DK |
| Have you ever had severe pains of the face or head? | Yes No DK |
| Do your gums bleed when you brush your teeth? | Yes No DK |
| Have you ever had gum treatments? | Yes No DK |
| Have you ever had an acute sore mouth? | Yes No DK |
| What was your last dental treatment and when? _____ | |
| Dentist's name: _____ | |
| Have you ever been given fluoride treatments by your dentist? | Yes No DK |
| When? _____ | |
| Are you taking or have you taken fluoride tablets? | Yes No DK |
| When? _____ | |

Fig. 15-2, cont'd. For legend see opposite page.

tion, erosion, calculus, hypoplasias, fractures, and stains, as well as for caries. Early discovery of dentifrice abrasion can prevent extensive tissue damage as can recognition of abrasion due to habits such as the opening of bobby pins with the teeth, of attrition caused by unusual food habits, of calcareous deposits, or of certain types of stains.

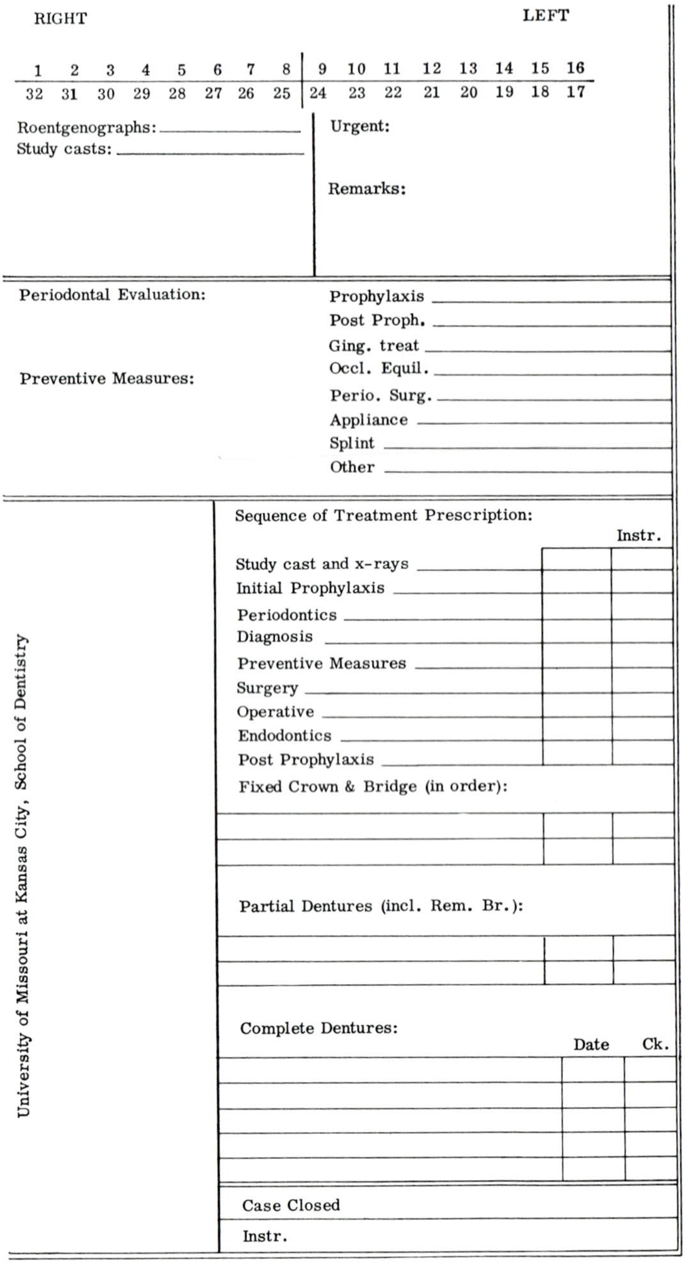

RIGHT | LEFT

| | | | | | | | | | | | | | | | |
|---|---|---|---|---|---|---|---|---|---|---|---|---|---|---|---|
| 1 | 2 | 3 | 4 | 5 | 6 | 7 | 8 | 9 | 10 | 11 | 12 | 13 | 14 | 15 | 16 |
| 32 | 31 | 30 | 29 | 28 | 27 | 26 | 25 | 24 | 23 | 22 | 21 | 20 | 19 | 18 | 17 |

Roentgenographs: ________
Study casts: ________

Urgent:

Remarks:

Periodontal Evaluation:

Preventive Measures:

Prophylaxis ________
Post Proph. ________
Ging. treat ________
Occl. Equil. ________
Perio. Surg. ________
Appliance ________
Splint ________
Other ________

Sequence of Treatment Prescription:

| | | Instr. |
|---|---|---|
| Study cast and x-rays | | |
| Initial Prophylaxis | | |
| Periodontics | | |
| Diagnosis | | |
| Preventive Measures | | |
| Surgery | | |
| Operative | | |
| Endodontics | | |
| Post Prophylaxis | | |

Fixed Crown & Bridge (in order):

Partial Dentures (incl. Rem. Br.):

Complete Dentures:

| | Date | Ck. |
|---|---|---|
| | | |
| | | |
| | | |
| | | |
| | | |

Case Closed

Instr.

University of Missouri at Kansas City, School of Dentistry

**Fig. 15-3.** Patient's record chart designed for preventive dentistry (University of Missouri at Kansas City).

Because of the great many changes that may be identified only with the aid of roentgenograms in the hard structures of the teeth and bones, intraoral or panagraphic x-ray examinations are essential. Study models are needed to aid in discovering potentially damaging occlusal discrepancies. Without pulp tests, diseases of the pulp may be overlooked.

The method of recording the patient's examination is important in guiding the dentist to a preventive approach. Two examples of dental records are shown in Fig. 15-3. Both of these forms are designed to direct priority in treatment programming to procedures preventing or controlling disease processes before repairing the results of prior disease. Of course, allowance is made for control of pain, acute infection, or other emergency conditions. The patient must be taught how to maintain oral hygiene and be given prophylactic treatment for caries, periodontal therapy including correction of occlusal disharmonies, and information on nutritional aspects of oral health at the beginning of his dental program. It is foolish to place and replace restorations until the patient is prepared for prevention and control of further dental disease. Almost 40 percent of dental restorations are replacements for earlier ones. We must prepare the patient as well as the tooth for restorative dentistry in a preventive program.

## LESIONS OF SOFT TISSUES

The dentist is responsible for prevention (and therapy) of *oral* disease, not simply dental or tooth disease. His primary region of responsibility extends from the vermilion borders of the lips to the anterior pillars of the fauces and includes the jaw bones, the salivary glands, and the temporomandibular joint. This does not preclude him from discovering a basal cell carcinoma on the face or from recognizing exophthalmos or cervical enlargement of lymphoid tissues. On the lips, solar cheilosis or hyperkeratosis may be discovered. Surgical procedures and protective measures against excessive exposure to solar radiation may be instituted in time to prevent carcinoma. Even if the patient is not seen early enough to find the precancerous lesions, carcinoma may be identified at an early stage and removed with

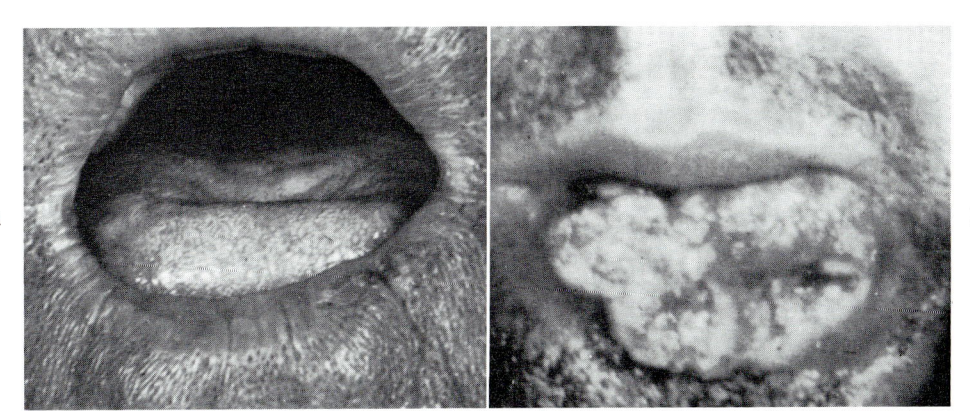

Fig. 15-4. **A,** Small relatively well-localized carcinoma evident midway between midline and commissure of lips in patient's left side. There are fissure and keratosis, both of which were chronic. A biopsy was necessary to make the diagnosis. **B,** Large fulminating invasive carcinoma of the lower lip with metastasis to the regional lymph nodes.

little or no mutilation and with complete protection from metastasis or recurrence. A small carcinoma of the lip is contrasted with a large fulminating labial carcinoma in Fig. 15-4. While the size of a carcinoma is not always a guide to its invasiveness or curability, in general a small lesion is a better candidate for effective therapy than a large one.

Intraorally the oral mucosa should be carefully examined for possible erosions, ulcerations, or lumps. Every deviation from the normal should be identified. This is the first stage in the prevention of destructive disease whether it be infectious, metabolic, traumatic, or neophytic in nature. *There is no substitute for careful clinical examination, visually and manually, at this stage of preventive clinical oral pathology.* If a lesion cannot be clinically identified with relative certainty, further steps should be taken. The time and size relationship of most carcinomas and emphasis of the importance of early diagnosis is shown in Fig. 15-5.

Oral cytology[4] has gained attention and some degree of popularity in recent years but one must be careful not to give it the role of the alpha and the omega in the diagnosis of oral lesions.[7] The technic for collecting cells and preparing the slides for oral exfoliative cytology is fairly easy to master. The critical problem is the information that can be obtained from the slide by the oral pathologist. It is no easy task to interpret an oral cytologic slide that demonstrates atypical cells. If the report is negative one is left with the question as to whether cells with malignant or premalignant changes were exfoliated into the saliva and removed from the mouth by its natural clearing mechanism. Moreover, if the report is positive or equivocal a biopsy is indicated. The real problem with oral exfoliative cytology is the false negative. In 82 oral carcinomas identified in 2,052 patients screened by exfoliative cytology and also biopsied, there were 14.6 percent false negatives in the exfoliative cytology smears.[8] In another group of 75 cases of oral carcinoma 10 false negatives were reported from smears.[3] Unfortunately, these patients with false negatives all would have been left untreated if the exfoliative cytology report had been accepted as final. The method of taking a biopsy specimen is not difficult to learn and practitioners of preventive dentistry should learn to use the scalpel for biopsy as they use

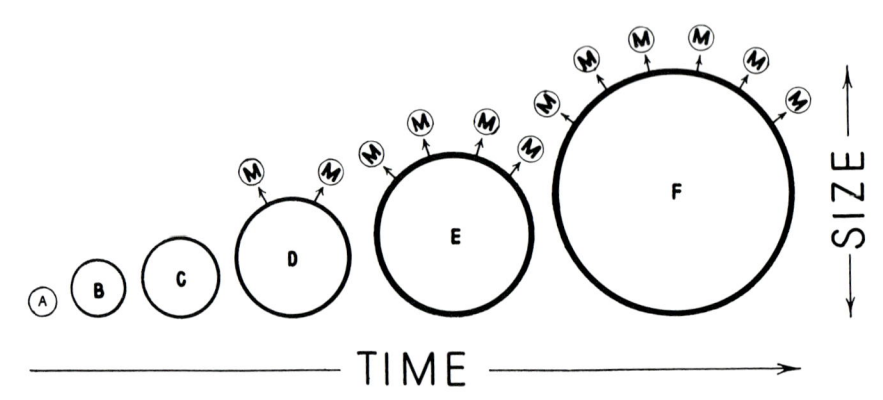

Fig. 15-5. Smaller carcinomas, **A**, usually have not metastasized or invaded the tissues extensively. With time the lesions usually increase in size, **B** to **F**, and are likely to have metastasized, **M**, and invaded the tissues to a greater degree. The dentist strives to recognize carcinoma as early as possible when therapy is more likely to be curative. No doubt there is a stage before **A** that we have not yet learned to recognize.

the explorer, the x-ray, and the pulp tester. Oral exfoliative cytology should not be belittled but rather should be placed in its proper place as an aid to diagnosis.

Prevention of deaths from oral cancer cannot depend on a single technic but begins with careful history taking and thorough clinical examination. Then and only then do biopsy and cytology become important; each has its place. The "yield" of oral cancer discovered by oral exfoliative cytology in unselected groups is extremely small. Using all aids available, only ten carcinomas were discovered in 19,128 persons examined in one state survey.[11] To depend on oral exfoliative cytology alone might give a false sense of security and lead to attempts to "automate" oral diagnosis by feeding into the machine inadequate data. On the other hand, to disregard the value of oral exfoliative cytology as an aid in diagnosis would be erroneous.

The importance of early diagnosis to prevent unnecessary mutilation or death from oral cancer cannot be overemphasized. Some 7,000 Americans die each year from cancer of the oral regions, and most of them die needlessly. Only a high index of suspicion, thorough and sharp diagnosis, and early and adequate treatment can prevent these deaths. But cancer is not the only dangerous oral disease that can be prevented or controlled by effective clinical oral pathology. Actinomycosis, blastomycosis, erythema multiforme, leukoplakia, noma, stomatitis venenata, and thrush, among others, may be local in origin and can be disfiguring or fatal. More benign local disturbances that challenge the dentist include cysts of odontogenic or nonodontogenic origin, various types of glossitis, gingival enlargements including epulis, granulomas, herpetic diseases, keratoses, lichen planus, mucoceles, pemphigus, stomatitis nicotina, and verruca vulgaris. These require preventive or control measures. The oral cavity may serve as a mirror, reflecting generalized or localized extraoral diseases when there are no other clinical signs apparent. These diseases include achlorhydria, Addison's disease, agranulocytosis, amyloidosis, anemias, argyrosia, carotenemia, chronic atrophic gingivitis and mucositis, diabetes mellitus, epizootic diseases, hemophilia, histoplasmosis, Hodgkin's disease, hormonal imbalances, infectious mononucleosis, metastatic tumors, leukemias, lupus erythematosus, metallic poisoning, osteitis deformans, osteitis fibrosa cystica, Plummer-Vinson syndrome, polycythemia, radiation illness, rubella, rubeola, sarcoidosis, scarlatina, scleroderma, smallpox, sprue, Steven-Johnson syndrome, thrombocytopenic purpura, vitamin deficiencies, and von Recklinghausen's neurofibromatosis. This is only a partial list of conditions identifiable in the oral cavity. While some of these diseases are relatively rare, there are numerous examples in the dental literature of discovery by dentists of these diseases in time to permit control or cure. For each reported case, there must be many more unreported cases where dentists have served their professional roles by discovering the oral lesions, by identifying the causes themselves, or by consulting and referring the patients for proper therapy.

The dentist has responsibility far beyond that of repair of defects caused by dental caries or injury produced by calculus, defective restorations or occlusal trauma. He needs to review his oral pathology, oral medicine, and oral diagnosis through up-to-date editions of the textbooks and to upgrade his knowledge by regular reading of current literature and by participation in continuing education courses. To rehabilitate a patient's mouth to a highly functional and esthetic level is a valuable service in which the dentist can take great pride. To discover thrombocytopenic purpura in a young child, early curable carcinoma of the tongue in a young man, early osteitis fibrosa cystica in a middle-aged woman, vitamin B-complex deficiency in an aging woman, or a metastatic jaw lesion from a supposedly controlled extraoral carcinoma in any patient is an extremely valuable professional service. Only the well-educated, well-trained, and alert professional man can perform this service which may prevent debilitation or which may save a life. This, too, is prevention, but knowledge of oral pathology can permit even greater service in preventing disease before it starts, for example, by preventing nutritional deficiency through teaching good nutritional practice, by preventing cancer through eliminating smoking and other oral irritants, or by preventing granulocytopenia by a knowledge of drug reactions. The first key is knowledge, the second is alertness, and the third is a philosophy directing one's practice toward prevention.

## CONCLUSION

Oral pathology contributes to preventive dentistry, first through contributing to the understanding of disease processes and then through clinical practice that embraces diagnosis, oral medicine, and stomatology. The dentist must take a careful history, make a thorough physical examination using roentgenograms and indicated laboratory aids, and then utilize his knowledge and reasoning ability to make a diagnosis when it can still prevent irreparable damage. Moreover, if he is to accept his full responsibility, he must teach his patients how to prevent disease.

## REFERENCES

1. Bernier, J. L.: The management of oral disease, ed. 2, St. Louis, 1959, The C. V. Mosby Co.
2. Colby, R. A., Kerr, D. A., and Robinson, H. B. G.: Color atlas of oral pathology, ed. 2, Philadelphia, 1961, J. B. Lippincott Co.
3. Gaitner, W. D.: Comparison of exfoliative cytodiagnosis and histodiagnosis of oral lesions; review of the literature and report of 75 cases, J. Oral Surg. 25:446-453, 1967.
4. Oral exfoliative cytology, Veterans Administration Cooperative Study, Washington, D. C., 1962.
5. Robinson, H. B. G.: The role of the dentist in the diagnosis and treatment of lesions of the oral mucosa, Oral Surg. 12:14, 1959.
6. Robinson, H. B. G.: The nature of the diagnostic process, Dent. Clin. N. Amer. March, 1963, p. 3.
7. Robinson, H. B. G.: Oral exfoliative cytology; a reinforcement of diagnosis, not a divining rod, Current Dental Comment 1:22-44, 1969.
8. Shklar, G., and others: Correlated study of oral cytology and histopathology; report of 2,052 oral lesions, Oral Surg. 25:61-70, 1968.
9. Symposium—applied preventive dentistry, The Curators, Columbia, Missouri, 1965, University of Missouri.
10. Thoma, K. H., and Robinson, H. B. G.: Oral and dental diagnosis, ed. 5, Philadelphia, 1960, W. B. Saunders Co.
11. Vickers, R. A., Gorlin, R. J., and Lovestedt, S. A.: Minnesota oral cancer detection, 1957-1961 —results, North-West Den. 44:339, 1965.

# Chapter 16 Radiation biology in dental practice

David Bixler

Introduction
Radiation—its effect on living tissue
    Factors modifying radiation effects
        Degree of penetration
        Type of tissue
        Amount of tissue exposure
        Reparative factor
    Terminology
Somatic effects of ionizing radiation
Chemical protection from radiation damage
Genetic effects of ionizing radiation
Conclusion

## INTRODUCTION

In order to achieve the ideal state of preventive dentistry, we must define what it is we are trying to prevent and then confirm that statement with reasons why we should do so. Hence, the purpose of the initial discussion in this chapter will be to provide the reader with a basic understanding of radiation biology and then present a picture of what it is in this area that we are attempting to prevent.

This chapter is not concerned with the reasons why we should use roentgenography in dentistry. There is almost universal agreement that the quality and standard of dental practice is immeasurably increased by its use. In fact it might be stated that, without its use, it is impossible to practice dentistry that provides total patient care.

As with many things, the use of x-rays in dentistry is accompanied by certain disadvantages, and it appears that "a little bit is good, but a lot more is not necessarily better." The prime purpose of this chapter is to bring evidence to the reader of the harmful aspects of x-radiation as valid reasons for its judicious use.

## RADIATION—ITS EFFECT ON LIVING TISSUE

The two principal points to be emphasized in this section are: (1) ionization is the underlying phenomenon by which radiation produces cellular changes; and (2) *all* ionizing radiation is assumed to be hazardous, but the degree of hazard varies materially.

Ionizing radiation affects tissue through a process whereby electrically stable atoms and molecules become electrically unbalanced. This process occurs when a quantum of ionizing radiation strikes a subatomic particle in one of the molecules

---

The author wishes to acknowledge the advice and assistance of Dr. James O. Beck, Department of Radiology, Indiana University School of Dentistry, in the preparation of this chapter.

of the cell. These subatomic particles are variously designated as protons, neutrons, electrons, and so forth. The subatomic particle may be displaced by the energy of this quantum, and if the particle carries an electric charge as do electrons and protons, a change in electric charge occurs and the molecule assumes a different electric charge. In other words, it becomes electrically unstable or reactive. The molecule is now described as ionized, and the basic principle may be summarized by saying that ionizing radiation creates ionized molecules. If an electron is displaced (and this is the most common situation), the molecule assumes a net positive charge. In living tissues there is a strong tendency for atoms and molecules to seek electric stability and the now positively charged molecule seeks out a negative charge with which to combine. As a result of such a combination, a new chemical may be formed within the cell, and the function of the cell in which this reaction occurs may be altered.

The basic effect of ionization may therefore be described as one of molecular alteration and creation of new chemicals. Examples of such reactions are illustrated in Fig. 16-1.

Since the human body is composed of billions of cells, and since there is usually an adequate supply of cells for replacement of dead or dying cells, the effects of ionizing radiation are not clinically apparent when it is confined to small numbers of cells. Subjective symptoms occur when the amount of radiation is sufficient to damage a relatively large number of cells such that the remaining cells cannot take over the functions of the damaged units in an adequate fashion.

A number of theories have been advanced to explain the effects of ionizing radiation on living tissue. These can be condensed into two principal ideas. The first may be called the principle of direct action. In this instance it is theorized that effects of the radiation are produced by damage to or destruction of a specific, vital molecule in the cell. For example, damage to the deoxyribonucleic acid (DNA) molecule, which makes up the functional part of the gene on the chromosome, results in permanent alteration of structure—a *mutation*. The second may be stated as the principle of indirect action. In this instance the radiation does not directly damage vital cell molecules, but instead may result in the formation of altered chemicals, which are toxic to its normal function, within the cell. These altered molecules indirectly produce cell damage and death. Both concepts acknowledge the possible formation of deleterious chemical products but only in the latter situation are the new chemicals formed by the radiation considered to be primarily important. Many workers subscribe to the idea that these injurious chemicals are highly reactive oxidants (peroxides) formed from the ionization of water and interfere with cell enzymatic reactions (Fig. 16-1). The importance of this idea in the concept of prevention of radiation damage by the administration of certain chemical compounds will be discussed later. Detailed summaries of the biological and cellular effects of ionizing radiation have been published; the reader is referred to these for additional information.[1, 2]

The reader will immediately recognize that the foregoing two ideas are not mutually exclusive. In fact, since it is known that the nucleus, which contains the genetic material, serves as the basis for all the processes associated with life, it has been suggested that *all* profound changes produced by x-radiation of any cell may be related to damage induced primarily in the nucleus. This damage is classified either as *mutations,* which are qualitative changes in individual genes, and/or

1. Ionization
$$H_2O \longrightarrow H_2O^+ + \text{electron} (-)$$

2. Activation
$$H_2O^+ \longrightarrow H^+ + OH^-$$

3. Chemical changes
$$OH^- + OH^- \longrightarrow H_2O_2$$
$$H^+ + O_2 \longrightarrow HO_2^-$$
$$OH_2^- + H^+ \longrightarrow H_2O_2$$

Fig. 16-1. Chemical transformations produced by ionizing radiation.

*structural changes,* which are large, major alterations in the chromosomes themselves and thereby may involve large numbers of genes. In view of this concept it would appear to be academic whether or not a cell is damaged by a direct "hit" to its genetic material or by some toxic chemical by radiation. The end result would be the same.

**Factors modifying radiation effects**

A number of variables involved in the clinical response to ionizing radiation will be mentioned and discussed briefly.

**Degree of penetration.** In general the speed of the radiation particle determines its damaging ability. The greater the speed, the greater will be the penetrating power. In terms of penetrating power, alpha rays have the least penetrating power, beta rays next, gamma rays and x-rays about the same, and "fast" neutrons have extremely high penetrating power.

**Type of tissue.** Not only may radiation have a differential effect upon a single cell, but it may also have a varying effect upon different tissues. This varying effect is closely related to the mitotic activity of the cell. Thus tissues with high rates of mitotic activity such as a hematopoietic tissue are more severely damaged by a given dose of x-rays than tissues with low mitotic rates such as central nervous system and muscle.

**Amount of tissue exposure.** Radiation of a small area of the body with a given dose of x-rays will produce a much smaller clinical response than the same dose spread over the entire body. In fact 500 R whole-body exposure is the $LD_{50}$ of man (50 percent of such radiated individuals die), whereas he may readily tolerate the local exposure of just the thyroid gland, for example, to as much as 5,000 R.

**Reparative factor.** Tissues vary in their ability to recover from the effects of ionizing radiation. Thus damage to certain tissues is irreparable.

A summary of the biologic reaction to ionizing radiation has appeared in the dental literature and is recommended for the interested reader.[3]

**Terminology**

A large number of new, descriptive terms have been formulated in the area of radiation biology. In general these new terms pertain to three areas: (1) the source of the radiation such as isotope and half-life, (2) the target of radiation such as RAD, REM, and LET, and (3) problems of nuclear warfare such as blast and fallout. Most of these new terms are beyond the scope of this chapter, but the reader may wish to refer to an excellent summary article of the new terminology by Aronow.[4] For our purposes we will need the definition of only the following few terms.

**roentgen** Unit of quantity of radiation, derived from the ionizing effect of x-rays in air, frequently abbreviated as R.

**milliroentgen** Designated as mR, representing one-thousandth of a roentgen.

**RAD** (**r**oentgen **a**bsorbed **d**ose) An attempt to differentiate between the penetrating effects of different kinds of radiation; for x-rays, 1 RAD equaling approximately 1 R.

**REM** (**r**oentgen **e**quivalent **m**an) Defined as the estimated amount of energy absorbed in tissue which is biologically equivalent in man to 1 R of gamma or x-rays, generally 1 R equaling 1 REM for man. (This term has been useful since some animal species are more resistant to a given form of radiation than others.)

**scatter radiation** Radiation that has been deviated in direction after passing through matter. To the clinician this is the same as *secondary radiation,* which is defined as radiation emitted by any radiated material.

The reader will recognize a subtle difference in these definitions which is not pertinent to our discussion here.

Since both the body cells (somatic cells) and the reproductive cells (genetic cells) contain genetic material, x-rays are capable of inducing changes in both types of cells. Damage to genetic material in the *body cells* produces the so-called somatic effects of radiation, and it is becoming increasingly evident that the effects that follow acute radiation for cancer can be traced to genetic damage in the body cells themselves. On the other hand genetic damage in the *reproductive* cells will only be manifest in subsequent generations and will appear as (1) increased mortality of zygotes due to the formation of dominant lethal and other detrimental genes and (2) alteration to a different form of one or more hereditary characteristics that thereafter are transmitted in their new form. It is most interesting to note that Neel,[5] reporting on survivors of the Hiroshima atomic blast, did not observe any significant changes in their offspring with the possible exception of a slightly altered sex ratio. This finding has been confirmed in human beings receiving other forms of radiation.[6] Neel concluded that the germ cell radiation from the atomic blast was certainly genetically significant and adequate for genetic change. Since none was observed, the hereditary changes that must have occurred were hidden (lethal or detrimental recessives) and as such will not be evident in the population for some generations.

Even though both the effect of radiation on the individual and the effect to his offspring may well have a common origin in the genetic material, it is nevertheless quite convenient and useful to consider these two categories separately. The principal reason is that recovery of the individual in the former category is possible, while effects of future generations are permanent.

## SOMATIC EFFECTS OF IONIZING RADIATION

It is convenient to think of the somatic effects of ionizing radiation as subdivided into two groups: those that are early or acute effects are characteristically the result of a single massive dose; those that are delayed or late effects may occur after a single dose or after the accumulation of many minor exposures. This latter group is of primary concern to the dentist since he is dealing with multiple small doses rather than single massive doses of radiation. The reader is referred to other textbooks on the subject of dental radiology for a more detailed discussion of acute radiation effects.[7-8]

In his everyday environment man finds himself surrounded by myriad potentially noxious and harmful agents, many of which may have selective effects in inducing congenital malformations in the fetus. In fact, it is remarkable that to date only one drug, thalidomide, has been clearly documented to be teratogenic in man. Irradiation of the fetus has also been purported to be teratogenic and, as with a number of potential human teratogens, the dose-effect relationship remains unclear. One reason for this is undoubtedly that human data are always more difficult to obtain but it is also true that a great number of reports claiming to show that x-rays are teratogenic have been incomplete, and hence practically useless, by failing to report the dosages received and developmental stage of the fetus radiated. The following, then, represents the author's summary and interpretation of the published literature on humans in this area.

1. X-ray doses much greater than 100 R, such as are used therapeutically, constitute a powerful teratogenic agent with deformities of the head, limbs, and spinal column reported.[9]
2. Doses less than 100 R, such as are used for diagnostic purposes, are not unequivocally without teratogenic effect, even though the proof of teratogenicity has yet to be accomplished.[10]

Jacobsen[11] reported that irradiation of the mouse embryo with only 5 R produced a significant increase in skeletal malformations. Furthermore, he feels these findings may be cautiously extrapolated to man since (1) there is a high degree of embryologic developmental similarity in man and mouse, and (2) radiation-induced defects are of similar types in these two organisms. This interpretation would place the nonteratogenic x-ray dosage at a very low level indeed. Nøkkentved[12] has reported on 152 pregnant women who received diagnostic pelvic radiation during the first 4 months of pregnancy. Incidence of malformations and height and weight data of children from these pregnancies were compared to those of children from 143 mothers who were not irradiated. The fetal dose was estimated to range between 220 mR (abdomen) and 7,130 mR (pelvimetry). An increased number of children with low birth weights and short stature were born to those mothers irradiated in the second month of pregnancy although this difference was not statistically significant. The total radiation given was not always able to be evaluated, so no conclusion was drawn in regard to a dose-effect relationship. However, the author concluded that even though no teratogenic effects were demonstrable, a somatic effect following irradiation is not excluded. These data are most interesting because they represent effects of low dose x-irradiation under routine conditions of pregnancy and would indicate that abdominal x-ray examination of fertile women should be made only in the first 2 weeks following a normal menstrual period.

These results pertain mostly to acute but relatively low dosage x-irradiation. The dentist should be aware of its potential dangers since he is employing both acute (to his patients) and chronic (to himself and his personnel) types of radiation, although probably at a much lower dosage level.

The important questions for our purposes are: (1) What are the effects of chronic, low-dosage radiation to somatic tissues? (2) How may these effects be avoided? The somatic tissues with which dentistry is most concerned are skin, eyes, bone, and glandular tissue such as pituitary, thyroid, and salivary glands. All of these structures may fall in the primary beam of x-rays during a routine roentgenographic, diagnostic dental procedure.

**Table 16-1.** *Dosage of radiation received by different tissues following routine dental diagnostic procedures*

| Tissue | Measured dose | Dose (in roentgens) |
|---|---|---|
| Eye | 1,500 mRAD | 1.5 |
| Thyroid gland | 500 mRAD | 0.5 |
| Submandibular glands | 2,000 mRAD | 2 |
| Maximal skin dose | 26,000 mRAD | 26 |
| Minimal bone and tooth dose | 90,000 and 180,000 mRAD, respectively | 90 and 180 |

No direct figures are available on the question of how much radiation produces how much effect on the tissues just mentioned. However, a number of studies have provided data obtained following various dosages of x-radiation. Bjarngard and associates[13] have measured doses to various organs during routine dental diagnostic roentgenographic procedures. The doses they reported are given in Table 16-1.

It is obvious that such figures, which indicate low tissue dosage, have little practical significance unless the conditions under which the radiation was given are known. O'Shaughnessy and Mitchell[14] have reported radiation doses received by various tissues when the various physical roentgenographic factors are systematically altered. Using ionization chambers in a cadaver and routine cone placement for a 16-film survey, they reported doses to pituitary and thyroid glands ranging from 32 to 112 mR (0.032 to 0.112 R) when no collimation was used. Combining the accepted technics of long cone, filtration, and collimation, no reading for any organ in the primary beam was greater than that for the thyroid, which was 2 to 5 mR (0.002 to 0.005 R). Essentially the same results were obtained in their study using 70, 80, and 90 kilovolt peak.

A study by the United States Public Health Service (Laboratory Evaluation of a Dental X-ray Unit Collimating Device, May, 1964) measured the tissue dose received from a 22-film series under the following conditions: (1) lead-lined long cone, (2) ultraspeed film, (3) 90 kvp machine, (4) 2¾ inch diameter beam, and (5) 2 mm. aluminum filtration. The results are reported in Table 16-2.

The results in Table 16-2 indicate that careful radiographic technic, and especially the use of the collimating device described in the article, may reduce local organ or tissue radiation to extremely low levels.

It appears then that, with the use of proper technics, the amount of radiation received by various organs and tissues during a full-mouth roentgenographic survey is extremely small. The question remains, is it small enough? Meyer and associates[15] have reported that 2,040 R produced degenerative changes in gingivae and interseptal bone of rats, while Chase and associates[16] reporting on thirteen patients receiving radiation therapy for oral cancer stated that 2,300 to 4,600 R over a period of 30 to 45 days increased the keratinized cells and reduced the total cells in the buccal mucosa of these patients. This would suggest that very high doses are needed to produce tissue damage of obvious clincal significance. Thus dental diagnostic roentgenograms would appear to be quite low. Wainwright[17] reported that the highest roentgen dose to any square centimeter of skin during a routine 14-film survey, using fast film, collimation, and filtration, was 0.8 R. It should be noted that

**Table 16-2.** *Radiation dose received by different tissues during routine dental x-ray examination when beam was collimating and noncollimating*

| Tissue | Without collimating device (in mR) | With collimating device (in mR) |
|---|---|---|
| Sublingual gland | 570 | 90 |
| Thyroid gland | 100 | 10 |
| Pituitary gland | 14 | 3 |
| Eye | 370 | 20 |
| Parotid gland | 240 | 40 |
| Skin next to bicuspids | 1,610 | 410 |

the maximum permissible dose (MPD) to the skin during a 1-year period of routine dental radiographic examinations is set at 10 R.

A more recent report by the Radiation Protection Committee of the American Academy of Oral Roentgenology[18] states that the maximum permissible exposure to whole body, blood-forming organs, and the lens of the eye is 0.1 R per week with no more than 5 R per year and no more than accumulative total of 5 R between 18 and 36 years of age. Considering the previously cited reports it would certainly seem as if routine dental diagnostic roentgenograms should not be a health hazard to either patients or personnel. But let us now consider some hazards of somatic radiation that are not well documented and to which, in our present state of knowledge, we can only allude.

A single report in the literature by Murano[19] indicates that very low x-ray dosage (30 R at the skin surface, which is probably attained in many offices using older equipment and technics) may stimulate the release of adrenocorticotropic hormone (ACTH) from the hypothalamohypophyseal system, which in turn will increase production of adrenocortical steroids. The significance of this finding remains to be shown, but many physiologists associate increased adrenocortical secretions with undesirable tissue reactions. A number of scientists are now actively pursuing the problem of "late" somatic effects, that is, those effects that accrue from either acute or chronic radiation but that do not appear until after the passage of many years.

Both aging and life shortening have been important topics considered at a United Nations Educational, Scientific, and Cultural Organization (UNESCO) sponsored symposium. At this meeting Harris[20] considered some of the factors that may be involved in cancer, leukemia, and life shortening. He concluded that somatic mutations, activation of latent viruses, and morphologic changes in specific tissues may all contribute to an increased risk to the aforementioned conditions following low-dosage radiation. Premature aging in particular was the subject of much discussion at this meeting. Casarett[21] hypothesized that premature aging following chronic irradiation was caused by nonspecific damage to endothelium of the fine vascular network. Such changes eventually result in arteriocapillary fibrosis, which in turn produces a progressive hypoxia and malnutrition of the dependent parenchymal cells. Thus the cycle of premature aging is initiated. On the other hand, Muller[22] concluded that radiation-induced life shortening is an expression of pointwise loss of individual cells, whose loss is caused by recessive-type genetic alterations resulting from mutation or chromosome loss. Such a conclusion is partially supported by the findings of Sasaki and associates,[23] who observed that radiation workers and radiologists show an excess of pseudodiploid cells, dicentrics, and other types of chromosomally altered cells in their blood. These individuals receive low-dosage, chronic-type radiation. Norman and associates[24] also reported significantly increased numbers of aneuploid cells and other chromosomal types indicative of major genetic change in radiation workers. Workers in such occupations also have been reported to have shortened life-spans.[25] Even though this latter finding has not been confirmed, environmental radiation most certainly is not the only chronic hazard to man's life-span. Tough and Court Brown[26] reported a significant increase in chromosome aberrations of the cells of men exposed to ambient benzene for periods ranging from 1 to 20 years.

Most scientists agree that radiation in sufficient dosage will produce cell death, although the exact mechanism—and there may well be more than one—is not universally agreed upon. Likewise most scientists agree that chronic, low-dosage radiation will produce cellular effects differing mostly from acute, high-dosage radiation in the degree of effectiveness in cell death. What most scientists do not agree upon is the radiation dosage that produces minimal and clinically unimportant effects although most would suggest that this is probably an extremely low dosage. Such thinking is reflected in the fact that the recommended maximum permissible dose for patients and technical personnel, as published by authoritative governmental agencies, has steadily decreased over the past 15 years. What was once thought to be a safe dose is no longer considered to be such. These changes would seem to suggest that, as more research data are obtained, lower and lower dosages of x-rays will be incriminated in producing deleterious biologic events.

In order to maintain these radiation problems in the proper perspective, it is worth noting an article by Richards.[27] He presented the main issues of tissue effects produced by low-level, chronic x-radiation and some of his conclusions merit emphasizing.

> Large numbers of patients have undergone repeated dental roentgenographic examinations in the past. The periods of time that have elapsed since then exceed the latent period for the occurrence of leukemia. Yet, in spite of this the incidence of leukemia has declined steadily for the past 20 years. The occurrence of leukemia as a result of dental x-radiation does not need to be feared greatly by the dentist or patient.

> Although some data indicate life-span shortening by chronic x-radiation, other studies have even shown increases in life-span under these conditions. A statistical study of the longevity of dentists indicated that dentists live almost 3 years longer than white nondentists. Apparently the dentist's life expectancy has not suffered from his occupational exposure to radiation.

## CHEMICAL PROTECTION FROM RADIATION DAMAGE

Various substances have been shown to alter lethal effects of ionizing radiation when they are present in the cell before or during irradation. These fall generally into two groups: (1) sensitizers and (2) protectors.

As a radiation sensitizer, oxygen is certainly the most important example and probably acts at two levels. First, in the aqueous medium of the cell it leads to the formation of $O_2^-$ and $HO_2$ (Fig. 16-1), as well as $H_2O_2$. Secondly, it may attack organic molecules directly leading to the formation of peroxy radicals, which prevent normal repair reactions. This sensitizing effect has been utilized by administering high pressure oxygen to patients receiving x-irradiation for neoplastic disease in an attempt to differentially increase radiosensitivity of the tumor relative to surrounding normal tissue.

Other sensitizers have been described such as the halogenated pyrimidine derivatives (BUdR) and IUdR). These compounds exert their radiosensitizing effect by being incorporated into the replicated DNA strands and thereby imparting structural weakness to the DNA chains at those points of incorporation. Persons receiving these drugs for therapeutic purposes have a known contraindication for x-irradiation and should receive the latter only under clearly indicated and highly controlled conditions.

During the past 10 to 15 years considerable interest has been shown in investigating ways in which radiation damage may be reduced or even prevented. Obviously such means would have great meaning to astronauts, atomic physicists, and individuals working with nuclear reactors. There is even the potential meaning of such protective agents for public health medicine in the event of nuclear war.

Generally the approach to chemical protection has been to look for agents that, when administered orally or parenterally, would lessen or prevent the effects of acute, whole-body radiation. The status of chemical radiation protection has been thoroughly reviewed by Bacq[28] in a detailed monograph; protective agents fall into two general groups. The first group includes diverse substances such as histamine, cyanides, catecholamines, p-aminopropriophenone (PAPP), and some anesthetic agents that are protective primarily by producing systemic hypoxia. The second group consists of thiols and disulfides; numerous studies have been performed that demonstrate their protectivity. The working hypothesis of such investigations has been based upon the idea that radiation produces toxic oxidizing agents in the cell (Fig. 16-1), and these agents will oxidize the sulfhydryl (-S-S-) groups of the protein chains of enzymes. When this occurs, enzymatic activity is lost and cell death follows. Hence any chemical agent that will protect these sulfhydryl groups will lessen or prevent the damage subsequent to cell radiation. Such compounds will most likely be thio-derivatives themselves and this is where most of the research attack has been concentrated. The following compounds have been shown to be effective in radiation protection: cystine, glutathione, methionine, thiourea, mercaptosuccinate, thiosulfate, and s,beta-aminoethylisothiuronium bromide (AET).

AET has shown significant ability to lessen the biologic effects of acute whole-body radiation in rats[29-31] and monkeys.[32] Cystine and glutathione also appear to be effective,[33, 34] while oxidized forms of these compounds are ineffective. On the other hand, the aminated form of cystine, cystamine, appears to be highly effective.[35, 36] More recently, the administration of AET with cystine has been reported to be more effective than either compound alone.[37] Although these compounds may give 30-day survival—the length of time beyond which radiated animals will live indefinitely—recent evidence has indicated that such "protected" animals may die a rather specialized form of death (after 4 months) because of the inability of these compounds to protect bone marrow.[38]

In an attempt to determine whether supportive care, chemical preradiation prophylaxis, or both treatments would be most effective in preventing radiation damage, Melville and associates[39] studied monkeys receiving 900 R in x-rays. They found that supportive care such as intravenous feeding and antibiotics prolonged survival time from 10 to 25 days in the untreated animals. However, supportive care plus several radioprotective agents administered just prior to radiation gave the longest survival time, 135 days. These protective agents were AET, cystine, and Nembutal, administered both intravenously and orally, 15 to 60 minutes prior to radiation. It should be noted that the acute radiation syndrome was *postponed* in the treated animals but *not* eliminated.

New and different chemical compounds have been studied, but as yet very little is known of their true effectiveness or mechanism of action in preventing the acute radiation syndrome. Some of these materials are yeast ribonucleic acid,[40] guanidoethyldisulfide,[42] and paraminopropiophenone.[41] A recent article by Rothe and associates[43] summarizes some of the current concepts regarding the mechanism of action of various radioprotective agents. From these reports it is obvious that chemical protection from radiation damage is still an experimental tool, and more studies must be forthcoming before the significance of this concept as a public health measure can be evaluated.

## GENETIC EFFECTS OF IONIZING RADIATION

It has been quite apparent, mostly as the result of governmental surveys, that human populations are becoming increasingly exposed to high energy radiation. This means that the effects of ionizing radiation in man are a composite of effects arising from several sources of radiation. The general categories usually listed are as follows.

1. *Natural.* This includes all radiation of the body from natural sources such as cosmic radiation and isotopic radiation from elements in the soil, air, and water.
2. *Industrial and man-made.* Such radiation includes radium-dial wristwatches, faulty TV tubes, radioactive fallout, and atomic pile sources.
3. *Therapeutic medical.* This radiation may be confined to a quite small area (x-radiation for thyroid carcinoma) or may cover a larger area as in treatment of acne or hemangiomas; generally this form is more of the acute type and local in coverage.
4. *Diagnostic medical and dental.*

Wuehrmann[44] extrapolated data of other authors and concluded that dentistry was contributing about 10 percent of the gonadal radiation that we are now receiving from background radiation (3.5 R in a 30-year period). It should be immediately obvious that the total of undesirable damage to the genetic material of man (his genetic "load") is a composite of radiation from these four categories.

For practical purposes, nothing can be accomplished to reduce the contribution of natural radiation. Similarly, it is unlikely, although desirable, that any significant reduction will occur in industrial and man-made radiation. Therapeutic medical radiation is necessary for the proper medical treatment of patients with a variety of diseases and tumors. However, in diagnostic medical and dental radiation it would seem that great strides could be made in both the professions of medicine and dentistry to reduce radiation exposure without lowering the standard of practice in either profession. Let us now consider, from a genetic viewpoint, why such a reduction may be required.

One must first recognize that much of the available information in this area stems from experiments performed on animals such as mice, rats, and even fruit flies. However, in most instances where comparable evidence has been obtained in man, the data are confirmatory. Hence scientists will undoubtedly continue to use animal experiments as guidelines for human studies. This approach is really not surprising when one considers that the genetic material of a fruit fly is chemically identical to that of man, and hence its response to radiation is undoubtedly comparable. A review article by Russell[45] on radiation gentics in the mouse supplies important information relative to radiation effects on germ cells. One of the first questions to be considered was, "Are offspring conceived, say, 18 months after radiation of the male as likely to bear a mutation as those conceived 3 months after radiation?" Their results indicated that there is no change in frequency with the passage of time even up to the end of reproductive life (2 years of age in the mouse). However, mature spermatozoa are somewhat more sensitive to radiation than young developing spermatozoa. It seems, then, that mutagenic events in the male or female persist and may well be carried on into the progeny. These observations also support the Atomic Energy Commission recommendation that workers involved in exposure to single high doses of radiation over short periods of time refrain from procreation for a few weeks. After this initial time has elapsed it appears that no genetic advantage may be gained by further delay.

Another most important question is, "Is there a safe *rate* at which radiation doses may be accumulated in order to minimize genetic alteration?" Russell's results[46] indicate that chronic, low-level radiation is considerably less mutagenic than acute, high-level radiation, and he hypothesizes that there may well be some repair or prevention of genetic damage at these lower rates. This finding was not previously demonstrated and introduces a factor of safety into the field of radiology that was not known to exist.

Finally, and of considerable importance to the dentist, is the evidence pertaining to the question, "Is there a threshold dose of radiation below which *no* mutagenic events occur?" A complete answer is not yet available for this question since the lowest levels of radiation produce so few mutant genes that a tremendous number of offspring must be observed and counted in order to obtain a true measure of the mutation frequency. Nevertheless, geneticists would agree that, so far, the evidence points to no threshold[46]; that is, each dose of radiation is responsible for some mutagenic event.

Since it appears that all radiation produces some genetic effect, and also that low *rates* appear to be much less mutagenic than the same total dose at a higher rate, the questions of obvious importance to the dentist are how much gonadal radiation is received by his dental patients and personnel during routine diagnostic roentgenographic procedures, and is this amount too great?

A number of studies have been reported on the amount of gonadal radiation received by dental patients. In 1955 Stanford and Vance[47] reported a 0.34 mR gonadal dose to males and 0.06 mR to females, using a 60 kvp, 10 mA machine, an 8-inch target-film distance and 1-second film exposure. This technic has been considerably improved in recent years and Murai and associates[48] reported gonadal doses estimated at $1.2 \times 10^{-3}$ mREM.

Sonnabend[49] claimed that proper use of ultraspeed film, intensifying screens and filtration could reduce gonadal exposure to a range of 0.01 to $0.10 \times 10^{-3}$ mR. Richards[50] has described the sources of gonadal radiation in the dental patient as scatter or secondary radiation from the radiated parts of the patient's head, radiated metal parts of cone and filters, and the focal spot of the x-ray tube. For this reason he advocated a short, open-ended, but shielded, cone for reduction of backscatter radiation. However, it would certainly appear that the previously cited papers indicate that very low gonadal doses may be obtained with technics that will give better film definition. It should be noted that Jung[51] has pointed out that gonadal doses as currently measured are actually "lap" doses and that the actual germ cell dose is something less than one-tenth of that which has been measured.

These results have been obtained with adults, but it would seem that gonadal radiation doses received by children are somewhat different, if for no other reason than the closer proximity of the gonads to the head and neck areas to be radiated. Jinks[52] reported that, by use of proper x-ray technics and a leaded cloth over the pelvic region, a 98.23 percent reduction in radiation to the child's reproductive organs can be achieved. Williamson and Williams[53] stated that the average gonadal dose to children, using a variety of x-ray technics, was 0.85 mR per pair of bite-wing exposures. The result obtained with a long-cone, fast-film technic, however, was 0.1 to 0.2 mR, which represented a considerable reduction. Since the area to be radiated represents a most important source of scatter radiation, which in turn is *the* source of gonadal radiation, Medwedeff[54] has proposed the use of additional collimation to the primary beam by a cone attachment that holds the film. He reported a 2,200 to 5,600 percent reduction in patient radiation when this device is used with ultraspeed film. An interesting summary of data pertaining to gonadal exposure obtained by various authors is presented by Wainwright.[55] This summary indicates a range of 0.005 to 15.0 mR per film according to various authors. However, the newer radiologic technics, and particularly ultraspeed film, would seem to invalidate results obtained as recently as 10 years ago. Wainwright[17] reported that the average gonadal dose per film using these newer technics was 0.05 mR.

No dentist should or needs to allow his dental patients to receive gonadal radiation doses anywhere near the recommended maximum dose of 500 mR during the reproductive years (10 to 40 years of age) as established by the National Science Foundation. However, Menczer[56] has reported that dentists in the Hartford, Connecticut, area in 1963 delivered from 8 to 88 mR to the gonads in routine surveys and their attitude toward potential radiation hazards was poor and unconcerned. Using Wainright's figure of 0.05 mR per film, this would allow the dentist to take 10,000 dental films during this 30-year period, or an average of more than three hundred per year! These figures should not encourage complacency. Many dentists are using faulty technics with faulty machines and so there is much room for improvement in order to reach Wainwright's figures. A number of articles have been published describing shielding specifications,[57,58] technic and machine modification in adults and children, which will produce the desired, absolute minimum of patient and personnel radiation. The reader is referred to these articles for details.

It is apparent from published data that the radiation given to gonadal tissues during routine dental radiography, provided the proper use is made of collimation, filtration, and high speed film, will not exceed that which is received from natural sources each day. However, many dentists do not feel that even this equivalency is assurance of safety and accordingly use leaded aprons on all children and patients in the reproductive age range. In fact, this is a pointed recommendation of the Council on Dental Research and the Council on Dental Materials and Devices of the American Dental Association. Probably complete prevention of radiation effects on genetic tissue, no matter how slight, can be achieved only by such approaches.

The available literature concerning the biologic effects of ionizing radiation clearly leads to the following conclusions.

Heavy doses of radiation such as 2,000 R to a limited area or 200 R whole body can readily produce clinically observable effects. Genetic tissue also undergoes significant alteration when exposed to such dosages.

Low doses of radiation such as are used every day in dentistry for diagnostic purposes do not produce clinically observable phenomena. There is some evidence that genetic alteration may occur, but even this may be reparable. Evidence for such effects as life-span shortening by chronic low-dosage radiation is presumptive and highly speculative.

Why does the dentist then need to be concerned? Primarily because in this low-dosage range there is little or no *evidence* for any kind of effect—good, bad, or indifferent. Thus the dentist may readily remove himself from the arguments concerning the harmful effects of ionizing radiation by using radiation doses that are the absolute minimum compatible with good radiography. The dental film then becomes the standard of good dental practice in radiography. If the dentist applies a minimum dose of x-rays that will just expose the film to proper diagnostic value (assuming at least a 5-minute developing time), he may feel assured that by any present-day standard he is protecting his patient. This is true preventive dentistry.

There is, however, an additional benefit that results from such a technic. Radiologists agree that the best diagnostic quality of x-ray film is obtained when that film is exposed to a minimum quantity of x-rays (*not* overexposed). Therefore the use of such a technic of minimum exposure gives him both quality diagnostic films and at least adequate patient protection.

## CONCLUSION

The effects of ionizing radiation on cells and tissues were briefly described with the emphasis placed upon x-radiation of both somatic and genetic tissues. Both acute and chronic radiation effects were discussed with definite emphasis upon the latter as pertaining to the practice of dentistry. In general, it was concluded that there may be no level of chronic, low-dosage radiation that does not produce some cellular effect. However, the evidence in this area is absent. The result presented indicates that the practicing dentist can and must be completely aware of potential problems in the use of x-radiation and how to avoid them. Only then can he truly be said to have a preventive practice.

## REFERENCES

1. Pollard, E. C.: The biological action of ionizing radiation, Amer. Sci. 57:206, 1969.
2. Little, J. B.: Cellular effects of ionizing radiation, New Eng. J. Med. 278:308, 1968.
3. Sears, T. P.: Biological reaction to ionizing radiation; atomic structure, J. Periodont. 34:174, 1963.
4. Aronow, S.: A glossary of radiation terminology, New Eng. J. Med. 266:1145, 1962.
5. Neel, J. V.: Changing perspectives on the genetic effects of radiation, Springfield, Illinois, 1963, Charles C Thomas, Publisher.
6. Schalte, P. J. L., and Sobele, F. H.: Sex ratio shifts among progeny from patients having received therapeutic x-irradiation, Amer. J. Human Genet. 16:26, 1964.
7. Wainwright, W. W.: Dental radiology, New York, 1965, McGraw-Hill Book Co.
8. Wuehrmann, A. H.: Radiation protection and dentistry, St. Louis, 1960, The C. V. Mosby Co.

9. Pollard, E. C.: The biological action of ionizing radiation, Amer. Sci. **57**:206, 1969.
10. Little, J. B.: Cellular effects of ionizing radiation, New Eng. J. Med. **278**:308, 1968.
11. Jacobsen, L.: Low dose x-irradiation and teratogenesis, Copenhagen, 1968, Munksgaard.
12. Nøkkentved, K.: Effect of diagnostic radiation upon the human fetus, Copenhagen, 1968, Munksgaard.
13. Bjarngard, B., and others: Radiation doses in oral radiography, Odont. Revy **10**:4, 1959.
14. O'Shaughnessy, P. E., and Mitchell, D. F.: Effect of altering physical roentgenographic factors on patient radiation dose levels, J.A.D.A. **69**:335, 1964.
15. Meyer, I., Shklar, G., and Turner, J.: Effects of 200 kv radiation and cobalt[60] radiation on the oral mucosa, gingiva and alveolar bone of experimental animals, J. Oral Surg., Anes. & Hosp. D. Serv. **21**:147, 1963.
16. Chase, L. P., Toto, P. D., and Magalotti, M. F.: Radiation-induced changes in the epithelium of the buccal mucosa, J. Dent. Res. **40**:929, 1961.
17. Wainwright, W. W.: How much radiation does the patient receive per set of dental radiographs? J. Calif. D. A. **39**:493, 1963.
18. Effective use of x-ray radiation in dentistry: a report of the Radiation Protection Committee of the American Academy of Oral Roentgenology, Oral Surg. **16**:294, 1963.
19. Murano, T.: Studies on the effects of x-ray irradiation on the area of the midbrain and the pituitary gland, J. Osaka City Med. Cent. **12**:1, 1963.
20. Harris, R. J. C., editor: Cellular basis and aetiology of late somatic effects of ionizing radiation, London, 1963, Academic Press.
21. Casarett, G. W.: Concept and criteria of radiologic aging. In Harris, R. G. C., editor: Cellular basis and aetiology of the late somatic effects of ionizing radiation, London, 1963, Academic Press.
22. Muller, H. J.: Mechanisms of life-span shortening. In Harris, R. J. C., editor: Cellular basis and aetiology of the late somatic effects of ionizing radiation, London, 1963, Academic Press.
23. Sasaki, M., Ottoman, R. E., and Norman, A.: Radiation-induced chromosome aberrations in man, Radiology **81**:652, 1963.
24. Norman, A., and others: Chromosome aberrations in radiation workers, Radiation Res. **23**:383, 1964.
25. Warren, S.: Longevity and causes of death from irradiation in physicians, J.A.M.A. **162**:464, 1956.
26. Tough, I. M., and Court Brown, W. M.: Chromosome aberrations and exposure to ambient benzene, Lancet **1**:684, 1965.
27. Richards, A. G.: How hazardous is dental roentgenography? Oral Surg. **14**:40, 1961.
28. Bacq, Z. M.: Chemical protection against ionizing radiation, Springfield, Illinois, 1965, Charles C Thomas, Publisher.
29. Doherty, D. G., and Burnett, W. T., Jr.: Protective effect of S, β-aminoethylisothiuronium: Br.HBr. and related compounds against x-radiation death in mice, Proc. Soc. Exper. Biol. Med. **89**:312, 1955.
30. Preston, R. L., Wells, A. F., and Ershoff, B. H.: Comparative effects of intraperitoneal and oral administration of AET on survival of x-irradiated rats, Radiation Res. **11**:255, 1959.
31. Shapiro, R., Doherty, D. G., and Burnett, W. T.: Chemical protection against ionizing radiation, III, mercaptoalkylguanidines and related isothiuronium compounds with protective activity, Radiation Res. **7**:22, 1947.
32. Crouch, B. G., and Overman, R. R.: Chemical protection against x-radiation death in primates, a preliminary report, Science **125**:1092, 1957.
33. Chapman, W. H., and Cronkite, E. P.: Further studies of beneficial effect of glutathione on x-irradiated mice, Proc. Soc. Exper. Biol. Med. **75**:318, 1950.
34. Patt, H. M., and others: Further studies on modification of sensitivity to x-rays by cysteine, Proc. Soc. Exper. Biol. Med. **73**:18, 1950.
35. Rugh, R.: Relative value of cysteamine and cystamine as radioprotective agents for fetal and adult mice, Amer. J. Physiol. **189**:31, 1957.
36. Bacq, Z. M.: Amines and particularly cysteamine as protectors against roentgen rays, Acta Radiol. **41**:47, 1954.

37. Melville, G. S., Jr., and others: Radioprotection in primates; a preliminary report, USAF Sch. Avia. Med. Rep. 61-3:1, 1961.
38. Pitcock, J. A., and Melville, G. S., Jr.: Subacute radiation death in chemically protected monkeys, USAF Sch. Aerospace Med. Rep. 61-105:5, 1961.
39. Melville, G. S., Jr., and others: Protection against ionizing radiation: x-irradiated monkeys receiving preirradation prophylaxis and postirradiation therapy, USAF Sch. Aerospace Med. 62:103, 1962.
40. Rounds, D. E.: Radioprotective agent; analysis of the potential antiradiation effect of nucleic acids on their precursors, USAF Sch. Aerospace Med. Rep. 61-58:1, 1961.
41. Shapiro, B., Schowartz, E. E., and Kollman, G.: Further studies on the distribution and metabolism of 2-mercaptoethylguanidine and bis (2-guanidoethyl) disulfide in mice, USAF Sch. Aerospace Med. 62-68:14, 1962.
42. Gray, L. H.: Proceedings of the Conference of Research on Radiotherapy of Cancer, New York, 1961, American Cancer Society.
43. Rothe, W. E., Grenan, M. M., and Wilson, S. M.: Radioprotective by pressor amidines, Nature (London) 198:403, 1963.
44. Wuehrmann, A. H.: Responsibility of the dental profession in reducing exposure to ionizing radiation, Oral Surg. 14:304, 1961.
45. Russell, W. L.: Studies in mammalian radiation genetics, Nucleonics 23:53, 1965.
46. Russell, W. L.: Is there a threshold dose for x-irradiation? In Sabels, F. H., editor: Repair from genetic radiation damage, Oxford, 1963, Pergamon Press.
47. Stanford, R. W., and Vance, J.: Quantity of radiation received by reproductive organs of patients during routine diagnostic x-ray examinations, Brit. J. Radiol. 28:266, 1955.
48. Murai, T., and others: The genetically significant radiation dose from dental x-ray diagnosis in Japan, Tokyo Med. D. Univ. 8:319, 1961.
49. Sonnabend, E.: Radiation tolerance of the patient in extraoral radiography, Int. Dent. J. 13:495, 1963.
50. Richards, A. G.: New method for reduction of gonadal irradiation of dental patients, J.A.D.A. 65:1, 1962.
51. Jung, T.: Gonadal doses resulting from panoramic x-ray examinations of the teeth, Oral Surg. 19:745, 1965.
52. Jinks, G. M.: Reduction of radiation dosage in dentistry for children, J. Dent. Child. 26:32, 1960.
53. Williamson, B. D. P., and Williams, A. B.: Gonadal exposure received by children during bitewing radiography, New Zealand D. J.: 55:180, 1959.
54. Medwedeff, F. M., and Knox, H.: Radiation reduction for children, J. Tennessee D. A. 42:321, 1962.
55. Wainwright, W. W.: Dental radiation dose: sensitometric method for determination of exposure-development factors, Oral Surg. 16:674, 1963.
56. Menczer, L. F.: Study of radiation exposure to gonads of preschool boys from diagnostic dental roentgenograms, J.A.D.A. 66:30, 1963.
57. Richards, A. G.: Shielding requirements for dental instillations, J.A.D.A. 64:788, 1962.
58. Trubman, A.: Radiation protection of dental presonnel, J.A.D.A. 65:751, 1962.

Chapter 17 The role of dental materials in preventive dentistry*

Simon Civjan

Introduction
Amalgam
    Biophysical considerations
Pure gold restorations
Gold alloy castings
    Biophysical considerations
Restorative resins
    Biophysical considerations
Dental cements
    Zinc phosphate cement
        Biophysical considerations
    Silicate cement
        Biophysical considerations
    Silicophosphate cement
Zinc oxide–eugenol cement
    Biophysical considerations
Calcium hydroxide
    Biophysical considerations
Resin cements
    Biophysical considerations
Cavity liners
    Biophysical considerations
Plastic implant materials
    Tissue adhesives
    Biostable polymers
    Synthetic cartilage
    Biodegradable polymers
Conclusion

## INTRODUCTION

It has been estimated that somewhere between 70 and 80 percent of all dental health service procedures involve the use of materials. When enamel and dentin are destroyed by caries, or when a tooth and its surrounding structures are lost through periodontal involvement, the remaining hard and soft tissues are replaced by materials that are intended to restore both function and esthetics. To ensure clinical success one should understand and consider the biologic and physical properties of materials as well as the manipulative effects of these properties. Improper selection and use of materials lead to clinical failures, early replacement of restorations, and refabrication of prosthetic appliances, not to mention the additional patient discomfort and expense. The role of materials in prevention, then, presents two facets; (1) materials restore function and esthetics and arrest further tissue destruction, and (2) when properly used, materials conserve the nation's critical dental manpower.

Investigations by Armstrong and Simon[1] and later by Phillips and others,[2] using radioactive isotopes as tracers, showed conclusively that all restorative materials leak at the margins. While some materials displayed more leakage than others, none of them was able to seal the tooth. These findings catalyzed investigators of dental materials to search for an ideal restorative material. The material being sought is one which, in addition to possessing a coefficient of thermal expansion equal to that of hard tooth structure, will withstand the stresses of mastication, be insoluble in the oral fluids, and have excellent color stability. It should also form a chemical

---

*The opinions expressed in this chapter are those of the author and do not reflect the policies of the Department of the Army or the Army Medical Department. This chapter was originally prepared by the late Colonel Peter M. Margetis, U. S. Army Dental Corps.

union with hydroxyapatite, or at least form some permanent bond with the hard tissues of the tooth. To date, although excellent progress has been made, efforts to develop such a material have not been successful.

The purpose of this chapter is to review a few of the basic concepts in the manipulation of the most commonly used materials, to include some recent advances in research, and to note pertinent relationships between materials and tissue receptivity.

## AMALGAM

Amalgam is the most widely used material in restorative dentistry. This is true partly because of its ease of manipulation, excellent adaptation to cavity walls, and adequate strength to withstand the stresses of mastication when placed in a properly prepared cavity. However, any deviation from accepted manipulative technics will result in clinical failure. Healey and Phillips[3] have shown that 40 percent of all such failures can be attributed to improper manipulation of the alloy.

A finished amalgam is a cored structure in which the core, primarily a silver-tin alloy, is strong and dimensionally stable, while the matrix, consisting of primarily mercury-tin and mercury-silver complexes, is weak and dimensionally unstable. Most acceptable amalgams are composed of approximately 50 percent alloy and 50 percent mercury, and any amalgam restoration with a final mercury content above 55 percent will show a significant loss in strength. By adhering to the proper mercury-alloy ratio, proper trituration, and good condensation technics, the mercury content in the finished restoration can be held at 45 to 50 percent. Fine-grained alloys seem to be preferred because they set faster, resulting in a higher compressive strength

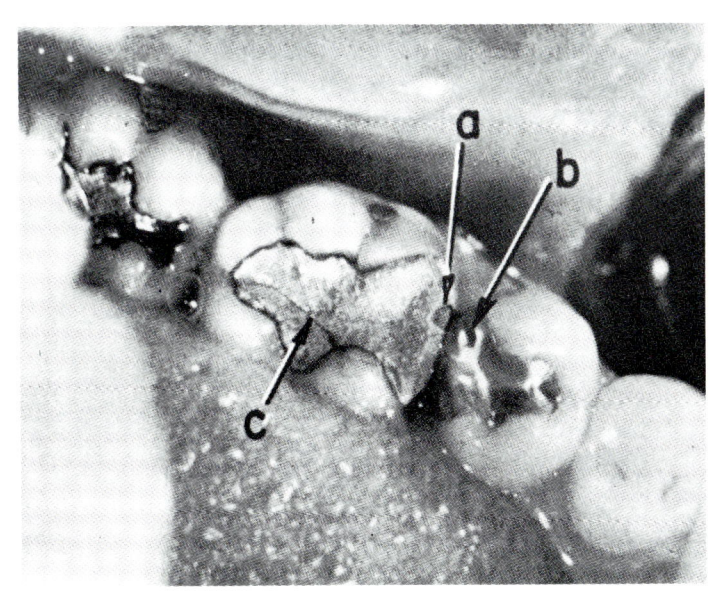

Fig. 17-1. Amalgam restorations after 1 year in mouth. Condition of restoration in first molar with high mercury content is in contrast to that in second bicuspid with a lower mercury content. Facets **a** and **b** show the effect of traumatic occlusion. A fracture is seen at **c**. (From Skinner, E. W., and Phillips, R. W.: The science of dental materials, ed. 5, Philadelphia, 1960, W. B. Saunders Co.)

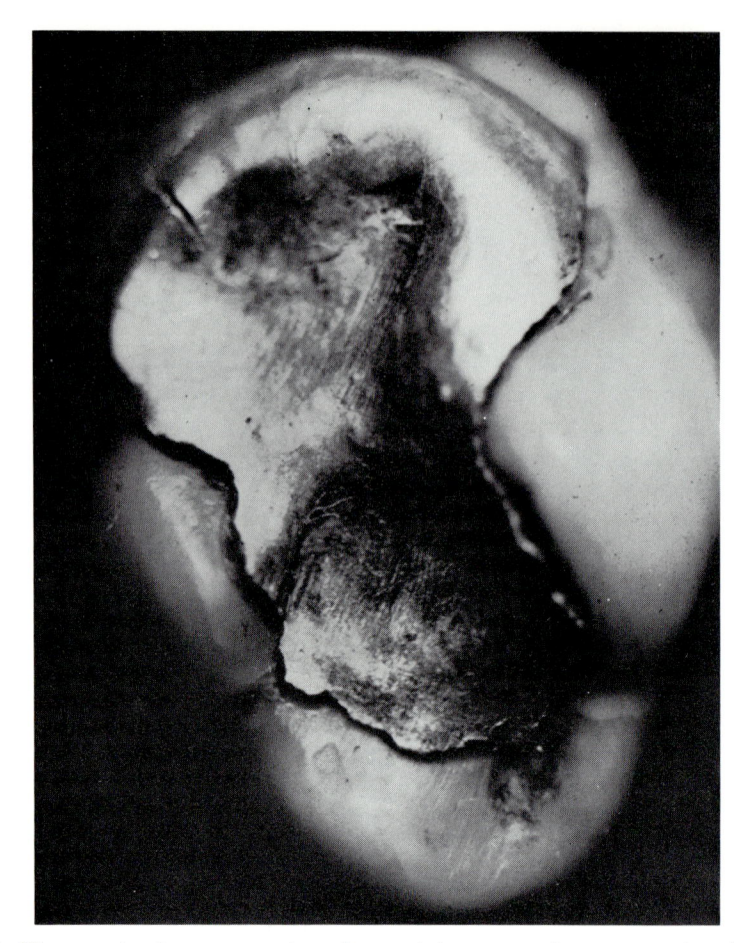

**372** *Improving dental practice through preventive measures*

**Fig. 17-2.** Photograph of an extracted tooth containing an amalgam restoration that has extruded from the cavity. One of the causes of such excessive expansion is contamination of a zinc-containing amalgam with moisture during mixing or during condensing in the cavity. (From Paffenbarger, G. C.: Ohio D. J. **33:**218, 1959.)

at the end of their first critical hour of life. Multiple mixes are mandatory for larger restorations. Leaving the triturated amalgam on the bracket table from 4 to 5 minutes before condensation will increase the final mercury content of the restoration up to 3 percent. Under no circumstances should fresh mercury be added to an already amalgamated alloy; such a practice will result in a marked loss in strength. The influence of the final mercury content in amalgam restorations is shown in Fig. 17-1. Proper condensing pressure is important for the removal of excess mercury and therefore for maximum strength and dimensional stability of the finished restoration. The Eames technic,[4] which utilizes approximately a 1:1 ratio of mercury to alloy, obviates the need to express excess mercury and renders the condensation less critical in that, ostensibly, excess mercury is not removed during condensation. The use of silver alloy in pellet form is widely used and is an aid in correct proportioning of alloy and mercury.

Contamination of the triturated amalgam by moisture either from mulling the

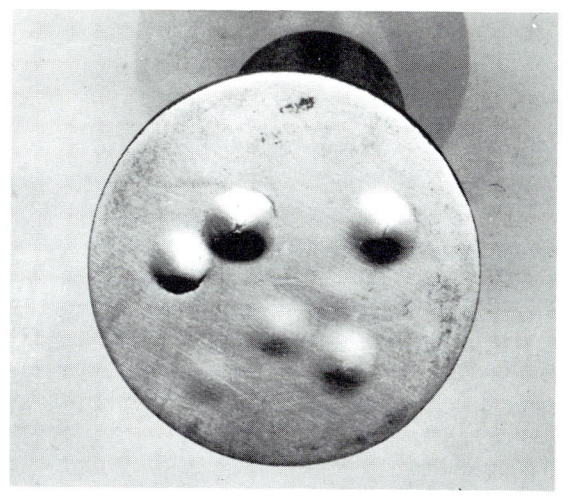

Fig. 17-3. Blisters formed on the surface of an amalgam disc, caused by escaping hydrogen as a result of moisture contamination. (Courtesy W. T. Sweeney, National Bureau of Standards.)

amalgam mass in the hand or from saliva accounts for many amalgam failures. Moisture contamination of a zinc containing amalgam results in delayed expansion of several hundred microns per centimeter and in blister formation because of evolution of hydrogen through the amalgam surface. Excessive expansion of an amalgam because of moisture contamination is shown in Fig. 17-2. Notice that the restoration has literally mushroomed from the prepared cavity. The formation of blisters is illustrated in Fig. 17-3. Protection of the amalgam from moisture contamination during condensation can best be accomplished by the use of a rubber dam.

Delayed expansion from moisture contamination is not as readily observed in amalgams made from nonzinc alloys. However, there is some indication that amalgams made from zinc-free alloys develop marginal failure more frequently than those containing zinc.

Although overtrituration can conceivably cause contraction of an amalgam during settling, far greater damage ensues if the amalgam is undertriturated. Hand and mechanical trituration have often been compared, and it has been shown that an acceptable restoration can be made using either method. However, mechanical trituration generally ensures a more homogeneous mix, and the short time required for trituration makes this method more desirable when multiple mixes are being utilized.

Corrosion resistance of a well-triturated, well-condensed, and properly finished silver amalgam restoration is quite good. However, even well-made amalgam restorations do tarnish and corrode in some mouths. The finishing of an amalgam restoration should not be attempted for a minimum of 24 hours following insertion and preferably not for several days. Such delay allows the amalgam to set completely and to reach maximum strength. In this manner the chances of removing particles of alloy from the matrix during polishing are minimized. Amalgams made with spherical alloy particles have recently become available commercially. It appears that such

**374** *Improving dental practice through preventive measures*

amalgams possess excellent physical properties and can adapt well to cavity walls with ony moderate packing pressures.

**Biophysical considerations**

It has been well demonstrated that a freshly placed amalgam exhibits marginal leakage with penetration of radioisotopes, not only into the dentin but also into the amalgam restoration proper. Mercury can also penetrate the dentinal tubules, causing a discoloration of the dentin. As the amalgam ages 6 months and longer, resistance to penetration increases. It has been postulated that this is probably caused by the marginal sealing effect of the corrosion products of amalgam. To protect the pulp from both thermal and galvanic shock, even if the cavity is only of moderate depth, the pulpal wall should be covered with a suitable liner or cement base prior to the insertion of the amalgam. Early marginal leakage can be drastically reduced by the use of varnish that extends to cavosurface borders of the preparation.

The toxicity of mercury has long been questioned, and although penetration into the dentinal tubules as well as into the pulp has been reported, it is doubtful that it would have any adverse systemic effect. Allergic responses to mercury, although not common, have been reported, and even a case of allergic reaction of the tongue caused by the silver in amalgam restorations was reported by Hitchen and Hall.[5] Zander[6] reported that gingival irritation from amalgam produced a chronic inflammation, while App reported that "Seven days after the insertion of amalgam restorations budding proliferation of the epithelium was evident in the subjacent connective tissue. A dense cellular infiltration extended from the oral epithelium to half the length of the dental epithelium. Hydropic degeneration though present in the surface dental epithelium was less than that found in silicate restorations."[7]

Waerhaug and Zander[8] have questioned the wisdom of extending restorations into the gingival sulcus.

## PURE GOLD RESTORATIONS

A gold foil restoration properly inserted into a carefully selected tooth is considered by many dentists as the finest type of restoration in clinical practice. Pure gold as a restorative material has been available in two forms—gold foil, both cohesive and noncohesive, and crystalline or mat gold. Recently, Baum[9] has introduced a third type—powdered or sintered gold. Although not widely used as yet, powdered gold appears to offer the following advantages: it has a better initial spreading quality than gold foil, which tends to draw and centralize toward the point of condensation; it has greater mass per unit volume than either foil or mat gold; and the greater density of the gold powder speeds condensation.

## GOLD ALLOY CASTINGS

Because of the many materials and factors involved in the making of a gold inlay or a crown, it is not possible to refer to the casting of either as a precision technique. However, meticulous attention to the impression and to the preparation of the die (if the indirect technic is used) coupled with an understanding of the physical interactions between the pattern and the investment (such as temperature rise and setting expansion forces) will result in a clinically acceptable casting.

The advantages and disadvantages of both the indirect and direct technics are well covered in the literature and therefore will not be discussed here.

Impression compound, still used by some dentists, does not reproduce surface detail with the same degree of accuracy as do some of the hydrocolloid and elastomeric impression materials. In addition, the thermal contraction of compound when cooled from its solidification to room temperature can be a source of inaccuracy in the die and ultimately in the final casting. Hydrocolloids and elastomeric impression materials, principally agar-base hydrocolloids and mercaptan rubbers, are generally preferred; however, alginate hydrocolloids and silicone rubbers can be used. The hydrocolloids retard the setting of gypsum products. To overcome this effect accelerators such as potassium sulfate are often added to the impression materials. With compatible die materials a better surface and perhaps greater reproduction of detail can be obtained when agar-base hydrocolloids are used, but distortions during gelation, removal, and stress relaxation contribute to dimensional instability of all hydrocolloid materials. It is therefore important that meticulous attention to details be exercised in the use of hydrocolloids. A stone surface produced by an incompatible reversible hydrocolloid impression material is shown in Fig. 17-4.

The mercaptan and silicone-rubber impression materials are widely used for single and multiple impressions of teeth that have been prepared for gold alloy castings. Care must be taken during the mixing of the rubber impression materials to ensure that the catalyst has been evenly distributed throughout the mass since an uneven or incomplete curing will result in a distorted impression. To alter the setting time of a mercaptan rubber impression material, add a drop of water to reduce the setting time and a drop of oleic acid to retard the set. The setting time of the silicone-base material can be altered by changing the amount of catalyst used.

Care must be taken not to remove the rubber impression too soon since the ma-

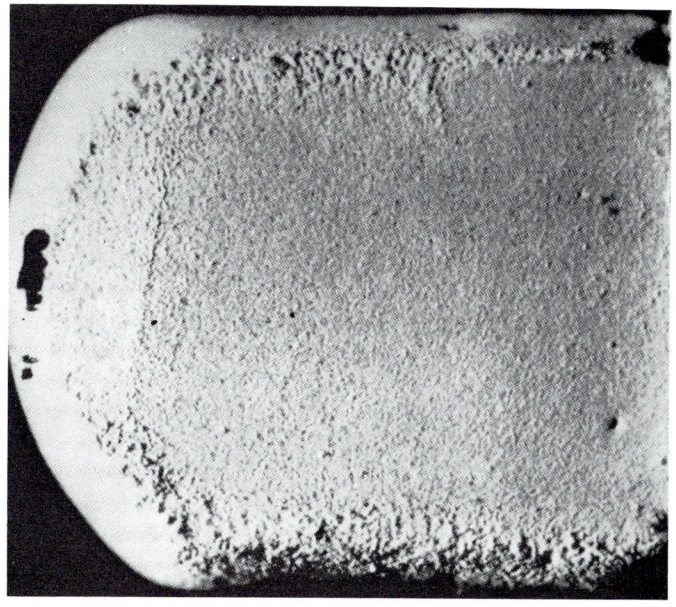

Fig. 17-4. Stone surface obtained after the stone had set in contact with the surface of a reversible hydrocolloid impression material. (From Skinner, E. W., and Phillips, R. W.: The science of dental materials, ed. 5, Philadelphia, 1960, W. B. Saunders Co.)

**376** *Improving dental practice through preventive measures*

terial may still lack the necessary strength and elasticity to eliminate or minimize distortion. By the same token, if insertion is unduly delayed, the curing will have progressed to a point where stress release upon removal of the tray or band will result in an undersized impression and die. Although excellent results can be obtained with both types of rubber impression materials, there are possibly some advantages that each material possesses over the other.

The surface reproduction or the registration of detail by both materials is excellent, although the mercaptan rubbers probably excel over the silicone materials in accuracy and dimensional stability. With the hydrocolloids as well as with the rubber-base materials, the die should be poured as soon as possible to ensure maximum accuracy. In pouring a die in an alginate impression, excessive vibration should be avoided to prevent stress release that may distort the impression and result in an inaccurate die or cast. The effect on the fit of a master casting on stone dies constructed from a polysulfide rubber impression of a master steel die at varying periods of removal of the impression is shown in Fig. 17-5.

The most common die materials in current use are improved stone (densite) and

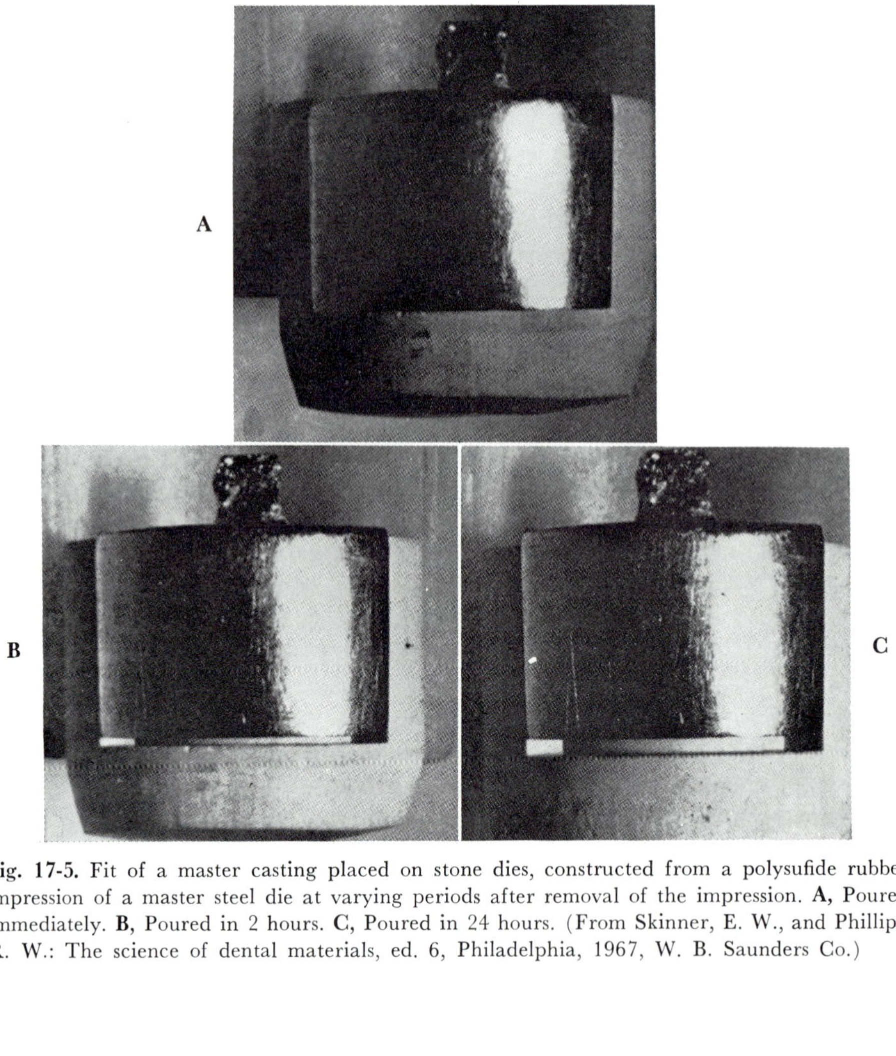

**Fig. 17-5.** Fit of a master casting placed on stone dies, constructed from a polysufide rubber impression of a master steel die at varying periods after removal of the impression. **A,** Poured immediately. **B,** Poured in 2 hours. **C,** Poured in 24 hours. (From Skinner, E. W., and Phillips, R. W.: The science of dental materials, ed. 6, Philadelphia, 1967, W. B. Saunders Co.)

resin, usually of the acrylic and the epoxy types. These newer products have in most instances replaced amalgam and silicophosphate cement in the preparation of dies.

The efficacy of silver-plating rubber-base impressions is doubtful since significant dimensional changes can take place in the impression during the 12 to 15 hours of required plating time. A die poured as soon as the impression is made will generally be more accurate than a die poured into an electroplated rubber impression. Improved stone, properly mixed, gives an excellent surface with sufficient hardness to allow the construction of wax patterns. A separating medium must be used to prevent the wax from adhering to the stone. Care should be taken in selecting the separating medium to avoid the accidental use of a wax solvent.

Within the past few years resin die materials for use with rubber impressions appear to be gaining in popularity in spite of the fact that there is some difficulty in their use. Because of their viscosity, the resins do not flow as readily into all recesses of a complex impression as does stone. Resin dies provide a hard surface and greater strength than do stone dies. Powdered aluminum has been added to epoxy resin in an effort to increase the hardness and abrasion resistance of the dies; however, sufficient data regarding metal-filled epoxy resin for die construction are not available at this time.

Wax is probably the most dimensionally unstable material used in clinical dentistry. There are two types of inlay wax: Type I wax, for use in the direct technic; and Type II wax, for use in the indirect technic. One of the most common sources of pattern distortion relates to the method by which the wax has been softened and the pattern cooled. The thermal conductivity of wax is low. Therefore adequate time at a constant temperature is needed for uniform softening or hardening. Many dentists soften inlay wax by heating the wax over an open flame. The practice should not be encouraged; if it is employed, however, the stick of wax should be held above the flame and rotated frequently so as not to allow the wax to melt. The use of a water bath for softening wax is also to be discouraged because the wax tends to become somewhat "granular" and loses its handling qualities. To minimize dimensional changes wax should be softened with dry heat at a constant temperature and inserted into the prepared cavity at as high a temperature as possible and under pressure. In the indirect technic the wax may either be melted and added in small increments or the plastic mass of wax can be compressed against the die and held under pressure until it hardens. Carving should be accomplished with a warm instrument to prevent the "drawing" of the wax and thereby introducing stresses that will affect the accuracy of the inlay. The addition of wax to the pattern before or after carving is not recommended. Such additions cause unequal rates of cooling in the solidified and melted wax and introduce stresses in the pattern. The dimensional changes caused by subsequent stress release will result in a loss of accuracy in the fit of the final product. In either the direct or indirect technic extreme care must be taken in spruing and in removing the pattern from the mouth or die. Single or double sprues may be employed, depending on the complexity of the pattern. Often in the direct technic the pattern is removed from the mouth and then sprued. Poor surface adaptation can occur when a pattern is constructed on a metal die because of the different cooling rates in the wax immediately next to the die and the wax on the surface of the pattern. The problem can be minimized by warming the die before construction of the wax pattern. Once sprued and removed, the wax pattern should not be touched and should be stored in an area protected from temperature changes.

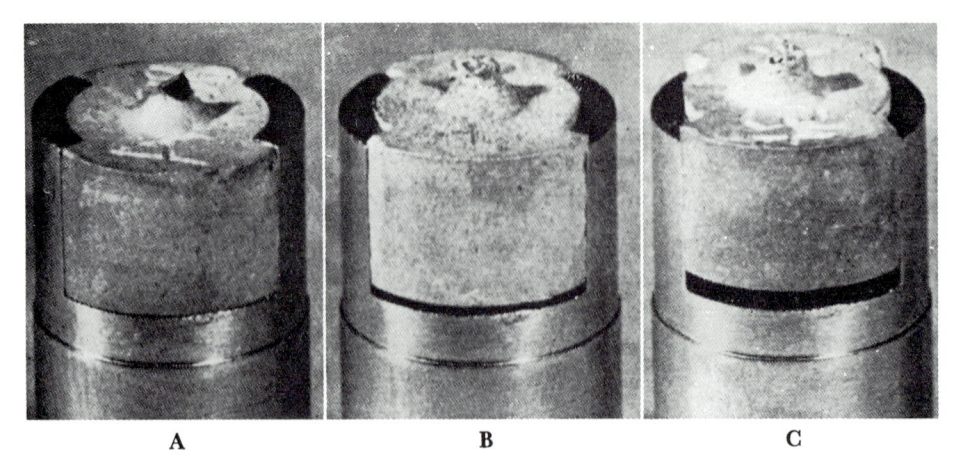

**Fig. 17-6.** Castings made from patterns prepared with melted wax, pooled under pressure. **A,** Pattern invested immediately. **B,** Pattern stored for 2 hours before investing. **C,** Pattern stored for 12 hours before investing. (From Skinner, E. W., and Phillips, R. W.: The science of dental materials, ed. 6, Philadelphia, 1967, W. B. Saunders Co.)

The pattern should be invested within 15 minutes and should not remain uninvested for over 30 minutes. The fit of castings made from melted wax, cooled under pressure, and invested after varying time intervals is shown in Fig. 17-6.

As indicated previously, the forces of the setting expansion of the investment on the wax pattern play an important role in the fit of the cast gold restoration. Casting investments for small gold castings are usually referred to as gypsum-bonded investments and are composed of three types of ingredients—refractory material, binder, and modifiers. The refractory material provides resistance to temperature and accounts in part for the expansion of the investment. The refractory material can be one of the allotropic forms of silicon dioxide such as quartz, cristobalite, tridymite, or a mixture of these forms. The binder holds the investment together and is a form of calcium sulfate hemihydrate. Modifiers include coloring agents, graphite or copper to prevent oxidation of the metal, potassium sulfate as an accelerator, borax as a retarder, and sodium chloride to decrease the shrinkage of the gypsum on heating. The role of investment is to compensate for the shrinkage of the wax and the gold by expanding the mold. The mold is expanded by a combination of normal setting and hygroscopic expansions or by thermal changes.

The American Dental Association Specification No. 2 for casting investment for dental gold alloys lists two types of investment for gold inlays—Type I (thermal), and Type II (hygroscopic). Type I relies mainly on thermal expansion of the mold after the investment is set. Since cristobalite produces a greater total thermal expansion than does quartz, cristobalite is the form of silica generally used in Type I investment. The Type II investment relies primarily on hygroscopic expansion, and quartz is the refractory generally used in this type of investment. Both investments contain calcium sulfate hemihydrate as the binder. Since alpha hemihydrate produces the higher hygroscopic expansion, either hydrocal or densite is used in Type II investments.

With both technics the initial step of investing the pattern is the same. If the thermal expansion technic is used, the investment is allowed to set without further

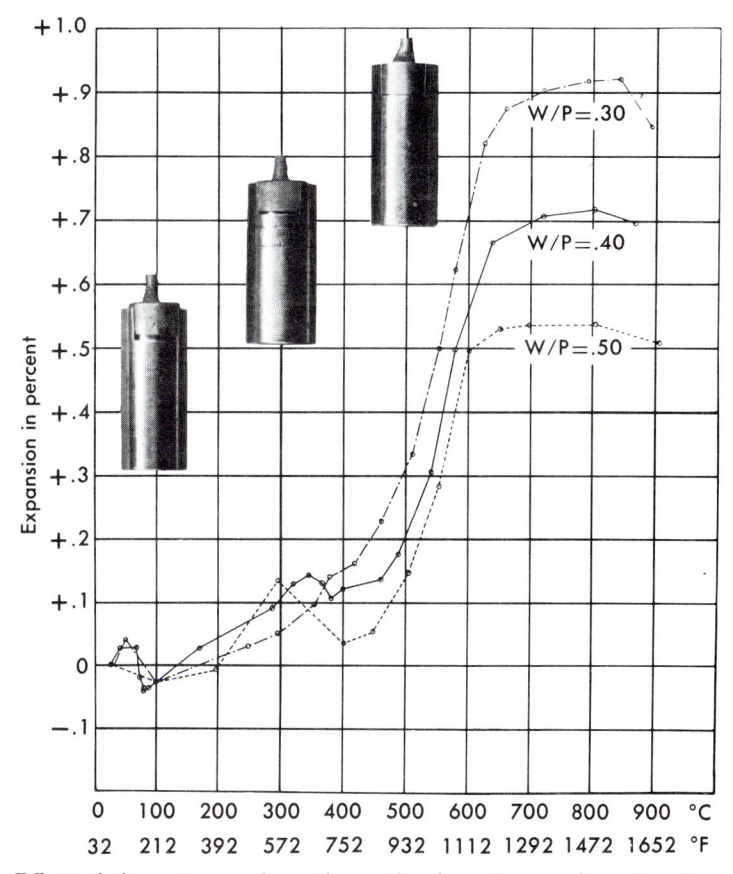

Fig. 17-7. Effect of the water-powder ratio on the thermal expansion of an investment containing 20 percent plaster of Paris and 80 percent quartz. (From Volland, R. H., and Paffenbarger, G. C.: J.A.D.A. 19:185, 1932.)

addition of water. The ring is then placed in an oven; the heat drives off the water, burns out the wax, and expands the mold. The casting is then made at a mold temperature of approximately 1300° F. The effect of the water-powder ratio on the thermal expansion of an investment is shown in Fig. 17-7. If the hygroscopic technic is used, one has the choice of the water bath immersion technic or the controlled water added technic. In the former the ring is immersed in a warm water bath at approximately 98° F., where it remains during setting. In the latter technic, after the pattern has been invested, a specific amount of water is added on the top of the investment. When hygroscopic expansion is used the wax is eliminated and the casting made at an approximate mold temperature of 900° F. In either the thermal or hygroscopic technic dimensional changes in the wax pattern occur during the setting of the investment. A typical pattern of distortion is shown in Fig. 17-8. One should distinguish between dimensional change and distortion of wax patterns. Dimensional change implies changes that are uniform in all directions and that affect the size but not the shape of the wax pattern, whereas distortion implies unequal changes that warp or distort the pattern.

The setting forces can be influenced by the water-powder ratio of the invest-

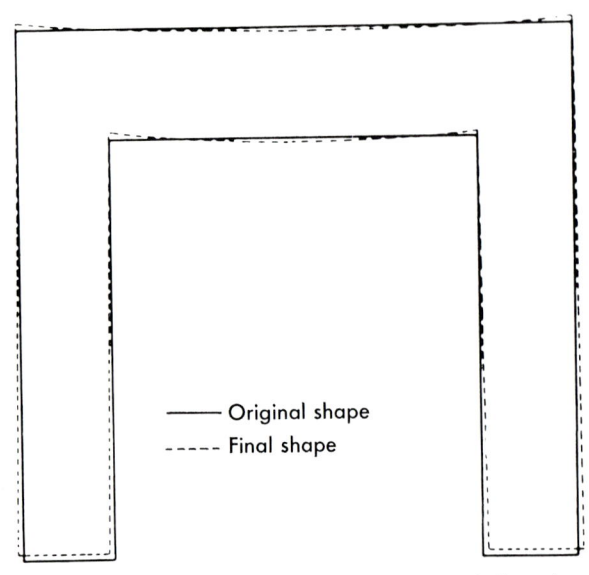

**Fig. 17-8.** Diagrammatic representation of the typical pattern of distortion. (From Mumford, G., and Phillips, R. W.: J. Dent. Res. 37:351, 1958. Reprinted by permission.)

ment, by the method of spatulation, by the type of investment ring used (such as metal or rubber), and by the position of the asbestos liner in the metal ring. Mold expansion by the thermal technic is influenced by the water-powder ratio as well as the type and amount of silica present in the investment. Setting expansion is affected by water-powder ratio, by spatulation rate and time, and by the water present in the wet asbestos liner. It is important to note that dimensional changes of the setting investment vary from place to place within the ring, from the top third to the middle and bottom thirds, and from the center to the sides of the ring. What clinical effects these often unpredictable changes have on the accuracy of the final gold casting have not been definitely established. However, should clinical failure ever be attributed to distortion by investment setting forces, one would think in terms of a casting investment with little or no setting expansion. Such an investment would rely solely on the thermal expansion of the mold.

The final step in the fabrication of gold inlays and crowns and other small dental gold alloy restorations or fixed prostheses is the casting of the metal into the mold. Casting defects can occur which may result in clinical failure. Casting defects can be classified in three main categories: (1) external defects, (2) internal defects, and (3) incomplete castings. The external defects can be further classified as local or general surface defects. The causes of the three main types of casting defects are many, but only the more common will be considered here. Nodules, or bubbles, of gold are caused by air bubbles in the investment and can be minimized by vacuum investing. This type of defect can usually be corrected when it appears on the surface of a casting. Removal of a bubble from a margin, however, usually violates the integrity of the margin and is not indicated. Fins or fin-like extensions on the surface of a casting can be caused by cracks in the investment from rapid heating of a thermal expansion investment. Back pressure porosity, one of the more common types seen in castings, may be both external and internal. This type of porosity is

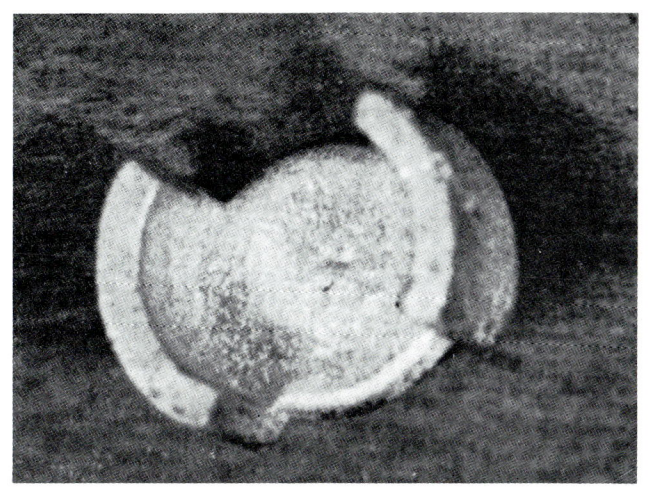

# The role of dental materials in preventive dentistry 381

**Fig. 17-9.** Rounded incomplete margins caused by insufficient casting pressure. (From Skinner, E. W., and Phillips, R. W.: The science of dental materials, ed. 5, Philadelphia, 1960, W. B. Saunders Co.)

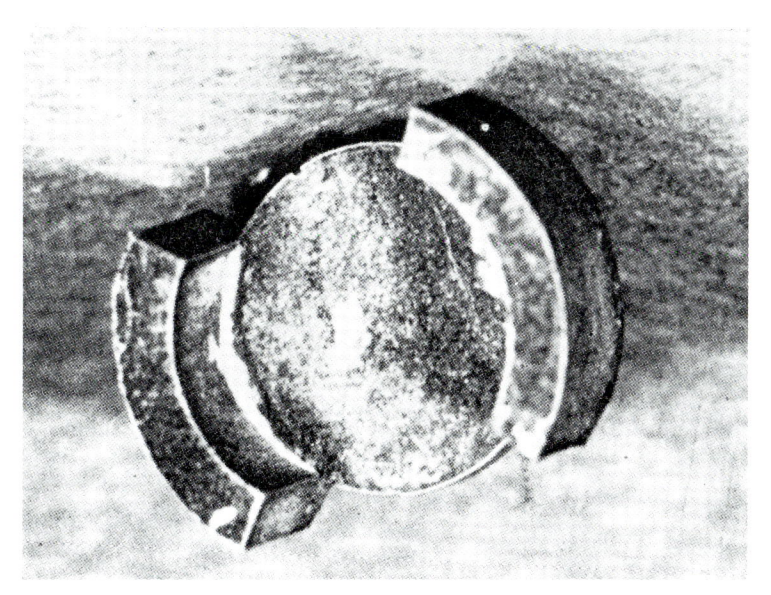

**Fig. 17-10.** A black-coated casting caused by either sulfur contamination or oxidation during melting. (From Skinner, E. W., and Phillips, R. W.: The science of dental materials, ed. 5, Philadelphia, 1960, W. B. Saunders Co.)

generally caused by an incomplete egress of gases from the investment, particularly the mold areas. Internal porosity, generally near the sprue, can occur when the sprue is too long or too thin and freezes before the casting. This is called shrinkage porosity. Another type of porosity, usually internal, is caused by occluded gases. Oxygen dissolved by some of the constituents of the gold alloy during the molten state is given off and trapped during solidification of the alloy. When the blow pipe is used, care should be taken to melt the metal with the reducing portion of the flame. Too low casting pressure can produce rounded and incomplete margins, as shown in Fig. 17-9. Generalized surface defects such as a blackening and roughening of the entire surface can be caused by prolonged heating of the mold at the burnout temperature. Prolonged heat soaking results in disintegration of the investment and sulfur contamination of the surface of the inlay. A black casting caused by sulfur contamination or oxidation during melting is shown in Fig. 17-10. In many instances the discoloration cannot be removed by pickling. Incomplete castings can be caused by casting into a mold that is too cold. As a result the metal will freeze before the mold is filled. Other causes for incomplete castings include low casting pressure and incomplete wax elimination from the mold. As mentioned earlier, by careful attention to each phase in the fabrication of small cast gold restorations successful castings can be made. Where hard metal is placed in apposition to the hard tooth structure, the margin of error, if one is to exist, must be small. Whereas with denture bases the resilient mucosa can to a degree accommodate dimensional changes in the denture, the hard structures of the tooth cannot accommodate discrepancies in the cast restoration. The weakest link perhaps in the success of a cast gold restoration is the solubility of the cement in the fluids of the oral cavity. Therefore the more accurate the fit of the inlay, the smaller will be the cement line exposed to the oral fluids.

**Biophysical considerations**

Unlike the amalgam restoration, gold appears to be tolerated by the soft tissues and produces no chronic inflammation in the adjacent gingival tissues. However, pulp injury, particularly in deeper cavity preparations, may result from the forces generated by malletting while seating the inlay during cementation. Another source

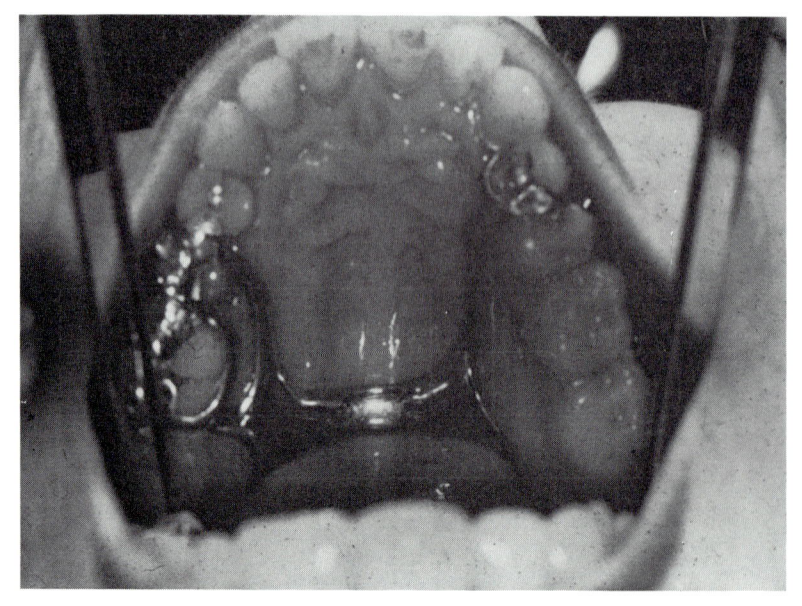

Fig. 17-11. Patient allergic to gold with gold alloy partial denture in place. (From Bernier, J. L.: Management of oral disease, ed. 2, St. Louis, 1959, The C. V. Mosby Co.)

of pulpal irritation stems from the fact that a thin mix of zinc phosphate cement is generally used for cementation. The excess acid not only increases pulpal irritation, but also increases the solubility of the cement. Dissolution of the cement may in turn expose the marginal areas to recurrent decay. The gold inlay, regardless of the cementing medium, exhibits marginal leakage that seems to increase slightly with the passage of time. Since varnishes reduce marginal leakage as well as acid penetration, a cavity varnish should be applied to the preparation especially before cementation of a larger casting.

Gold foil restorations, like cast gold, possess high biologic receptivity; like other restorative materials, however, they exhibit marginal percolation when subjected to thermal changes. The malleting of a gold foil restoration can cause pulpal irritation. The severity of such irritation is partly related to the depth of the cavity. Because of the large pulps and thin layers of dentin in children's teeth, gold foil restorations for children are contraindicated in most instances. Allergic responses to gold are uncommon but have been reported.

An allergic response to a gold partial denture frame is shown in Figs. 17-11 and 17-12. When the gold partial denture frame was removed the symptoms regressed. Upon reinsertion of the appliance symptoms reappeared within several days. A new appliance was fabricated with a chromium-cobalt alloy that was well tolerated by the patient.

**RESTORATIVE RESINS**

Restorative resins were introduced shortly after the close of World War II and were greeted by the profession with great enthusiasm. However, the enthusiasm

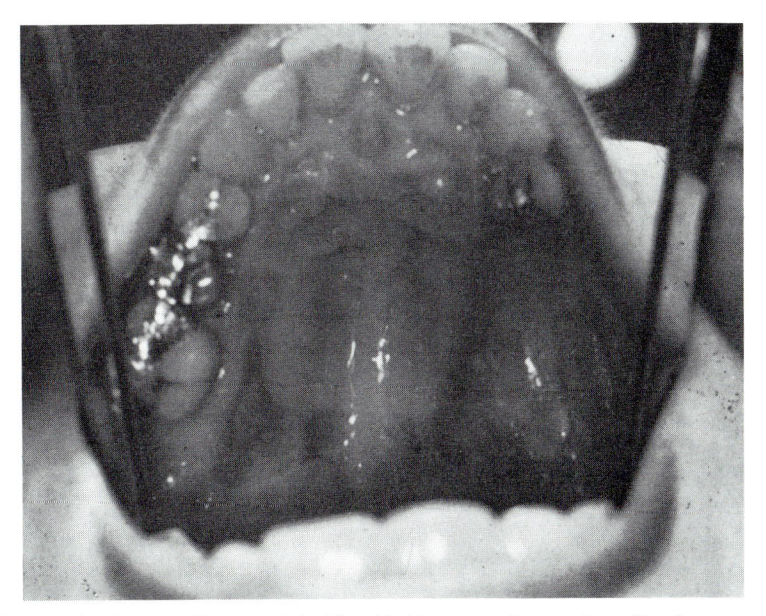

Fig. 17-12. Partial denture illustrated in Fig. 17-11 removed, exposing allergic response to the gold alloy partial denture frame. Notice that the allergic reaction was elicited only in those areas where the tissue was in intimate contact with gold alloy. (From Bernier, J. L.: Management of oral disease, ed. 2, St. Louis, 1959, The C. V. Mosby Co.)

dwindled rapidly when clinical failures with the early autopolymerizing restorative resins were reported. These initial failures were probably caused not only by the materials but also by the dentist's lack of knowledge and experience in the use of restorative resins. Although the current restorative resins have been vastly improved and their manipulative technics modified, they remain perhaps the most controversial restorative materials in use today.

The powder, or polymer, of these materials is poly(methyl methacrylate) and generally contains benzoyl peroxide as the initiator and pigments, as well as opacifiers, for proper shading. The liquid is methyl methacrylate monomer and usually contains hydroquinone as an inhibitor and dimethyl-*p*-toluidine as an accelerator. Some of the resins contain small amounts of a cross-linking agent.

The polymer and monomer are mixed according to the technic for insertion preferred by the dentist. There are two main technics. The first is the pressure, or compression, technic. In this method the powder and liquid may be mixed on a slab. To minimize entrapment of air, it is preferable to add the polymer to the monomer in a dappen dish without mixing. The dish is tapped on the table several times to ensure complete saturation of the polymer. The material is then carried to the cavity. A matrix band or strip is secured tightly in position until polymerization is completed.

The second is the nonpressure technic. In this method the restoration is formed by placing monomer-polymer mixtures in small successive increments into the prepared cavity with the tip of a fine sable brush. Two dappen dishes are utilized, one containing the monomer and the other containing the polymer. The cavity is painted with the monomer. The tip of the brush is first dipped in the monomer and then brought in light touch with the powder. The small globule, or bead, of monomer-polymer mixture is then carried to and deposited in the cavity. This cycle is repeated until the cavity is properly filled, preferably somewhat overfilled. At this stage tinfoil or some other inert material is placed over the restoration to prevent evaporation of the monomer and is left there until polymerization is complete.

Immediately after hardening, the restoration should be only prefinished with sharp instruments. Final finishing is accomplished approximately 24 hours later. Although both technics can yield good results, the brush method is perhaps less technic-sensitive and appears to result in better adaptation to the cavity walls. Regardless of the technic used, shrinkage occurs during polymerization to a greater degree than that exhibited by silicate cements.

Restorative resins have several highly desirable properties. They possess high esthetic qualities, have a low thermal conductivity, and are insoluble in the fluids of the mouth. On the other hand, they have low resistance to abrasion, low compressive strength, and a high coefficient of thermal expansion. The development of an ideal restorative material, as mentioned in the introduction to this chapter, is the object of many investigations today. Most investigators are using synthetic resins as a starting point. Many avenues have been explored in order to obtain a more permanent mechanical or chemical bonding, or adhesion, between the restoration and hard tooth structure. Effects of surface active comonomers and other tooth structure surface conditioners have been studied. A reduction of the high coefficient of thermal expansion has been accomplished by the use of mineral fillers such as fused silica.

**Biophysical considerations**

There have been conflicting reports in the literature concerning the effect of restorative resins on the pulp. Some investigators maintain that pulp response is rather mild and usually reversible. Others cite severe inflammatory changes with ensuing abscess formation and total pulp necrosis. Radioactive tracer studies show that restorative resins, along with other restorative materials, exhibit marginal leakage. Perhaps one of the most severe drawbacks of restorative resins is their high coefficient of thermal expansion, which accounts for a high degree of marginal percolation. It is perhaps through this route that mouth fluids, microorganisms, and debris gain access to the cavity and cause pulpal irritation and recurrent caries.

Resin materials do not possess bactericidal properties; attempts to overcome this deficiency by the addition of antibacterial agents have not been successful. The addition of fluorides has not been successful either. The materials as they exist today should only be considered for use in limited stress or nonstress areas where esthetics is a prime consideration.

## DENTAL CEMENTS

Dental cements have a wide application in the practice of dentistry. It has been estimated that between 50 and 60 percent of all restorations in one way or another involve their use and that 10 percent of all permanent restorations are cement. In general, the cements lack strength, shrink on setting, and are soluble in the fluids of the oral cavity. Many of them cause pulpal irritation. All cements have low thermal conductivity and thereby protect the pulp from thermal shock.

Cements are usually classified according to their composition and both their primary and secondary uses. Different authors have suggested various classifications. The following is a suitable classification of cements for general use: (1) restorative cements for permanent and temporary restorations; (2) cementing agents for luting cast metallic restorations; (3) insulating bases for protection against thermal, chemical, and mechanical irritation; and (4) therapeutic cements for pulp capping and obturation of root canals and for use as surgical dressings.

Because of limited space, only the most commonly used cements will be considered in this chapter.

**Zinc phosphate cement**

Zinc phosphate cement powders are chiefly composed of calcined zinc oxide and magnesium oxide in a ratio of approximately 9:1. The liquid contains approximately 50 percent phosphoric acid, 18 percent buffers, usually zinc and/or aluminum salts, and approximately 32 percent water. The liquid is hygroscopic; its container should be kept tightly stoppered, for any gain or loss of water affects the physical properties of the cement. An increase in the water content of the liquid reduces the setting time, whereas a loss of water tends to retard the set. An accelerated set will not give the dentist or the assistant sufficient time to incorporate the optimum amount of powder in a given amount of liquid. The chemical reaction between the powder and the liquid results in the formation first of a zinc acid phosphate and, later, as more powder is incorporated and the set progresses, the more stable tertiary zinc phosphate salt. The reaction is exothermic; consequently, the mixing slab should be cool. Small increments of powder should be added to the liquid with thorough spatulation over a wide area of the slab. This method helps retard the set and allows incorporation of more powder into the liquid, which improves the physical properties of the final product.

**Biophysical considerations.** Any pulpal damage that may result from zinc phosphate cement is caused by residual free phosphoric acid. The pH of the cement, particularly during its first hours, is low, with values ranging from 1.5 to 6.0. There is a divergence of opinion as to when the mix reaches neutrality; some investigators contend that neutralization is never achieved. It is obvious that the remaining thickness of dentin between the cavity and the pulp is a critical factor in regard to pulpal damage.

To improve durability of zinc phosphate cement restorations, practitioners often add amalgam alloy filings to their cement mixes. Research by Mahler and Armen[10] and by Wolcott and associates[11] substantiates the efficacy of this approach.

The addition of antibiotics to zinc phosphate cements in an effort to establish long-term bacteriostatic properties has not been fruitful. Attempts to impart anticariogenic properties to the cement by addition of fluorides have not been successful either.

Copper cements, once widely used in dentistry, particularly in pedodontics, are rapidly vanishing from the scene because of their severe pulp response. Their popularity stemmed from the belief that they possessed lasting germicidal properties, but such belief has not been substantiated.

**Silicate cement**

In spite of the fact that silicate cement is soluble, brittle, and irritating to the pulp, its superior esthetic properties and ease of manipulation have made it the material of choice for the restoration of anterior teeth in nonstress-bearing areas over a period of many years. Like other cements, silicates are supplied to the user in the form of a powder and a liquid. A typical powder consists of 40 percent silica, 30 percent alumina, 20 percent sodium or calcium fluoride, and 10 percent calcium oxide. The composition of the liquid is generally phosphoric acid 50 percent, water 40 percent, aluminum phosphate and zinc phosphate salts 10 percent. When the powder and liquid are mixed the liquid wets the powder, forming silicic acid. The set cement presents a cored structure consisting of unreacted portions of the powder particles embedded in a silicic acid gel. The unreacted (core) particles are strong, dimensionally stable, and insoluble in mouth fluids, while the gel matrix is weak, dimensionally unstable, and soluble in saliva. It is therefore obvious that a high powder-liquid ratio is mandatory if the operator expects to exploit the full capabilities of a silicate cement restoration. A silicate cement showing powder particles as the core embedded in the gel matrix is shown in Fig. 17-13.

In mixing silicate cement, a chilled slab is used to prevent premature gel formation, but it should not be chilled below the dew point because moisture condensation from the air will accelerate the set. It is also important to remember that changes in the water content of the liquid has an effect on the physical properties of the set cement. Since the hygroscopic liquid is sensitive to changes in relative humidity, the bottle should be kept tightly stoppered. The powder-liquid ratio recommended by the manufacturer should be followed. Generally, 50 percent of the powder should be incorporated into the liquid initially and mixed for 30 seconds; the remaining 50 percent is added in two or three increments during the last 30 seconds of mixing. The mixing is accomplished by using a folding motion of the

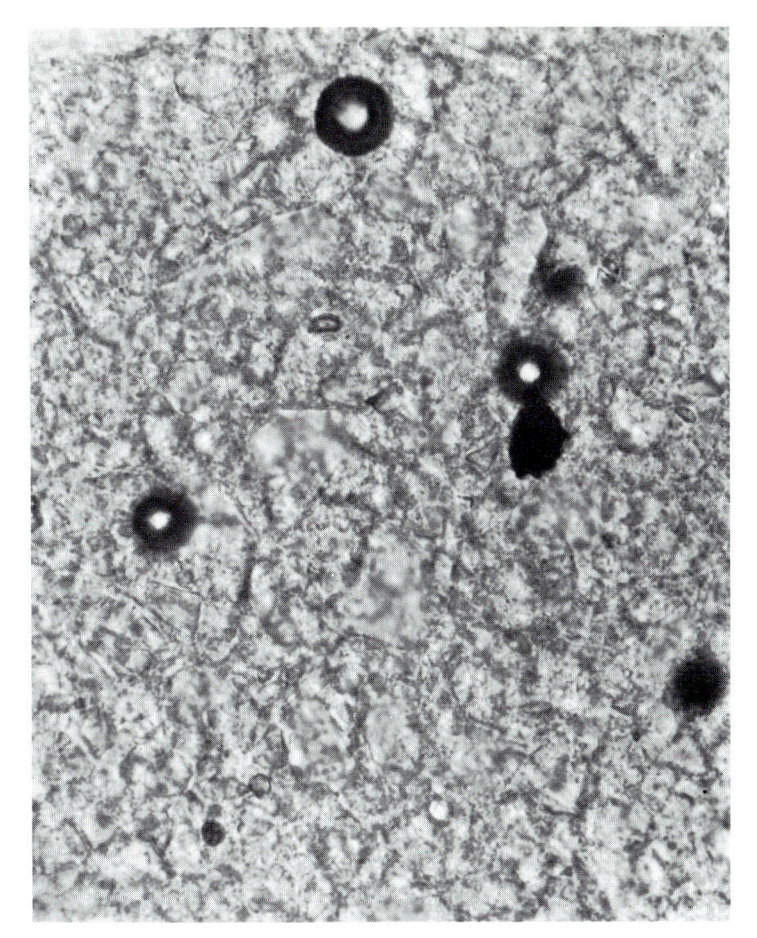

Fig. 17-13. Photomicrograph of a hardened silicate cement, showing the powder particles embedded in matrix formed by the reaction between the surface of the particles of silicate cement powder and the silicate cement liquid. The sphere-like shapes are air bubbles incorporated during spatulation of the powder-liquid mixture. (From Paffenbarger, G. C., Schoononer, I. C., and Souder, W.: J.A.D.A. 25:32, 1938.)

spatula, which can be referred to as vertical spatulation as opposed to the rotary spatulation employed in the mixing of zinc phosphate cements. In addition to employing vertical spatulation, silicate cement should be mixed on a very small area of the slab to keep from exposing a broad surface of the unset hygroscopic cement to the atmosphere. Within limits, the more powder that can be incorporated into a given amount of liquid the stronger and less soluble will be the cement. In addition, such a cement will shrink less and will have greater stain resistance. The practice of increasing the setting time by prolonged mixing or by a lowered powder-liquid ratio is contradicted. Prolonged mixing will disturb the matrix and will not only reduce the strength of the cement but will produce a restoration with poor optical properties.

The silicate cement should be inserted into the cavity immediately after mixing. This is important because the gel, which began forming when the powder and the liquid were first brought into contact, should not be disturbed by undue or delayed manipulation. Prolonged manipulation will break down the gel structure and will adversely affect the properties and the clinical course of the restoration. The freshly inserted silicate cement is held in place under pressure with a cellulose strip until the cement is set. Upon removal of the strip, the restoration is further protected from a change in water content with a coat of cocoa butter or varnish. Ideally, at this point, the patient should be returned to the waiting room for at least 1 hour before any prefinishing procedures are accomplished. The final finishing of the restoration should not be attempted for at least 48 hours, preferably not for several days.

Within the past few years methods for the mechanical mixing of silicates have been introduced. Available data do not show any significant difference in properties between mechanically mixed silicates and manually mixed silicates. To increase strength, reduce solubility; to improve abrasion resistance, silicate cement powders containing glass fibers have been formulated. To date, silicate cements containing glass fibers do not show any significant improvements over the more conventional products.

**Biophysical considerations.** Swartz and Phillips[12] showed by the use of radioisotope tracer technics that, in most instances, silicate cement restorations exhibited gross marginal leakage. It was further demonstrated that the marginal leakage did not show any significant change with the passage of time. Nevertheless, margins of silicate cement restorations show little recurrent caries. This unique anticariogenicity is caused by the fluoride uptake by enamel from the silicate cement, which reduces the solubilility of the enamel.

Zander[6] and App[7] have both reported the effect of silicate cement on the gingiva. More marked hydropic degeneration of the surface dental epithelial cells than was noted with amalgam restorations was noted with silicates 30 days after insertion. As with amalgam, chronic inflammation of the gingival sulcus epithelium was produced by silicate cement restorations.

The damaging effect of silicate on the pulp, particularly in deep cavity preparations, is well documented in the literature. Chronic inflammation may persist for periods of up to a year with abscess formation and ultimate pulp necrosis. As with zinc phosphate, the severity of the inflammatory response is related to cavity depth. The acid content of the silicic acid gel formed during the setting of silicate cements is probably the cause of pulpal irritation. A varnish, liner, and/or base should be used under silicate cement restorations for maximum pulp protection. Since varnishes may impede fluoride uptake by enamel, they should be applied to the dentin only.

### Silicophosphate cement

Silicophosphate cement, also referred to as zinc silicate and zinc silicophosphate cement, is a hybrid material in that its powder is a mixture of zinc oxide, magnesium oxide, and silicate cement powders. The liquid is essentially the same as for silicate cement. The silicophosphates therefore combine the properties of silicate and zinc phosphate cements. Some dentists use silicophosphates for permanent cementation of jacket crowns. The cements have also been used as die materials and as temporary restorations. The fluoride of their silicate component offers protection to the adjacent tooth structure by decreasing the solubility of enamel. Since the silicophosphate cement powder is predominantly silicate, the cement is mixed and handled in the manner described for silicate cement.

## Zinc oxide–eugenol cement

Zinc oxide–eugenol cements were introduced late in the nineteenth century and have been continually improved during the intervening years. In the beginning, zinc oxide–eugenol cements were used solely for temporary restorations. At the present time they are additionally used in temporary and permanent cementation of crowns and bridges, as root canal sealers, as tissue packs in periodontal surgery and in pulp capping, and as bases under permanent restorations. A typical commercial zinc oxide–eugenol cement powder is composed of nearly 70 percent zinc oxide, 29 percent rosin, and small amounts of zinc acetate and/or zinc stearate. The rosin improves the mixing properties of the cement, and zinc salts act as accelerators. The liquid consists of approximately 85 percent eugenol and 15 percent olive oil. The olive oil aids mixing and reduces any burning sensation caused by the eugenol. The setting of zinc oxide–eugenol, as shown by Copeland and associates,[13] is a result of both chemical and physical processes. The zinc oxide and eugenol react chemically to form a chelate compound, zinc eugenolate. The zinc eugenolate crystals then form a matrix to which unreacted eugenol is adsorbed, while the unreacted zinc oxide is dispersed throughout the mass as a filler. The setting time of zinc oxide–eugenol cement is accelerated by zinc salts, water, a small particle size of zinc oxide, and a high powder-liquid ratio. A smaller particle size also tends to reduce solubility.

In mixing of zinc oxide and eugenol, the slab should not be chilled below the dew point since water condensation will accelerate the set. High humidity will also reduce setting time to the point where the cement may set while still on the glass slab or the mixing pad.

Compressive strengths in excess of 5,000 pounds per square inch have been reported for zinc oxide–eugenol cements mixed at a high powder-liquid ratio. In an effort to improve the strength, abrasion resistance, and other properties, various agents have been added to both the powder and the liquid with varying degrees of success. The addition of plastics such as poly(methyl methacrylate) and polystyrene to the eugenol may improve the strength somewhat. Civjan and Brauer[14, 15] and others[16, 17] added *o*-ethoxybenzoic acid (EBA) to the eugenol and fused quartz, alumina, rosin, hydrogenated rosin, and acrylic resin to the powder. Strengths approaching those of zinc phosphate cement were obtained, although results of clinical trials[15] did not correlate with laboratory data on solubility and disintegration or abrasion. However, the formulations did show promise for use as cementing media, bases, and pulp capping agents.

**Biophysical considerations.** Radioactive tracer studies have shown that zinc oxide–eugenol cements do not exhibit as much leakage as do the zinc phosphate cements. Also, pulpal studies indicate that, of all restorative materials, zinc oxide–eugenol cements possess the highest biologic receptivity. It is perhaps for these reasons that some practitioners prefer using zinc oxide–eugenol cements for final cementation of crowns and fixed prostheses. The wide use of zinc oxide–eugenol materials ranging from temporary restorations to impression pastes explains the continued attention they are receiving from dental materials investigators.

## Calcium hydroxide

Calcium hydroxide mixed with distilled water is an excellent pulp capping agent and, when used as such, stimulates formation of reparative dentin. Calcium hydroxide in a methyl cellulose base, or suspensions of calcium hydroxide and zinc oxide in solutions of resins such as polystyrene or poly(methyl methacrylate) or in volatile solvents such as chloroform or methyl ethyl ketone are used as liners and are effective in protecting the pulp against irritation by silicate cement. Generally, in deep cavity preparations, where there may be nonhemorrhagic microscopic pulp exposures it is advisable to cover the calcium hydroxide with zinc phosphate cement prior to inserting the restoration.

**Biophysical considerations.** The exact mechanism by which calcium hydroxide induces or stimulates the growth of repair dentin has not been clearly elucidated. It appears that part of its role is to keep the immediate area in an alkaline state, which is necessary for dentin formation. Whatever else its role may be, it does not appear that the calcium hydroxide enters into the actual formation of the dentin bridge.

**Resin cements**

Resin cements were introduced in 1952. The powder is poly(methyl methacrylate) to which quartz or calcium carbonate or other inorganic materials have been added as fillers. The liquid is methyl methacrylate. Accelerators and inhibitors normally found in autopolymers are present in the polymer and the monomer of the resin cements. The cements may be mixed either in the usual manner on a glass slab or in a small jar or dappen dish as in the mixing of denture base or repair resins. The powder-liquid ratio, although important, is not as critical as for zinc phosphate cement. A cool mixing slab should be used in order to prolong the initiation stage since resin cements normally have a very short working time. The rate of addition of the powder to the liquid is not critical. Resin cements shrink during polymerization, but this deficiency is partly compensated for by the fact that cementation usually involves thin films. Although poly(methyl methacrylate) is quite insoluble in mouth fluids, the resin cements exhibit about the same solubility as the zinc phosphate cements. The solubility of the resin cements is probably caused by their high filler and plasticizer content. Resin cements cannot be used over zinc oxide–eugenol materials because the eugenol inhibits polymerization.

**Biophysical considerations.** The biophysical considerations of resin cements are much the same as those discussed earlier in the chapter. The lack of popularity of resin cements probably stems from their rather short working time and the difficulty of removing the excess hardened cement, or "flash," from the margins of the restoration, interproximal spaces, and gingival crevice.

## CAVITY LINERS

Cavity varnishes, often referred to as cavity liners, have been used for years for sealing the dentinal tubules in prepared cavities. They are usually composed of natural or synthetic resins dissolved in such solvents as acetone, chloroform, alcohol, benzene, and ether. Additives such as zinc oxide, calcium hydroxide, and polystyrene are included in some formulations. These preparations are applied to the cavity by brushes, wire loops, or cotton pledgets. Their mode of action involves the rapid evaporation of the solvent, leaving a thin film of material to serve as a barrier for pulpal protection. Because the films deposited on the cavity walls are thin and often discontinuous, several layers are recommended for increased effectiveness. The varnish films act as semipermeable membranes that selectively limit ionic penetration.

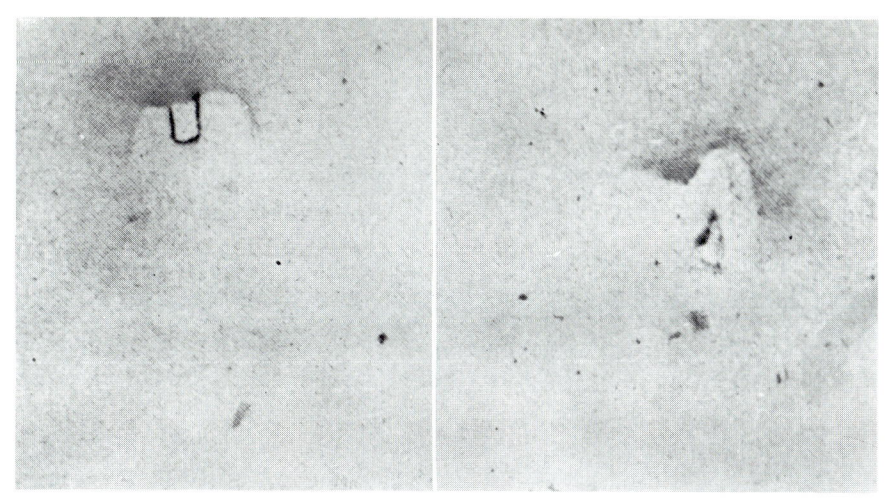

Fig. 17-14. Radioautograms showing leakage around the amalgam restoration, with and without the use of a cavity varnish. Severe leakage around restoration at left is typical of the conventional in vivo 48-hour old amalgam. No leakage is seen on restoration at right where a cavity liner was first applied before insertion of the restoration. (From Skinner, E. W., and Phillips, R. W.: The science of dental materials, ed. 5, Philadelphia, 1960, W. B. Saunders Co.)

## Biophysical considerations

The efficacy of a cavity varnish in minimizing fluid penetration in a newly placed amalgam is illustrated in Fig. 17-14. Cavity liners are also very effective in reducing the amount of acid penetration into dentin under silicate cement restorations. It is also interesting to note that cavity liners under silicate cements inhibit the beneficial effect of fluoride in decreasing enamel solubility. It would seem quite obvious that the marginal areas where the fluoride in the silicate would exert its anticariogenic effect on enamel should not be coated with varnish.

Because of their poor sealing and often irritating qualities, definitive restorative materials should seldom be used without a liner or a base.

## PLASTIC IMPLANT MATERIALS

Not too many years ago dentists and physicians desiring to investigate the use of plastic materials for the replacement or repair of tissues and organs injured or lost as a result of trauma or disease were limited to industrial and commercial products. Recent advances in surgery have shown a need for materials designed for specific applications. The wide range of mechanical properties available in polymers made them attractive candidates for dental and medical uses. However, mechanical properties alone give no assurance that a polymer may be successfully used in the body. Biologic receptivity is indispensable for the long-term utilization of a surgical repair material.

Surgical repair polymers may belong to one of two general types: biostable or biodegradable. In the former the interaction between the host and the implant is expected to be minimal, and the implant is expected to maintain its integrity for a lifetime. In the latter the implant material is expected to degrade at a desirable rate, and the products of degradation excreted through the normal excretory routes with none of the materials accumulating in tissues or organs.

The effect of polymers in the tissues may be divided into two types—local effects surrounding the polymer implant, and more remote or systemic effects. Among the possible local effects are acute inflammatory responses, as well as tumor induction and carcinogenesis. Of the more remote and systemic polymer effects may be listed antigenicity, hypertension and nephritis, and polymer deposition in various internal organs, resulting in tumors. The stability of a polymer depends on the structure of the polymer and the chemical environment in which the polymer is placed (the tissues). Because of the complexity of the problem, the development of tailor-made polymeric materials for a specific application in dentistry and medicine must of necessity involve the efforts of multidisciplined groups.

Present cooperative investigations at the United States Army Institute of Dental Research, the United States Army Medical Biomechanical Research Laboratory, and the Division of Surgical Research, Walter Reed Army Institute of Research, include tissue adhesives and other biodegradable and biostable polymers for specialized applications.

**Tissue adhesives**

The ability of rapidly polymerizing alkyl alpha cyanoacrylates to adhere to moist surfaces has excited considerable medical interest. These resins appeared promising as hemostatic agents and tissue adhesives for closure of wounds in place of or in conjunction with conventional surgical sutures. Medical and dental evaluation of the methyl alpha cyanoacrylates has revealed that the resin can adhere to a variety of tissues, with healing ensuing at the bonded site. It was further shown that the monomer and polymer elicited an acute inflammatory response and that the polymer disappeared after a time from its initial point of application, indicating that biodegradation had occurred. Leonard and associates,[18] in order to elucidate structure-tissue interaction and ultimately develop a less toxic adhesive, undertook the synthesis and biologic evaluation of the homologous series of the alkyl alpha cyanoacrylates. It was postulated that the higher homologues would exhibit higher biologic receptivity and would degrade at a slower rate because of their more hydrophobic nature. Further work substantiated these predictions. The butyl and isobutyl derivatives seem to be well tolerated and are being applied experimentally for wound closures in oral surgery, periodontal surgery, and in surgically injured livers and intestines. Attempts to induce hemostasis indicate that these compounds can stop capillary and venous bleeding. The results obtained in the patient with arterial bleeding are equivocal. In addition to these surgical applications, Civjan, Margetis, and Reddick[19, 20] are investigating filled alkyl alpha cyanoacrylates for use in restorative dentistry.

**Biostable polymers**

Leonard and associates synthesized a terpolymer composed of a biostable polymer of butyl acrylate, methyl methacrylate, and methacrylamide, which may be reinforced and vulcanized.[21] In conjunction with organic reinforcing agents, polymeric materials having a range of mechanical properties, from stiff and rigid to soft and elastomeric, can be designed for possible use in internal body and maxillofacial prostheses. Maxillofacial prostheses in the form of a thin terpolymer skin placed over a foamed silicone filler are shown in Fig. 17-15. McFall and associates[22] recently reported the use of the terpolymer foam in experimental orofacial surgery. The ter-

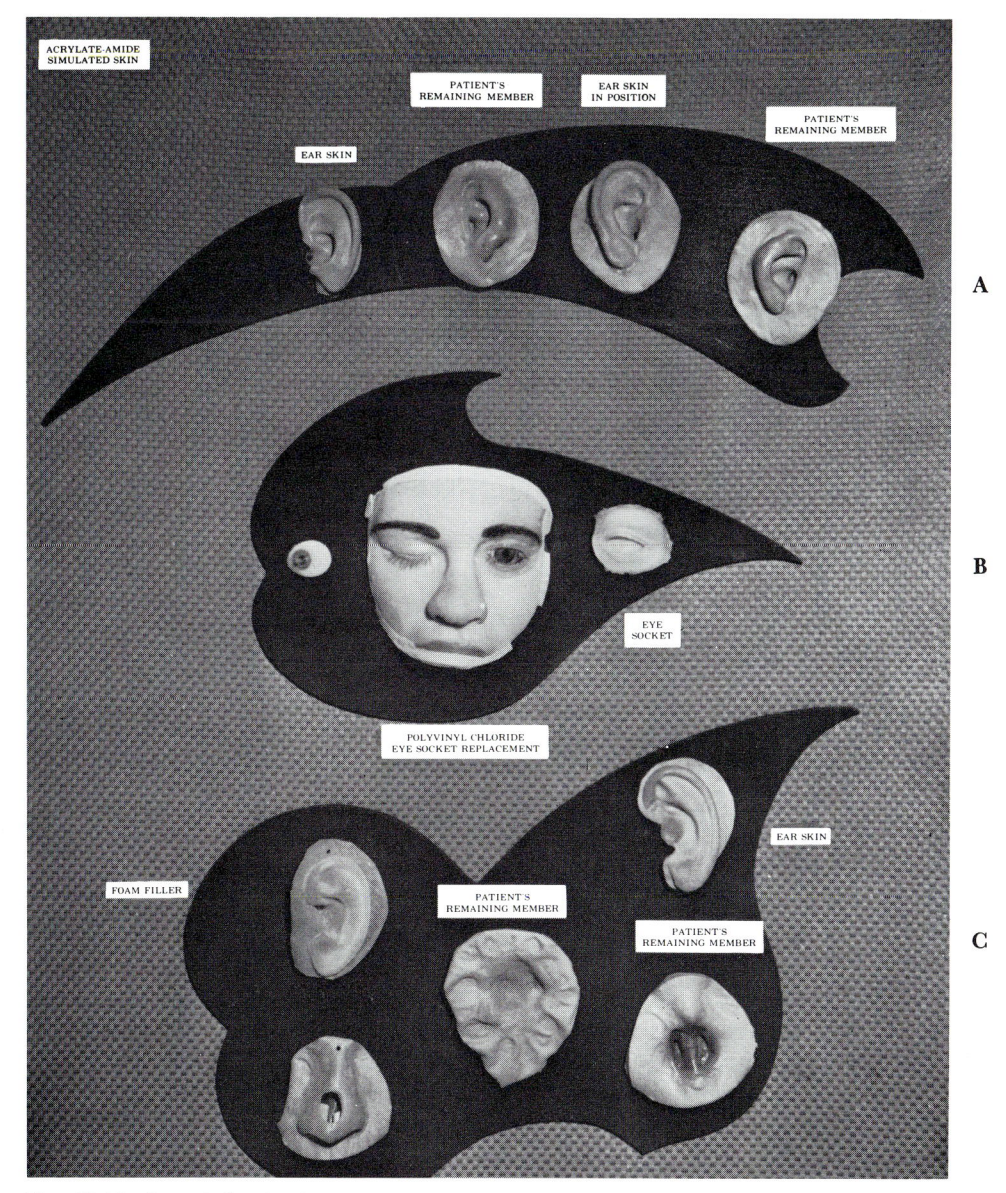

Fig. 17-15. A and C, Simulated ear and nose skins with foam fillers fabricated from a terpolymer composed of a biostable polymer of butyl acrylate, methyl methacrylate, and methacrylamide. B, Polyvinyl chloride facial prosthesis including ocular prosthesis. (From United States Army Medical Biomechanical Research Laboratory.)

polymer has also been used with encouraging results in the fabrication of arterial sections, the trachea, and bile ducts.

## Synthetic cartilage

Efforts are being made to synthesize hydrophilic polymers with frictional characteristics and mechanical properties similar to those of cartilage. Polymers prepared from glycol methacrylates are currently being investigated.

## Biodegradable polymers

The United States Army Medical Biomechanical Research Laboratory is synthesizing biodegradable polymers such as L (+) polylactic acid for use in composite artificial arteries and burn dressings. To date, the polymer has been prepared in both radioactive ($C^{14}$ tagged) and nonradioactive forms. The rates of degradation in vivo have been studied by implantation of radioactive polymers in rats and by measuring the disappearance rate of radioactivity. Histologic studies have indicated that the polymer and its degradation products are well tolerated. Use of the polymer in orofacial surgery is being studied at the United States Army Institute of Dental Research.

## CONCLUSION

Good dentistry is a major method of prevention. The vast majority of all oral health service procedures involves the use of materials. When the hard tooth structures are destroyed by caries or when the surrounding tissues are destroyed by periodontal disease, functional and esthetic restoration or replacement of lost hard and soft tissues helps prevent further destruction. Research in dental materials has evolved a series of scientific principles that underlie manipulative technics. An understanding and proper application of these principles will determine to a great extent the professional success of the dentist. On the other hand, the improper selection and use of materials or a disregard of biophysical relationships will lead to clinical failures. Every step in the use of materials must therefore be accompanied by meticulous care and attention to details, for only through intelligent and conscientious practice can the biomechanical oral procedures become not only restorative but preventive as well.

## REFERENCES

1. Armstrong, W. W., and Simon, W. J.: Penetration of radiocalcium at the margins of filling materials; a preliminary report, J.A.D.A. 43:684, 1951.
2. Phillips, R. W., and others: Adaptation of restorations *in vivo* as assessed by $Ca^{45}$, J.A.D.A. 62:23, 1961.
3. Healey, H. J., and Phillips, R. W.: A clinical study of amalgam failures, J. Dent. Res. 28:439, 1949.
4. Eames, W. B.: Preparation and condensation of amalgam with low mercury-alloy ratio, J.A.D.A. 58:78, 1959.
5. Hitchen, A. D., and Hall, D. C.: Allergic lesions of the tongue due to silver content of amalgam fillings, Dent. Pract. 14:1943, 1963.
6. Zander, H. A.: Effect of silicate cement and amalgam on the gingiva, J.A.D.A. 55:11, 1957.
7. App, G. R.: Effect of silicate, amalgam, and cast gold on the gingiva, J. Prosth. Dent. 11:522, 1961.
8. Waerhaug, J., and Zander, H. A.: Reaction of gingival tissue to self-curing acrylic restorations, J.A.D.A. 54:760, 1957.
9. Baum, L.: Gold foil (filling golds) in dental practice, Dent. Clin. N. Amer., March, 1965, p. 199.
10. Mahler, D. B., and Armen, G. K., Jr.: Addition of amalgam alloy to zinc phosphate cement, J. Prosth. Dent. 12:157, 1962.
11. Wolcott, R. B., Shiller, W. R., and Kraske, L. M.: Clinical evaluation of temporary restorative materials, J. Prosth. Dent. 12:782, 1962.
12. Swartz, M. L., and Phillips, R. W.: *In vitro* studies on the marginal leakage of restorative materials, J.A.D.A. 62:142, 1961.

13. Copeland, H. I., Jr., and others: Setting reaction of zinc oxide and eugenol, J. Res. National Bureau of Standards 55:134, 1955.
14. Civjan, S., and Brauer, G. M.: Physical properties of cements based on zinc oxide, hydrogenated rosin, o-ethoxybenzoic acid and eugenol, J. Dent. Res. 43:281, 1964.
15. Civjan, S., and Brauer, G. M.: Clinical behavior of o-ethoxybenzoic acid-eugenol-zinc oxide cements, J. Dent. Res. 44:80, 1965.
16. Brauer, G. M., McLaughlin, R., and Huget, E. F.: Aluminum oxide as a reinforcing agent for zinc oxide-eugenol-o-ethoxybenzoic acid cements, J. Dent. Res. 47:622, 1968.
17. Brauer, G. M., Huget, E. F., and Termini, D. J.: Plastic reinforced EBA cements as restorative materials, I.A.D.R. 47:104, 1969.
18. Leonard, F.: Advances in the uses of plastic materials for implants. Paper presented at the American Association for the Advancement of Science symposium on materials, science in dentistry, medicine and pharmacy, December, 1965.
19. Civjan, S., Margetis, P. M., and Reddick, R. L.: Properties of n-butyl-α-cyanoacrylate mixtures, J. Dent. Res. 48:536, 1969.
20. Civjan, S., Margetis, P. M., and Reddick, R. L.: Properties of alkyl-α-cyanoacrylate restorative materials, I.A.D.R. 47:144, 1969.
21. Leonard, F., Nelson, J., and Brandes, G.: Vulcanizable saturated acrylate elastomers, Indust. Eng. Chem. 50:1053, 1958.
22. McFall, T. A., Henefer, E. P., and Clinton, E. E.: Study of acrylate-amide foam in experimental orofacial surgery, J. Oral Surg. 23:108, 1965.

## ADDITIONAL READINGS

Asgar, K., Mahler, D. B., and Peyton, F. A.: Hygroscopic technique for inlay casting using controlled water additions, J. Prosth. Dent. 5:711, 1955.
Barber, D., Lyell, J., and Massler, M.: Effectiveness of copal resin varnish under amalgam restorations, J. Prosth. Dent. 14:533, 1964.
Bowen, R. L.: Dental filling material comprising vinyl-silane treated fused silica and a binder consisting of the reaction product of bisphenol and glycidyl acrylate, United States Patent No. 3066112, Nov. 27, 1962.
Brauer, G. M., White, E. E., and Moshonas, M. G.: The reaction of metal oxides with o-ethoxybenzoic acid and other chelating agents, J. Dent. Res. 37:547, 1958.
Brekhus, P. J., and Armstrong, W. D.: Civilization—a disease, J.A.D.A. 23:1459, 1936.
Cameron, J. L., and others: The degradation of cyanoacrylate tissue adhesive I, Surgery 58:424, 1965.
Eames, W. B., Skinner, E. W., and Mizera, G. T.: Amalgam strength values relative to mercury percentages and plasticity, J. Prosth. Dent. 11:765, 1961.
Frykholm, K. O., and Obeblad, E.: Studies on the penetration of mercury through dental hard tissues using Hg$^{203}$ in silver amalgam fillings, Acta Odont. Scand. 13:157, 1955.
Gilmore, W. H., Schnell, R. J., and Phillips, R. W.: Factors influencing the accuracy of silicone impression materials, J. Prosth. Dent. 9:304, 1959.
Guide to dental materials, ed. 4, Chicago, 1968-1969, American Dental Association.
Going, R. E., and Massler, M.: Influence of cavity liners under amalgam restorations on penetration by radioactive isotopes, J. Prosth. Dent. 11:298, 1961.
Going, R. E., Massler, M., and Dute, H. L.: Marginal penetration of dental restorations by different radioactive isotopes, J. Dent. Res. 39:273, 1960.
Mahler, D. B., and Ady, A. B.: The influence of various factors on the effective setting expansion of casting investments, J. Prosth. Dent. 13:365, 1963.
Mang, S. L., and others: Antibacterial action of certain fluoride-containing dental restorative materials, J. Dent. Res. 38:88, 1959.
Margetis, P. M., and Hansen, W. C.: Changes in agar-agar type duplicating material and agar-agar on heating and storage, J.A.D.A. 54:737, 1957.
Massler, M. P.: Biologic considerations in the selection and use of restorative materials, Dent. Clin. N. Amer., March, 1965, p. 131.
Menegale, C., Swartz, M. L., and Phillips, R. W.: Adaptation of restorative materials as influenced by roughness of cavity walls, J. Dent. Res. 39:825, 1960.

Mumford, G. M., and Phillips, R. W.: Dimensional change in wax patterns during setting of gypsum investments, J. Dent. Res. **37**:351, 1958.

Mumford, G. M., and Phillips, R. W.: Measurement of thermal expansion of cristobalite type investments in the inlay ring: preliminary report, J. Prosth. Dent. **8**:860, 1958.

Nelson, R. J., Wolcott, R. B., and Paffenbarger, G. C.: Fluid exchange at the margins of dental restorations, J.A.D.A. **44**:288, 1952.

Norman, R. D., Phillips, R. W., and Swartz, M. L.: Fluoride uptake by enamel from certain dental materials, J. Dent. Res. **39**:11, 1960.

Norman, R. D., Swartz, M. L., and Phillips, R. W.: Additional studies on the solubility of certain dental materials, J. Dent. Res. **38**:1038, 1959.

Palmer, D. W., Roydhouse, R. G., and Skinner, E. W.: Asbestos liner and casting accuracy, D. Progress **1**:155, 1961.

Peyton, F. A., editor: Restorative dental materials, ed. 3, St. Louis, 1968, The C. V. Mosby Co.

Phillips, R. W.: Cavity varnishes and bases, Dent. Clin. N. Amer., March, 1965, p. 159.

Phillips, R. W.: Dental cements: a comparison of properties, J.A.D.A. **66**:496, 1963.

Phillips, R. W.: Failure of materials in restorative dentistry, J. S. Calif. Dent. Ass. **24**:19, 1956.

Phillips, R. W.: Some current observations on restorative materials, Aust. D. J. **9**:258, 1964.

Phillips, R. W., and Boyd, D. A.: Importance of the mercury-alloy ratio to the amalgam filling, J.A.D.A. **34**:451, 1947.

Phillips, R. W., and Love, D. R.: The effect of certain additive agents on the physical properties of zinc oxide–eugenol mixtures, J. Dent. Res. **40**:294, 1961.

Phillips, R. W., and Schnell, R. J.: Electroformed dies from thiokol and silicone impressions, J. Prosth. Dent. **8**:992, 1958.

Phillips, R. W., and Swartz, M. L.: Effect of certain restorative materials on solubility of enamel, J.A.D.A. **54**:623, 1957.

Schnell, R. J., and Phillips, R. W.: Dimensional stability of rubber base impressions and certain other factors affecting accuracy, J.A.D.A. **57**:39, 1958.

Sciaky, I., and Pisanti, S.: Localization of calcium placed over amputated pulps in dog's teeth, J. Dent. Res. **39**:1128, 1960.

Seltzer, S., and Bender, I. B.: The dental pulp, Philadelphia, 1965, J. B. Lippincott Co.

Skinner, E. E., and Cooper, E. N.: Desirable properties and use of rubber impression materials, J.A.D.A. **51**:523, 1955.

Skinner, E. W., and Phillips, R. W.: The science of dental materials, ed. 6, Philadelphia, 1967, W. B. Saunders Co.

Swartz, M. L.: Dental cements and restorative resins, Dent. Clin. N. Amer., March, 1965, p. 169.

Swartz, M. L., and Phillips, R. W.: Influence of manipulative variables on the marginal adaptation of certain restorative materials, J. Prosth. Dent. **12**:172, 1962.

Swartz, M. L., and Phillips, R. W.: Permeability of cavity liners to certain agents, J. Dent. Res. **39**:1232, 1960.

Swartz, M. L., and Phillips, R. W.: Residual mercury content of amalgam restorations and its influence on compressive strength, J. Dent. Res. **35**:458, 1956.

Thanik, K. D., Boyd, D. A., and Huysen, G. V.: Cavity base materials and the exposed pulp marginal blood vessels, J. Prosth. Dent. **12**:165, 1962.

Symposium on dental materials, Dent. Clin. N. Amer., March, 1965.

Waerhaug, J.: Effect of zinc phosphate fillings on gingival tissues, J. Periodont. **27**:284, 1956.

Wilson, C. J., and Ryge, G.: Clinical study of dental amalgam, J.A.D.A. **66**:763, 1963.

Wilson, R. T., Phillips, R. W., and Norman, R. D.: Influence of certain condensation procedures upon the mercury content of amalgam restorations, J. Dent. Res. **36**:458, 1957.

Woodward, S. C., and others: Histotoxicity of cyanoacrylate tissue adhesive in the rat, Ann. Surg. **162**:113, 1965.

# Chapter 18 Physical fitness and dynamic health

## Thomas K. Cureton, Jr.

Dentistry and physical unfitness
    Dentistry and chronic ailments
        Prevention is needed
    Why dentists are involved in physical fitness
    Health and fitness related to teeth
    Medical examinations and exercise
Prevention of chronic ailments by protective physical fitness work
    The deeper meaning of physical fitness and dynamic health
    Improvement of the maximal oxygen intake of middle-aged men
Positive physical fitness—practical dynamic health rules
    The health values of exercise
    The positive fitness approach
Physical deterioration (unfitness) is the greatest disease
    The evidence that deterioration disease is the greatest disease
    Poor physical fitness, aging, poor nutrition, and ecologic maladjustment are intertwined
How much exercise is enough? What is the best program for a busy professional man?
    The variety of programs; some are dangerous
    Cardiovascular fitness is related to habitual energy output (calories per week)
    Energy cost of adult physical activities
    Exhibits of evaluation of several programs of exercise
        Weight training is compared with running (walk-jog-run)
        Comparison of Cureton's low gear program with isometric exercises and tennis
        Golfers and fitness class middle-aged men evaluated

## DENTISTRY AND PHYSICAL UNFITNESS
### Dentistry and chronic ailments

Various studies have shown dentistry to be a very confining occupation, and it ranks at the top for chronic ailments: heart disease, varicose veins, nervous disorders, eye fatigue, fatigue at the end of the day, and arthritic-rheumatic disorders.[1-3] The country as a whole is unhealthy too, according to various reports, suffering from lack of exercise, too much food and drink, contamination of the air and the waters, crowded conditions in the cities, excessive additives to the food, stale and processed food rather than fresh food, and deterioration diseases in general—heart disease (noninfectious, CHD) and psychosomatic nervous disorders head the list of diseases. A Washington report[4] states that mental health requires $421 million for 1970, health planning and services, $196.9 million, hospital construction $254 million, regional medical support programs $50 million, drugs and alcohol "facilities" $12 million, new mental health construction $29.2 million, and migrant health $8.1 million. The drift is to build more and more hospitals across the country, with the expectancy of more and more people in them and more and more people to man them—with costs skyrocketing. The other alternative is to work harder and harder on cheaper *preventive* programs, the chief of which is physical fitness. There is some general dissatisfaction over what the country is getting for such enormous expenditures. Forbes[5] has indicated this in two national reports and has further postulated that more effort in physical fitness, control of accidents, and some simplification of living habits with reduction of alcohol, cigarettes, and drugs would produce better results for less cost.

**Prevention is needed.** These trends mean also that the incidence of infectious disease has been going down, while deterioration disease has gone up and up, so much so that it is quite out of hand. There is a great physiologic failure among Americans, most of it preventable. Such prevention will depend upon one's choices, mainly what one does himself about it. Fitness programs have become more popular, and joggers, home exercisers, increased school programs, and adult programs are now more numerous than ever.[6-8] Educational and protective programs are needed.

The second aspect is related to dentists maintaining their fitness—to look better, to feel better, and to fight off the ravages of deterioration disease that may prevent their working. I have found that, as a group, dentists do very poorly on physical fitness tests (Table 18-1).

The experimental group of dentists, 100 in number, averaged 44.5 years of age, 69.76 inches tall, and 172.6 pounds in weight. In the physical ability tests, 37.3 percent could not step up and down for 5 minutes on a 17-inch bench; 36.4 percent could not jump over 15 inches in the vertical jump; and 80 percent were below 12 on the 18-Item Motor Test (average male adult standard in the U.S.A.).

It is shown in Table 18-1 that, by comparison with the adult fitness tables (Cureton's University of Illinois Tables for Adults), the sample of 100 dentists averaged above average in none of the 28 tests given on the physical fitness profile for adults.

## Why dentists are involved in physical fitness

A family dentist may have an important influence on children by emphasizing physical fitness; it is one major factor related to developing a good set of teeth and gums. Steinman, Brassett, and Tartaryn[9] reported an experiment that has implications along this line.

A study was made of the effect of exercise vs. the effect of immobilization (in cages) on the production of dental caries in rats. Twenty-eight white rats were divided into two groups and given exactly the same diets for about three-fourths of their lives. The exercised rats were allowed to run for 4 hours each day in a series of bouts (16 minutes at a time, followed by 8 minutes of rest), and to run a total of 4 hours per day. The immobilized group was confined in cages that permitted little movement. The results showed that the exercised rats had 61 caries (4.3 per animal) and that the confined rats had 192 caries (14.0 per animal). The exercised group of rats had fewer caries by approximately 1 to 3; exercise seemed to be the deciding factor in building resistance to the formation of dental caries.

## Health and fitness related to teeth

Good health has a relationship to good teeth and gums. Price, an anthropologist, has reported that two principal causal sets of factors other than hereditary determine

**Table 18-1.** *Results of objective physical fitness tests of dentists**

|  | Units | Range | Mean | Standard score |
|---|---|---|---|---|
| 1. *Quiet sitting blood pressures* | mm. Hg |  |  |  |
|    Systolic blood pressure |  | 105–190 | 131 | 37 |
|    Diastolic blood pressure |  | 60–122 | 84.1 | 31 |
|    Pulse pressure |  | 14–97 | 46.5 | 46 |
| 2. *Quiet sitting brachial pulse waves* |  |  |  |  |
|    (Sphygmograms, indicating stroke volume of heart by heartograms) |  |  |  |  |
|    Pulse rate, sitting | Beats/min. | 51–128 | 78.1 | 51 |
|    Area (by plainemter) | Sq. cm. | 0.10—0.50 | 0.272 | 36 |
|    Systolic amplitude, sitting | Cm. | 0.63—1.56 | 1.01 | 33 |
|    Systolic amplitude, standing | Cm. | 0.22—1.40 | 0.71 | 52 |
|    Diastolic surge, sitting | Cm. | 0 to 0.53 | 0.007 | 28 |
|    Angle of ejection, sitting | Degs. | 9.0 to 52° | 18.0° | 23.5 |
|    Amplitude after 1 min. run in place at 180 steps/min. | Cm. | 0.30 to 2.22 | 1.05 | 36 |
| 3. *Vital capacity and breath holding* |  |  |  |  |
|    Vital capacity residual | Cu. in. | 82 to —117 | —32.3 | 42 |
|    Breath holding after 1′ step test, 30/min. | Cu. in. | 6 to 46 | 16.4 | 49 |
| 4. *Flexibility of the chest and spine* |  |  |  |  |
|    Trunk extension backward | In. | 5.8-22.4 | 14.4 | 50 |
|    Trunk flexion forward | In. | 24—7.8 | 14.6 | 34 |
|    Chest expansion | In. | 1.7—5.1 | 3.24 | 50 |
| 5. *Metropolitan Life Ins. Co. index* |  |  |  |  |
|    Fat (by calipers over skin folds) | mm. | 60-197 | 129.1 | 54 |
|    Exp. chest girth—normal abdominal girth | In. | —3.0 to 8.6 | 4.15 | 50 |
| 6. *Strength* (by dynamometers) |  |  |  |  |
|    Right hand grip | Lb. | 52-140 | 97.6 | 33 |
|    Left hand grip | Lb. | 52-126 | 87.8 | 32 |
|    Back strength | Lb. | 150-500 | 337.4 | 47 |
|    Leg strength | Lb. | 270-600 | 431.7 | 48 |
|    Total strength | Lb. | 588-1215 | 950.6 | 44 |
|    Strength weight | Lb. | 4.1-7.8 | 5.52 | 38 |
| 7. *Cardiovascular adjustments to exercise* |  |  |  |  |
|    Terminal pulse rate | Beats/min. | 138-192 | 169.6 | 50 |
|    5 min. step test | Counts | 138-213 | 178.1 | 48 |
|    Systolic blood pressure after 5 min. step test | mm. Hg | 100-227 | 154.3 | 48 |
|    Diastolic blood pressure after 5 min. step test | mm. Hg |  |  |  |
|    Drop in diastolic blood pressure after exercise | mm. Hg | —23 to 22 | —1.4 | 38 |

*From Cureton, T. K.: Health and physical fitness of dentists (with Implications), J. Dent. Med. 16:211-223, 1961.

good teeth, namely (1) mobility and (2) eating raw, uncooked, and unprocessed food.[11] He depicts the inhabitants of the Swiss mountains without draft animals habitually practicing strenuous physical tasks on a diet of black bread made from unbolted rye flour, cheese, fresh cow's milk, and goat's milk, with meat about once a week—the combined effect resulting in almost perfect immunity to dental caries. This example and a number of others are contrasted with more populated and sophisticated regions around Saint-Moritz, where bread made from refined flour, jams, canned goods, much meat, and little milk generally resulted in poor teeth.

Cheraskin and Ringsdorf of the University of Alabama Medical Center in Birmingham have published a chart showing the age of the body related to the number of the teeth.[12] Beginning at about 6 years of age (Fig. 18-1) and continuing up to about 24, the teeth increase in number; then there is a slow decline until approximately age 70, when the teeth are fully deteriorated by average. This curve is remarkably similar to the curve of motor fitness determined by the 18-Item Motor Fitness Test to 2200 men and boys (Cureton's 18-Item Motor Test, Fig. 18-2); the curves have the same general shape.[13] While causal connection cannot be guaranteed from such a comparison, physical fitness is approximately similar to age of the teeth at various stages of life. It is probable that the major factors which undermine health and fitness in general undermine both teeth and motor fitness. It is generally accredited to aging, but it has been shown that, after 25 years, physical fitness can be markedly improved so that the curve descends more gradually and extrapolation causes it to reach the base axis at approximately 120 years. It is also contended that adults who maintain their fitness throughout life have much better teeth than individuals who do not maintain fitness. There is some reality to the association, but as yet no study has carried the physical conditioning program throughout life for any established group of people. Generalizations up to now hinge on a number of known individual examples.

**Medical examinations and exercise**

Normally medical examinations are expected to be helpful but people are suspicious of them, partly because of excessive costs. Millions of people exercise without them, still we say "See your doctor first." The dentist may be able to determine the state of relative deterioration (by the teeth)[12] but the physician is generally best to test the dynamics of the body.[13] Any trained person can make physiologic determinations of normal people to help understand them and guide their fitness (but not test for infectious disease). To understand a person the health habits must be appraised on a day-to-day basis, not just by a yearly medical examination. What the person can do with his body is important to test out balance, flexibility, agility, strength, power, and endurance. If there has been an infarct or blood clot a cardiographer can usually find it and define it, but most will recommend exercise of the cautious, nonviolent type anyway. If extreme S-T segment depression is present in stress tests, then medical control may be indicated, but still most of these cases can exercise in moderation. The real problem is that such "medical indicators" come too late; there should be exercise of a regular type to prevent such deviations. It is also important to classify people according to low gear, middle gear, or high gear possibilities, and guide them into effective exercise and improved health practices. Most people need help. But the solution is not with drugs or immobility, nor to develop fear of exertion, but to introduce a reasonable set of rules and guide the individuals in their

*Physical fitness and dynamic health* 401

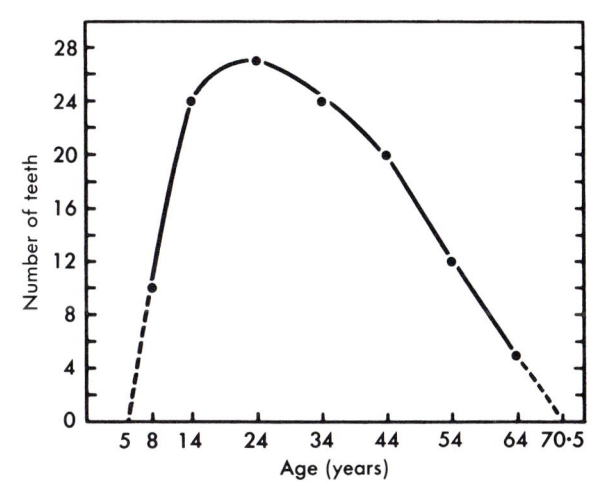

Fig. 18-1. Relation of age to tooth loss. Continuous line, data; interrupted lines, extrapolations. (From Cheraskin, E., and Ringsdorf, W. M., Jr.: Ageing by the teeth, Lancet 1:580, 1969.)

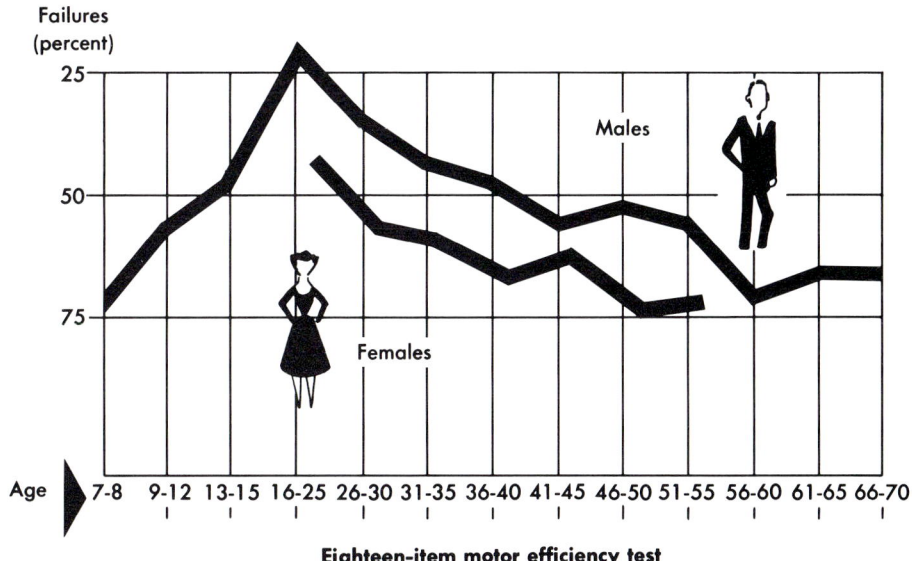

**Eighteen-item motor efficiency test**

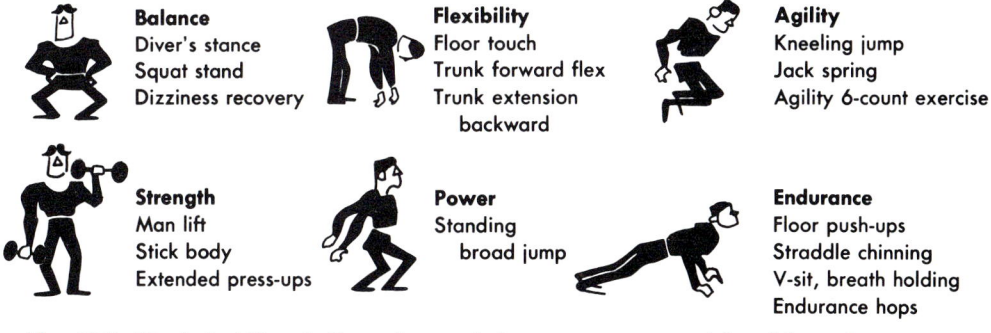

**Balance**
Diver's stance
Squat stand
Dizziness recovery

**Flexibility**
Floor touch
Trunk forward flex
Trunk extension backward

**Agility**
Kneeling jump
Jack spring
Agility 6-count exercise

**Strength**
Man lift
Stick body
Extended press-ups

**Power**
Standing broad jump

**Endurance**
Floor push-ups
Straddle chinning
V-sit, breath holding
Endurance hops

Fig. 18-2. Physical ability declines after peak in teens, as measured by eighteen-item motor efficiency test. (From Cureton, T. K.: Pageant, February, 1959.)

application at home, in the gym or pool, or on the roads and sidewalks, parks, and playgrounds. People do not understand the positive aspects of exercise for their benefit, nor do they comprehend many of the possible dangers; some instruction is necessary. They should also be introduced to self-tests of a rather simple type (for balance, flexibility, agility, strength, power, and endurance) so they may develop some ideational standards as to their abilities and needs. Good tables exist, and there are thousands of physical education instructors trained in this type of work. The needs should be pinpointed and counteracted by the proper application of exercise.

## PREVENTION OF CHRONIC AILMENTS BY PROTECTIVE PHYSICAL FITNESS WORK
### The deeper meaning of physical fitness and dynamic health

Increased automation (work and transportation done by machines), and overheated offices and homes are, over a period of time, very destructive to circulation and to health; the prevention is simply more daily movement and more time spent in cooler quarters. While some improvements in joint mobility can be effected with short programs of 15 to 30 minutes per day, such programs are entirely inadequate to greatly increase the uptake of sugar and other carbohydrates and to use them up and to reduce the lipids (fats, cholesterol, triglycerides, and lipoprotein giant molecules) that slowly clog up the body and cause debility and death. At least 40,000,000 Americans suffer from this "creeping death." Immobility for hours at a time is in itself a devastating chronic disease cause.[14, 15]

Studies of middle-aged men to estimate the effect of a physical training program to eliminate or reduce such ailments have been made by Holmes[16] and by Joseph.[17] Both studies indicate that such ailments can be reduced. The Holmes study was a longitudinal study spread over 8 years. The men were tested at the beginning and at the end on a wide variety of physical fitness tests and were also asked to fill in a checklist, indicating every ailment of the recurring type. The 76 men involved in the study were classified into three groups: (1) those who habitually carried out strenuous exercise regularly, (2) those who practiced moderate exercise rather intermittently, and (3) those who were almost completely sedentary. The strenuous exercise group reduced their chronic complaints and ailments the most compared to the other two groups, which were not very different from each other. The strenuous exercise group reduced the complaints of aching backs, swollen joints, and painful feet. Moderate negative correlations were found with the scores on the objective tests. Joseph's study also found that the men improved over as short a period as 6 months. A list of such chronic ailments is shown in Table 18-2, excluding the virile infectious diseases.

---

Dr. Hans Kraus, Associate Professor of Medicine and Rehabilitation at New York University, claims that physically inactive people are more likely to suffer from organic troubles, diabetes, and psychiatric illnesses than active people. He came to the conclusion that physically active people suffer less and live longer, and he advises doctors to prescribe physical exercises, as well as medicine, to keep patients healthy.

Dr. Hans Kraus, *Vigor* **8**:36, 1955.

**Table 18-2.** *What is the field of physical fitness? What reversals of deterioration trends are possible by fitness programs?*\*

| Disease | Number of men, women, and children afflicted at any one time in one year |
|---|---:|
| Allergies, nasal drip, watery eyes | 30,000,000 |
| Arthritis (several types, including shrinkage and dehydration of the tissues) | 10,000,000 |
| Cancer (several types due to viruses, irradiation, repeated injury, and failure of adaptation to stress) | 6,000,000 |
| Childbirth deaths | 600,000 |
| Diabetes and "tendency toward diabetes, high blood sugar" | 10,000,000 |
| Emphysema, cataarh, repetitious coughing | 900,000 |
| Gallstones, kidney stones | 20,000,000 |
| Hemorrhoids | 30,000,000 |
| Heart disease (CHD and angina pectoris) | 17,000,000 |
| Hypertension or hypotension | 8,000,000 |
| Impotency, repetitious failure | 30,000,000 |
| Poor heart stroke (low velocity and acceleration) | 40,000,000 |
| Obesity (more than 10 pounds overweight) | 40,000,000 |
| Metabolic and nutritional disorders | 30,000,000 |
| Psychosomatic, psychological, temperament disorders | 25,000,000 |
| Ulcers, gout | 10,000,000 |
| Stroke (apoplexy) | 300,000 |
| Deteriorated eyesight, hearing, taste, feeling, etc. | 20,000,000 |
| Weak bones, broken bones (ankles, wrists, hips, knees, clavicles, etc.) | 1,000,000 |
| Motor morons (who cannot pass more than 6 items on the 18-Item Motor Test) | 25,000,000 |
| Deteriorated, uncorrected teeth | 50,000,000 |

\*Data from various health groups were consulted, also U. S. Public Health Statistical Reports, data from the National Aging Institute, and mental health data.

Table 18-2 is an approximate list, as some of the disorders are not recognized in modern medical or public health statistics, such as the motor morons or the poor heart stroke. Nevertheless, from the point of view of physical unfitness these ailments are real enough. They are also mainly preventable or correctable, although such data are hard to find and data are not kept on many exercise-fitness programs considered longitudinally. The figures are round figures arrived at by considering the public health reports and from smaller sample studies, adjusted pro rata to the whole population.

The positive factors needed to balance the score for health include: (1) a daily, adequate workout to 30 minutes beyond the point of sweating, (2) a plan for pacing the day, alternation of work and rest, such as stretching, movement, (3) improved nutrition to counteract the dietary insufficiency that almost everyone has, (4) improved environmental conditions (cooler rooms, air movement, filtered air, cleanliness), (5) attention to the necessity for relaxation, and (6) less exposure to contamination and infectious disease. Physical fitness in its full concept requires attention to all of these positive factors.

A special report by Time-Life points out that "despite dramatic advances made against infections, a man of 25 can expect to live only 8 years longer than his grandfather did, and after 50 years of age the advantage is small if any. The present life

**404**  *Improving dental practice through preventive measures*

expectancy in the United States is 18th for men and 10th for women; and if present trends continue, within 10 years we shall be about 38th in rank order for men."[6] More and more money spent for medical attention does not seem to solve the problem, as people abuse themselves by violating the rules for fitness and dynamic health. The hazards of enforced immobility are well researched; air force pilots, dentists, doctors, shoemakers, bench workers, electrical factory workers, bankers, desk workers, traffic controllers, "spotted" policemen, bank tellers, and similar occupa-

**Occupational death rates from coronary disease**

| | |
|---|---|
| Agricultural workers | 32 |
| Coal miners below ground | 40 |
| | 100 |
| Banking and insurance officials | 183 |
| Anglican clergy | 218 |
| Physicians and surgeons | 368 |
| Average death rate from coronary disease all males 20-65 | 100 |

Fig. 18-3. Incidence of coronary heart disease and occupation. (From Stewart, I. McD.: Coronary disease and modern stress, Lancet 2:867, 1950.)

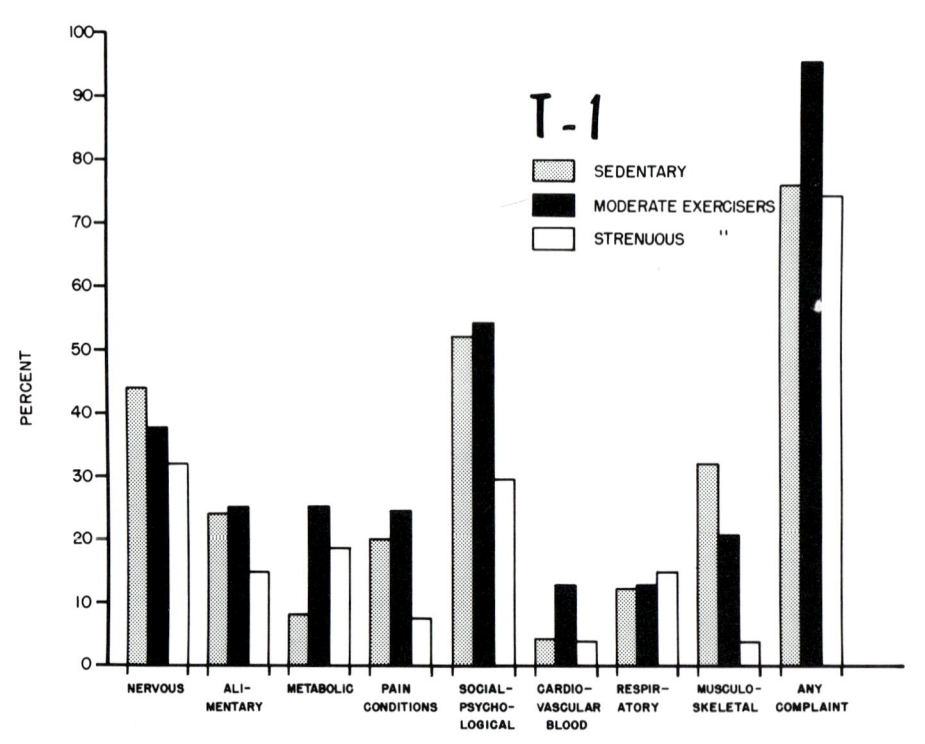

Fig. 18-4. Reduction of chronic ailments over 8 years in sedentary, moderate, and strenuously exercised middle-aged men. (From Holmes and Cureton: Physical fitness research laboratory, 1969.)

tions are the worst for "occupational disease." To guarantee that one's vulnerability goes up five to ten times, one simply takes one of these jobs for his confinement[18] (Fig. 18-3). Then physical deterioration is guaranteed.

The declining slopes represent the amount of deterioration by average. Lack of oxygen may cause aging of the cells, as claimed by one important researcher.[19] The accumulated wastes of the body, lack of change of body fluids, low metabolic rate, and poor circulation are related to poor nutrition. Proper alternation of sleep, work, rest, and nutrition, with interspersed periods of relaxation, seem to be related to improved physical fitness tests.

One study has shown that, over a period of 8 years, there is a marked reduction of chronic ailments by middle-aged men following a led and professionally directed physical fitness program[16] (Fig. 18-4). Another study has shown that anxiety states were changed by the same program and over a span of 8 years the men who were consistent followers of the fitness work improved their psychologic states.[22] Women too, who typically have even greater anxiety than men in the 45 to 55 year age group, improved their nervous state and reduced their total peripheral resistance.[23] This also means that they improved their circulation; temperature, pulse, and respiration are inversely related to circulation.

The list of chronic ailments is stupendous; Table 18-2 indicates some overlapping, of course, because each person has several such deterioration diseases, especially the middle-aged.

## Improvement of the maximal oxygen intake of middle-aged men

Fig. 18-5 shows the results of training fifteen men in a longitudinal experiment. They averaged 40.2 yrs. of age (range 33 to 48); they ran over a cross-country course at the University of Illinois for 5 months, four to five times per week. The distance was 3.5 miles. At the beginning of the experiment most of them could not run more than a mile but gradually improved. In the 2-mile run for time given after

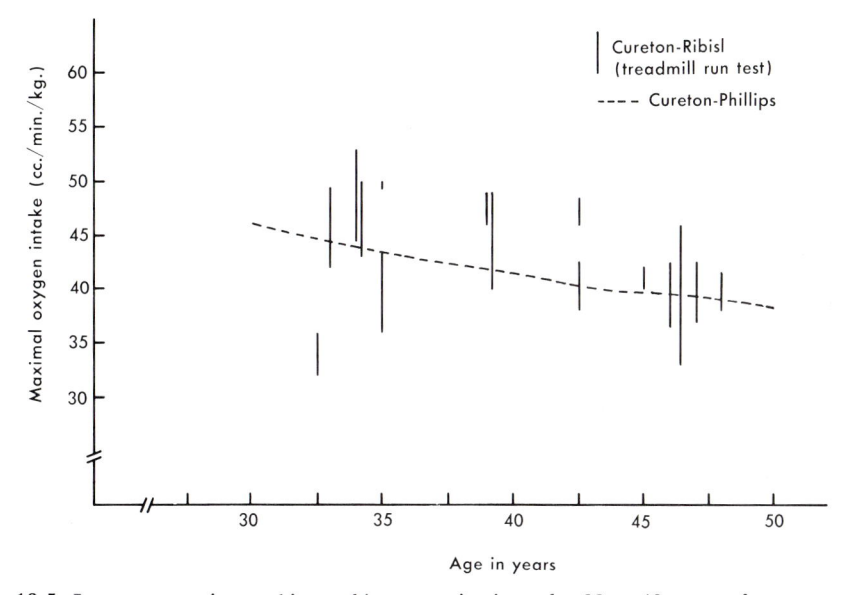

Fig. 18-5. Improvement in aerobic working capacity in males 33 to 48 years of age.

the first two months, the improvement was from 17:42.1 to 14:41.5, an average reduction in time of approximately 3 minutes. Concomitantly the improvement in "peak" oxygen intake was from 40.12 to 45.54 ml./kg./min., a statistically significant difference greater than the .01 level. Other significant changes were in maximum pulmonary ventilation (13.9 liters/min.), and in maximal oxygen pulse (2.13 ml./beat). Each of these measures normally declines with advancing age, so the improvements may be interpreted as "reversing the aging trend."

## POSITIVE PHYSICAL FITNESS—PRACTICAL DYNAMIC HEALTH RULES
### The health values of exercise

Science is coping with the problems of exploding population, adulteration and staleness of foods, and only 4 percent of the adult population exercising enough (Gallup Poll) to do any real good. But research has rolled on in the past 20 years; there have accumulated many studies showing the health value of exercise, in terms of better flexibility and balance, better strength and agility, and better endurance and circulatory-respiratory fitness (athletic power excepted). In several recent works the value of progressive, relatively hard, high calorie type exercise is documented.* One report, summarized in the world congress at Hanover (1966), reports various studies which show the value of proper exercise to develop increased general resistance to fatigue, irradiation, cold and heat, and even nervous irritation.[30] Studies have also shown that anxiety (which can kill) can be minimized[23, 31] and mental depression reduced and virtually prevented as long as the fitness program is applied. Physical fitness programs in the field of mental health are making much use of exercise work and balanced (paced) living.[32]

There are many short-term (3 to 9 month) studies, and a few of longer duration (8 years) that show impressive psychologic and physiologic benefits, sufficient to make it worthwhile.[33, 34] It is also clear that it takes a good deal of work, as much as an hour per day, to get good results—approximating 300 to 500 calories equivalent of work per day for the average sedentary adult.[27, 35] High correlation has been shown between the calories of work per week and the cardiorespiratory ratings; six workouts per week are better than three. Endurance work (long, continued) is better than short, violent efforts; results are better in a relatively cool environment than in a hot environment. Moreover, massage and "isometric" programs have very little effect upon the metabolism and blood fatigue indicators (of stress).[36, 37] Golf and weight lifting are less effective for circulatory-respiratory improvements than jogging or continuous endurance work, interval work, and test-exercises (partly for motivation).[38, 39]

### The positive fitness approach

Physical fitness is the opposite of having many ailments and associated complaints; it is also characterized most by a positive outlook on work and health, with constant seeking of the ways which lead to relatively higher energy, health, and freedom from chronic disease and hypochondriacal complaining. It is also typified by a mental attitude to make a place for exercise and positive living in the scheme of life; a determination to "balance the day" maintains a sound basis of energy for all of the intellectual, social, and business activities of life.

---

*See references 24, 26, 28, and 29.

In physical fitness work the following definite goals are established.[7]
1. To train the body and mind so as to cultivate a greater margin of resistance (stamina, fortitude) to the wearing, tearing, fatiguing influences of life
2. To follow the rules which lead to relatively better adjustment to the stress of work, leading to greater relaxation and relative efficiency in living—to permit getting more work done
3. To check out the body's abilities (balance, flexibility, agility, strength, power, and endurance), knowing that mind and body are one and that one reflects the other; and the taking of tests leads to awareness of weak or failing areas, so that particular protective measures can be followed (a well-developed profile system has been developed by the author)
4. To learn how to exercise in the continuous, rhythmical system: (a) low gear, 30 minutes; (b) middle gear, 45 minutes; (c) high gear, 1 hour with a challenge test; thus building up the calorie expenditure from 100 to 200 to 300 to 500 calories per workout, at least three times per week
5. To be medically examined, immunized, and protected in accordance with modern public health and medical knowledge, including dental examinations
6. To become familiar with the known curves of physical deterioration (and physiologic aging) and to work out ways to resist such deterioration at any age whatever by leading a balanced life and by maintaining good nutrition and a dynamic exercising approach; always persisting to be better than average (which is not very good today)
7. To become aware of "the science of exercise and dynamic health," in addition to doctoring with pills, rest, and medical inspection

Rules for protection are necessary and should be known to all beginners. While it is not generally possible for a medical doctor to tell if one is in danger of dropping dead, or to know if one is really going to exercise too hard, it is best to have a medical examination before taking up a new exercise program if one has been sedentary a number of years or has recently been very sick.

Some rules that have been worked out from experience with middle-aged people in exercise programs are the following.

1. *Warm-up*—take it easy, walk before you run; get up a sweat slowly before exerting violently

2. *Regulation of dosage*—build up the intensity of work from 15 to 20 minutes of warm-up, climb to a peak in the next 30 minutes, and taper off for at least 10 minutes before stopping

3. *Progressively, more and more work*—improvement will depend on doing more and more work as the weeks and months pass

4. *Recuperation*—keep moving but at a slower pace; breathe deeply with forced inhalations; stretch, shake the limbs, and finally take a cold shower

5. *Work all parts of the body*—begin with a walk, then add walking calisthenics movements while walking; then do exercises for the waist, abdomen, and lower back; then add enough jogging or interval training work to reach the 300 to 500 calorie level after a few weeks

6. *Heart protection*—get a medical examination and put an electrocardiogram on file, and other cardiovascular tests if possible; avoid sudden, violent exertions; always observe the warm-up rule

7. *Deep breathing with forced exhalation*—throughout the exercise itself, take

long deep breaths and force them out a bit harder than normal; this helps the pulmonary circulation

8. *Use of fat, fuel*—work moderately for a long time, as all endurance exercisers do (5 calories per minute × 60 minutes = 300 calories); the longer the work, the more fuel burned

9. *Eliminate defective areas*—do not tolerate poor scores in balance, flexibility, agility, strength, power, or endurance; work to do something remedial for any such inadequacy

10. *Posture*—depends upon strength enough to resist gravity pull; the posture muscles should be strengthened: neck, shoulder retractors, abdominal retractors, glutei (to hold pelvis in position), and foot supinators

11. *Flexibility*—practice flexibility (stretching) of any tired muscle; fight off the aging tendency to lose flexibility in all joints

12. *Strength*—may be improved by working at hard or fast work, and also by using resistance devices to use muscles to at least half their maximal strength capacity

13. *Circulation*—the key to middle-aged fitness; depends upon enough rhythmical, continuous movement; good exercises include walking, swimming, cycling, skating, skiing, dancing, and continuous rhythmical calisthenics for at least an hour per day

14. *Use your own muscles*—avoid passive procedures, such as massage and heat treatments, and all types of machines that do the work for you

15. *Time of workout*—is best on an empty stomach, 3 to 4 hours after the last meal; there may be some advantage to exercising at midday, to break the tension of a long indoor day

16. *Take cool baths*—take cool baths except just before going to bed; these are best after a good workout when body heat is up; view the fitness bath as an adjunct to the exercise and as exercise in itself

17. *Fortify the diet*—in hard exercise, there is abnormal use of vitamins C and $B_1$ and some proteins, and more fuel in general; so it may be advantageous to fortify the diet with these as extra vitamins; and use more vegetable and nut oil fats rather than fried (hard) fat, as the typical diet is deficient in polyunsaturated oils and may also be deficient in iodine[79]

18. *Protective foods*—include abundant amounts of red, yellow, and green vegetables in the diet

19. *Check and clean teeth*—needed regularly to forestall decay, uncleanliness, bad breath and to emphasize prevention

20. *Recreational diversions*—are needed to balance the life, to live in a rhythm of work, rest, nutrition, relaxation, and diversion; an alternation of work and play is needed for relaxation and to prevent mental staleness

21. *Never give up*—no matter how old, never give up; there is always a way

## PHYSICAL DETERIORATION (UNFITNESS) IS THE GREATEST DISEASE
### The evidence that deterioration disease is the greatest disease

The greatest disease, so far relatively ineffectually treated, in American society today is deterioration disease. It can be reduced by sufficient exercise, obeying the rules of health, avoiding exposure and contamination, and adopting a reasonable and balanced regimen of life. The curves of deterioration turn downward at about

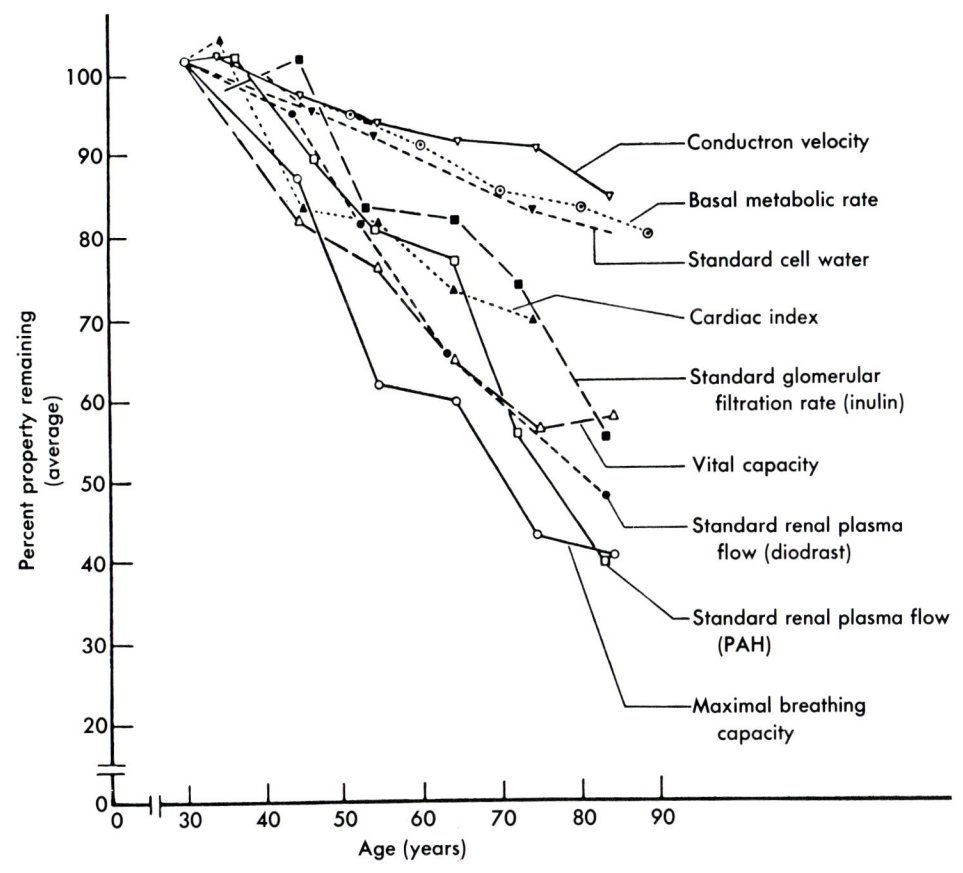

Fig. 18-6. Deterioration of physical fitness tests with age. (From Starr and Wood: Circulation 23:714-732, 1961.)

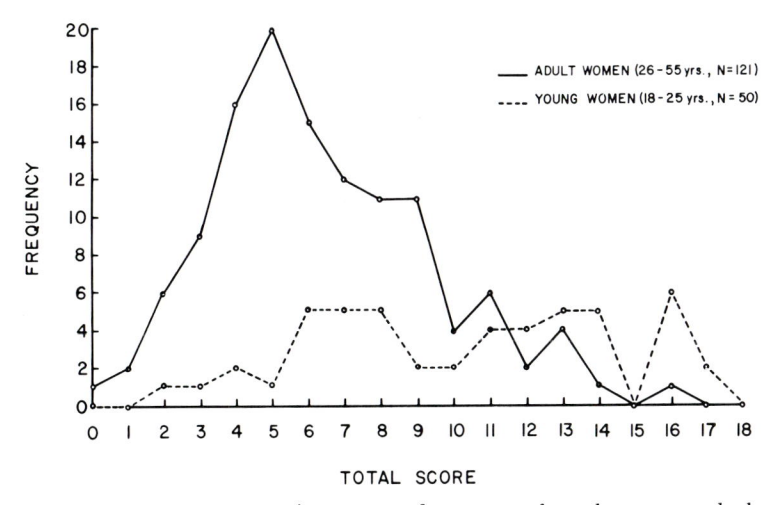

Fig. 18-7. Eighteen-item motor efficiency test—frequency of total scores made by women. (From Physical Fitness Research Laboratory, University of Illinois, Urbana.)

26 to 30 years of life in almost every important parameter of health. Circulation, for instance, deteriorates about 60 percent from 18 to 36 years of age as determined by Geiger counter tests made on workers in an aviation plant (25 to 10 c.c. per unit of muscle mass).[40] The physiologic age of the heart has been calculated by Starr and Wood[8] (Fig. 18-6) at the University of Pennsylvania; almost all of the circulatory-respiratory items follow the downward trend of the vigor of the heart stroke tested by the ballistocardiogram method. I demonstrated with 2200 men and 660 women that the all-around performance ability by the 18-Item Motor Test[7] improved in youth, leveled off between 14 and 25 years of age in the adolescence period, and deteriorated after 26 years of age[41] (Fig. 18-7). The heart stroke depends considerably upon the condition of the heart in terms of nutritive state, nervous sympathetic stimulation through the accelerator nerves, which are more active in the trained state compared to the sedentary state, and activity of the hormones from the adrenal glands. Persistent endurance exercise induces a larger heart stroke and a greater minute volume of blood flow.[42] Even the deterioration of the peripheral nerve propagation speed has been shown to parallel the blood flow and the flow of plasma through the kidneys.[43] The loss of energy that accompanies aging is pitiful, although it is reversible to some considerable extent through the physical fitness process, which is my fundamental thesis. Nathan W. Shock[43] of the government's aging center has documented the declining curves of energy and fitness tests, and there are now many research studies showing the reversal of these same items by physical training and improved nutritional processes.[45, 46] The physiologic aging of the body can be prevented to an extent of 50 to 80 percent of the amount of deterioration if one devotes himself to an adequate program.

### Poor physical fitness, aging, poor nutrition, and ecologic maladjustment are intertwined

Poor fitness has many causes, including aging, poor nutrition, and ecologic maladjustment or maladaptation. Unfitness is caused by lack of vigorous physical activity, gluttony, nervous tension (leading to overeating, overdrinking, oversmoking), lowered resistance because of poor nutrition (lack of protective foods high in vitamins C, P, K, and E), lack of vitaminization in general, lack of balance in foods, or lack of one or more of the seven major food groups. It cannot be said that chronologic aging alone is the cause of rapid deterioration after 25 years of age; the percentage of body fat rises steadily from 25 to 55 years of age from 10 to 30 percent in American business men.[47] A projection of the "trained" $O_2$ intake data to the base axis strikes the base axis at 120 years whereas, otherwise, with many detrimental influences at work and poor living habits in general being the prevalent social custom in overcrowded cities, the actual curve strokes the base axis at approximately 72.

People do not have to live in smog areas but they do, and little is done to correct the situation in Los Angeles, Chicago, or New York. London has made better progress. Most people settle for pretty low fitness standards and know very little about such standards for endurance, for circulation, for resistance to chronic ailments, or even for physical ability. Television, automobiles, the overabundant news media, the "spectatoritis" everywhere, lead to poor health; then the majority turn to tranquilizers, or even more potent drugs or alcohol to restore their health. It is all a bit pitiful and ridiculous! The morale for healthful vigor fades away in pursuit of wealth and position, or complete capitulation to destructive social habits (parties, gambling, knitting bees or drinking away the little spare time available). Most of the unfitness is cultivated. Improvement of living habits is the need. Let's not blame so much of it on our ancestors or our government. The important thing is the understanding of each person and his individual resolve to do something about it.

Poor nutrition is prevalent and almost everyone has nutritional deficiencies; many are just cultivated in terms of taste and habit rather than careful scientific governance. The mode, especially among women, is to "diet," which means semistarvation; yet the classic semistarvation data show that heavy penalties are paid in reduced vigor, failure of the heart, loss of hair, lowered resistance to the elements and stresses in general, and low-grade sex life.[48, 49] In young children poor nutrition stunts the growth of the brain, and in adults it leads to low morale for fitness and gradual withdrawal from vigorous activity. The healthiest people eat well and exercise relatively hard. Excessive smoking, alcohol, and semistarvation and/or lack of nutritional balance hurt human efficiency, and tensions mount. It is recognized in the area of mental health that vitamin B complex plays a very important role, and even schizophrenia has been overcome by massive doses of vitamins; but deficiencies are correlative with being forgetful, irritable, quarrelsome, apathetic, confused, restless, and anxious.[50, 51]

Recent testimony before Congress by representatives of the American Medical Association indicated that if people would only exercise, keep as slim as reasonable for their body type, reduce the excesses of eating, smoking, and drinking, and carefully regulate weight, they would extend longevity by ten years at least and probably even more if the progress in immunization continues. We emphasize health appraisal and sufficient exercise.[52]

McFarland, of the Harvard School of Public Health, has drawn a powerful case for the progressive choking off of the body's oxygen supply as a theory of aging, even more logical than just wearing out of cytoplasm or progressive intestinal putrefaction as aging theories.[21] There is a progressive decline of maximal oxygen intake as determined by Robinson[53] from childhood to old age, and Dill and Ross have followed the decline of this test for 30 years in a group of top runners, to find that the ones who kept up their running and strenuous exercises of the endurance type the most declined the least in the test, and vice versa.[54]

A most important angle is how people feel. A typical statement is, "I do not feel like exercising, nor do I have time, but my experience has been that I always feel better for hours afterward, and my conscience is relieved, as I know that I need it." If oxygen is pressured into the body, dramatic improvements result in the feeling tone and mental functioning of older people.[55]

Relief from chronic ailments is being studied more fully. Undoubtedly this is an immediately experienced practical benefit in the experience of most, as various testimonial studies show. Letounov,[56] Mateef,[57] and Zimkin and Korobkov[30] have put forth data to show the protective and preserving value of systematic physical training.

Many types of benefits are claimed, such as relief from mental depression and relief from insomnia and worry. Anxiety seems to be reduced in most who consistently follow fitness programs. Gross change of body shape is an unsound view, as extreme dieting may do damage; it is best to regulate weight by exercise. Jokl[11] states that there is no validity to the fact that extremely virulent infections are pre-

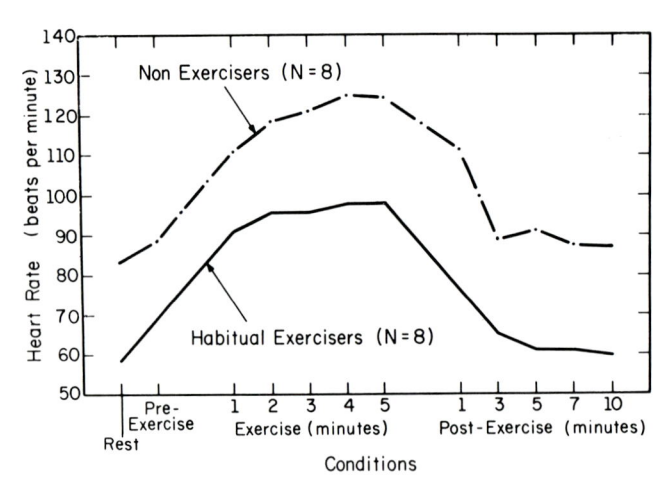

**Fig. 18-8.** Changes in heart rate during exercise. (Jette and Cureton, 1969.)

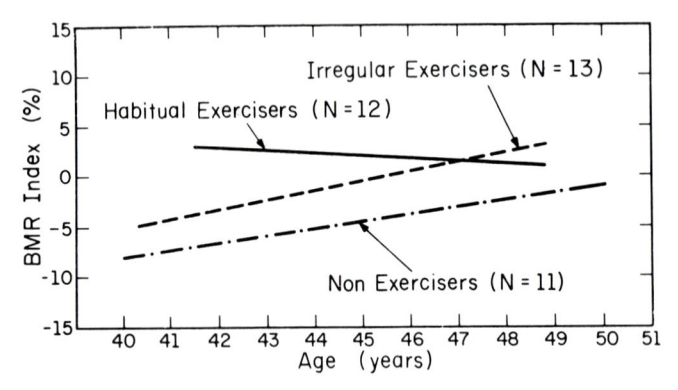

**Fig. 18-9.** Changes with age in BMR index. (Jette and Cureton, 1969.)

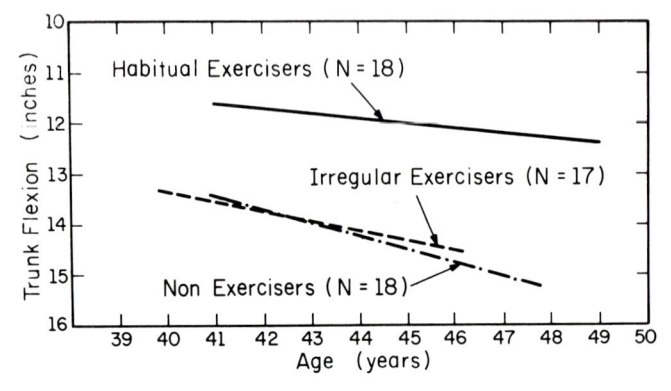

**Fig. 18-10.** Changes with age in trunk flexion. (Jette and Cureton, 1969.)

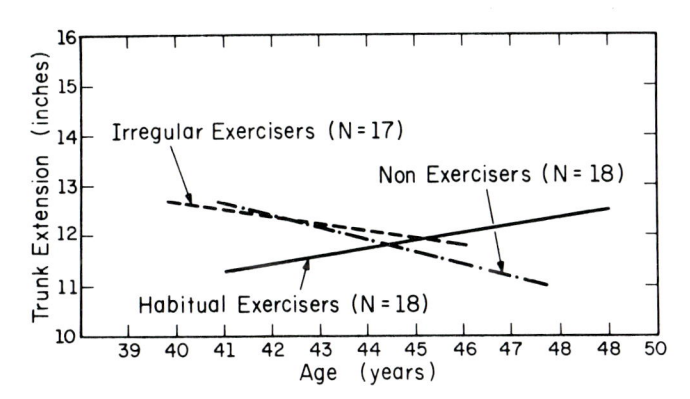

Fig. 18-11. Changes with age in trunk extension. (Jette and Cureton, 1969.)

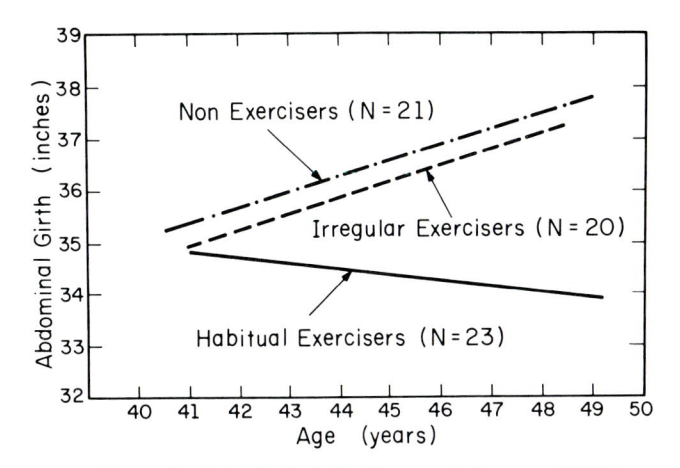

Fig. 18-12. Changes with age in abdominal girth. (Jette and Cureton, 1969.)

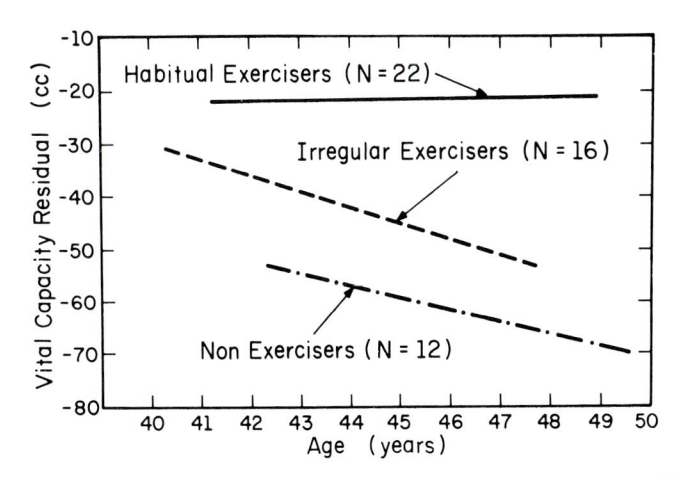

Fig. 18-13. Changes with age in vital capacity residual. (Jette and Cureton, 1969.)

vented or eliminated by exercise, but the natural immunity that exists in some people is so far unexplained with any exactness. Sufficient exposure can result in an infection even in the fittest person.

Older people apparently need more exercise than they get. There is now experimentation in gerontologic institutions on this, but the results are not fully in; however, improved psychologic attitudes and perceptions are reported.[59, 60] It is certainly true that people over 60 years of age can be physically trained to their great improvement in motor fitness, circulatory fitness, and confidence.[61, 62] More and more research will develop in this area. Older people do not live or die by their strength but much more by whether they will develop blood clots or not. Even in this area, exercise has been shown to reduce the tendency to cramps (intermittent claudication) and blood clots.[63] Spieth[64] points out that the functional decline is not caused by genuine aging. While there are marked physiologic and psychologic deteriorations observable in many adults after 35 years of age, these seem to be reversible to some real extent in as short a period as 8 weeks, although longer and higher calorie level

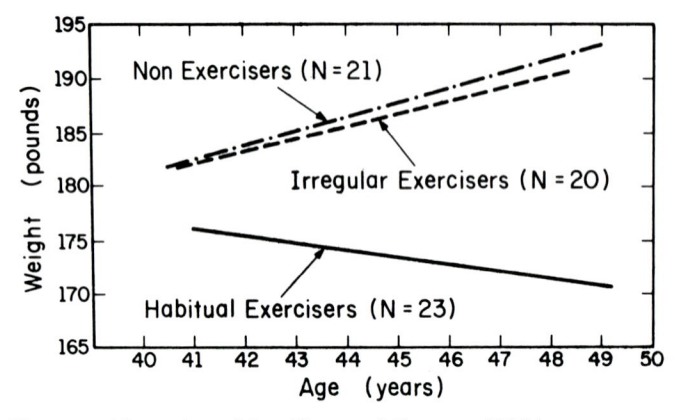

Fig. 18-14. Changes with age in weight. (Jette and Cureton, 1969.)

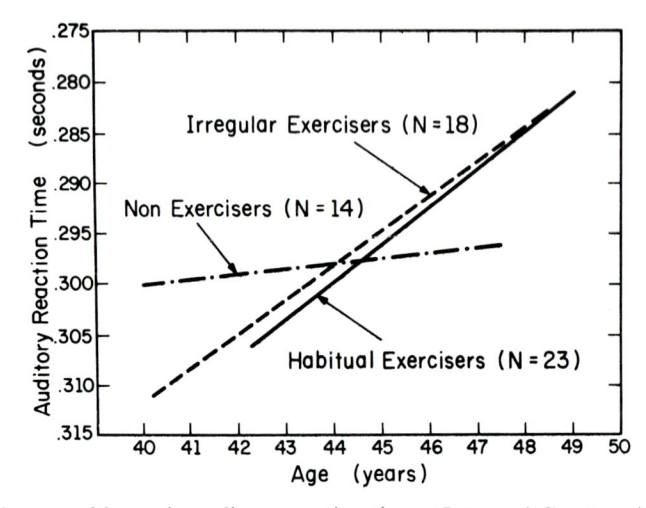

Fig. 18-15. Changes with age in auditory reaction time. (Jette and Cureton, 1969.)

work show more impressive improvements.[33] An inspirational theme is "creative aging," the title of Bortz' book in which he makes it plain that there are many factors at work to destroy man, but "the therapy of work" is put forth as a great positive force which should be more fully used.

## HOW MUCH EXERCISE IS ENOUGH? WHAT IS THE BEST PROGRAM FOR A BUSY PROFESSIONAL MAN?
### The variety of programs; some are dangerous

There are many programs but there is no easy way, and no machine or other person can do the work for you. It will take time, patience, and unusual understanding and devotion to succeed. But if you are persistent, it will pay great dividends; there will be protection in some degree from dehydration, shrinkage, and loss of mobility that accompany physiologic aging.

It takes 2 to 3 months to induct an "out of condition" adult into an hour of exercise per day with safety and with reasonably good physical and mental adjustments to the work. The introduction should be "nonheroic" in that all extreme "show-off" exercises or competitions should be carefully avoided. The work load should be relatively low and cautiously approached in the first few weeks for an "out of condition" person. In this low gear stage the work should be easy, rhythmic, and always done with adequate breathing. The aim should be to work the whole body over thoroughly with moderate effort exercises and considerable rhythmic (repeated) stretching. There should be avoidance of extreme breathlessness, tensions, or super-strength efforts.

The fact that quite a few people die from shovelling snow or carrying objects that are very heavy for longer than a minute is well known. The fact is also known that moderately paced walking or swimming, cycling, and rhythmic activity in general are quite harmless. High speed and power efforts may cause minute ruptures in the muscles, especially "shin-splints" in the forelegs, and minute ruptures in the shoulder ligaments. Older people usually do better by themselves, in a self-motivated program, not led by young, fit leaders, nor should they try to keep up with any unusual motivation scheme until they are quite fit. No highly motivated scheme is safe for men over 35 years of age.

Every 2 or 3 months the work should be gradually increased, meaning more and more total work; attention should be paid to elements of balance, flexibility, strength, power, and endurance. Jogging alone is not enough. Every part of the body should be conditioned, and the various parts are very specific in their needs. No oversimplified scheme of a few minutes per day, such as 6 seconds per day, will work, considering the metabolic needs, circulation, and total calories.

Begin by walking for a month or two, then add in addition a simple set of exercises to use each major part of the body[80] (Fig. 18-16). Some exercises can be performed by a beginner in about 30 minutes. It is not enough but it is important not to go too hard, to do the exercises slowly at first, and to learn them properly. Then after the "first month" set gets rather easy, progress to do two for each part of the body. This will take about 45 minutes. When this gets relatively easy, then do three for each part of the body and progress downward through the sheet doing all three columns in about an hour. Do them faster than before if you feel up to it.[80]

Then you should join a class led by a competent instructor if this is possible. If it is not, then you can arrange for a demonstration of low gear, middle gear, and

# CURETON'S PROGRAM OF DAILY RHYTHMIC EXERCISES FOR BODY CONDITIONING

| BODY SEGMENT AND PRINCIPAL MUSCLE GROUPS USED | EASY EXERCISES FOR FIRST MONTH | MODERATE EXERCISES FOR SECOND MONTH | HARD EXERCISES FOR THIRD MONTH AND LATER | ALLOTTED TIME |
|---|---|---|---|---|
| NECK, SHOULDERS, UPPER BACK AND CHEST; NECK AND SHOULDER RETRACTORS, ARM ELEVATORS AND CHEST ELEVATORS | Standing, arms extended along sides, flex arms to chest. Rhythmically swing arms downward, forward, upward over head, as far back as possible. With upward motion, take a deep breath, fill lungs with air and stretch chest. | Standing, swing both arms across the front of the body in full arm circles. Rhythmically rise on the balls of the feet with each upward movement of the arms, taking regular full, deep breaths. | Standing with legs wide apart, alternately cross over arms, touching hand as far as possible to the floor outside of foot. Whip arm back and forth. While doing exercise, suck in and blow out air forcefully. | Perform each set of exercises for 5 minutes, breathing deeply. Rest, take 10 full breaths, then start exercises for next muscle group. |
| BACK REGION, BUTTOCKS AND UPPER LEGS; HAMSTRINGS, GLUTEI AND SACROSPINALIS | Lying on stomach with hands tucked under the thighs and with back arched and head up, flutter-kick continuously, moving the legs 8 to 10 inches apart. Kick from the hips with a slight bend in the knees. | Two exercises: 1) Back toward floor, supporting body on hands and heels, whip midsection up and down in rapid movement. 2) Lying on stomach with hands behind the neck, arch body, raising chest and legs off the floor 15 times. | Lying on stomach with hands behind neck, exercise in four counts: a) arch back, legs and chest off floor; b) extend arms fully forward; c) return hands to neck; d) flatten body to floor and relax one second. Repeat exercise 15 times. | Perform each set of exercises for 5 minutes, breathing deeply. Rest, take 10 full breaths, then start exercises for next muscle group. |
| ABDOMINAL REGION; THIGH FLEXORS, QUADRICEPS AND ABDOMINALS | Two exercises: 1) Kneeling on both hands and knees, inhale, pull knee toward floor, then suck in abdomen toward the spine—hold for a few seconds. 2) Sitting, alternately raise right and left knees toward the chest. | Two exercises: 1) Lying on back, raise legs to vertical position, then slowly lower them to the floor 20 times. 2) In four counts: a) raise legs 18 inches; b) spread legs apart; c) return legs together; d) lower legs to floor. 20 times. | Two exercises lying on back: 1) Raise legs to vertical position, then slowly lower them to the floor 20 times. 2) In four counts: a) raise legs 18 inches; b) spread legs apart; c) return legs together; d) lower legs to floor. 20 times. | Perform each set of exercises for 5 minutes, breathing deeply. Rest, take 10 full breaths, then start exercises for next muscle group. |
| WAIST AND SIDES OF THE BODY; LATERAL MUSCLES OF THE TRUNK AND LEGS | Lying full length, right side of the body on the floor, whip left leg up and down in rapid motion 12 inches as high as possible. Repeat exercise with left side of body down, raising right leg off floor 50 times. | Lying full length, right side of the body on the floor, whip left leg up and down in rapid motion as high as possible. Repeat exercise with left side of body down, raising right leg off floor 30 times. | With right side of body down, rigidly supported off floor by extended right arm and foot, raise left leg up to horizontal and down 30 times. Repeat exercise with left side of body, raising right leg off the floor 30 times. | Perform each set of exercises for 5 minutes, breathing deeply. Rest, take 10 full breaths, then start exercises for next muscle group. |
| HANDS, ARMS AND SHOULDERS; ARM EXTENSORS AND FLEXORS AND ENTIRE SHOULDER GIRDLE | Two exercises: 1) Lying on back, grasp one knee and while resisting with hip muscle, pull knee toward chest. Repeat exercise with other knee. 2) With chest down, resting on both hands, do full-length push-ups to 10 times. | Two exercises: 1) Chest down, resting on both hands, do full-length push-ups up to 20 times or more. 2) Chin the bar, lifting body weight off the floor, 10 times. | Two exercises: 1) Chest down, resting on both hands, do full-length push-ups up to 20 times or more. 2) Chin the bar, lifting body weight off the floor, 12 times or more. | Perform each set of exercises for 5 minutes, breathing deeply. Rest, take 10 full breaths, then start exercises for next muscle group. |
| FEET, LEGS AND ANKLES; ARCH SUPPORTERS, FOOT SUPINATORS, FOOT EXTENSORS, LEG EXTENSORS AND THIGH EXTENSORS | Three exercises: 1) Walk in circle on outside edges of feet. 2) Facing wall, lean forward, hands on wall, and push up and down on toes. 3) In extended push-up position, feet pointed in, bounce body weight on ankles to stretch joints. | Hop on both feet up to 100 times; change to straddle hop, up to 100 times; change to alternate stride hop, up to 100 times; hop on right foot 50 times; hop on left foot 25 times. | Hop on both feet 200 times; change to straddle hop, 200 times; change to alternate stride hop, 200 times; do up to 50 full-squat jumps, touching fingers to floor each time and springing 4 inches to upright position. | Perform each set of exercises for 5 minutes, breathing deeply. Rest, take 10 full breaths, then start exercises for next muscle group. |
| CIRCULATORY AND RESPIRATORY ENDURANCE; ARMS, LEGS, TORSO AND HEART, BLOOD VESSELS AND LUNGS | Walk one mile each day, taking long strides and deep breaths. Or swim, cycle, row, bowl, skate, ski, dance, play handball, golf or any other activity to use the various muscle groups, increase efficiency and develop endurance. | Walk-jog-walk-run-walk 2 miles each day. Or swim, cycle, row, bowl, skate, ski, dance, play handball, golf or any other activity which puts various muscles of the body to test, increases agility and develops greater | Walk a mile, run a mile, walk 1/4 mile, sprint 200 yards and walk 1/2 mile each day; breathe deeply, stretch chest. Or, to develop maximum motor ability and endurance, strenuously engage in an activity described at left. | Do above exercises for 30 minutes to warm up specific muscles. Then add exercises for endurance, including walking or game (left) for 30 minutes. |

O-1435

**Fig. 18-16.** Cureton's program of daily rhythmic exercises for body conditioning. (From White, W. H.: Exercise to keep fit, Health, January 17, 1955.)

high gear progression. Beginners do only low gear; people of average ability do low gear and middle gear; and people who have been accustomed to training may do low, middle, and high gear all in the same workout period to guarantee a gradual buildup with proper graduated warm-up.

The program should be varied to include balance, flexibility, agility, strength, power, and endurance tests and exercises. Self-tests can easily be learned.[68]

Perhaps something is better than nothing but there are many advertised schemes and devices which do not work, and they usually fall far short of what is needed on a calorie basis: vibration devices, motorized equipment, isometric devices and exercises, and heat exposure methods, light treatments, and massage. Usually these produce inadequate physiologic effects. Rollers, vibrators, and weight resistance devices should be considered adjunctive to the full use of one's own muscles in a way to increase the circulation and metabolic cost week to week in a progressive way. The same submaximal program, done day by day in the same way, will not produce satisfactory results. The level sought is a factor to consider but top athletes are typically putting in 2 to 5 hours per day to achieve top fitness. Many people in the world work all day long at hard work, as do coal miners, farmers, and many types of laborers, and have fewer heart attacks.

The best program for the white-collar sedentary worker is a gradually progressive rhythmic type program and not games. The latter are too intermittent, too infrequently played, and require such an amount of time for organization and officiating that few adults can participate enough to get fit, although some games like handball, tennis, and soccer are very good when played several times per week. Even then the games do not produce the circulatory-respiratory fitness that characterizes the endurance running, swimming, rowing, cycling, skating, skiing, and dancing.[37, 65-68]

Gradually one might take self-testing stunts, and learn to check up on many types of fitness. There *are* many types of fitness, and most are quite specific. Fat is not a measure of flexibility; nor is strength a measure of circulatory-respiratory fitness; nor is balance a measure of endurance. The greatest need for most overweight adults is to work long enough at moderate exercise, in a continuous or interval training manner to work off 300 to 500 calories of body heat per day. This takes approximately an hour. Several shorter programs have been found to be lacking from this calorie cost point of view, and several of the more statical (on the spot) tensing type programs are also found to be deficient in inducing much circulatory-respiratory fitness. Table 18-3 shows the standard score improvements obtained from various experimental programs completed under my supervision at the University of Illinois. At the top are the tests used for evaluation; the subheadings at the side name the researcher and also the type of program followed during the time of the study (usually 4 to 6 months of participation). It is seen from this table that swimming and endurance training (jogging) are best, done in a progressive athletic training way. The Health Walker (by Battle Creek Equipment Company) is good too; walk uphill on the portable treadmill for 30 minutes five days per week. Thirty minutes of volleyball and 30 minutes of calisthenics, or vice versa, are fairly good. Handball and physical activity (mixed calisthenics, jogging, and a game) are intermediate. Weight lifting, prescribed exercise, and volleyball are only fair.

Some improvement can be made with only a walking program or with 3 to 15 minutes of "brisk" running in place along with a few calisthenics exercises, done faster and a bit longer as time goes along.

**Table 18-3.** *Rank of physical activities for improving middle-aged men (26-60 years)*

| Rank | Activity | Time spent (days/week) | Number tests averaged | S.S. average improvement | Weeks of training |
|---|---|---|---|---|---|
| 1 | Progressive swimming training | 1 hr./day 5/wk. | 8 | 21.37 | 10 |
| 2 | Nonstop running 10 miles/hr. | 30 min. 5/wk. | 7 | 20.43 | 10 |
| 3 | Battle Creek Health Walker (14 percent grade) | 30 min. 5/wk. | 8 | 20.20 | 8 |
| 4 | Calisthenics and volleyball | 30 min. 3/wk. | 6 | 11.57 | 16 |
| 5 | Handball | 50 min. 3/wk. | 7 | 11.26 | 24 |
| 6 | Mixed volleyball and conditioning exercises | 50 min. 3/wk. | 7 | 10.91 | 16 |
| 7 | Rowing machine | 15 min. 5/wk. | 8 | 8.62 | 8 |
| 8 | Prescribed exercises | 60 min. 5/wk. | 7 | 8.53 | 20 |
| 9 | Weight lifting | 50 min. 4/wk. | 7 | 7.54 | 10 |
| 10 | Mixed gym work | 1 hour 3/wk. | 10 | 5.70 | 20 |
| 11 | Mixed instructional swimming | 1½ hrs. 5/wk. | 4 | 4.84 | 5 |
| 12 | Badminton | 50 min. 3/wk. | 5 | 0.91 | 16 |
| 13 | Weight lifting (13 lifts) | 50 min. 3/wk. | 2 | −2.59 | 16 |
| 14 | Mixed alternating individual exercise (squash, calisthenics, swim) | 1 hr./day 5/wk. | 6 | −6.83 | 8 |
| 15 | Volleyball | 50 min. 3/wk. | 10 | −7.90 | 20 |

*in cardiovascular fitness tests*

| Research study | Number of subjects | Net estimated calories per workout | Calories per week | Fat change | Change in maximal O$_2$ intake |
|---|---|---|---|---|---|
| Nakamura (1951) | 1 | 500 | 2500 | 90 to 75 mm. 73 to 85 S.S. (12 S.S.) | |
| Kristufek (1951) | 1 | 400 | 2000 | 130 to 108 mm. 55 to 66 S.S. (11 S.S.) | 48 to 69 c.c./min./Kg. 1.81 to 2.42 L./min. 40 to 55 S.S. |
| Herden (1956) | 4 | 300 | 1500 | Av. of cheeks and rear thigh (10.8 S.S.) | |
| Hopkins (1951) | 16 | 200 | 600 | 0 | |
| Bryant (1950) | 9 | 240 | 720 | Not taken | |
| Herkimer (1949) | 12 | 300 to 500 | 900 to 1500 | 9.4 S.S. | |
| Domke (1955) | 3 | 225 | 1125 | 5.33 S.S. | |
| Wolfson (1949) | 9 | 200 | 1000 | 8.0 S.S. | |
| Brodt (1950) | 6 | 100 | 400 | Gained 4.5 mm. 0 S.S. | |
| Wells (1950) | 10 | 200 | 600 | −3 S.S. | |
| Harrison (1950) | 8 | 100 | 750 | 0 | |
| Sterling (1956) | 22 | 100 | 300 | 0 | |
| Wilson (1947) | 16 | 100 | 300 | Not taken | |
| Campney (1953) | 1 | 200 | 1000 | 110.3 to 94 mm. 65 to 75 S.S. (10 S.S.) | 2.57 to 2.43 L./min. (−3 S.S.) |
| Wolbers (1949) | 9 | 100 | 300 | 163 to 156 mm. 37 to 39 S.S. (2 S.S.) | |

Table 18-4 compared a vibrating table, an exercycle, and a resistance bicycle with free exercise (jogging and calisthenics mixed), 30 minutes per day, three days per week. The data are for middle-aged women. The calorie cost progresses from left to right across the table, the jogging mixed with free exercises being the best (most calorie expenditure). Of course, these figures can be increased for men doing the exercises more vigorously, but even so the energy expenditure is small, compared with many other known and tested programs. A first level of evaluation is to show that the pulse rate is reduced; a second level of evaluation is to show that the stroke volume (by heartograph) area is increased, and the diastolic blood pressure after 1 and 6 minutes of exercise is lowered after 8, 12, 16, 20, and 24 weeks of practice (progressive pulse ratio test with blood pressures); and a third level of evaluation would involve a loss of fat and "fat weight" and a gain in lean body mass, and lowered triglycerides (blood fat) and possibly lower cholesterol values, and better endurance tests (five-minute step test, 14 inches for women and 17 inches for men, with blood pressures taken before and after the test; or a mile run and/or 5-item muscular endurance test).

In research accomplished, golf is considered much overrated as a fitness program.[38] Social activities like bowling, social dancing, bowling on the green, quoits, deck tennis, shuffleboard, and similar low calorie recreations have been shown to contribute little to reduction of lipids or the development of heart force and other circulatory-respiratory and metabolic needs.

The objection to Canadian 5-BX and 10-BX (BX = Basic Exercise) is not the exercises but to the low total calories of work. Energy cost values are given in Table 18-7. Normally progression should be from light (low gear) to moderate (middle gear) to heavy (high gear) exercises.

In Cureton's Progressive Exercise Series the approximate calorie cost value is the following.[37]

1. *Low gear*—av. 1.693 Liters/min. of oxygen
    30 min. work totaling 108.3 calories (net)
    Total of 216.6 calories per hour
2. *Middle gear*—av. 1.693 Liters/min. oxygen
    380.9 cal. (net) for 45 min.
    482.2 cal. per hour
3. *High gear*—av. 2.38 Liters/min. oxygen
    706 calories per min. for full hour

If the same amount of work is done day after day, week after week, month after month, and this averages less than 200 calories, the result will surely be disappointing. In such submaximal work there will be quite typically statistically insignificant changes in critical fitness tests such as maximal oxygen intake capacity, basal metabolic rate (which improves in very unfit people), muscular endurance, and reduction of fat, triglycerides, and cholesterol in the blood serum. Nor are the changes in heart force or velocity or acceleration at all impressive. However, changes in balance, flexibility, and agility may come readily from playing games. Harder work is usually required to improve strength, power, and speed. Long work, an hour per day (20 minutes of warm-up, plus 30 minutes of progressively harder work toward or to the "peak," plus 10 minutes taper-down work), is needed to influence the lipids, which have more to do with longevity, long-range health, and youthfulness than do skill and strength.

Table 18-4. *Metabolic analysis of four types of exercises*

| Average of four women | Vibrating table N = 4 ||| Exercycle N = 4 (relaxed, without resistance) |||| Resistance bicycle N = 4 |||| Free exercise N = 4 ||||
|---|---|---|---|---|---|---|---|---|---|---|---|---|---|---|---|
| | Quiet | Exercise | Recovery | Quiet | Exercise | Recovery | | Quiet | Exercise | Recovery | | Quiet | Exercise | Recovery | |
| R. Q. | .77 | .79 | .80 | .86 | .88 | .87 | | .89 | .99 | 1.06 | | .85 | 1.03 | 1.10 | |
| Uncorrected | | | | | | | | | | | | | | | |
| Ventilation—total | 30.85 | 34.25 | 37.72 | 42.55 | 78.30 | 70.39 | | 51.98 | 153.49 | 116.38 | | 54.41 | 192.5 | 117.5 | |
| Ventilation—L./min. | 3.09 | 3.43 | 3.20 | 4.26 | 7.83 | 4.69 | | 5.20 | 23.17 | 8.86 | | 5.44 | 30.05 | 10.14 | |
| True $O_2$ | 4.74 | 4.43 | 4.68 | 3.82 | 4.42 | 3.84 | | 3.41 | 4.38 | 3.13 | | 4.00 | 4.12 | 3.36 | |
| $CO_2$ | 3.64 | 3.51 | 3.78 | 3.31 | 3.77 | 3.35 | | 3.09 | 4.41 | 3.32 | | 3.39 | 4.11 | 3.43 | |
| Net $O_2$ L./min. | .123 | .016 | −.0002 | .136 | .150 | .037 | | .150 | .740 | .118 | | .190 | .895 | .107 | |
| Net $O_2$ L./min./kg. | .0082 | −.0001 | −.0001 | .0022 | .0024 | .0003 | | .0022 | .0112 | .0018 | | .0028 | .0132 | .0016 | |
| Net calories | | | | | | | | | | | | | | | |
| Cal./hr./kg. | .584 | −.044 | .002 | .632 | .707 | .096 | | .668 | 3.38 | .432 | | .796 | 3.86 | .477 | |
| Cal./hr./$M^2$ | 21.57 | 1.55 | .06 | 24.02 | 26.69 | 3.67 | | 25.94 | 130.68 | 16.49 | | 30.92 | 126.38 | 18.55 | |
| Pulse rate | 68.5 | 68. | 71. | 87. | 94. | 88. | | 91. | 131. | 107. | | 76. | 123. | 98. | |
| Systolic B.P. | 124.6 | 127.4 | 125.8 | 119. | 126. | 122. | | 116. | 144. | 112. | | 116. | 155. | 123. | |
| Diastolic B.P. | 68.9 | 73. | 72.5 | 68. | 65. | 70. | | 71. | 78. | 80. | | 79. | 77. | 78.5 | |
| Pulse pressure | 55.7 | 54.4 | 53.3 | 51. | 61. | 52. | | 45. | 66. | 32. | | 37. | 78. | 44.5 | |
| Total cal. cost | | | | | | | | | | | | | | | |
| Per minute | .013 calories/min. ||| .871 calories/min. |||| 4.24 calories/min. |||| 5.93 calories/min. ||||
| Per hour | 0.78 calories/hr. ||| 52.26 calories/hr. |||| 254.4 calories/hr. |||| 355.8 calories/hr. ||||

*Physical fitness and dynamic health*

422  *Improving dental practice through preventive measures*

**Table 18-5.** *Training effects of health-walker: comparison of the improvements in selected cardiovascular variables with those recorded in various other training programs*

| Name | Type of program | Number of subjects | Brachial pulse wave ||||| Schneider index | Five-minute step test | Barach index |
|------|-----------------|:------------------:|:----:|:------------------:|:-------------------:|:----------------:|:---------------:|:---------------:|:---------------------:|:------------:|
|      |                 |                    | Area | Systolic amplitude | Diastolic amplitude | Diastolic surge | Rest to work ratio |              |                       |              |
| Hopkins   | Volleyball and calisthenics | 16 | 17.88 | 17.88 | 9.31  | 19.5   | −5.44 | 10.31 |         | |
| Wolbers   | Volleyball         | 9  | 2.67  | 4.33  | 3.22  | −4.11  | 1.44  | 7.22  | −22.67  | |
| Harrison  | Swimming           | 8  | 5.5   |       |       |        |       | 3.75  | 5.28    | |
| Domke     | Rowing machine     | 3  | 9.0   | 7.33  | 8.33  | 21.67  |       | −3.0  | 13.33   | 3.67 |
| Bryant    | Handball           | 9  | 7.78  | 12.89 | 20.01 | 10.45  | 3.78  | 12.78 | 11.11   | |
| Kristufek | Endurance training | 1  | 25.0  | 15.0  | 20.0  |        | 40.0  | 12.0  | 18.0    | 13.0 |
| Herden    | Health-walker      | 2  | 20.5  | 15.5  | 25.0  | 28.5   | 20.0  | 16.0  | 19.5    | 16.5 |
| Brodt     | Weight lifting     | 6  | 7.17  | 1.0   | 9.17  | 21.15  | 4.83  | 12.5  | 7.17    | |
| Campney   | Physical activity  | 1  | 3.0   | −2.0  | −1.0  | −39.0  | 0     | 15.0  | −24.0   | |
| Nakamura  | Swimming           | 1  | 37.0  | 34.0  | 40.0  | 5.0    | 9.0   | 20.0  | 20.0    | 6.0 |
| Wolfson   | Prescribed exercise| 9  | 2.11  | 11.33 | 1.0   | 24.44  | .11   | 12.22 |         | |
| Herkimer  | Physical activity  | 12 | 13.5  | 14.17 | 16.83 | 8.58   | 7.83  | 6.67  | 8.8     | |

Note: Average standard score improvement used for comparison.

The improvements in cardiovascular status are very important, judged to be much more so from the point of view of health and longevity, even more than strength. Table 18-5 gives the results of a number of separate studies in which various activities were used to improve cardiovascular fitness. The standard score improvements, as averaged, are given. It is plain that the continuous, rhythmical activities approached in a progressive way, with gradually longer and harder work, produced the best results—swimming, jogging, and mixture of running and calisthenics, 30 minutes or more each workout day. Five days were better generally than 3 days per week.

**Cardiovascular fitness is related to habitual energy output (calories per week)**

Table 18-3 shows that the activity groups which averaged 1500 calories expenditure per week in the activity mentioned averaged out the best in a series of cardiovascular tests; the value given is an average standard score (number of tests aver-

**Table 18-6.** *Caloric expenditure classification of work and exercise*

| 2.5 cal./min. (150 cal./hr.) | 2.5-4.9 cal./min. (150-299 cal./hr.) | 5.0-7.4 cal./min. (300-449 cal./hr.) | 7.5 cal./min. (450 cal./hr.) |
|---|---|---|---|
| *Very light* | *Light* | *Moderate* | *Strenuous* |
| Standing at ease | Personal care | Walking, moderate to fast | Running |
| Lying | Walking slowly | Walking, moderate up-hill | Walking fast up hill |
| Sitting | Standing, using arm movement | | Climbing a ladder |
| Sitting, using arm movements | Housework, except stooping and bending | Housework, stooping and bending | Skiing |
| Reading | | Swimming | Walking in snow |
| Writing | Light gardening | Heavy gardening | Digging |
| Sewing | Driving car or motorcycle | Tennis | Sawing wood |
| Typing | | Dancing (*some may be L or S) | Planing wood |
| Knitting | Golfing | Bicycling | Shoveling |
| Light machine work | Carpentry work | Bowling | Carrying load upstairs |
| Light assembly line | Gymnastic exercises, except hopping | Gymnastic exercises, hopping and swinging arms | Playing football |
| *Talking on phone | Mixing cement | | Chopping with an axe |
| Playing musical instrument (*except organ) | Playing with child | Stacking firewood | Horseback riding |
| | Pee-wee golfing | Using pickaxe | *Iceskating |
| | *Playing organ | Pushing wheelbarrow | *Basketball (some may be L or M) |
| | *Driving go-cart | *Washing car | |
| | *Fair rides | *Washing windows | |
| | *Playing baseball | *Roller skating | |
| | *Playing ping-pong | *Mowing lawn (not motorized) | |
| | | *Moving furniture | |
| | | *Badminton | |
| | | *Lifting weights | |
| | | *Pull-ups | |

Note: 75 steps up are equal to 1 minute of strenuous activity.

Used by Bureau of Nutrition, California State Department of Public Health, in research on obesity and leanness. (Adapted from Passmore and Durnin (Human energy expenditure, Physiol. Rev. 35:801, 1955.)
*Added for School of Public Health research project.

424 *Improving dental practice through preventive measures*

**Table 18-7.** *Energy cost of various physical activities (Physical Fitness Research*

|  | Mowing lawn |||
|  | 1188 sq. ft. (10 min. exercise)—1 grad. student (male) |||
|  | Light rotary power mower | Cylinder hand mower | Heavy rotary power mower |
| --- | --- | --- | --- |
| Subject |  |  |  |
| Age (years) | 26 | 26 | 26 |
| Height (in.) | 72 | 72 | 72 |
| Weight (lb.) | 160 | 160 | 160 |
| Weight (Kg.) | 72.6 | 72.6 | 72.6 |
| $O_2$ intake (net $O_2$ requirement) |  |  |  |
| Liters/min. | 1.639 | 2.227 | 1.947 |
| L./min./Kg. | .0226 | .0307 | .0268 |
| Net calories | 36.82 | 73.85 | 59.10 |
| Cal./min. | 3.68 | 7.39 | 5.91 |
| Cal./hr. (rate) | 220.8 | 443.4 | 354.6 |
| $O_2$ debt (liters) | 0.04 | 0.76 | 1.32 |

*Net $O_2$ intake, exercise.

aged, and average converted to S.S.). The results show that progressive training in swimming ranks at the top (21.37 S.S. improvement), then nonstop running, 30 minutes on the Battle Creek Walker, and mixed calisthenics and volleyball—and the lowest were self-directed participation in mixed sports-exercises three times per week, weight lifting, and badminton.

**Energy cost of adult physical activities**

Tables 18-6 and 18-7 show the energy cost of some activities commonly practiced by adults, as determined partly at my laboratory. The calorie per hour rate varies from 52.62 cal./hr. to 620.5 cal./hr. While there are exceptions for those who really "go after it" the calorie expenditure is extremely small and inadequate for most people. In the first place only 4 percent of the general public take regular exercise; and most of them choose low calorie activities (bowling, golf, volleyball for fun, a bit of social dancing). To get fit requires that one choose to participate in regular exercise for 30 minutes to an hour per day, and the level of fitness obtained is quite proportional to the habitual energy expenditure per day, per week, or per month. When one exercises 3 days per week, that is about half a program compared to what is needed. More improvement has been proved to be associated with greater frequency of participation.* Very typically isometric programs do not change the constituents of the blood or metabolism.[71, 72] Weight lifting programs are poor for developing or maintaining cardiovascular fitness.[37, 39] Held tensions tend to block the circulation and build up high oxygen debt, just the opposite of the aerobics championed by Lt. Col. Cooper, in the U. S. Air Force Program.[73]

Continuous training has been compared with interval training and burst repetitions. On an equal work basis there is little advantage.[74] The continuous endurance

*See references 33, 35, 69, and 70.

*Laboratory, University of Illinois)*

|  | Exercycle |  |  |  | Handball |
|---|---|---|---|---|---|
| Slimnastics Mean—2 college women | 1 grad. student (male) mean of 2 tests—15 minutes each |  | 1 young woman—30 minutes | Mean of 4 middle-aged women—15 minutes | Mean of 4 grad. students (male) 15 minutes |
|  | Moderate | Severe | Relaxed | Relaxed |  |
| 23.5 | 26 | 26 |  | 39.5 | 27.75 |
| 66.75 | 71 | 71 |  | 63.3 |  |
| 126.77 | 155 | 155 |  | 141.4 |  |
| 57.5 | 70.3 | 70.3 |  | 64.1 |  |
| 1.470 | 1.765 | 2.700 |  | .150* |  |
| .0255 | .0251 | .0384 |  | .0024* | .027 |
| 166 | 127.5 | 186 | 64.63 | 13.05 | 155.12 |
| 7.35 | 8.5 | 12.4 | 2.15 | 0.87 | 10.34 |
| 441 | 510 | 744 | 129.26 | 52.52 | 620.5 |
| 2.36 | 2.0 | 5.0 |  |  |  |

worker who works for an hour or more puts out more total energy. Running a mile as a single event approximates 120 calories. Jogging 4 miles is approximately 400 calories. From the point of view of burning up food, reducing fat, training the "extra capillarization" of the heart, and keeping the oxygen debt down, aerobic exercise has the advantage for health.[75-78]

### Exhibits of evaluation of several programs of exercise

Many programs of exercise have been evaluated at the University of Illinois Physical Fitness Research Center and Institute by the scientific staff. The heartograph (Cameron Heartometer Co., Chicago, Ill.) has usually been involved but many other types of tests have been used.[7, 13]

**Weight training is compared with running (walk-jog-run).** The data in Table 18-8 were obtained by Du Toit.[39] The results show that running influences cardiovascular fitness much more than weight training. In jogging there is more energy expended and greater improvements.

**Comparison of Cureton's low gear program with isometric exercises and tennis.** Table 18-9 gives the results of Cureton's Low Gear Program, 1 hour per day, evaluated at 650.25 calories per day (previously described).[68] Eight minutes of isometric exercise per day were evaluated at 32.10 calories. With a pound of fat equated to approximately 4380 calories, it is impractical to reduce weight by isometrics. Tennis was relatively good, evaluated at 593.10 calories for an hour of play.

**Golfers and fitness class middle-aged men evaluated.** Table 18-10 shows the way a group of twenty middle-aged golfers (average age 39.38 years) compared with ten middle-agers in the fitness class group under an instructor. By comparison of the means the two groups were statistically insignificantly different by average in body measurements (fat) and weights (186.73 vs. 179.06 lbs., golfers vs. controls, respectively). Both groups were sedentary at the start of the experiment. At the

Table 18-8. Cardiovascular measures on experimental subjects

| | Pulse rate $T_1$ | Pulse rate $T_2$ | Systolic blood pressure $T_1$ | Systolic blood pressure $T_2$ | Diastolic blood pressure $T_1$ | Diastolic blood pressure $T_2$ | Systolic amplitude of pulse wave $T_1$ | Systolic amplitude of pulse wave $T_2$ | Area under pulse wave $T_1$ | Area under pulse wave $T_2$ | Pulse pressure $T_1$ | Pulse pressure $T_2$ | Pulse pressure × pulse rate $T_1$ | Pulse pressure × pulse rate $T_2$ | T-wave amplitude $T_1$ | T-wave amplitude $T_2$ | Basal $O_2$ consumption $T_1$ | Basal $O_2$ consumption $T_2$ | |
|---|---|---|---|---|---|---|---|---|---|---|---|---|---|---|---|---|---|---|---|
| **Weight training subjects** | | | | | | | | | | | | | | | | | | | |
| Si | 60 | 52 | 115 | 108 | 78 | 80 | .76 | .85 | .23 | .25 | 37 | 28 | 2220 | 1456 | .20 | .29 | 340 | 350 | |
| Ca | 60 | 60 | 103 | 102 | 80 | 78 | .89 | .95 | .20 | .23 | 28 | 24 | 1680 | 1440 | .29 | .28 | 335 | 345 | 120 Net calories per hour |
| La | 70 | 72 | 120 | 118 | 80 | 80 | .80 | .90 | .24 | .26 | 40 | 38 | 2800 | 2736 | .23 | .25 | 380 | 360 | |
| So | 62 | 60 | 105 | 106 | 78 | 82 | .90 | .99 | .21 | .22 | 27 | 24 | 1674 | 1440 | .23 | .28 | 390 | 295 | |
| Mi | 56 | 56 | 108 | 106 | 70 | 70 | 1.10 | 1.10 | .25 | .26 | 38 | 36 | 2128 | 2016 | .28 | .29 | 145 | 150 | |
| He | 60 | 60 | 110 | 108 | 80 | 78 | .82 | .80 | .18 | .19 | 30 | 30 | 1800 | 1800 | .20 | .22 | 246 | 240 | |
| Be | 60 | 60 | 112 | 110 | 76 | 74 | .83 | .81 | .20 | .21 | 36 | 36 | 2160 | 2160 | .23 | .23 | 260 | 270 | |
| Ki | 64 | 60 | 108 | 105 | 78 | 75 | .87 | .89 | .18 | .20 | 30 | 30 | 1920 | 1800 | .14 | .15 | 295 | 305 | |
| Mean | 61 | 60 | 110 | 106 | 77 | 77 | .87 | .91 | .21 | .22 | 33 | 28 | 2045 | 1769 | .21 | .24 | 311 | 264 | |
| **Running subjects** | | | | | | | | | | | | | | | | | | | |
| As | 84 | 72 | 140 | 135 | 90 | 84 | .85 | 1.50 | .20 | .40 | 50 | 51 | 4200 | 3672 | .18 | .21 | 200 | 220 | |
| Ba | 60 | 48 | 132 | 122 | 95 | 80 | 1.00 | 1.20 | .20 | .28 | 37 | 42 | 2220 | 2016 | .30 | .45 | 230 | 320 | |
| Co | 80 | 80 | 126 | 125 | 93 | 80 | .53 | .59 | .12 | .17 | 33 | 45 | 2640 | 3600 | .37 | .41 | 327 | 380 | 800 Net calories per hour |
| Es | 68 | 60 | 112 | 115 | 90 | 80 | .97 | — | .16 | — | 22 | 35 | 1496 | 2100 | .10 | .18 | 210 | 270 | |
| Ve | 66 | 58 | 120 | 125 | 100 | 90 | 1.02 | 1.20 | .25 | .31 | 20 | 35 | 1320 | 2030 | .10 | .18 | 350 | 350 | |
| Li | 68 | 64 | 106 | 112 | 76 | 86 | .80 | 1.01 | .20 | .25 | 30 | 26 | 2040 | 1664 | .10 | .20 | 252 | 280 | |
| Nu | 70 | 60 | 106 | 116 | 70 | 65 | .80 | 1.10 | .20 | .30 | 36 | 51 | 2520 | 3060 | .20 | .30 | 250 | 275 | |
| Wr | 64 | 60 | 116 | 120 | 88 | 82 | 1.01 | 1.36 | .25 | .30 | 28 | 38 | 1792 | 2880 | .15 | .19 | 145 | 190 | |
| Mean | 70 | 62 | 119 | 121 | 88 | 81 | .87 | 1.14 | .20 | .29 | 32 | 40 | 2153 | 2353 | .21 | .27 | 245 | 286 | |

**Table 18-9.** *Cardiovascular indices on experimental subjects*\*

|  |  | Resting pulse rate $T_1$ $T_2$ | Systolic blood pressure (sitting) $T_1$ $T_2$ | Diastolic blood pressure (sitting) $T_1$ $T_2$ | Brachial pulse wave area (sitting) $T_1$ $T_2$ | Progressive pulse ratio $T_1$ $T_2$ | Schneider test score $T_1$ $T_2$ | Calorie cost |
|---|---|---|---|---|---|---|---|---|
| Progressive exercise | JV | 74  68 | 111  121 | 82  76 | .18  .31 | 2.6  2.0 | 16  19 |  |
| Low gear (Cureton) | ES | 92  86 | 105  123 | 84  75 | .13  .17 | 2.5  2.1 | 8   12 | 650.25 |
|  | Mean | 83  77 | 108  122 | 83  76 | .16  .24 | 2.6  2.1 | 12  16 |  |
| Isometric subjects | NP | 74  78 | 113  122 | 88  81 | .15  .17 | 2.5  2.2 | 15  16 |  |
|  | JJ | 80  80 | 110  114 | 85  82 | .20  .22 | 2.6  2.3 | 16  15 | 32.10 |
|  | Mean | 77  79 | 112  118 | 87  82 | .18  .20 | 2.6  2.3 | 16  16 |  |
| Tennis subjects | AD | 96  89 | 118  123 | 82  81 | .17  .12 | 2.5  2.5 | 15  15 |  |
|  | WD | 68  72 | 109  121 | 84  81 | .18  .24 | 2.7  2.4 | 17  18 | 593.10 |
|  | Mean | 82  81 | 114  122 | 83  81 | .18  .18 | 2.6  2.5 | 16  16.5 |  |
|  | Units | Beats/min. | mm. Hg | mm. Hg | Sq. cm. | Av. ratio | Points | Net calories |

\*After Kapilian, R. H.: University of Illinois, 1969.

428  *Improving dental practice through preventive measures*

**Table 18-10.** *Golfers vs. fitness group*

| Variable | Units | Golfers | Fitness group |
|---|---|---|---|
| **Physical characteristics** | | | |
|   Age | years | 39.38 | 39.00 |
|   Height | inches | 70.30 | 69.22 |
|   Weight | lb. | 184.03 | 173.40 |
|   Body surface area | sq. m. | 2.01 | 1.97 |
| **Treadmill walk (10 min., 8.6% grade, 4 m.p.h.)** | | | |
|   Peak gross $O_2$ intake | ml./Kg./mm. | 29.56 | 30.41 |
|   Pre-heart rate (sitting) | beats/min. | 74.84 | 65.50 |
|   Presystolic blood pressure (sitting) | mm. Hg | 126.74 | 118.50 |
|   Prediastolic blood pressure (sitting) | mm. Hg | 83.89 | 73.20 |
|   Terminal heart rate | beats/min. | 156.95 | 136.60 |
|   Terminal systolic blood pressure | mm. Hg | 184.63 | 167.40 |
|   Terminal diastolic blood pressure | mm. Hg | 69.38 | 70.12 |
| **3-minute step test (30 steps/min., 17 in. bench)** | | | |
|   Pre-heart rate (sitting) | beats/min. | 74.50 | 64.60 |
|   Presystolic blood pressure (sitting) | mm. Hg | 123.50 | 121.40 |
|   Prediastolic blood pressure (sitting) | mm. Hg | 85.20 | 77.80 |
|   Terminal heart rate | beats/min. | 169.50 | 145.80 |
|   Terminal systolic blood pressure | mm. Hg | 177.10 | 172.80 |
|   Terminal diastolic blood pressure | mm. Hg | 65.50 | 58.40 |
|   Sum of 3 recovery heart rates | beats/min. | 173.60 | 134.60 |

| Energy cost → | Units | Golf | Exercises 45' |
|---|---|---|---|
| Note: *Values for N:* | cal./Kg./hr. | 3.27 | |
|   Golfers, N = 20 (Except TMW = 19) | cal./hr., net | 196.00 | |
|   Fitness, N = 10 | net cal. | | 650.25 |
|   Term DBP: TMW, Golf = 13, Fit = 8 | cal./Kg. | | 8.93 |
|   St. T, Golf = 12, Fit = 5 | cal./sq. m. | | 335.18 |

end of five months of golf (3 times per week) and fitness (3 times per week) the two groups were significantly different in many tests, the fitness group having improved much more than the golfers. This work was carried out by Getchell[38] under my supervision and with the help of the Physical Fitness Research Laboratory Staff, University of Illinois.

**REFERENCES**

1. Biller, F. E.: Occupational hazards in dental practice, Oral Hygiene **36:**194, 1946.
2. Austin, L. T., and Krueger, G. O.: Common ailments of dentists, a statistical study, J.A.D.A. **35:**797, 1947.
3. Bernstein, A., and Balk, J. L.: The common diseases of practicing dentists, J.A.D.A. **46:**525-529, 1953.
4. Special Report on the Health Budget Crisis, Washington, D. C.: Washington Report on Medicine and Health, Washington, D. C., 1969, National Press Building.
5. Forbes, W. H.: Life span longer abroad despite spending by U. S., The Milwaukee Journal, September 5, 1967.
6. Life-Time Special Report: The healthy life, New York, 1966, Life-Time Book Division.
7. Cureton, T. K., Jr.: The physiological effects of exercise programs in adults, Springfield, Illinois, 1969, Charles C Thomas, Publisher.

8. Starr, I., and Wood, F. C.: Twenty-year studies with the ballistocardiograph, Circulation 23:714-723, 1961.
9. Steinman, R. R., Brassett, M., and Tartaryn, P.: Comparison of caries incidence in exercised and immobilized rats, J. Dent. Res. 90:218, 1961.
10. Cureton, T. K., Jr.: Health and physical fitness of dentists (with implications), J. Dent. Med. 16:211-223, 1961.
11. Missenard, A.: In search of man (heredity, climate and diet), New York, 1965, Hawthorn Books, Inc.
12. Cheraskin, E., and Ringsdorf, W. M., Jr.: Aging by the teeth, Lancet 1:580, 1969.
13. Cureton, T. K., Jr.: Physical fitness workbook, ed. 3, St. Louis, 1947, The C. V. Mosby Co.
14. Olson, E. V.: The hazards of immobility, Amer. J. Nurs. 67:780-797, 1967.
15. Asher, R. A.: Dangers of going to bed, Brit. Med. J. 2:967, 1947.
16. Holmes, H. Z.: Effects of training on chronic health complaints of middle-aged men, Urbana, Illinois, 1969, University of Illinois (doctoral dissertation).
17. Joseph, J. J.: The effects of exercise and sedentary living on middle-aged adults, Amer. Corrective Ther. J. 22:2-7, 1968.
18. Stewart, McD. G.: Coronary disease and modern stress, Lancet 2:867-870, 1950.
19. Tappel, A. L.: Where old age begins, Nutrition Today, December, 1967.
20. Jacobs, E. A., and others: $O_2$ for old age, Newsweek, October 13, 1969.
21. McFarland, R. A.: Experimental evidence of the relationship between aging and oxygen want—in search of a theory of aging, Ergonomics Research Society Lecture, 1963.
22. Jette, M. J.: A study of long-term physical activity in sedentary middle-aged men, Urbana, Illinois, 1969, University of Illinois (doctoral dissertation).
23. Popejoy, I.: The effects of a physical fitness program on selected psychological and physiological measures of anxiety, Urbana, Illinois, 1967, University of Illinois (doctoral dissertation).
24. Levi, L.: Life stress and urinary excretion of adrenaline and noradrenaline. In Raab, W., editor: Prevention of ischemic heart disease, Springfield, Illinois, 1966, Charles C Thomas, Publisher.
25. Betz, R. L.: A comparison between personality traits and physical fitness tests of males, Urbana, Illinois, 1956, University of Illinois (doctoral dissertation).
26. Skinner, J. S., Holloszy, J. O., and Cureton, T. K., Jr.: Effects of a program of endurance exercises on physical work, Amer. J. Cardiol. 14:747-752, 1964.
27. Skinner, J. S., Holloszy, J. O., and Cureton, T. K., Jr.: Effects of six months program of endurance exercise on the serum lipids of middle-aged men, Amer. J. Cardiol. 14:761-770, 1964.
28. Raab, W., editor: Prevention of ischemic heart disease, Springfield, Illinois, 1966, Charles C Thomas, Publisher.
29. Karvonen, M., and Barry, A. J.: Physical activity and the heart, Springfield, Illinois, 1967, Charles C Thomas, Publisher.
30. Zimkin, N. V., and Korobokov, A. V.: The importance of physical exercise as a factor of increasing resistance of the body to unfavorable influence under conditions of modern civilization. In Lubke, H., editor: Weltkingress fur Sportmedicin, vol. XVI, Koln, 1966, Deutscher Arzte-Verlag.
31. Cureton, T. K., Jr.: Improvement of psychological states by means of exercise-fitness programs, J. Ass. Phys. Ment. Rehab. 17:14-25, 1963.
32. Van Vleet, P. P.: Some effects of physical education therapy on the personality characteristics of schizophrenic patients, Berkeley, California, 1950, University of California (doctoral dissertation).
33. Pollock, M. L., Cureton, T. K., Jr., and Greninger, L.: Effects on working capacity, cardiovascular function and body composition of adult men, Med. Sci. Sport 1:70-74, 1969.
34. Cureton, T. K., Jr., and Phillips, E. E.: Physical fitness changes in middle-aged men attributable to equal eight-week periods of training, non-training and re-training, J. Sport Med. 4:1-7, 1964.

35. Campbell, D.: Influence of several physical activities on serum cholesterol concentrations in young men, J. Lipid Res. **6**:478-480, 1965.
36. Editorial: Is massage good for you? Fitness for Living **2**:60, 1968.
37. Kapilian, R. H.: The effects of rhythmical, progressive exercises, isometric exercises, and tennis on the cardiovascular system of young men, Urbana, Illinois, 1969, University of Illinois (doctoral dissertation).
38. Getchell, L. H., Jr.: An analysis of the effects of a season of golf on selected cardiovascular, metabolic and muscular fitness measures on middle-aged men, and the caloric cost of golf, Urbana, Illinois, 1965, University of Illinois (doctoral dissertation).
39. DuToit, S. F.: Running and weight training effects upon the cardiac cycle, Urbana, Illinois, 1966, University of Illinois (doctoral dissertation).
40. Jones, H.: It is the blood flow, Time, October 5, 1952.
41. Jokl, E.: Exercise, training and cardiac stroke force. In Raab, W., editor: Prevention of ischemic disease, Springfield, Illinois, 1966, Charles C Thomas, Publisher.
42. Honet, J. C., Jebsen, R. H., and Tenckhoff, H. A.: Motor nerve condition velocity in chronic renal insufficiency, Arch. Phys. Med. **47**:647-652, 1966.
43. Shock, N. W.: Physical activity and the rate of aging, Canadian International Report, October 11, 1966.
44. Holloszy, J. S., and others: Effect of physical conditioning on cardiovascular function, Amer. J. Cardiol. **14**:761, 1964.
45. Fox, S. M., and Skinner, J. S.: Physical activity and cardiovascular health, Amer. J. Cardiol. **14**:731, 1964.
46. Cureton, T. K., Jr.: Exercise and fitness, Chicago, 1960, The Athletic Institute.
47. Brozek, J.: Changes in body composition during maturity, Fed. Proc. **11**:784, 1952.
48. Keys, A., and others: The biology of human starvation, Minneapolis, 1950, University of Minnesota Press.
49. Keys, A.: Psychological aspects of nutrition with special reference to experimental psychodietetics, Third International Congress of Nutrition, The Hague, 1955.
50. Gwinup, G.: The sensible way to diet, Look **33**:84-90, 1969.
51. Brozek, J.: Personality of young and middle-aged men, J. Geront. **7**:410, 1952.
52. Swartz, F. C.: Report to Congress, 1969.
53. Robinson, S.: Experimental studies of physical fitness in relation to age, Arbeitphysiology **10**:251, 1938.
54. Dill, D. B., and Ross, J. C.: A longitudinal study of 16 champion runners, J. Sport Med. **7**:4-27, 1967.
55. Jacobs, E. A., and others: Hyperoxygenation effect on cognitive functioning of the aged, New Eng. J. Med. **281**:753, 1969.
56. Letounov, S.: The importance of physical education and sport as preventive measures for healthy and sick persons, J. Sport Med. **9**:142-151, 1969.
57. Mateef, D.: Morphological and physiological factors of aging and longevity. In The Athletic Institute: Health and fitness in the modern world, Chicago, 1960, The Institute.
58. Mayer, J.: Exercise and weight control. In The Athletic Institute: Exercise and fitness, Chicago, 1960, The Institute.
59. Barry, A. J., and others: The effects of physical conditioning on older individuals, II, motor performance and cognitive functioning, J. Geront. **21**:192-199, 1966.
60. Barry, A. J., and others: The effects of physical conditioning on older individuals, I, work capacity, circulatory-respiratory function and the work electrocardiogram, J. Geront. **21**:182-191, 1966.
61. Cureton, T. K., Jr.: A case study of Joie Ray (60-70 years), J. Phys. Ment. Rehab. **18**:64-72, 1964.
62. Cureton, T. K., Jr.: A case study of Sydney Meadows, J. Phys. Ment. Rehab. **19**:36-43, 1965.
63. Skinner, J. S., and Strandness, D. E., Jr.: Exercise and intermittent claudication, the effect of repetition and intensity of exercise, Circulation **36**:15-22, 1967.
64. Spieth, W.: Cardiovascular health status, age and psychological performance, J. Geront. **19**:277, 1964.

65. Cureton, T. K., Jr.: Physical fitness improvement of a middle-aged man, with brief reviews of related studies, Res. Quart. **23:**149-160, 1952.
66. Cureton, T. K., Jr.: The relative value of various exercise programs to protect adult human subjects from degenerative heart disease. In Raab, W., editor: Prevention of ischemic heart disease, Springfield, Illinois, 1966, Charles C Thomas, Publisher.
67. Cureton, T. K., Jr.: Improvements in cardiovascular condition of humans associated with physical training, persistently performed sports and exercises, Proc. Coll. Phys. Ed. Ass. **60:**82-104, 1957.
68. Cureton, T. K., Jr.: Physical fitness and dynamic health, New York, 1965, The Dial Press.
69. Gettman, L. R.: Effects of different amounts of training on cardiovascular and motor fitness of men, Urbana, Illinois, 1967, University of Illinois (master's thesis).
70. Greninger, L. C.: Effects of frequency of running on the progressive pulse ratio and other cardiovascular-respiratory measures of adult men, Urbana, Illinois, 1967, University of Illinois (master's thesis).
71. Vanderhoof, E. R., Imig, C. J., and Hines, H. M.: Effect of muscle strength and endurance development on blood flow, J. Appl. Physiol. **16:**873-877, 1961.
72. McArdle, W. D., and Foglia, G. F.: Energy cost and cardiorespiratory stress of isometric and weight training exercises, J. Sport Med. **9:**23, 1969.
73. Cooper, K. H.: Aerobics, New York, 1968, M. Evans & Co., Inc.
74. Haskell, W. L.: The effects of three endurance training programs on energy metabolism, Urbana, Illinois, 1965, University of Illinois (doctoral dissertation).
75. Eckstein, R. W.: Effect of exercise and coronary artery narrowing on coronary collateral circulation, Circ. Res. **5:**230-235, 1957.
76. Cotes, J. E., Davies, C. M. T., and Healy, M. J. R.: Factors relating to maximal oxygen uptake in young adult male and female subjects, J. Physiol. **189:**79-80, 1967.
77. Knuttgen, H. G.: Physical working capacity and physical performance, Med. Sci. Sport **1:**1-8, 1969.
78. Taylor, H. L.: Exercise and metabolism. In Johnson, W. R., editor: Science and medicine of exercise and sports, New York, 1960, Harper & Row, Publishers.
79. Williams, R.: Nutrition in a nutshell, New York, 1962, Doubleday & Co., Inc.
80. Cureton, T. K., Jr.: Program of daily rhythmic exercises for body conditioning, Sports Illustrated, January 17, 1955.

# Index

## A

Abrasiveness of dentifrices, 160, 350
Absorption of fluoride, 101
Abutment teeth and partial dentures, 305-306, 315
Acid production
 and cariogenic foods, 41-43
 and fluoride, 94-95
Acid solubility of enamel, 40-41
Acidogenic organisms and rampant dental caries, 81
Acrylic resin and periodontal disease, 218
Alcoholic (chronic), 40
Alumina (levigated) in dentifrices, 160
Amalgam restoration
 biophysical consideration, 374
 contamination of, 372
 corrosion of, 373
 as dental restoration, 371-374
 effect on gingiva, 374
 expansion of, 372
 overtrituration of, 372
Ameloblasts
 effect of fluoride on, 93
 effect of nutrition on, 40
Ammonia compound in dentifrices, 170
Aneuploid cells, 362
Ankylosis, 190
Anoxia and dental disease, 45
Anterior crossbite, 203
Antibacterial properties of saliva, 82
Antibiotics
 in dentifrices, 171
 in oral surgery, 330
 and periodontal disease, 217
 in zinc phosphate cements, 386
Antienzymes in dentifrices, 171
Antihistamine drugs in rampant dental caries, 87-88
Applegate-Kennedy Classification System for partial dentures, 307
Ariboflavinosis, 39
Arrestment of dental caries
 and phosphate-fluoride systems, 133
 and stannous fluoride, 25
Arthritis and vitamin D, 54
Audiovisual programming, 18-21
Automatic filmstrip projector, 18-21

Auxiliaries
 in nutrition counselling, 32
 and patient education, 16-18

## B

Basic four food groups, 36-39
 bread-cereal group, 38
 meat group, 37
 milk group, 37
 vegetable-fruit group, 38
Between-meal eating and dental caries, 38-39, 41-43, 82-83
Blood, fluoride in, 94, 104-106, 107
Bone meal and dental caries, 96
Bottle caries, 82
Breakfast cereals, fluoridation in, 112
Bruxism and occlusion, 220
Butter in nutrition, 37

## C

Calcification
 effect of fluoride on, 93
 imperfect, 40
 and nutrition, 40
Calcium
 and fluoride metabolism, 97, 98
 interference of, in dentifrices, 161
 in nutrition, 30, 39, 41, 43
 in periodontal disease, 209
 requirement, 37
Calcium fluoride in fluoride tablets, 96-99
Calcium hydroxide
 biophysical considerations, 390
 properties of, 390, 391
 in rampant dental caries, 84
Calcium phosphates in dentifrices, 161
Calcium pyrophosphate in dentifrices, 168
Calculus
 and gingival inflammation, 210
 and plaque, 210
 as precursor of periodontal disease, 209
 prevention of, 158, 164-166, 170, 172, 209-211
Caloric need, 38
 and obesity, 51-53
Candy
 and dental caries, 38, 42
 in nutrition, 38

433

Carbohydrates
    and cariogenic foods, 44, 54
    and dental caries, 42-54
    in dietary improvement, 51-53
    and dietary phosphates, 43-44
    and food retention, 54
    and natural inhibitors of acid production, 54
    and rampant dental caries, 81-82
Carbonate and dental caries, 75-76
Caries activity tests
    case histories, 9
    disclosing tablets, 11
    educational benefits, 8
    glucose clearance test, 11
    Green test, 11
    *Lactobacillus* plate count determination, 11
    and nutritional counselling, 11-16
    and patient education, 16-22
    and preventive dentistry laboratory, 10
    in rampant dental caries, 84-86
    salivary flow determination, 11
    salivary viscosity determination, 11
    Snyder test, 11
    Wach test, 11
Cariogenic foods
    and acid production, 41-43
    and rampant dental caries, 84-86
Cavity liners (varnishes)
    biophysical considerations, 391
    composition of, 390
Cells
    activities of, 31
    requirements of, 31, 32
Cements
    classification, 385
    copper, 386
    resin, 390
    silicate, 386
    silicophosphate, 388
    zinc oxide–eugenol, 389
    zinc phosphate, 385
Cementum, 161, 168
Centric jaw relation, 227-228
Chalk in dentifrices, 160-161
Chelation, 68
Chewing gum
    clinical results of use, 112
    fluoridated, 112
Chlorophyll in dentifrices, 170
Chromosomes, 356
Chronic endemic dental fluorosis
    clinical appearance, 93
    and communal fluoridation, 92
    effect on ameloblasts, 93
    effect on odontoblasts, 93
    and enamel hypoplasia, 93
    from fluoride tablets, 103
    pathology of, 93
    and topical fluorides, 94
Cleft lip, 44-45
Cleft palate, 44-45
Communication and preventive dentistry, 7
Comprehensive dentistry, 3
Congenital errors of development, mechanisms of, 44-45
Counselling in self-care, 4
Crown-root ratio, 306

D

Decalcification from phosphate fluoride systems, 131
Delayed eruption, 41, 195
Demineralization
    and rampant dental caries, 84-86
    and stannous fluoride, 23, 84
Dental care of indigent population, 96
Dental caries
    and acid demineralization, 80-81, 131
    and acid solubility of enamel, 40
    activity tests, 8-11, 82-83, 86
    arrestment of, 23-24, 127, 133
    and between-meal eating, 38-39, 41-43, 82-83
    and bone meal, 96
    and carbonate, 75-76
    and cariogenic foods, 41-44, 53
    and chelation, 68
    and chronic endemic dental fluorosis, 92
    and communal fluoridation, 25, 81-82, 92
    control of, in children, 185
    and dental materials, 2
    and dentifrices, 157-174
    and dietary phosphate, 43-44
    and enamel pigmentation, 23-24
    etiology of, 59, 66-70
    and fermentable carbohydrates, 41-44, 53, 81
    and fluoride, 22-25, 30-41
    and fluoride tablets, 96-102
    and food retention, 83
    and high calcium–low phosphorus diets, 40
    initiation of, 41, 80
    mechanism of, 67-70
    and mineralization, 40-41
    and mouthwashes, 133-136
    and nursing bottle, 82, 182
    and nutrition, 30-57
    and oral pathology, 346
    and orthodontics, 10
    and partial dentures, 398
    pathogenesis of, 66-69
    and plaque, 80-84, 85
    progression of, 41
    proteolytic concept, 69
    rampant, 9, 80-89
    resistance to, 41, 70-77
    saliva in, 81-89
    and topical fluorides, 22-25, 84, 92-145
    and trace elements, 41
    and use of pilocarpine, 87-88
    use of zinc oxide and eugenol in, 83-84
    and Vipeholm study, 42
    and vitamin D deficiency, 41-43
    and zirconium silicate prophylaxis paste, 4, 22-25, 84
Dental disease and anoxia, 45
Dental education, 2

Dental practice, 1-2
Dental profession, attitude of, 5
Dentifrices
   abrasiveness of, 160, 350
   and activity affected by calcium, 161
   ammonia compound in, 170
   antibiotics in, 171
   binding agents in, 162
   calcium phosphates in, 161
   calcium pyrophosphate in, 168
   chlorophyll in, 170
   choice of, 167
   composition of, 159
   containing antienzymes, 171
   containing chalk, 161
   containing sodium monofluorophosphate, 170
   containing stannous fluoride, 168
   consumer properties of, 161
   damage to oral tissues from, 165
   effect of on bacterial count, 171
   foaming agents in, 161
   function of, 158
   humectants in, 162
   in gingival health, 158, 163, 165
   inactivation of fluoride and tin by components, 168
   interference of calcium, 161
   levigated alumina in, 160
   liquid form, 159
   neutral, 171
   patient reaction to, 162
   polishing agent in, 159
   powder form, 159
   and prevention of pellicle, 163-166
   in reducing calculus, 172
   in reducing mouth odors, 158
   and removal of oral debris, 165
   reservoir of tin in, 169
   and salt and soda, 162-163
   stomatitis, 165
   use of
      after meals, 172
      by cigar and cigarette smokers, 168
      in control of caries in adults, 169
      in fluoride areas, 169
      with prophylaxis paste, 169
      with toothbrush, 158, 164, 172
Dentist
   and health tables, 399
   health of, 398
   role of
      in nutrition counselling, 32
      in producing malocclusions, 240
Denture-supporting tissues
   physical conditioning, 278
   surgical correction, 278-279
   systemic measures for, 278
Dentures
   damage to from dentifrices, 168
   and preventive dentistry, 7, 273-295
Deoxyribonucleic acid (DNA), 363
Diagnosis
   and oral pathology, 345-348

Diagnosis—cont'd
   and oral surgery, 328
   and partial dentures, 301
Diagnostic zones, 346
Diet
   and immediate dentures, 285
   in oral surgery, 338
Diet counselling
   and dental caries, 11-16
   patient education, 16-22
Diet history, 32, 45-49
Diet requirements
   and chronic alcoholic, 39
   composition of, 33
   daily allowances, 34-35
   and four basic food groups, 30-39
   ideal, 33
   meat group, 37-38
   and mental deficiency, 39
   milk group, 37
   and mineralized tissues, 40-44
   and nutritional deficiencies, 39
   and rampant dental caries, 80-89
   and relation to oral cavity, 39-45
   and soft tissues, 39-40
Diet survey
   evaluation, 12-16, 45-49, 84
   instructions, 12-16, 45-49
Dietary supplementation, 53-54
Disclosing solution for identification of plaque, 212
Disclosing tablets, 9

E

Ectopic eruption, etiology and treatment, 191, 192
Education, dental
   and automatic filmstrip projector, 18-21
   and caries activity tests, 8-11
   communication of nutritional knowledge, 57
   and dental radiographs, 17
   and diet counselling, 17
   direct techniques, 16-17
   and electromatic slide viewer, 18-21
   and filmstrip, 19
   and immediate dentures, 285
   indirect techniques, 17-21
   objective of, 16
   and pamphlets, 21
   and partial dentures, 300
   and periodontal disease, 211
   and public relations, 16
   recall procedures, 25-28
   and record device, 18
   slides, 22
   and study models, 17
   and tape recorder, 21
   telephone procedures, 25
   and toothbrushing technique, 17
   and topical fluoride, 22-25
   and use of auxiliaries, 17
   visual aids, 17
Electric toothbrushes, 173, 213

# 436  Index

Electromatic slide viewer, 20
Enamel
  acid solubility of, 40-41
  composition, 60-65
  crystallographic nature of, 61-65
  decalcification from phosphate-fluoride systems, 131
  fluoride content of, 60
  fluoride uptake from phosphate-fluoride systems, 130
  structure of, 65-66
Enamel hypoplasia, causes of, 93
Enamel matrix, effect of nutrition on, 40
Endodontic therapy and partial dentures, 304
Enolase, effect of fluoride on, 99
Erythroplasia, 341
Eruption, delayed, 41
Exercise and physical fitness, 397-428
Exfoliative cytology, 353
Extraction and indirect dental health education, 17

## F

Factors in rampant dental caries, 88
Fats in nutrition, 37, 51-52
*Fifty-two Pearls and their Environment,* 18
Filmstrips, 19-21
Fluoridation
  and chronic endemic dental fluorosis, 92
  comparison with fluoride tablets, 102
  comparison with topical fluorides, 24-25, 112, 121, 122-125, 126, 132, 133
  cost of, 95
  and dental plaque, 94
  effect on acid production, 94
  effectiveness of, 93
  as function of temperature, 93
  and hydroxyapatite, 94
  and indigent dental care, 96
  mechanism of action, 94-96
  population served by, 95
  and rampant dental caries, 81-82
  and use of topical stannous fluoride, 23-24
Fluoride
  absorption of, 101
  and acid production, 94-95
  in blood, 95, 107, 111
  in breakfast cereals, 111
  and calcification, 71-75
  in chewing gum, 112
  and crystal size of hydroxyapatite, 40, 73
  in dental plaque, 94
  in dentifrices, 157-174
  effectiveness, 112, 113, 121, 122-126, 136-139
  effects of
    on ameloblasts, 93
    on enolase, 94
    on magnesium, 94
    on oral flora, 94
  in enamel, 41, 95, 107
  in food, 98
  and formation of fluoroapatite, 94
  metabolism of, 95, 96, 98, 101, 109, 111

Fluoride—cont'd
  in milk, 111
  in mouthwashes, 133-136
  in placenta, 107
  in prenatal tablets, 106-109
  in prophylactic pastes, 134-135
  in rampant dental caries, 84
  relation to chronic endemic dental fluorosis, 94
  in saliva, 94
  in skeleton, 107, 112
  in table salt, 109-111
  tablets
    advantages of, 105
    and calcium, 98
    clinical effects of, 96-99, 102-105
    comparison with communal fluoridation, 102
    composed of calcium fluoride, 96
    composed of sodium fluoride, 97-105
    and concentration in blood, 100-102
    and content in food, 96
    disadvantages of, 102
    effect of in adults, 101
    effect on vitamin utilization, 103
    excretion in urine, 96, 98-100
    frequency of ingestion, 105
    metabolism of, 96-100, 103-105
    and multiple daily doses, 101
    in presence of vitamins, 96-100, 103-105
    recommended levels, 102
    retention of fluoride in teeth from, 98
    and skeletal retention of fluoride, 96
    use in a single dose, 98, 101, 102
  during tooth development and maturation, 39, 40-41
  as topical agent, 22-25, 92-148
Fluoride-phosphates, 23, 25, 130
  in caries arrestment, 133
  clinical studies, 130
  decalcification of enamel from, 131
  effectiveness in fluoride areas, 132
  enamel uptake from, 130
  mechanism of action, 131-135
Fluoroapatite
  formation during fluoridation, 94
  formation from fluoride tablets, 91
  solubility of, 72, 94
Foaming agents in dentifrices, 161
Folic acid, 45
Food
  clearance from mouth, 41
  and fluorides, 40-41
  retention in mouth, 41-46
Food habits, 11
Food traps and partial dentures, 298-299
Fulcrum line, 299
Full dentures
  centric jaw relation, 281-282
  choice of prosthesis, 274-275
  evaluation of patient, 274-277
  factors to consider in removing teeth, 275-277
  function of, 273-274

Full dentures—cont'd
  and impression, 279-281
  and nutrition, 278
  and occluding vertical dimension, 281
  and periodontium, 276
  posterior tooth selection and arrangement, 282-284
  preparing denture-supporting tissues, 278-279
  and recording interjaw relations, 281-282
  and resilient liners, 284-285
  and supporting bone, 276-277
  and tooth, 275-276

G

Genetics and orthodontics, 229
Gingiva
  and dentifrices, 158, 159, 160, 163, 165
  effects of
    amalgam restoration, 374
    silicate cements, 388
    stannous fluoride, 127
Gingivitis
  etiology of, 208
  and oral dental restoration, 218
  and preventive dentistry, 3, 4
Glucose clearance test, 9
Gold alloy casting
  advantages of, 374
  allergic response to, 374-375
  biophysical considerations, 380-382
  casting of, 379
  as dental restoration, 374
  and die materials, 375
  disadvantages of, 374
  and internal porosity, 380, 381
  and investment, 377
  and patterns, 378
  and surface defects, 380, 381
  and use of compound impression material, 374, 375
  and use of wax, 376
Gold foil as dental restoration, 374
Guiding plane, 306

H

Halitosis and dentifrices, 158
Human relations and preventive dentistry, 7
Humectants in dentifrices, 162
Hydrocolloids, 374, 375
  and surface reproduction, 375
Hydroxyapatite
  crystal size, 40, 73
  and fluoridation, 72-75, 94

I

Immediate dentures
  care of, 290-292
  care of mouth in, 289-290
  and diet, 54-57, 288
  eating habits, 54-57, 288
  insertion and removal procedures, 286-287
  knowledge of, 286
  and patient education, 285-286

Immediate dentures—cont'd
  and postinsertion therapy, 294-295
  preventive features of, 285
  salivation, 288-289
  and speech, 289
  and tongue, 287-288
Imperfect calcification, 40
Impression
  border edges, 280-281
  intimate contact, 280
  maximum extension, 279-280
  and tissue control, 279
Incisal rest, 314
Indigent population, 96
Infectious hepatitis and oral surgery, 330
Inflammation, cause of in periodontal disease, 208
Inlays and periodontal disease, 218
Interceptive orthodontics
  advantages, 241
  disadvantages, 245
Interdental cleansing, 214
Investment material
  distribution of, 382
  and setting forces, 373
  thermal expansion of, 381
  and water-powder ratio, 381
Iodized salt, 49
Ionizing radiation, effects of, 355, 358
Iron in nutrition, 35
Iron (ferric) fluoride as topical agent, 118, 120, 125
Irradiation, effect of on salivary glands, 87
Irrigators, dental, 17

L

Laboratory tests in oral pathology, 345
*Lactobacillus* in rampant dental caries, 84
Lava pumice, 4
Lead fluoride as topical agent, 128, 130
Leukoplakia, 341
Lingual reciprocal arm, 305
Local anesthetics in oral surgery, 334
Local factors and periodontal disease, 208

M

Magnesium
  effect of fluoride on, 94
  in nutrition, 40, 43
Malignant disease
  in oral pathology, 347-351
  and oral surgery, 339
Malocclusions, 237; *see also* Orthodontics
  and arch length inadequacies, 238
  and breast feeding, 239
  and mouth breathing, 237
  and periodontal disease, 220
  and premature loss of teeth, 239
  and retained primary teeth, 240
  produced by dentist, 240
Mastickes, 159
Meat group, composition of, 37-38
Menopause, 88

Mental stress and rampant dental caries, 88-89
Mentally deficient patient, diet for, 39
Mercaptan impression material, 375
    surface reproduction of, 375, 376
Mercury, toxicity of, 374
Metabolism of fluoride, 96, 98, 101, 109, 111
Milk
    fluoridated, 111
    as food group, 37
    suggested levels in nutrition, 36
Mineralization
    and fluoride in, 40
    and nutritional effects, 40-45
    and teeth, 30, 40-45
    calcification, 40-45
    hydroxyapatite, 40
    imbalances in, 40
Mineralized tissues
    deficiencies of, 40
    nutritional influences during tooth development, 40-44
Minerals
    in dietary improvement, 49
    in nutrition, 30, 35, 37-44
Molybdenum in nutrition, 41
Mouthwashes
    clinical studies, 132-136
    fluoride in, 133-136
    toxicity of, 136
Multivitamins in nutrition, 33, 54
Mutations, 356

# N

Natural inhibitors, 53
Neuromuscular problems and orthodontics, 233
Niacin in nutrition, 35
Nursing bottle caries, 82
Nutrition
    ariboflavinosis as defect, 39
    and between-meal eating, 38, 39, 41-43
    and calcification, 40
    calcium in, 30, 39, 41, 43
    and calories, 38, 51, 53
    carbohydrates in, 44, 52, 54
    and cariogenic foods, 44, 54
    and cellular function, 31
    and congenital errors of development, 44
    counselling of patient, 11-16
    and deficiencies, 39
    and diet history, 32
    diet survey instructions, 12-14
    diet survey sheet, 12, 13
    diet supplementation, 53, 54
    and dietary allowances, 33
    effect of, with loss of teeth, 54
    and enamel matrix, 40
    evaluation of, 45
    and fat consumption, 37, 52
    and fermentable carbohydrates, 41-45
    folic acid in, 35, 45
    and four basic food groups, 36-39
    and full dentures, 224

Nutrition—cont'd
    goals of, 30
    and ideal diet, 33-39
    influence of during tooth maturation, 41
    iron in, 35
    lactose in, 43
    magnesium in, 40, 44
    meat group, 37-38
    milk group, 37
    and mineralization, 30, 40-44
    and mineralized tissues, 40-44
    minerals in, 35-50
    multivitamins in, 33, 54
    natural sugars in, 52-53
    niacin in, 35
    and obesity, 51-53
    and optimal nurture, 30-32
    phosphorus in, 30-44
    and periodontal disease, 44
    and poor dietary practices, 31
    postdevelopmental effects of, 41-44
    and prevention of disease, 30-33
    during pregnancy, 51
    protein in, 37-50
    and rampant dental caries, 82-83
    recommended daily allowances, 33-37
    relation to oral cavity, 30-45
    riboflavin in, 35, 45
    role of dentist in, 32
    selenium in, 41
    substitute foods, 14
    techniques of teaching in dental office, 32
    thiamine in, 35, 36
    and trace elements, 40
    tryptophane in, 44
    use of fluoride in, 30-41
    vanadium, 41
    vegetable-fruit group, 38
    and vegetarian diets, 35
    and vitamin A, 34, 37, 38, 40, 44, 45
    vitamin B complex, 37, 44, 45
    vitamin C, 35, 38, 40, 44
    vitamin D, 30, 34, 37, 40, 41, 44

# O

Obesity, 51-53
Occluding vertical dimension, 281
Occlusal adjustment, 4
Occlusal rest, 314
Occlusion
    and bruxism, 220
    and erythroplasia, 341
    and leukoplakia, 341
    and malignant disease, 339
    and partial dentures, 306
    and periodontal disease, 220
Odontoblasts
    effect of fluoride on, 93
    effect of nutrition on, 40
Oleomargarine, 37
Operative dentistry
    diagnosis and treatment of enamel caries, 249-252

Operative dentistry—cont'd
  extension for prevention, 254-255
  finishing the restoration, 258-259
  and preventing defective restorations, 252-253
  and preventing loss of pulp vitality, 261-264
  and preventing loss of teeth, 265-268
  and preventing periodontal involvement, 260-261
  and preventing physical failure of restoration, 259-260
  and preventing recurrent caries, 253-254
  and preventive dentistry, 248-270
  and preparing enamel walls, 255-256
  and pulpotomy, 264-265
  and use of cavity varnish, 257
  use of fluorides in, 256
Optimal nurture, 30-32
Oral flora and fluoridation, 94
Oral hygiene
  and abnormal swallowing, 236
  and arch length inadequacies, 238
  and deleterious habits, 235
  environmental factors, 232
  interceptive, 231
  and mouth breathing, 237
  and periodontal disease, 83, 212
  and rampant dental caries, 81-82
  and tongue thrust, 236
  and trauma to jaws, 232
Oral pathology
  clinical history, 345
  and dental caries, 346
  and dentifrice abrasion, 348
  diagnosis in, 345-350
  and diagnostic zones, 346
  and laboratory tests, 345
  lesions of soft tissues, 351
  and malignant disease, 347
  and oral exfoliative cytology, 353
  and pain, 346
  and patient record chart, 351
  and periodontal disease, 346
  and radiographs, 345
  and systemic diseases, 347
Oral surgery
  and antibiotics, 330
  and apprehension, 335
  to correct facial deformities, 338
  and infectious hepatitis, 330
  and leukoplakia, 341
  in minimizing prosthetic failures, 338
  and orofacial trauma, 336
  and pain, 335
  and postoperative care, 330
  and preoperative evaluation, 331
  and prevention
    of adverse reactions to local anesthetics, 334-336
    of ameloblastomas, 330
    of cysts, 330
    of deaths from malignant disease, 339
    of errors, 328, 329
    of major surgical problems, 329

Oral surgery—cont'd
  and prevention—cont'd
    of operative and postoperative complications, 331-334
    of postoperative hemorrhage, 336-338
  and radiographs, 333
  space infections, 330
  and sterilization, 329
Orthodontics; *see also* Malocclusions
  and dental caries, 10
  genetic factors in, 229
  interceptive, 240
  in monozygotic twins, 233
  and muscular pattern, 233
  and neuromuscular problem, 233
  and periodontal disease, 220
  prevalence of, 229

P
Pain
  and oral pathology, 346
  in oral surgery, 335
  and preventive dentistry, 3
  and rampant dental caries, 80-81
Partial dentures
  and abutment teeth, 305-306, 315
  and adult space maintainers, 298-300
  and artificial teeth, 324
  and bone maintenance, 306
  and caries, 298
  classification of, 307
  construction program, 314
  continuum between easy and difficult caries, 307
  and contour of natural tooth, 301
  and crown-root ratio, 306
  and crowns of teeth, 301
  and dental caries, 298
  diagnosis for, 301
  and endodontic therapy, 304
  and examination record, 302
  and food traps, 298, 299
  and free-end saddle, 299
  and fulcrum line, 299
  guiding planes, 306
  and home-care program, 323
  impression procedure, 320
  and investing tissue, 306
  mouth preparation, 314
  and nonretentive arm, 305
  path of insertion, 305
  and patient education, 300
  and periodontal disease, 276, 298
  premature occlusion, 307
  and prescription program, 301
  and recall system, 325
  rest preparations, 314
  and soft tissues, 307
  and stannous fluoride, 301
  support for, 307
  surgical therapy for, 307
  surveying in, 304
  surveyor spindle, 307
  and terminology, 298

Partial dentures—cont'd
  and tooth sensitivity, 315
  and treatment program, 313
  types, 298
  units of, 316
Pedodontics
  and ankylosis, 190
  and anterior crossbite, 203
  and delayed eruption, 195
  and dental aberrations, 190
  and dental caries, 185
  early diagnosis, 178
  and ectopic eruption, 191
  and nursing bottle caries, 182
  objectives of, 177
  and operative dentistry, 189
  oral findings in, 180
  and partial dentures, 298
  and premature loss of primary teeth, 198
  preventing initiation of dental caries, 187
  preventive management in, 184
  and recall evaluation, 206
  technique of examination in, 179
Periodontal disease
  and acquired pellicle, 209
  and acrylic resin, 218
  and antibiotics, 217
  and calculus, 209
  and dental floss, 214
  and dental restorations, 218
  etiology of, 208
  and inflammation, 208
  and interdental cleansing, 214
  and local factors, 208
  and neglect, 208
  and nutrition, 44
  and oral hygiene, 82, 212
  and orthodontics, 220
  and partial dentures, 218
  and patient education, 211
  and plaque, 209, 212
  prevention of, 211
  and systemic factors, 216
  and toothbrushing, 212
  and trauma from occlusion, 220
  and water irrigation, 214
  and vaccines, 218
Periodontics, 4
Phosphorus
  and dental caries, 43-44
  in nutrition, 30-44
  and saliva, 88
Physical fitness
  and cardiovascular fitness, 423-428
  and chronic ailments, 397, 402-405
  and dentist's health, 398
  and dynamic health, 406-408
  and exercise, 406, 415
  and improvement in oxygen intake, 405-406
  and magnitude of chronic disease, 397
  and mechanics of circulation, 412-415
  and need for prevention, 398
  and physical deterioration, 408-415

Physical fitness—cont'd
  and principles of exercise, 406
  program for, 406
  and teeth, 398
  and tension, 403
Pigmentation, effect of stannous fluoride on, 25
Pilocarpine, use of for rampant dental caries, 9, 87
Placenta
  concentration of fluoride in, 107
  passage of fluoride, 106
Plaque
  and calculus formation, 211
  composition of, 82, 209
  control of, 215
  effect of fluorides on, 94
  and periodontal disease, 211
  in rampant dental caries, 80-81
Plastic implant materials
  and biodegradable polymers, 394
  and biostable polymers, 392
  effects of on tissues, 392
  and synthetic cartilage, 393
  as tissue adhesive, 392
  use of, 391, 392
Polishing agents in dentifrices, 162
Pontics and periodontal disease, 218
Potassium fluoride
  in chewing gum, 116
  in mouthwash, 135
  as topical agent, 126, 128
Potassium fluorostannite, 128, 130
Pregnancy and nutrition, 51
Premature loss of teeth
  causes of malocclusion, 239
  effects of, 239
  and space maintenance, 239
Prenatal fluorides
  and placental barrier, 106
  clinical results, 106-108
  concentration in blood, 107
  concentration in hard tissues, 107
  concentration in placenta, 107
  concentration in soft tissues, 107
  interference by calcium, 110
  mechanism of action, 106
  metabolism of fluoride from, 106, 108
  and placental barrier, 106
  usefulness of, 109
Preventive dentistry
  attitude of dental profession, 5
  and between-meal eating, 38, 39, 41-43
  and calculus prevention, 158
  and caries activity tests, 8-11, 86
  counselling, 4
  definition of, 1-6
  and dental caries resistance, 41
  and dental materials, 318-347
  and dentures, 7
  and diet counselling, 11
  and facial habits, 11
  and fluoride during tooth development, 30-41

Preventive dentistry—cont'd
  and full dentures, 273-295
  and gingivitis, 3, 4, 215
  and human relations, 7
  and immediate dentures, 285-295
  and nutritional counselling, 32
  occlusal adjustment, 4, 220
  in office practice, 7-28
  and operative dentistry, 248-270
  and oral pathology, 345-354
  and oral surgery, 328-343
  and orthodontics, 10, 229
  and partial dentures, 10, 297
  and patient communication, 7
  and patient education, 16
  and pedodontics, 177
  and periodontics, 4, 208-224
  and prophylaxis, 4, 23
  and public health dentistry, 3
  and rampant dental caries, 80-81
  and social dentistry, 3
  stannous fluoride–calcium pyrophosphate dentifrice, 23, 168
  and topical fluorides, 22-25, 92
  treatment plan, 3
  and use of toothbrush, 158
  and use of toothpick, 158
Prophylaxis, 4, 23
  oral disclosing solution, 212
  paste (stannous fluoride), 23-25, 168
  and patient education, 211
  and periodontal disease, 211
  and plaque, 211
  during recall procedures, 27
Protein
  in delayed eruption, 41
  in periodontal disease, 44
Public health dentistry, 3
Public relations and patient education, 16

# R

Radiation
  and cell death, 362
  chemical protection from, 362
  and chemical transformation, 355
  and collimation, 366
  dosage received by different tissues, 359
  and effect on aging, 361
  effect on aneuploid cells, 362
  effect on chromosomes, 356
  effect on DNA, 356
  and effect on life shortening, 361
  effect on living tissue, 355
  factors modifying radiation effects, 356
  and formation of oxidants, 357
  and genetic changes, 362
  and gonadal effects, 366
  and ionizing radiation, 355
  and mutations, 357
  and somatic effects, 359
  terminology, 357
  and ultraspeed film, 365
Radiographs
  and dental health education, 17

Radiographs—cont'd
  and oral pathology, 345
  and oral surgery, 333
Rampant dental caries, 9, 80-81
  and acidogenic organisms, 81
  and calcium hydroxide, 84
  and caries activity tests, 8, 86
  causes, 81
  and communal fluoridation, 81
  control, 82
  definition, 80
  dental plaque in, 80-85
  and diet control, 84
  and familial factors, 88
  and food clearance from mouth, 82
  and frequency of food ingestion, 82-84
  and individual control measures, 83
  and *Lactobacillus*, 84
  oral hygiene in, 85
  pain in, 86
  patient counselling in, 87
  and patient recall, 83
  planning in, 83
  prevalence of, 80
  process, 81
  psychologic factors, 88
  and restorative procedures, 87
  saliva in, 87
  and sucrose, 81-82
  systemic factors, 88
  treatment planning in, 83
  use of fluorides, 84
  use of pilocarpine, 87
  and use of stannous fluoride–calcium pyrophosphate dentifrice, 83-85
  use of zinc oxide–eugenol, 83
  use of zirconium silicate prophylaxis paste, 84
Recall system
  file system in, 26
  methods of, 25, 206
  in patient education, 25-28
  reference filing, 26
  requirements for, 27
  treatments during, 27
  use of, in rampant dental caries, 84, 87
Recommended daily dietary allowance, 33-37
Record device and automatic filmstrip projector, 18
Resilient liners, 284-285
Resins
  and bacterial properties, 385
  biophysical considerations, 385
  biophysical properties of, 386
  cements, 385
  mixing of, 385
  polymer in, 383, 384
  powder in, 384
  properties of, 384
  as restorative materials, 383-385
Restorative dentistry
  in pedodontic practice, 189
  and periodontal disease, 218
  in rampant dental caries, 87

## S

Saliva
- acid-buffering capacity, 82
- antibacterial properties, 82
- and antihistamine drugs, 87
- effect on
  - of calcium and phosphate ions, 88
  - of fluoride, 94
  - following irradiation, 87
  - following oral surgery, 87
  - following menopause, 87
  - of pilocarpine, 87
- and rampant dental caries, 87
- and rate of flow, 11, 82, 87
- and tranquilizing drugs, 87
- and vitamin B complex deficiency, 87
- and xerostomia, 82
- viscosity determination, 11, 87

Salivary flow determination, 11
Salivary viscosity determination, 11
Salt
- consumption of, 109-110
- fluoridated, 109-111
- fluoride content of, 110
- and soda as dentifrice, 162

Sea salt, 109
Selenium in nutrition, 41
Silicate cements
- biophysical considerations, 388
- composition of, 386
- effect on gingiva, 388
- effect on pulp, 388
- hardening of, 387
- insertion in cavity, 387
- mixing of, 386
- use of, 386

Skeleton, fluoride in, 107, 111
Social dentistry, 13
Sodium fluoride
- in adults, 113
- in chewing gum, 112
- comparison to stannous fluoride, 114-116, 127
- in fluoride tablets, 97-105
- in mouthwashes, 133, 135-140
- in prophylactic pastes, 134-135, 136-139
- as topical agent, 22-25, 112

Sodium monofluorophosphate
- in dentifrice, 170
- in mouthwash, 135
- as topical agent, 128, 130

Sodium silicofluoride as topical agent, 128, 130
Soft tissues
- metabolic status, 39
- and oral disease, 39-40

Space infections, 330
Space maintenance
- and partial dentures, 298
- in preventing malocclusions, 239

Stannous chlorofluoride as topical agent, 128-130
Stannous fluoride, 4, 22-25
- for adults, 126, 127

Stannous fluoride—cont'd
- application of, 126
- in calcium pyrophosphate dentifrice, 168
- and caries arrestment, 23, 24, 127
- in chewing gum, 112
- comparison to sodium fluoride, 124-126, 127
- effect on gingivitis, 127
- and enamel pigmentation, 23, 24, 127
- laboratory studies of, 113
- and partial dentures, 301
- in prophylactic paste, 134-139
- in rampant dental caries, 84
- as topical agent, 112
- use of
  - in fluoride areas, 121, 122-123, 126, 127
  - during recall procedures, 27
  - in single application, 127

Stomatitis caused by dentifrices, 165
Stress
- in nutrition, 39
- in rampant dental caries, 88

Study models, 17
Substitute foods in relation to dental caries, 15
Sucrose
- in foods, 15
- in rampant dental caries, 81-82, 165

Surveying
- and partial dentures, 201
- spindle, 305

Systemic disease in oral pathology, 347
Systemic factors
- of periodontal disease, 216
- of rampant dental caries, 88

## T

Thiamine in nutrition, 35, 36
Thumb-sucking
- characteristics of, 235
- correction of, 235
- and orthodontics, 235

Toothbrushing
- in calculus prevention, 172
- and dentifrices, 164
- design of, 172
- effects of, 172
- and electric toothbrush, 173, 213
- and patient education, 172
- technique for topical application, 135
- types, 172, 212

Toothpick, 158
Topical fluorides
- benefits of, 22-25
- and caries arrestment, 23, 24
- and enamel demineralization, 23, 24
- and enamel pigmentation, 23, 24
- and ferric fluoride, 128, 130, 135
- fluoride-phosphate compounds, 22-25, 130, 133
- frequency of application, 22-25
- indications, 22-25
- multiple uses, 22-25, 136-139
- and partial dentures, 301

Topical fluorides—cont'd
  and potassium fluoride, 129, 130, 135
  in preventive dentistry, 4, 22-25, 164-165
  for rampant dental caries, 84
  and sodium fluoride, 22-25, 112-113, 135, 136
  and sodium monofluorophosphate, 128, 130, 135
  and sodium silicofluoride, 128, 130
  and stannous chlorofluoride, 128, 130
  and stannous fluoride, 22-25, 128, 130
  and stannous fluoride–calcium pyrophosphate dentifrice, 25, 168
  and stannous fluoride–lava pumice prophylactic paste, 24, 25, 134-135
  taste of, 24, 25
  use of
    by adults, 25, 136-139
    in areas with fluoridated water, 25, 112, 121, 122-125, 136-139
    by children, 22-25
  and zirconium tetrafluoride, 128, 130, 135
Tranquilizer drugs in rampant dental caries, 87
Treatment planning
  caries susceptibility tests in, 83
  in rampant dental caries, 83

U
Ultraspeed film, 365
Urine, fluoride in, 96, 98-100

V
Vaccines and periodontal disease, 218
Vipeholm study, 42-43
Visual aids, 16-22
Vitamin
  A, 34, 37, 38, 40, 44, 45
  B complex, 37, 44, 45

Vitamin—cont'd
  C, 35, 38, 40, 44, 217
  D, 30, 34, 37, 40, 41, 44
  and fluoride tablets, 96-100, 103-105
  and fluorosis, 103
  and gingivitis, 45
  and periodontal disease, 44-45

W
Wach test, 9
Water irrigation and periodontal health, 214
Wax pattern
  carving of, 377
  distortion of, 377-379
  in gold alloy restorations, 377
  and surface adaptation, 376, 377
  and thermal conductivity, 377

X
Xerostomia, 82

Z
Zinc oxide–eugenol
  biophysical considerations, 389
  cement, 389
  composition of, 389
  compressive strength, 389
  mixing of, 389
  in rampant dental caries, 83
  sealing of, 389
  use of, 389
Zinc phosphate cements
  and antibiotics, 385
  biophysical considerations, 386
  composition, 385
  mixing of, 385
  reactions of, 385, 386
Zirconium silicate, 4, 22-25
Zirconium tetrafluoride as topical agent, 128